# Medical Terminology

## A Living Language

### THIRD EDITION

**BONNIE F. FREMGEN, Ph.D**

**SUZANNE S. FRUCHT, Ph.D**

PEARSON

Prentice Hall

Upper Saddle River, New Jersey 07458

**Library of Congress Cataloging-in-Publication Data**

Fremgen, Bonnie F.
  Medical terminology : a living language / Bonnie F. Fremgen, Suzanne S. Frucht.—3rd ed.
    p. ; cm.
  Includes bibliographical references and index.
  ISBN 0-13-184910-7
  1. Medicine—Terminology. I. Frucht, Suzanne S. II. Title.
  [DNLM: 1. Medicine—Terminology—English. W 15 F869m 2005]
  R123.F697 2005
  610'.1'4—dc22

2004044265

**Publisher:** Julie Levin Alexander
**Publisher's Assistant:** Regina Bruno
**Senior Acquisitions Editor:** Mark Cohen
**Development Editor:** Jill Rembetski, Triple SSS Press Media Development
**Associate Editor:** Melissa Kerian
**Editorial Assistant:** Jaquay Felix
**Director of Marketing/Marketing Manager:** Karen Allman
**Channel Marketing Manager:** Rachele Strober
**Marketing Coordinator:** Janet Ryerson
**Director of Production and Manufacturing:** Bruce Johnson
**Managing Editor for Production:** Patrick Walsh
**Production Liaison:** Julie Li
**Production Editor:** Amy Gehl, Carlisle Publishers Services
**Media Editor:** John Jordan
**Manager of Media Production:** Amy Peltier
**New Media Project Manager:** Stephen J. Hartner
**Manufacturing Manager:** Ilene Sanford
**Manufacturing Buyer:** Pat Brown
**Creative Director:** Cheryl Asherman
**Senior Design Coordinator:** Maria Guglielmo
**Interior Designer:** Mary Siener
**Cover Designer:** Joseph DePinho
**Composition:** Carlisle Publishers Services
**Printing and Binding:** The Banta Company
**Cover Printer:** Lehigh Press

*Dedication*

*To my husband for his love and encouragement.*
*Bonnie Fremgen*


*To my husband, Rick, and my daughter,*
*Kristin, for their love, support, and friendship.*
*Suzanne Frucht*

Notice: The authors and the publisher of this volume have taken care that the information and technical recommendations contained herein are based on research and expert consultation, and are accurate and compatible with the standards generally accepted at the time of publication. Nevertheless, as new information becomes available, changes in clinical and technical practices become necessary. The reader is advised to carefully consult manufacturers' instructions and information material for all supplies and equipment before use, and to consult with a health care professional as necessary. This advice is especially important when using new supplies or equipment for clinical purposes. The authors and publisher disclaim all responsibility for any liability, loss, injury, or damage incurred as a consequence, directly or indirectly, of the use and application of any of the contents of this volume.

Pearson Education LTD.
Pearson Education Australia PTY, Limited
Pearson Education Singapore, Pte. Ltd
Pearson Education North Asia Ltd
Pearson Education Canada, Ltd.

Pearson Educación de Mexico, S.A. de C.V.
Pearson Education—Japan
Pearson Education Malaysia, Pte. Ltd
Pearson Education, Upper Saddle River, NJ

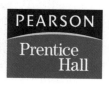

10 9 8 7 6 5 4 3 2 1
ISBN 0-13-184910-7

## Brief Contents

## Streamlined Organization

14 chapters make this book the perfect "fit" for a one-term course.

## Professional Profile Boxes

Chapter openers profile different health professions—providing career overview and real-world insight.

---

### Chapter 5
### Cardiovascular System

#### Learning Objectives

*Upon completion of this chapter, you will be able to:*

- Recognize the combining forms, prefixes, and suffixes introduced in this chapter.
- Gain the ability to pronounce medical terms and major anatomical structures.
- List the major organs of the cardiovascular system and their functions.
- Describe the flow of blood through the heart and the body.
- Explain how the electrical conduction system controls the heartbeat.
- Build cardiovascular system medical terms from word parts.
- Define vocabulary, pathology, diagnostic, and therapeutic medical terms relating to the cardiovascular system.
- Recognize types of medication associated with the cardiovascular system.
- Interpret abbreviations associated with the cardiovascular system.

**MedMedia**
www.prenhall.com/fremgen
Additional interactive resources and activities for this chapter can be found on the Companion Website. For animations, audio glossary, and review, access the accompanying CD-ROM in this book.

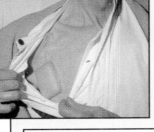

#### Professional Profile

**Cardiovascular Professionals**

Cardiology technologists, electrocardiogram technicians, and cardiac sonographers are all involved in the diagnosis and treatment of heart and blood vessel disease. The results of the tests and procedures they conduct are vitally important for the diagnosis and treatment of cardiovascular disease. These health care professionals are found wherever procedures to study the functioning of the cardiovascular system are performed. This includes hospitals, physicians' offices, cardiac rehabilitation programs, and diagnostic centers.

**Cardiology Technologist**

- Assists with invasive heart procedures
- Includes cardiac catheterizations and angioplasty procedures
- Must complete an accredited 2-to 4-year program

**Electrocardiogram Technician**

- Conducts tests to record the electrical activity of the heart
- Includes electrocardiography (EKGs), Holter monitoring, and stress testing
- May complete a 1-year certification program or receive on-the-job training

**Cardiac Sonographer**

- Uses ultrasound to produce a moving image of the heart for diagnostic purposes
- Graduates from a 1-year certification, 2-year associate's degree, or 4-year baccalaureate program

*For more information regarding these health careers, visit the following websites:*
Alliance of Cardiovascular Professionals at **www.acp-online.org**
American Society of Echocardiography at **www.asecho.org**

#### Chapter Outline

Overview
Anatomy and Physiology
Word Building
Vocabulary
Pathology
Diagnostic Procedures
Therapeutic Procedures
Pharmacology
Abbreviations
Chapter Review
Pronunciation Practice
Case Study
Chart Note Transcription
Practice Exercises
Professional Journal

---

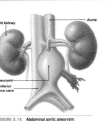

FIGURE 5.16   Abdominal aortic aneurysm.

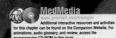

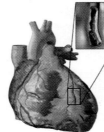

FIGURE 5.17   Coronary artery disease due to atherosclerosis.

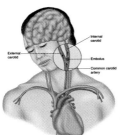

FIGURE 5.18   Embolus.

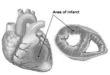

FIGURE 5.19   Cross section of myocardial infarction.

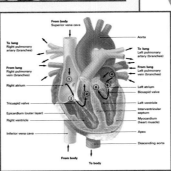

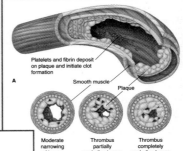

Platelets and fibrin deposit on plaque and initiate clot formation

Smooth muscle   Plaque

Moderate narrowing of lumen    Thrombus partially occluding lumen    Thrombus completely occluding lumen

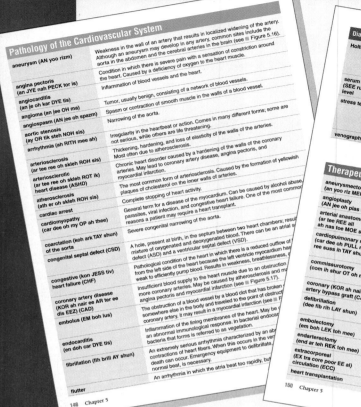

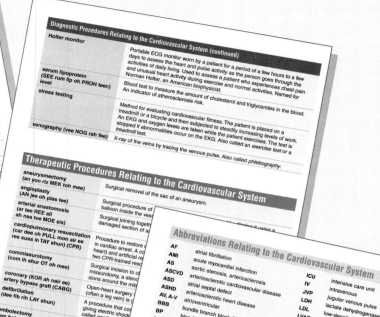

## Pathology of the Cardiovascular System

| | |
|---|---|
| aneurysm (AN yoo rizm) | Weakness in the wall of an artery that results in localized widening of the artery. Although an aneurysm may develop in any artery, common sites include the aorta in the abdomen and the cerebral arteries in the brain (see ■ Figure 5.16). |
| angina pectoris (an JYE nah PECK tor is) | Condition in which there is severe pain with a sensation of constriction around the heart. Caused by a deficiency of oxygen to the heart muscle. |
| angiocarditis (an je oh kar DYE tis) | Inflammation of blood vessels and the heart. |
| angioma (an jee OH ma) | Tumor, usually benign, consisting of a network of blood vessels. |
| angiospasm (AN jee oh spazm) | Spasm or contraction of smooth muscle in the walls of a blood vessel. |
| aortic stenosis (ay OR tik steh NOH sis) | Narrowing of the aorta. |
| arrhythmia (ah RITH mee ah) | Irregularity in the heartbeat or action. Comes in many different forms; some are not serious, while others are life threatening. |
| arteriosclerosis (ar tee ree oh skleh ROH sis) | Thickening, hardening, and loss of elasticity of the walls of the arteries. Most often due to atherosclerosis. |
| arteriosclerotic heart disease (ASHD) (ar tee ree oh skleh ROT ik) | Chronic heart disorder caused by a hardening of the walls of the coronary arteries. May lead to coronary artery disease, angina pectoris, and myocardial infarction. |
| atherosclerosis (ath er oh skleh ROH sis) | The most common form of arteriosclerosis. Caused by the formation of yellowish plaques of cholesterol on the inner walls of arteries. |
| cardiac arrest | Complete stopping of heart activity. |
| cardiomyopathy (car dee oh my OP ah thee) | General term for a disease of the myocardium. Can be caused by alcohol abuse, parasites, viral infection, and congestive heart failure. One of the most common reasons a patient may require a heart transplant. |
| coarctation of the aorta (koh ark TAY shun) | Severe congenital narrowing of the aorta. |
| congenital septal defect (CSD) | A hole, present at birth, in the septum between two heart chambers; result mixture of oxygenated and deoxygenated blood. There can be an atrial septal defect (ASD) and a ventricular septal defect (VSD). |
| congestive heart failure (CHF) (kon JESS tiv) | Pathological condition of the heart in which there is a reduced outflow of from the left side of the heart because the left ventricle myocardium has weak to efficiently pump blood. Results in weakness, breathlessness, |
| coronary artery disease (KOR ah nair ee AR ter ee dis EEZ) (CAD) | Insufficient blood supply to the heart muscle due to an obstruction more coronary arteries. May be caused by atherosclerosis and ma angina pectoris and myocardial infarction (see ■ Figure 5.17). |
| embolus (EM boh lus) | The obstruction of a blood vessel by a blood clot that has broken somewhere else in the body and traveled to the point of obstruct coronary artery, it may result in a myocardial infarction (see ■ F |
| endocarditis (en doh car DYE tis) | Inflammation of the lining membranes of the heart. May be an abnormal immunological response. In bacterial endoca bacteria that forms is referred to as vegetation. |
| fibrillation (fih brill AY shun) | An extremely serious arrhythmia characterized by an ab contractions of heart fibers. When this occurs in the ve death can occur. Emergency equipment to defibrillate normal beat, is necessary. |
| flutter | An arrhythmia in which the atria beat too rapidly, bu |

## Diagnostic Procedures Relating to the Cardiovascular System (continued)

| | |
|---|---|
| Holter monitor | Portable ECG monitor worn by a patient for a period of a few hours to a few days to assess the heart and pulse activity as the person goes through the activities of daily living. Used to assess a patient who experiences chest pain and unusual heart activity during exercise and normal activities. Named for Norman Holter, an American biophysicist. |
| serum lipoprotein (SEE rum lip oh PROH teen) level | Blood test to measure the amount of cholesterol and triglycerides in the blood. An indicator of atherosclerosis risk. |
| stress testing | Method for evaluating cardiovascular fitness. The patient is placed on a treadmill or a bicycle and then subjected to steadily increasing levels of work. An EKG and oxygen levels are taken while the patient exercises. The test is stopped if abnormalities occur on the EKG. Also called an *exercise test* or a *treadmill test*. |
| venography (vee NOG rah fee) | X-ray of the veins by tracing the venous pulse. Also called *phlebography*. |

## Therapeutic Procedures Relating to the Cardiovascular System

| | |
|---|---|
| aneurysmectomy (an yoo riz MEK toh mee) | Surgical removal of the sac of an aneurysm. |
| angioplasty (AN jee oh plas tee) | Surgical procedure of balloon inside the ve |
| arterial anastomosis (ar tee REE all ah nas toe MOE sis) | Surgical joining togeth damaged section of a |
| cardiopulmonary resuscitation (car dee oh PULL mon air ee ree suss in TAY shun) (CPR) | Procedure to restore in cardiac arrest. A co heart) and artificial re two CPR-trained resc |
| commissurotomy (com ih shur OT oh mee) | Surgical incision to c missurotomy, a stenc sions around the mit |
| coronary (KOR ah nair ee) artery bypass graft (CABG) | Open-heart surgery (often a leg vein) is p |
| defibrillation (dee fib rih LAY shun) | A procedure that co giving electric shock called *cardioversion* |
| embolectomy (em boh LEK toh mee) | Removal of an emb |
| endarterectomy (end ar teh REK toh mee) | Excision of the dise to remove atherosc |
| extracorporeal (EX tra core poor EE al) circulation (ECC) | During open-heart can be oxygenated |
| heart transplantation | Replacement of a |

## Abbreviations Relating to the Cardiovascular System

| | | | |
|---|---|---|---|
| AF | atrial fibrillation | ICU | intensive care unit |
| AMI | acute myocardial infarction | IV | intravenous |
| AS | aortic stenosis, arteriosclerosis | JVP | jugular venous pulse |
| ASCVD | arteriosclerotic cardiovascular disease | LDH | lactate dehydrogenase |
| ASD | atrial septal defect | LDL | low-density lipoproteins |
| ASHD | arteriosclerotic heart disease | LVAD | left ventricular assist device |
| AV, A-V | atrioventricular | LVH | left ventricular hypertrophy |
| BBB | bundle branch block (L for left; R for right) | MI | myocardial infarction, mitral insufficiency |
| BP | blood pressure | mm Hg | millimeters of mercury |
| bpm | beats per minute | MR | mitral regurgitation |
| CABG | coronary artery bypass graft | MS | mitral stenosis |
| CAD | coronary artery disease | MVP | mitral valve prolapse |
| cath | catheterization | NSR | normal sinus rhythm |
| CC | cardiac catheterization, chief complaint | P | pulse |
| CCU | coronary care unit | PAC | premature atrial contraction |
| CHF | congestive heart failure | PDA | patent ductus arteriosus |
| CoA | coarctation of the aorta | PTCA | percutaneous transluminal coronary angioplasty |
| CP | chest pain | | |
| CPK | creatine phosphokinase | PVC | premature ventricular contraction |
| CPR | cardiopulmonary resuscitation | S1 | first heart sound |
| CSD | congenital septal defect | S2 | second heart sound |
| CV | cardiovascular | SA, S-A | sinoatrial |
| DVT | deep vein thrombosis | SGOT | serum glutamic oxaloacetic transaminase |
| ECC | extracorporeal circulation | SK | streptokinase |
| ECG, EKG | electrocardiogram | tPA | tissue-type plasminogen activator |
| ECHO | echocardiogram | Vfib | ventricular fibrillation |
| GOT | glutamic oxaloacetic transaminase | VLDL | very low density lipoproteins |
| HDL | high-density lipoproteins | VSD | ventricular septal defect |
| HTN | hypertension | VT | |

## Word Tables

A logical, revised format reorganized for a streamlined presentation as an easier study tool. Color-coded design eases the learning process.

## Med Term Tips

This popular feature offers tidbits of noteworthy information about medical terms that engage learners.

## Pharmacology Relating to the Cardiovascular System

| | |
|---|---|
| antiarrhythmic (an tye a RHYTH mik) | Reduces or prevents cardiac arrhythmias. |
| anticoagulant (an tye koh AG you lant) | Prevent blood clot formation. |
| antihypertensive (an tye hye per TEN sive) | Lowers blood pressure. |
| antilipidemic (an tye lip ih DEM ik) | Reduces amount of cholesterol and lipids in the bloodstream. Treats hyperlipidemia. |
| cardiotonic (card ee oh TAHN ik) | Increases the force of cardiac muscle contraction. Treats congestive heart failure. |
| diuretic (dye ou RET ik) | Increases urine production by the kidneys, which works to reduce plasma and therefore blood volume. This results in lower blood pressure. |
| thrombolytic (throm boh LIT ik) | Dissolves existing blood clots. |
| vasoconstrictor (vaz oh kon STRICK tor) | Contracts smooth muscle in walls of blood vessels. Raises blood pressure. |
| vasodilator (vaz oh DYE late or) | Relaxes the smooth muscle in the walls of arteries, thereby increasing diameter of the blood vessel. Used for two main purposes: increasing circulation to an ischemic area and reducing blood pressure. |

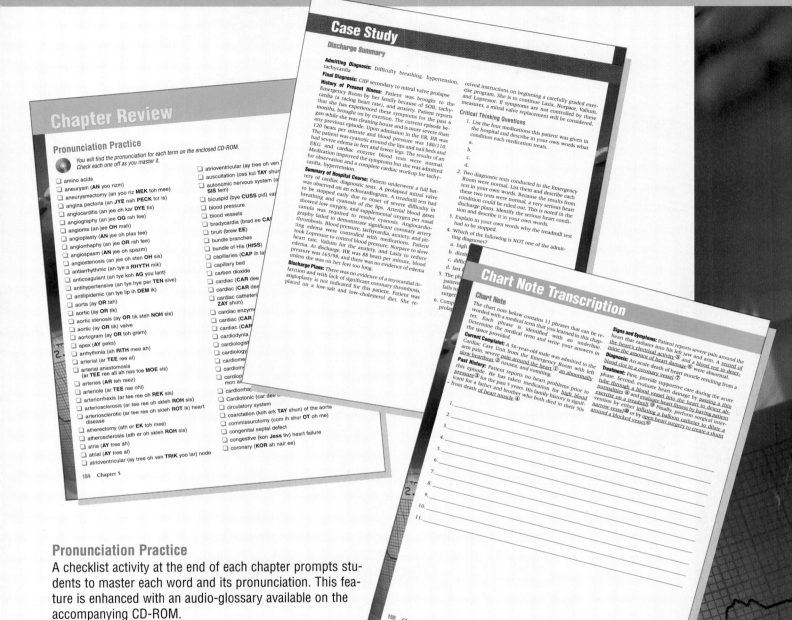

## Pronunciation Practice
A checklist activity at the end of each chapter prompts students to master each word and its pronunciation. This feature is enhanced with an audio-glossary available on the accompanying CD-ROM.

## Case Study
These scenarios use critical thinking questions to help students develop a firmer understanding of the terminology in context.

## Chart Note Transcription
This exercise provides a slice of real life and asks students to replace lay terms in a medical chart with the proper medical term. This builds both retention and familiarizes students with documentation.

# Additional Exercises

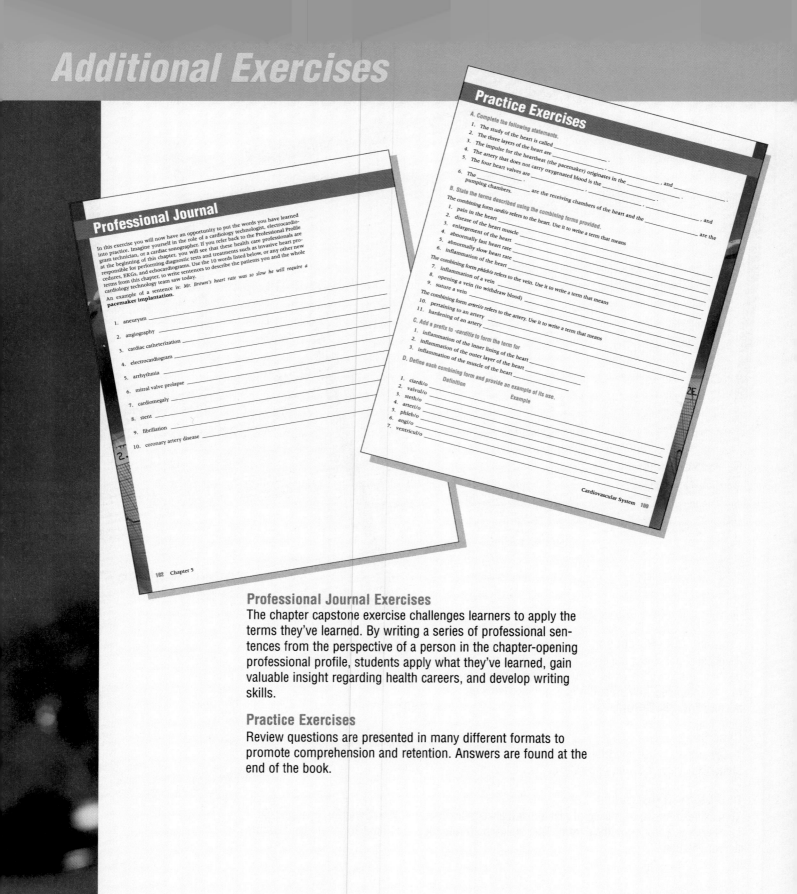

## Professional Journal

In this exercise you will now have an opportunity to put the words you have learned into practice. Imagine yourself in the role of a cardiology technologist, electrocardiogram technician, or a cardiac sonographer. If you refer back to the Professional Profile at the beginning of this chapter, you will see that these health care professionals are responsible for performing diagnostic tests and treatments such as invasive heart procedures, EKGs, and echocardiograms. Use the 10 words listed below, or any other new terms from this chapter, to write sentences to describe the patients you and the whole cardiology technology team saw today.

An example of a sentence is: *Mr. Brown's heart rate was so slow he will require a* **pacemaker implantation**.

1. aneurysm
2. angiography
3. cardiac catheterization
4. electrocardiogram
5. arrhythmia
6. mitral valve prolapse
7. cardiomegaly
8. stent
9. fibrillation
10. coronary artery disease

162   Chapter 5

## Practice Exercises

**A. Complete the following statements.**
1. The study of the heart is called _____.
2. The three layers of the heart are _____, _____, and _____.
3. The impulse for the heartbeat (the pacemaker) originates in the _____.
4. The artery that does not carry oxygenated blood is the _____.
5. The four heart valves are _____.
6. The _____, _____, and _____ are the
   pumping chambers. _____ and _____ are the receiving chambers of the heart and the _____.

**B. State the terms described using the combining forms provided.**
The combining form *cardi/o* refers to the heart. Use it to write a term that means
1. pain in the heart _____
2. disease of the heart muscle _____
3. enlargement of the heart _____
4. abnormally fast heart rate _____
5. abnormally slow heart rate _____
6. inflammation of the heart _____
The combining form *phleb/o* refers to the vein. Use it to write a term that means
7. inflammation of a vein _____
8. opening a vein (to withdraw blood) _____
9. suture a vein _____
The combining form *arteri/o* refers to the artery. Use it to write a term that means
10. pertaining to an artery _____
11. hardening of an artery _____

**C. Add a prefix to *-carditis* to form the term for**
1. inflammation of the inner lining of the heart _____
2. inflammation of the outer layer of the heart _____
3. inflammation of the muscle of the heart _____

**D. Define each combining form and provide an example of its use.**

|  | Definition | Example |
|---|---|---|
| 1. cardi/o |  |  |
| 2. valvul/o |  |  |
| 3. steth/o |  |  |
| 4. arteri/o |  |  |
| 5. phleb/o |  |  |
| 6. angi/o |  |  |
| 7. ventricul/o |  |  |

Cardiovascular System   189

## Professional Journal Exercises
The chapter capstone exercise challenges learners to apply the terms they've learned. By writing a series of professional sentences from the perspective of a person in the chapter-opening professional profile, students apply what they've learned, gain valuable insight regarding health careers, and develop writing skills.

## Practice Exercises
Review questions are presented in many different formats to promote comprehension and retention. Answers are found at the end of the book.

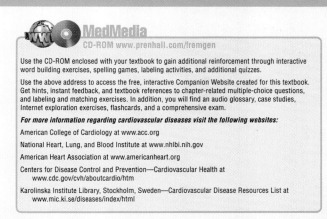

Use the CD-ROM enclosed with your textbook to gain additional reinforcement through interactive word building exercises, spelling games, labeling activities, and additional quizzes.

Use the above address to access the free, interactive Companion Website created for this textbook. Get hints, instant feedback, and textbook references to chapter-related multiple-choice questions, and labeling and matching exercises. In addition, you will find an audio glossary, case studies, Internet exploration exercises, flashcards, and a comprehensive exam.

***For more information regarding cardiovascular diseases visit the following websites:***

American College of Cardiology at www.acc.org

National Heart, Lung, and Blood Institute at www.nhlbi.nih.gov

American Heart Association at www.americanheart.org

Centers for Disease Control and Prevention—Cardiovascular Health at
www.cdc.gov/cvh/aboutcardio/htm

Karolinska Institute Library, Stockholm, Sweden—Cardiovascular Disease Resources List at
www.mic.ki.se/diseases/index/html

## MedMedia

Included at the beginning of each chapter, this feature prompts readers to use the various media components on the accompanying CD-ROM and Companion Website. MedMedia serves as a gateway to deeper understanding.

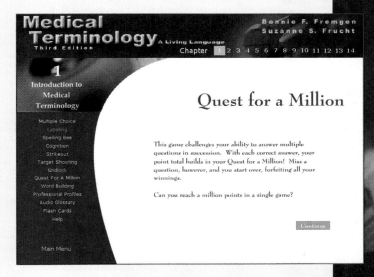

## CD-ROM

A free CD-ROM is included with every text, and provides a wide variety of interactive games, animations, videos, an audio glossary, as well as exercises such as labeling, word building, spelling, and more. A custom flashcard generator is also available on the CD-ROM–allowing students to select glossary terms and printout flashcards for any or all terms for study.

## Online Learning

This text breaks new ground by offering online options in both a free-access Companion Website as well as premium-level distance learning courses. The Companion Website (www.prenhall.com/fremgen) serves as a text-specific, interactive online workbook and includes a variety of quizzes, links, and an audio glossary. Instructors adopting this textbook for their courses have free access to an online Syllabus Manager with a host of features that facilitate the students' use of this Companion Website and allow faculty to post their syllabi online for their students. Finally, those instructors wishing to facilitate online courses will be able to access OneKey, our premium online course management option, which is available in WebCT, Blackboard or CourseCompass formats. For more information or a demonstration of our online course please visit www.prenhall.com/OneKey.

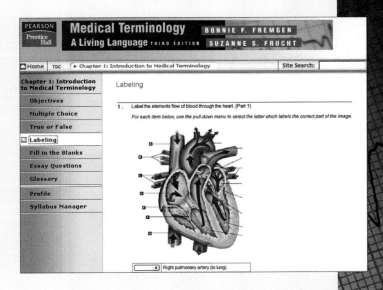

# Brief Contents

# Contents

# Preface

## To the Student

Welcome to the fascinating study of medical language—a vital part of your preparation for a career as a health professional. Throughout your career, in a variety of settings, you will use your understanding of medical terminology to communicate with other health professionals and patients. Employing a carefully constructed learning system, *Medical Terminology: A Living Language* is designed to guide you toward gaining a successful grasp of medical language, while giving you a real-world glimpse of its application within many different health care professions.

The book will introduce you to the basic rules for using word parts to form medical terms. The use of phonetic pronunciation throughout the book will help you to easily say a word by spelling out the word part according to the way it sounds. You will find this integrated approach will help you learn by applying medical terminology to anatomy and physiology content by body system. Throughout the text there are many features and real-life photographs and illustrations to enhance your comprehension of the material. A variety of end-of-chapter exercises allow you to review and master the content as you go along. An interactive CD-ROM and online study guide come free with the text and provide additional reinforcement of what you have learned in each chapter. The CD-ROM also includes the pronunciation of each bold term found in the text.

## Chapter Organization

Each chapter begins with a Professional Profile feature that gives you a brief glimpse into the training and duties of a specific health career. Every chapter also begins with learning objectives that present the chapter goals and an outline to give you a quick overview of the chapter's contents.

### Introductory Chapters

Chapter 1 contains information necessary for an understanding of how medical terms are formed. This includes learning about word roots, combining forms, prefixes, and suffixes, and general rules for building medical terms. You will also learn about terminology for medical records and the different health care settings. In Chapter 2, you will learn about terminology relating to the body structure, including organs and body systems. Here you will first encounter a feature found in each remaining chapter, Word Building tables, which list medical terms and their respective word parts. Throughout each chapter are also Med Term Tips, which are intended to stimulate your interest by describing quick facts about medical terms.

### Anatomy and Physiology Chapters

Chapters 3 through 13 are organized by body system. Each chapter begins with an overview of the organs in the system and is followed by lists of combining forms, prefixes, and/or suffixes with their meanings. The anatomy and physiology section is divided into the various components of the system, and each subsection begins with a list of key medical terms. Key terms are boldfaced and accompanied by a pronunciation guide the first time they appear in the narrative. A Word Building table and medical terms with pronunciations follow each anatomy and physiology section. For ease of learning, the medical terms are divided into four separate sections: vocabulary, pathology, diagnostic procedures, and therapeutic procedures. The new terms presented in the chapter are completed in a pharmacology and abbreviations section. The chapter review section includes a wide variety of exercises that both test your understanding and challenge you to apply the terms you have learned.

### Special Topics Chapter

Chapter 14 contains timely information and appropriate medical terms relevant to the following medical specialties: pharmacology, mental health, diagnostic imaging, rehabilitation services, surgery, and oncology. Knowledge of these topics is necessary for the well-rounded health care worker.

### Appendices

The appendices contain helpful reference lists of word parts and definitions. This information is intended for quick access. There are four main topics in the appendix: Abbreviations; Combining Forms; Prefixes; and Suffixes. The Combining Forms, Prefixes, and Suffixes Appendices present terms going from English to medical terms and then from medical terms to English. Finally, all of the key terms appear again in the glossary at the end of the text.

# To the Instructor

The third edition of *Medical Terminology: A Living Language* uses an integrated approach for teaching medical terminology to the health care student. It assists students in mastering terminology and incorporating this knowledge through an understanding of anatomy and physiology. In this way, beginning students learn the purpose and use of the medical terms to which they are being introduced.

## Features of the New Edition

This edition contains many new features that facilitate student mastery, while maintaining the best features of the second edition. Each chapter is arranged in a similar format and the content has been reorganized with an emphasis on maintaining consistency and accuracy. All terms have been reevaluated to ensure they remain in current use and terms that reflect new technologies and procedures have been added.

- Professional Profile boxes highlight different career options to help students become more familiar with the health care field, and the Professional Journal exercise at the end of each chapter challenges students to write sentences from the perspective of that professional.
- Word Building tables within each chapter put much needed emphasis on building words rather than rote memorization.
- Learning objectives are listed at the beginning of each chapter and outline the chapter's goals for students.
- Med Term Tips help pique student interest by presenting quick facts about medical terminology.

- Chapter 14, the special topics chapter, covers medical terminology that is specific to a variety of health care fields, including pharmacology, mental health, diagnostic imaging, rehabilitation services, surgery, and oncology.
- Full-color, realistic photographs and illustrations of body systems, organs, and pathological conditions bring medical terminology to life and make learning more fun and effective.
- The Pronunciation Practice feature that appears at the end of each chapter also serves as a quick reference summary of the chapter key terms.
- Abbreviations used in the medical field are integrated in each chapter and are also listed for handy reference in an appendix. Pronunciations are based on *Dorland's Illustrated Medical Dictionary*, 29th edition.

## End-of-Chapter Activities

The end-of-chapter activities have been significantly expanded in this edition and answers at the end of the text provide immediate feedback. Activities include:

### Pronunciation Practice

This feature includes an alphabetical listing of each term from the chapter with its see-and-say pronunciation. Students are encouraged to listen to the audio pronunciation of each term on the accompanying CD-ROM and check off each term as they master how to say it correctly.

### Case Studies

Students see practical application of medical terminology for each body system by reading a realistic case scenario and responding to critical thinking questions about it.

### Chart Note Transcription

Students read a patient scenario and then replace the phrases used to describe maladies, procedures, tests, and conditions with the accurate medical terms.

### Practice Exercises

These include a variety of questions that allow students to test their knowledge of chapter material.

### Professional Journal

This new feature, linked to the Professional Profile content at the beginning of each chapter, serves as a capstone exercise, challenging students to use specified vocabulary words from the point of view of different health care professionals in a writing exercise.

# Teaching and Learning Package

To enhance the teaching and learning process, an attractive media-focused supplements package for both students and faculty accompanies *Medical Terminology: A Living Language.* The full complement of supplemental teaching materials is available to all qualified instructors from your Prentice Hall Health sales representative.

## Student CD-ROM

The student CD-ROM is packaged **FREE** with every copy of the textbook. It includes:

- Custom flashcard generator that allows students to easily create custom study aids for additional practice
- Audio glossary that allows students to practice and listen to correct pronunciations of terms presented in the text
- Career profile videos that dynamically enrich and augment material covered in each chapter-opening profile
- Interactive exercises, games, and activities that quiz students on spelling, word building concepts, anatomy, and more.

## Online Learning and Instruction

### Companion Website and Syllabus Manager®

Students and faculty will both benefit from the **FREE** Companion Website at www.prenhall. com/fremgen. This website serves as a text-specific, interactive online workbook to *Medical Terminology: A Living Language.* Featuring an automatic scoring and feedback function, the Companion Website is organized in correspondence with the chapters of the text. Highlights include:

- A variety of multiple-choice, true/false, labeling, and fill-in-the-blank quizzes
- Internet links that relate to chapter content
- An audio glossary with pronunciations of key terms
- Case studies that allow students to apply their knowledge of the chapter content

The website instantly tabulates student results and allows those results to be sent to instructors via e-mail. Instructors adopting this textbook for their courses have **FREE** access to an online Syllabus Manager with a variety of features that facilitate the students' use of this Companion Website and allow faculty to post their syllabi online for their students. For more information or a demonstration of Syllabus Manager®, please contact your Prentice Hall sales representative or visit www.prenhall. com/demo, click on Companion Websites, and select Syllabus Manager Tour.

## Distance Learning Options

Those instructors wishing to facilitate online courses will be able to access OneKey our premium online course management option, which is available in WebCT, Blackboard, or CourseCompass formats. These online courses include interactive learning modules, tests, PowerPoint lectures, video clips, animations, and full course management tools. For more information or a demonstration of our online course systems, please contact your Prentice Hall sales representative or visit www.prenhall.com/onekey.

## Instructional Tools

### Instructor's Resource Guide with Test Bank and PowerPoint Lecture on CD-ROM

This guide contains a wealth of material to help faculty plan and manage the medical terminology course. It includes handouts, lecture suggestions and outlines, learning objectives, a complete test bank, and content correlations to the instructional media materials.

Packaged along with the printed instructor's guide, a CD-ROM provides many resources in an electronic format. First, the CD-ROM includes the complete 490-question test bank that allows instructors to generate customized exams and quizzes. Second, it includes a comprehensive, turn-key lecture package in PowerPoint format. The lectures contain discussion points along with embedded color images from the textbook as well as bonus animations and videos to help infuse an extra spark into the classroom experience. Instructors may use this presentation system as it is provided, or they may opt to customize it for their specific needs.

# Reviewers

Richard T. Boan, PhD
Coordinator
Allied Health Sciences
Midlands Technical College
Columbia, SC

Susan W. Boggs, RN, BSN, CNOR
Program Coordinator
Surgical Technology
Piedmont Technical College
Greenwood, SC

Gloria H. Coats, RN, MSN
Nursing Instructor
Modesto Junior College
Modesto, CA

Theresa H. deBeche, RN, MN, CNS
Head, Division of Nursing and Allied Health
Louisiana State University at Eunice
Eunice, LA

Brenda L. Gleason, MSN
Assistant Professor
Nursing
Iowa Central Community College
Fort Dodge, IA

Marcie C. Jones, BS, CMA
Program Director, Medical Assisting
Gwinnett Technical Institute
Lawrenceville, GA

Norma Longoria, BS, COI
Instructor
Health & Medical Administrative Service
Nursing/Allied Health Division
South Texas Community College
McAllen, TX

Katrina B. Myricks
Instructor
Business and Office Technology
Holmes Community College
Ridgeland, MS

Tina M. Peer, BSN, RN
Nursing and Allied Health Instructor
College of Southern Idaho
Twin Falls, ID

Sister Marguerite Polcyn, OSF, PhD
Professor of Health Education
Lourdes College
Sylvania, OH

LuAnn Reicks, RNC, BS, MSN
Professor/Practical Nursing Coordinator
Iowa Central Community College
Fort Dodge, IA

Connie Smith, RPh
Coordinator, Advanced Practice Experience
Instructor
University of Louisiana at Monroe School of Pharmacy
Monroe, LA

Karen Snipe, CPhT, ASBA, MAEd
Pharmacy Technician Program Coordinator
Trident Technical College
Charleston, SC

Janet Stehling, RHIA
Instructor
Health Information Technology
Mclennan College
Lorena, TX

Marilyn Turner, RN, CMA
Program Director, Medical Assisting
Allied Health Department Chair
Ogeechee Technical College
Statesboro, GA

Leesa Whicker, BA, CMA
Instructor
Central Piedmont Community College
Charlotte, NC

# About the Authors

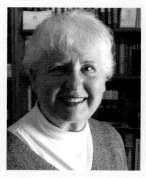

## Bonnie F. Fremgen

PhD, is a former associate dean of the Allied Health Program at Robert Morris College. She has taught medical law and ethics courses as well as clinical and administrative topics. In addition, she has served as an advisor for students' career planning. She has broad interests and experiences in the health care field, including hospitals, nursing homes, and physicians' offices.

Dr. Fremgen holds a nursing degree as well as a master's in health care administration. She received her PhD from the College of Education at the University of Illinois. She has performed postdoctoral studies in Medical Law at Loyola University Law School in Chicago.

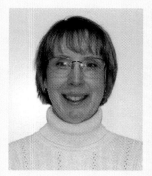

## Suzanne S. Frucht

is an Assistant Professor of Physiology at Northwest Missouri State University (NWMSU). She received a BA in biological sciences in 1975 and a BS in physical therapy in 1977, both from Indiana University. She worked full-time as a physical therapist in various health care settings, including acute care hospitals, extended care facilities, and home health from 1977 to 1991.

Dr. Frucht received a MS degree in biological sciences from NWMSU in 1987. Based on her health care experience and graduate degree, she was invited to teach medical terminology part-time in 1988. Discovering a love for the challenge of teaching at the college level she joined the NWMSU biology faculty full-time in 1991. While continuing to work full-time on the faculty she obtained a PhD from the University of Missouri–Kansas City in molecular biology and biochemistry in 1999.

Today, she teaches a varied course load including medical terminology, human anatomy, human physiology, and animal anatomy and physiology. Most recently, she was voted to receive the 2003 Governor's Award for Excellence in Teaching. To remain up-to-date in health care she continues to work as a PT on an occasional basis and takes continuing education courses to maintain her physical therapy license.

# Medical Terminology

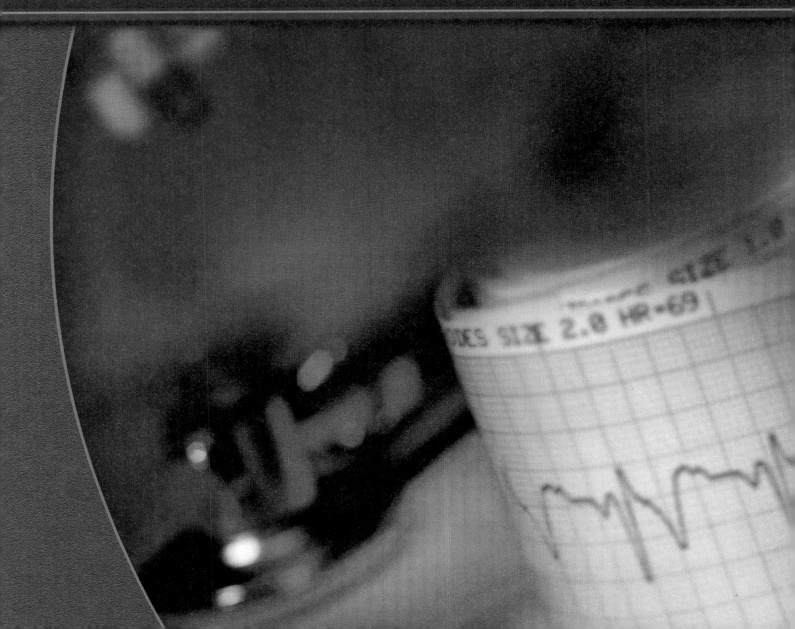

# Chapter 1

# Introduction to Medical Terminology

## Learning Objectives

*Upon completion of this chapter, you will be able to:*

- Discuss the four parts to medical terms.
- State the importance of correct spelling of medical terms.
- Recognize word roots and combining forms.
- Identify the most common prefixes and suffixes.
- Define word building.
- State the rules for determining singular and plural endings.
- Discuss the importance of using caution with abbreviations.
- Recognize the documents found in a medical record.
- Recognize the different health care settings.
- Understand the importance of confidentiality.

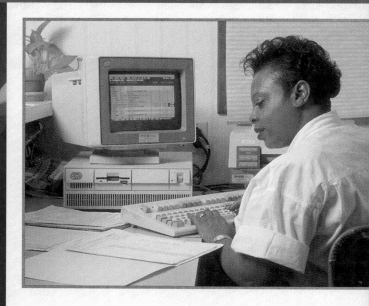

## MedMedia
www.prenhall.com/fremgen

Additional interactive resources and activities for this chapter can be found on the Companion Website. For animations, audio glossary, and review, access the accompanying CD-ROM in this book.

## Professional Profile

### Health Information Management

Health information management workers maintain accurate, orderly, and permanent records of each patient's condition and treatment. They also prepare patient information for release as appropriate to health personnel, insurance companies, researchers, lawyers, and the courts. They work in acute and long-term care facilities, health maintenance organizations, clinics, physicians' offices, public health departments, and insurance companies.

### Registered Health Information Administrator (RHIA)

- Directs the functioning of a health information department
- Graduates from an accredited 4-year bachelor's degree program in health information administration
- Passes national certification examination

### Registered Health Information Technician (RHIT)

- Makes certain that medical records are complete and accurate
- Graduates from an accredited 2-year associate's degree program in health information technology
- Passes national certification examination

### Certified Coding Specialist (CCS)

- Classifies medical information using an established coding system for billing and insurance purposes
- Graduates from an accredited 2-year associate's degree program in health information technology
- Passes national certification examination

### Medical Transcriptionist

- Transcribes dictated medical notes
- Completes a vocational education program or receives on-the-job training
- May opt to take an examination to become a certified medical transcriptionist (CMT)

***For more information regarding these health careers, visit the following websites:***
American Association for Medical Transcription at **www.aamt.org**
American Health Information Management Association at **www.ahima.org**

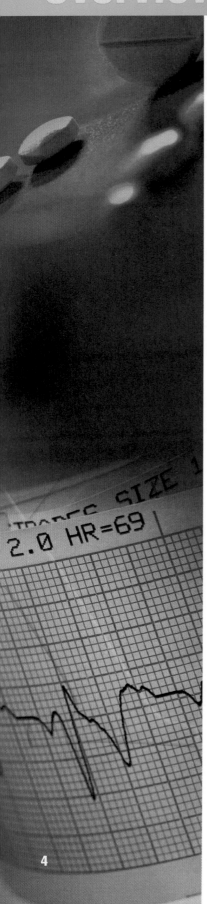

# Overview

Learning medical terminology can initially seem like studying a strange new language. But once you understand some of the basic rules as to how medical terms are formed using word building, it will become much like piecing together a puzzle. The general guidelines for forming words; an understanding of word roots, combining forms, prefixes, and suffixes; pronunciation; and spelling are discussed in this chapter. Chapter 2 introduces you to terms used to describe the body as a whole. Chapters 3 through 13 each focus on a specific body system and present new combining forms, prefixes, and suffixes, as well as exercises to help you gain experience building new medical terms. Finally, Chapter 14 includes the terminology for several important areas of patient care. In addition, "Med Term Tips" are sprinkled throughout all of the chapters to assist in clarifying some of the material. New medical terms discussed in each section are listed separately at the beginning of the section and each chapter contains numerous pathological, diagnostic, treatment, and surgical terms. You can use these lists as an additional study tool for previewing and reviewing terms.

Understanding medical terms requires you to be able to put words together or build words from their parts. It is impossible to memorize thousands of medical terms; however, once you understand the basics, you can distinguish the meaning of medical terms by analyzing their prefixes, suffixes, and word roots. Remember that there will always be some exceptions to every rule, and medical terminology is no different. We will try to point out these exceptions. Most medical terms, however, do follow the general rule that there is a **word root** or fundamental meaning for the word, **prefixes** and **suffixes** that modify the meaning of the word root, and sometimes a **combining vowel** to connect other word parts. You will be amazed at the seemingly difficult words you will be able to build and understand when you follow the simple steps in word building.

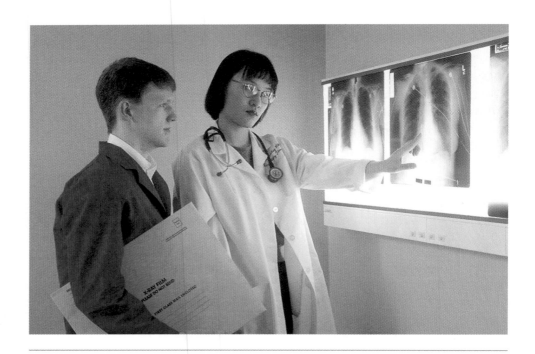

# Building Medical Terms from Word Parts

Four different word parts or elements are used to construct medical terms:

1. The **word root** is the foundation of the word.  cardi = heart
2. A **prefix** is at the beginning of the word.  pericardium = around the heart
3. A **suffix** is at the end of the word.  carditis = inflammation of the heart
4. The **combining vowel** is a vowel (usually *o*) that links the word root to another word root or a suffix.  cardiomyopathy = disease of the heart muscle

The following sections on word roots, combining vowels and forms, prefixes, and suffixes will consider each of these word parts in more detail and present examples of some of those most commonly used.

## Word Roots

The main part of the word, or word root, is the foundation of a medical term. This provides us with the general meaning of the word. The word root often indicates the body system or part of the body that is being discussed, such as *cardi* for heart. At other times the word root may be an action. For example, the word root *cis* means to cut (as in surgery).

A term may have more than one word root. For example, **osteoarthritis** (oss tee oh ar **THRY** tis) combines the word root *oste* meaning bone and *arthr* meaning the joints. When the suffix *-itis*, meaning inflammation, is added, we have the entire word, meaning an inflammation involving bone at the joints.

## Combining Vowel/Form

To make it possible to pronounce long medical terms with ease and to combine several word parts, a combining vowel is used. This is most often the vowel *o*. Combining vowels are utilized in two places: between two word roots or between a word root and a suffix.

To decide whether or not to use a combining vowel between a word root and suffix, first look at the suffix. If it begins with a vowel, do not use the combining vowel. If, however, the suffix does not begin with a vowel, then use a combining vowel. For example:

To combine *arthr* with *-scope* will require a combining vowel: **arthroscope** (**AR** throh scope). But to combine *arthr* with *-itis* does not require a combining vowel: **arthritis** (ar **THRY** tis).

The combining vowel is typically kept between two word roots, even if the second word root begins with a vowel: for example, **gastroenteritis** (gas troh en ter **EYE** tis) is correct instead of gastrenteritis. As you can tell from pronouncing these two terms, the combining vowel makes the pronunciation easier.

New word roots are typically presented as a **combining form**. This consists of the word root and its combining vowel written in a word root/vowel form, for example, *cardi/o*. Since it is often simpler to pronounce word roots when they appear in their combining form, this format is used throughout this book.

### Common Combining Forms

Some commonly used word roots in their combining form, their meaning, and examples of their use follow. Review the examples to observe when a combining vowel was kept and when it was dropped according to the rules presented above.

| Combining Form | Meaning | Example (Definition) |
|---|---|---|
| aden/o | gland | adenopathy (gland disease) |
| carcin/o | cancer | carcinoma (cancerous tumor) |
| cardi/o | heart | cardiac (pertaining to the heart) |
| chem/o | chemical | chemotherapy (treatment with chemicals) |
| cis/o | to cut | incision (process of cutting into) |
| dermat/o | skin | dermatology (study of the skin) |
| enter/o | small intestines | enteric (pertaining to the small intestines) |
| gastr/o | stomach | gastric (pertaining to the stomach) |
| gynec/o | female | gynecology (study of females) |
| hemat/o | blood | hematic (pertaining to the blood) |
| hydr/o | water | hydrocele (protrusion of water [in the scrotum]) |
| immun/o | immune | immunology (study of immunity) |
| laryng/o | voice box | laryngeal (pertaining to the voice box) |
| morph/o | shape | morphology (study of shape) |
| nephr/o | kidney | nephromegaly (enlarged kidney) |
| neur/o | nerve | neural (pertaining to a nerve) |
| ophthalm/o | eye | ophthalmic (pertaining to the eye) |
| ot/o | ear | otic (pertaining to the ear) |
| path/o | disease | pathology (study of disease) |
| pulmon/o | lung | pulmonary (pertaining to the lungs) |
| rhin/o | nose | rhinoplasty (surgical repair of the nose) |
| ur/o | urine, urinary tract | urology (study of the urinary tract) |

### Prefixes

A new medical term is formed when a prefix is added to the front of the term. Prefixes frequently give information about the location of an organ, the number of parts, or the time (frequency). For example, the prefix *bi-* stands for two of something, such as **bilateral** (bye **LAH** ter al), which means having two sides. However, not every term will have a prefix.

**MED TERM TIP** Remember to break down every word into its components (prefix, word root/combining form, and suffix) when you are learning medical terminology. Do not try to memorize every medical term. Instead, figure out how the word is formed from its components. In a short time you will be able to do this automatically when you see a new term.

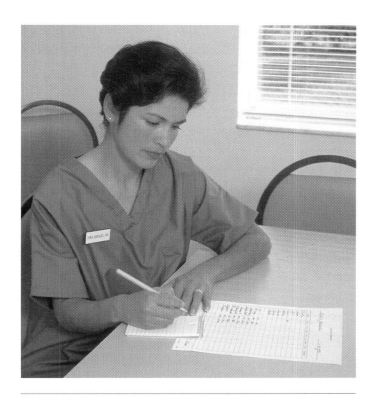

## Common Prefixes

Some of the more common prefixes, their meanings, and examples of their use follow. When written by themselves, prefixes are followed by a hyphen.

| Prefix | Meaning | Example (Definition) |
|---|---|---|
| a- | without, away from | aphasia (without speech) |
| an- | without | anoxia (without oxygen) |
| ante- | before, in front of | antepartum (before birth) |
| anti- | against | antibiotic (against life) |
| auto- | self | autograft (a graft from one's own body) |
| brady- | slow | bradycardia (slow heartbeat) |
| dys- | painful, difficult | dyspnea (painful breathing) |
| endo- | within, inner | endoscope (instrument to view within) |
| epi- | upon, over | epigastric (upon or over the stomach) |
| eu- | normal, good | eupnea (normal breathing) |
| hetero- | different | heterograft (a graft from another person's body) |
| homo- | same | homozygous (having two identical genes) |
| hydro- | water | hydrotherapy (water therapy) |
| hyper- | over, above | hypertrophy (overdevelopment) |
| hypo- | under, below | hypoglossal (under the tongue) |
| infra- | under, beneath, below | infraorbital (below, under the eye socket) |
| inter- | among, between | intervertebral (between the vertebrae) |
| intra- | within, inside | intravenous (inside, within a vein) |

| | | |
|---|---|---|
| macro- | large | macrocephalic (having a large head) |
| micro- | small | microcephalic (having a small head) |
| neo- | new | neonate (newborn) |
| pan- | all | pancarditis (inflammation of all the heart) |
| para- | beside, beyond, near | paranasal (near or alongside the nose) |
| per- | through | percutaneous (through the skin) |
| peri- | around | pericardial (around the heart) |
| post- | after | postpartum (after birth) |
| pre- | before, in front of | prefrontal (in front of the frontal bone) |
| pseudo- | false | pseudocyesis (false pregnancy) |
| retro- | backward, behind | retrograde (movement in a backwards direction) |
| sub- | below, under | subcutaneous (under, below the skin) |
| super- | above, excess | supernumerary (above the normal number) |
| supra- | above | suprapubic (above the pubic bone) |
| tachy- | rapid, fast | tachycardia (fast heartbeat) |
| trans- | through, across | transurethral (across the urethra) |
| ultra- | beyond, excess | ultrasound (high-frequency sound waves) |

## Number Prefixes

Some common prefixes pertaining to the number of items or measurement, their meanings, and examples of their use follow.

| Prefix | Meaning | Example (Definition) |
|---|---|---|
| bi- | two | bilateral (two sides) |
| di- | two | diplegic (paralysis of two extremities) |
| hemi- | half | hemiplegia (paralysis of one side/half of the body) |
| mono- | one | monoplegia (paralysis of one extremity) |
| multi- | many | multigravida (woman pregnant more than once) |
| nulli- | none | nulligravida (woman with no pregnancies) |
| poly- | many | polyuria (large amounts of urine) |
| quad- | four | quadriplegia (paralysis of all four extremities) |
| semi- | partial, half | semiconscious (partially conscious) |
| tri- | three | triceps (muscle with three heads) |
| uni- | one | unilateral (one side) |

## Suffixes

A suffix is attached to the end of a word to add meaning, such as a condition, disease, or procedure. For example, the suffix *-itis*, which means inflammation, when added to *cardi-* forms the new word **carditis** (car **DYE** tis), which means inflammation of the heart. Every medical term must have a suffix. The majority of the time, the suffix is added to a word root, as in carditis above. However, terms can also be built from a suffix added directly to a prefix, without a word root. For example, the term **dystrophy** (**DIS** troh fee), which means abnormal development, is built from the prefix *dys-* (meaning abnormal) and the suffix *-trophy* (meaning development).

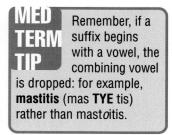

**MED TERM TIP** Remember, if a suffix begins with a vowel, the combining vowel is dropped: for example, **mastitis** (mas **TYE** tis) rather than mast*o*itis.

# Common Suffixes

Some common suffixes, their meanings, and examples of their use follow. When written by themselves, suffixes are preceded by a hyphen.

| Suffix | Meaning | Example (Definition) |
|---|---|---|
| -algia | pain | gastralgia (stomach pain) |
| -cele | hernia, protrusion | cystocele (protrusion of the bladder) |
| -cise | cut | excise (to cut out) |
| -dynia | pain | cardiodynia (heart pain) |
| -ectasis | dilatation | bronchiectasis (dilated bronchi) |
| -ectopia | displacement | corectopia (pupil of the eye not centered) |
| -gen | that which produces | mutagen (that which produces mutations) |
| -genesis | produces, generates | osteogenesis (produces bone) |
| -genic | producing | carcinogenic (producing cancer) |
| -ia | state, condition | hemiplegia (condition of being half paralyzed) |
| -iasis | abnormal condition | lithiasis (abnormal condition of stones) |
| -ism | state of | hypothyroidism (state of low thyroid) |
| -itis | inflammation | cellulitis (inflammation of cells) |
| -logist | one who studies | cardiologist (one who studies the heart) |
| -logy | study of | cardiology (study of the heart) |
| -lysis | destruction | osteolysis (bone destruction) |
| -malacia | abnormal softening | chondromalacia (abnormal cartilage softening) |
| -megaly | enlargement, large | cardiomegaly (enlarged heart) |
| -oma | tumor, mass | carcinoma (cancerous tumor) |
| -osis | abnormal condition | cyanosis (abnormal condition of being blue) |
| -pathy | disease | myopathy (muscle disease) |
| -plasia | development, growth | dysplasia (abnormal development) |
| -plasm | formation, development | neoplasm (new formation) |
| -ptosis | drooping | proctoptosis (drooping rectum) |
| -rrhage | excessive, abnormal flow | hemorrhage (excessive bleeding) |
| -rrhea | discharge, flow | rhinorrhea (discharge from the nose) |
| -rrhexis | rupture | hysterorrhexis (ruptured uterus) |
| -sclerosis | hardening | arteriosclerosis (hardening of an artery) |
| -stenosis | narrowing | angiostenosis (narrowing of a vessel) |
| -therapy | treatment | chemotherapy (treatment with chemicals) |
| -trophy | nourishment, development | hypertrophy (excessive development) |
| -uria | condition of the urine | hematuria (blood in the urine) |

## Adjective Suffixes

The following suffixes are used to convert a word root into an adjective. These suffixes usually are translated as *pertaining to*.

| Suffix | Meaning | Example (Definition) |
|--------|---------|----------------------|
| -ac | pertaining to | cardiac (pertaining to the heart) |
| -al | pertaining to | duodenal (pertaining to the duodenum) |
| -an | pertaining to | ovarian (pertaining to the ovary) |
| -ar | pertaining to | ventricular (pertaining to a ventricle) |
| -ary | pertaining to | pulmonary (pertaining to the lungs) |
| -eal | pertaining to | esophageal (pertaining to the esophagus) |
| -iac | pertaining to | chondriac (pertaining to cartilage) |
| -ic | pertaining to | gastric (pertaining to the stomach) |
| -ical | pertaining to | neurological (pertaining to the study of the nerves) |
| -ile | pertaining to | penile (pertaining to the penis) |
| -ior | pertaining to | superior (pertaining to above) |
| -ory | pertaining to | auditory (pertaining to hearing) |
| -ose | pertaining to | adipose (pertaining to fat) |
| -ous | pertaining to | intravenous (pertaining to within a vein) |
| -tic | pertaining to | acoustic (pertaining to hearing) |

## Surgical Suffixes

The following suffixes indicate surgical procedures:

| Suffix | Meaning | Example (Definition) |
|--------|---------|----------------------|
| -centesis | puncture to withdraw fluid | arthrocentesis (puncture to withdraw fluid from a joint) |
| -ectomy | surgical removal | gastrectomy (surgically remove the stomach) |
| -ostomy | surgically create an opening | colostomy (surgically create an opening for the colon through the abdominal wall) |
| -otomy | cutting into | thoracotomy (cutting into the chest) |
| -pexy | surgical fixation | nephropexy (surgical fixation of a kidney) |
| -plasty | surgical repair | dermatoplasty (surgical repair of the skin) |
| -rrhaphy | suture | myorrhaphy (suture together muscle) |

## Procedural Suffixes

The following suffixes indicate procedural processes or instruments:

| Suffix | Meaning | Example (Definition) |
|--------|---------|----------------------|
| -gram | record or picture | electrocardiogram (record of heart's electricity) |
| -graph | instrument for recording | electrocardiograph (instrument for recording the heart's electrical activity) |
| -graphy | process of recording | electrocardiography (process of recording the heart's electrical activity) |
| -meter | instrument for measuring | audiometer (instrument to measure hearing) |
| -metry | process of measuring | audiometry (process of measuring hearing) |
| -scope | instrument for viewing | gastroscope (instrument to view stomach) |
| -scopy | process of visually examining | gastroscopy (process of visually examining the stomach) |

## Word Building

Word building consists of putting together several word elements to form a variety of terms. The combining form of a word may be added to another combining form along with a suffix to create a new descriptive term. For example, adding *hyster/o* (meaning uterus) to *salping/o* (meaning fallopian tubes) along with the suffix *-ectomy* (meaning surgical removal of) forms **hysterosalpingectomy** (hiss ter oh sal pin **JEK** toh mee), the removal of both the uterus and the fallopian tubes. You will note that the combining vowel *o* is dropped when adding the suffix *-ectomy* since two vowels are not necessary.

# Pronunciation

You will hear different pronunciations for the same terms depending on where people were born or educated. As long as it is clear which term people are discussing, differing pronunciations are acceptable. Some people are difficult to understand over the telephone or on a transcription tape. If you have any doubt about a term being discussed, ask for the term to be spelled. For example, it is often difficult to hear the difference between the terms **abduction** and **adduction**. However, since the terms refer to opposite directions of movement, it is very important to double check if there is any question about which term was used.

Each new term in this book is introduced in boldface type, with the phonetic or "sounds like" pronunciation in parentheses immediately following. The part of the word that should receive the greatest emphasis during pronunciation appears in capital letters: for example, **pericarditis** (per ih car **DYE** tis). Toward the end of chapters 2-14 is a Pronunciation Practice exercise. This is a list of all the key terms from the chapter. Each term is also pronounced on the CD-ROM. Listen to each word, then pronounce it silently to yourself or out loud. Check each term off the list as you master it. This list may also serve as a review list for all the terms introduced in each chapter.

# Spelling

Although you will hear differing pronunciations of the same term, there will be only one correct spelling. If you have any doubt about the spelling of a term or of its meaning, always look it up in a medical dictionary. If only one letter of the word is changed, it could make a critical difference for the patient. For example, imagine the problem that could arise if you note for insurance purposes that a portion of a patient's **ileum**, or small intestine, was removed when in reality he had surgery for removal of a piece of his **ilium**, or hip bone.

Some words have the same beginning sounds but are spelled differently. Examples include the following:

**Sounds like *si***

| | |
|---|---|
| psy | **psychiatry** (sigh **KIGH** ah tree) |
| cy | **cytology** (sigh **TALL** oh gee) |

**Sounds like *dis***

| | |
|---|---|
| dys | **dyspepsia** (dis **PEP** see ah) |
| dis | **dislocation** (dis low **KAY** shun) |

# Singular and Plural Endings

Many medical terms originate from Greek and Latin words. The rules for setting up the singular and plural forms of some words follow the rules of these languages. For example, the heart has a left atrium and a right atrium for a total of two *atria*, not two *atriums*. Other words, such as *virus* and *viruses*, are changed from singular to plural by following English rules. Each medical term needs to be considered individually when changing from the singular to the plural form. The following examples illustrate how to form plurals.

| Words ending in | Singular | Plural |
| --- | --- | --- |
| -a | vertebra | vertebrae |
| -ax | thorax | thoraces |
| -ex or -ix | appendix | appendices |
| -is | metastasis | metastases |
| -ma | sarcoma | sarcomata |
| -nx | phalanx | phalanges |
| -on | ganglion | ganglia |
| -us | nucleus | nuclei |
| -um | ovum | ova |
| -y | biopsy | biopsies |

# Abbreviations

Abbreviations are commonly used in the medical profession as a way of saving time. However, some abbreviations can be confusing, such as *SM* for simple mastectomy and *sm* for small. Use of the incorrect abbreviation can result in problems for a patient, as well as with insurance records and processing. If you have any concern that you will confuse someone by using an abbreviation, spell out the word instead. It is never a good idea to use one's own abbreviations. Throughout the book abbreviations are included, when possible, immediately following terms. In addition, a list of common abbreviations for each body system is given in each chapter. Finally, the Abbreviations Appendix provides a complete alphabetical listing of all the abbreviations used in this text.

# The Medical Record

The medical record or chart documents the details of a patient's hospital stay. Each health care professional who has contact with the patient in any capacity completes the appropriate report of that contact and adds it to the medical chart. This results in a permanent physical record of the patient's day-to-day condition, when and what services he or she received, and the response to treatment. Each institution adopts a specific format for each document and its location within the chart. This is necessary because each health care professional must be able to locate quickly and efficiently the information he or she needs in order to provide proper care for the patient. The medical record is also a legal document. Therefore, it is essential that all chart components be completely filled out and signed. Each page must contain the proper patient identification information: the patient's name, age, gender, physician, admission date, and identification number.

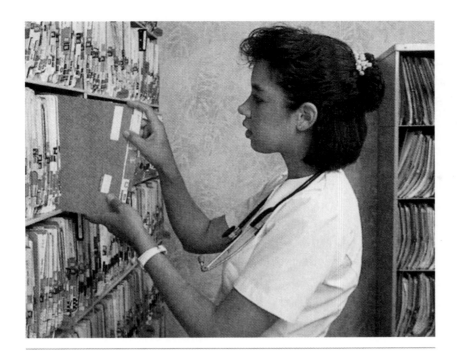

While the patient is still in the hospital, the unit clerk is responsible for placing documents in the proper place. After discharge, the medical records department ensures that all documents are present, complete, signed, and in the correct order. If a person is readmitted, especially for the same diagnosis, parts of this previous chart can be pulled and added to the current chart for reference. Physicians' offices and other outpatient care providers such as clinics and therapists also maintain a medical record detailing each patient's visit to their facility.

A list of the most common elements of a hospital chart with a brief description of each follows.

**History and Physical**—Written or dictated by the admitting physician; details the patient's history, results of the physician's examination, initial diagnoses, and physician's plan of treatment

**Physician's Orders**—A complete list of the care, medications, tests, and treatments the physician orders for the patient

**Nurse's Notes**—Record of the patient's care throughout the day; includes vital signs, treatment specifics, patient's response to treatment, and patient's condition

**Physician's Progress Notes**—The physician's daily record of the patient's condition, results of the physician's examinations, summary of test results, updated assessment and diagnoses, and further plans for the patient's care

**Consultation Reports**—The report given by a specialist whom the physician has asked to evaluate the patient

**Ancillary Reports**—Reports from various treatments and therapies the patient has received, such as rehabilitation, social services, or respiratory therapy

**Diagnostic Reports**—Results of all diagnostic tests performed on the patient, principally from the lab and medical imaging (for example, X-rays and ultrasound)

**Informed Consent**—A document voluntarily signed by the patient or a responsible party that clearly describes the purpose, methods, procedures, benefits, and risks of a diagnostic or treatment procedure

**Operative Report**—Report from the surgeon detailing an operation; includes a pre- and postoperative diagnosis, specific details of the surgical procedure itself, and how the patient tolerated the procedure

**Anesthesiologist's Report**—Relates the details regarding the drugs given to a patient, the patient's response to anesthesia, and vital signs during surgery

**Pathologist's Report**—The report given by a pathologist who studies tissue removed from the patient (for example, bone marrow, blood, or tissue biopsy)

**Discharge Summary**—A comprehensive outline of the patient's entire hospital stay; includes condition at time of admission, admitting diagnosis, test results, treatments and patient's response, final diagnosis, and follow-up plans

## Health Care Settings

The use of medical terminology is widespread. It provides health care professionals with a precise and efficient method of communicating very specific patient information to one another, whether they are in the same type of facility or not. Descriptions follow of the different types of settings where medical terminology is used:

**Acute Care or General Hospitals**—These hospitals typically provide services to diagnose (laboratory, diagnostic imaging) and treat (surgery, medications, therapy) diseases for a short period of time. In addition, they usually provide emergency and obstetrical care.

**Specialty Care Hospitals**—These hospitals provide care for very specific types of diseases. A good example is a psychiatric hospital.

**Nursing Homes or Long-Term Care Facilities**—These facilities provide long-term care for patients who need extra time to recover from an illness or injury before they return home, or for persons who can no longer care for themselves.

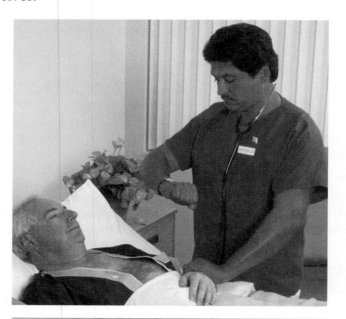

**Ambulatory Care, Surgical Centers or Outpatient Clinics**—These facilities provide services that do not require overnight hospitalization. The services range from simple surgeries to diagnostic testing or therapy.

**Physicians' Offices**—Individual or groups of physicians providing diagnostic and treatment services in a private office setting.

**Health Maintenance Organizations**—A group of primary-care physicians, specialists, and other health care professionals who provide a wide range of services in a prepaid system.

**Home Health Care**—Agencies that provide nursing, therapy, personal care, or housekeeping services in the patient's own home.

**Rehabilitation Centers**—These facilities provide intensive physical and occupational therapy. They include inpatient and outpatient treatment.

**Hospices**—An organized group of health care workers who provide supportive treatment to dying patients and their families.

# Confidentiality

Anyone who works with medical terminology and is involved in the medical profession must have a firm understanding of confidentiality. Any information or record relating to a patient must be considered privileged. This means that you have a moral and legal responsibility to keep all information about the patient confidential. If you are asked to supply documentation relating to a patient, the proper authorization form must be signed by the patient. Give only the specific information that the patient has authorized. The Health Insurance Portability and Accountability Act of 1996 (HIPAA) set federal standards that provide patients with more protection of their medical records and health information, better access to their own records, and greater control over how their health information is used and to whom it is disclosed.

# Final Word

If you have any doubt about the meaning or spelling of a word, look it up in your medical dictionary. Medical personnel who have been practicing in their profession for many years still need to look up a few words. The student who is just learning medical terminology needs to look up words even more frequently.

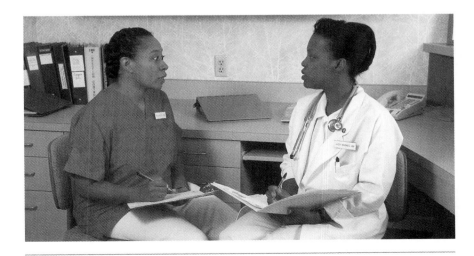

# Chapter Review

## Practice Exercises

### A. Complete the following statements.

1. The combination of a word root and the combining vowel is called a(n) _____ .

2. The vowel that connects two word roots or a suffix with a word root is usually a(n) _____ .

3. A word part used at the end of a word root to change the meaning of the word is called a(n) _____ .

4. A(n) _____ is used at the beginning of a word to indicate number, location, or time.

5. Although the pronunciation of medical terms may differ slightly from one person to another, the _____ must never change.

6. The four components of a medical term are _____ , _____ , _____ , and _____ .

### B. Define the following combining forms.

1. aden/o _____
2. carcin/o _____
3. cardi/o _____
4. chem/o _____
5. cis/o _____
6. dermat/o _____
7. enter/o _____
8. gastr/o _____
9. gynec/o _____
10. hemat/o _____
11. hydr/o _____
12. immun/o _____
13. laryng/o _____
14. morph/o _____
15. nephr/o _____
16. neur/o _____
17. ophthalm/o _____
18. ot/o _____
19. pulmon/o _____
20. rhin/o _____
21. ur/o _____

### C. Define the following suffixes.

1. -plasty _____
2. -stenosis _____
3. -itis _____
4. -al _____

5. -algia _____

6. -otomy _____

7. -megaly _____

8. -ectomy _____

9. -rrhage _____

10. -centesis _____

11. -gram _____

12. -ac _____

13. -malacia _____

14. -ism _____

15. -rrhaphy _____

16. -ostomy _____

17. -pexy _____

18. -rrhea _____

19. -scopy _____

20. -oma _____

**D. Join a combining form and a suffix to form words with the following meanings.**

1. study of lungs _____

2. pain relating to a nerve _____

3. nose discharge or flow _____

4. abnormal softening of a kidney _____

5. enlarged heart _____

6. cutting into the stomach _____

7. inflammation of the skin _____

8. surgical removal of the voice box _____

9. inflammation of the joint _____

10. gland disease _____

**E. Write a prefix for each of the following expressions.**

1. within, inside _____

2. large _____

3. before/in front of _____

4. around _____

5. new _____

6. without _____

7. half _____

8. painful, difficult _____

9. above _____

10. over, above _____

11. many _____

12. slow _____

13. self _____

14. across _____

15. two _____

**F. Circle the prefix in the following terms and define the prefix.**

1. tachycardia _____

2. pseudocyesis _____

3. hypoglycemia _____

4. intercostal _____

5. eupnea _____

6. postoperative _____

7. monoplegia _____

8. subcutaneous _____

**G. Change the following singular terms to plural terms.**

1. metastasis _____

2. ovum _____

3. diverticulum _____

4. atrium _____

5. diagnosis _____

6. vertebra _____

**H. Using the suffix -*ology*, meaning *the study of*, write a term for each of the following medical specialties.**

1. heart _____

2. stomach _____

3. skin _____

4. eye _____

5. urinary tract _____

6. kidney _____

7. blood _____

8. females _____

9. nerve _____

**I. Build a medical term by combining the word parts requested in each question.**

For example, use the combining form for *spleen* with the suffix meaning *enlargement* to form a word meaning *enlargement of the spleen* (answer: *splenomegaly*).

1. combining form for *heart* _____

   suffix meaning *abnormal softening* _____

   term meaning *softening of the heart* _____

2. word root form for *stomach* _____

   suffix meaning *to surgically create an opening* _____

   term meaning *creating an opening into the stomach* _____

3. combining form for *nose* _____

   suffix meaning *discharge or flow* _____

   term meaning *flow from the nose* _____

4. prefix meaning *over, above* _____

   suffix meaning *nourishment, development* _____

   term meaning *overdevelopment* _____

5. combining form meaning *disease* _____

   suffix meaning *the study of* _____

   term meaning *the study of disease* _____

6. word root meaning *gland* _____

   suffix for *tumor/mass* _____

   term meaning *gland tumor or mass* _____

7. combining form meaning *stomach* _____

   combining form meaning *small intestines* _____

   suffix meaning *study of* _____

   term meaning *study of stomach and small intestines* _____

8. word root meaning *ear* _____

   suffix meaning *inflammation* _____

   term meaning *ear inflammation* _____

9. prefix meaning *water* _____

   suffix meaning *treatment* _____

   term meaning *water treatment* _____

10. combining form meaning *cancer* _____

    suffix meaning *that which produces* _____

    term meaning *that which produces cancer* _____

# Professional Journal

In this exercise you will now have an opportunity to put the words you have learned into practice. Imagine yourself in the role of a registered health information technician. If you refer back to the Professional Profile at the beginning of this chapter, you will see that this health care professional is responsible for checking that health care records are accurate and complete. Double check the 10 sentences below to find terms that are either misspelled or used incorrectly and correct them.

*Example*: A gastroscopy was inserted into the patient's stomach to look for an ulcer.

The suffix *-scopy* means *a procedure of visually examining inside an organ*, while the suffix *-scope* refers to the *instrument used to examine inside an organ*. This sentence is referring to the instrument being inserted into the stomach, so the correct sentence is *A gastroscope was inserted into the patient's stomach to look for an ulcer*.

1. The patient was diagnosed with a stomach ulcer that required a gastrektomy.

2. The child was suspected of having a bladder infection and was referred to a urologist.

3. The tingling in her hand was diagnosed as neuralgia.

4. Listening to the patient's chest revealed wheezing within her lungs, leading to the diagnosis of an interpulmonary infection.

5. The nose damage from being hit by a soccer ball will require rhinplasty to correct.

6. A laryngotomy was performed to remove small nodules from the voice box.

7. Nephrorrhea was performed to sew up the tear in the kidney.

8. The severe, itching skin rash was diagnosed as dermatitis.

9. The patient had bradycardia and required medicine to slow down his heart rate.

_____

_____


10. The opthalmologist conducted an eye exam.

_____

_____


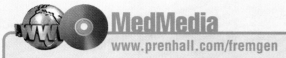

**MedMedia**
www.prenhall.com/fremgen

Use the CD-ROM enclosed with your textbook to gain additional reinforcement through interactive word building exercises, spelling games, labeling activities, and additional quizzes.

Use the above address to access the free, interactive Companion Website created for this textbook. Get hints, instant feedback, and textbook references to chapter-related multiple-choice questions, as well as labeling and matching exercises. In addition, you will find an audio glossary, case studies, and Internet exploration exercises.

# Chapter 2

# Body Structure

## Learning Objectives

*Upon completion of this chapter, you will be able to:*

- Recognize the combining forms and prefixes introduced in this chapter.

- Gain the ability to pronounce medical terms.

- Discuss the organization of the body in terms of cells, tissues, organs, and systems.

- Define the four types of tissues.

- List the major organs found in the 12 organ systems.

- Describe the anatomical position.

- Define the body planes.

- Define directional and positional terms.

- List the body cavities and their contents.

- Locate and describe the nine anatomical divisions of the abdomen.

- Locate and describe the four clinical divisions of the abdomen.

- Build body structure medical terms from word parts.

- Interpret abbreviations associated with body structure.

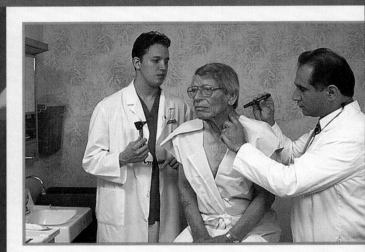

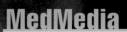

## MedMedia
www.prenhall.com/fremgen
Additional interactive resources and activities for this chapter can be found on the Companion Website. For animations, audio glossary, and review, access the accompanying CD-ROM in this book.

## Professional Profile

### Medical Care

Physicians oversee patient care. They examine patients, diagnose diseases, order treatments, perform surgery, and educate patients on health issues. Physician assistants (PAs) and certified medical assistants (CMAs) assist physicians in direct patient care. PAs perform many of the tasks previously performed only by physicians. CMAs have a variety of duties ranging from front office management to routine medical duties.

### Doctor of Medicine (MD)

- Also known as allopathic physicians
- Graduates from an approved 4-year medical school
- Passes national board examination and completes 3- to 8-year residency

### Doctor of Osteopathy (DO)

- Osteopathic physicians emphasize the role of the musculoskeletal system in the health of the body
- Graduates from an approved 4-year osteopathic school
- Passes national board examination and completes internship and residency

### Physician Assistant (PA)

- Performs tasks such as conducting physical examinations, ordering tests and treatments, making diagnoses, counseling patients, assisting in surgery, and writing prescriptions
- Works under the supervision of a physician
- Graduates from 2-year physician assistant program
- Passes national certification examination

### Certified Medical Assistant (CMA)

- Duties may include record keeping, billing, preparing insurance forms, taking vital signs, and stocking examination rooms
- Works under the supervision of a physician
- Completes an accredited 1-year certificate or 2-year associate's degree clinical medical assistant program and passes a certification exam

*For more information regarding these health careers, visit the following websites:*
American Academy of Physician Assistants at **www.aapa.org**
American Association of Colleges of Osteopathic Medicine at **www.aacom.org**
American Association of Medical Assistants at **www.aama-ntl.org**
Association of American Medical Colleges at **www.aamc.org**

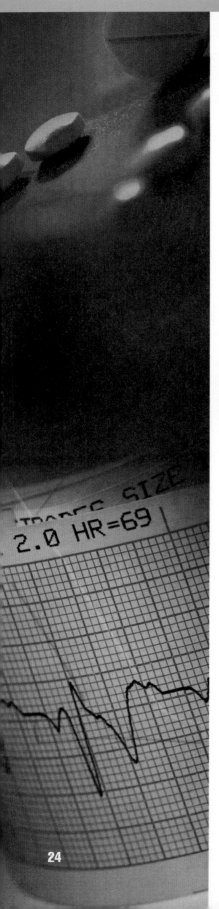

### Combining Forms Relating to Body Structure

| | | | |
|---|---|---|---|
| abdomin/o | abdomen | muscul/o | muscle |
| adip/o | fat | neur/o | nerve |
| anter/o | front | organ/o | organ |
| caud/o | tail | oste/o | bone |
| cephal/o | head | pelv/o | pelvis |
| chondr/o | cartilage | poster/o | back |
| crani/o | skull | proxim/o | near to |
| cyt/o | cell | somat/o | body |
| dist/o | away from | spin/o | spine |
| dors/o | back of body | super/o | above |
| epitheli/o | epithelium | system/o | system |
| hist/o | tissue | thorac/o | chest |
| infer/o | below | ventr/o | belly |
| later/o | side | viscer/o | internal organ |
| medi/o | middle | | |

**MED TERM TIP** Remember that the prefixes and suffixes introduced in Chapter 1 will be used over and over again in your medical terminology course. A few of these are frequently used in body structure terms. Examples of these prefixes are included in the Prefixes Relating to Body Structure table.

### Prefixes Relating to Body Structure

| Prefix | Meaning | Example | Definition |
|---|---|---|---|
| epi- | above | epigastric | above the stomach |
| inter- | between | intervertebral | between the vertebrae |
| intra- | within | intramuscular | within the muscle |
| peri- | around or about | pericardium | around the heart |
| post- | behind or after | postnasal | behind the nose |
| retro- | behind or backward | retrosternal | behind the sternum |
| sub- | under or below | substernal | below the sternum |
| supra- | above | suprasternal | above the sternum |
| trans- | through or across | transurethral | across the urethra |

## Organization of the Body

**cell**      **organs**      **tissues**

**organism**      **systems**

Before taking a look at the whole human body, we need to examine its parts. The human **organism** consists of **cells, tissues, organs,** and **systems.** These components are arranged in a hierarchical manner. That is, cells come together to form tissues, tissues come together to form organs, organs come together to form systems, and all the systems come together to form the whole organism.

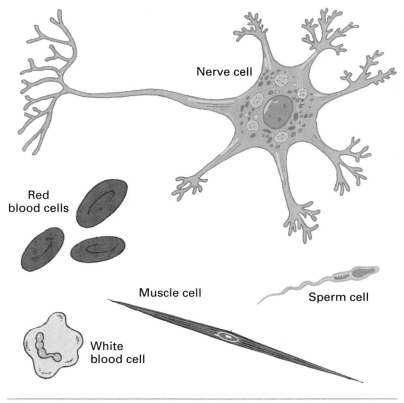

**FIGURE 2.1** Examples of cells found in the human body.

## Cells

### cytology

The cell is the basic unit of all living things. In other words, it is the fundamental unit of life. All the tissues and organs in the body are composed of cells. Individual cells perform functions for the body such as reproduction, respiration, metabolism, and excretion. Special cells are also able to carry out very specific functions, such as contraction by muscle cells and electrical impulse transmission by nerve cells. The study of cells and their functions is called **cytology** (sigh **TALL** oh jee). Figure 2.1 illustrates several types of cells.

## Tissues

| | | |
|---|---|---|
| **adipose tissue** | **epithelial tissue** | **neurons** |
| **bone** | **histology** | **skeletal muscle** |
| **brain** | **mucous membranes** | **skin** |
| **cardiac muscle** | **muscle tissue** | **smooth muscle** |
| **cartilage** | **nerves** | |
| **connective tissue** | **nervous tissue** | |

**Histology** (hiss **TALL** oh jee) is the study of tissue. A tissue is formed when like cells are grouped together to perform one activity. For example, nerve cells, also called **neurons** (**NOO** rons), combine to form nerve fibers. Neurons have the ability to communicate between cells and conduct impulses throughout the body. The knee-jerk reaction that occurs when a physician taps the patellar tendon and the muscles in the leg extend the leg is an example of neurons responding to stimuli.

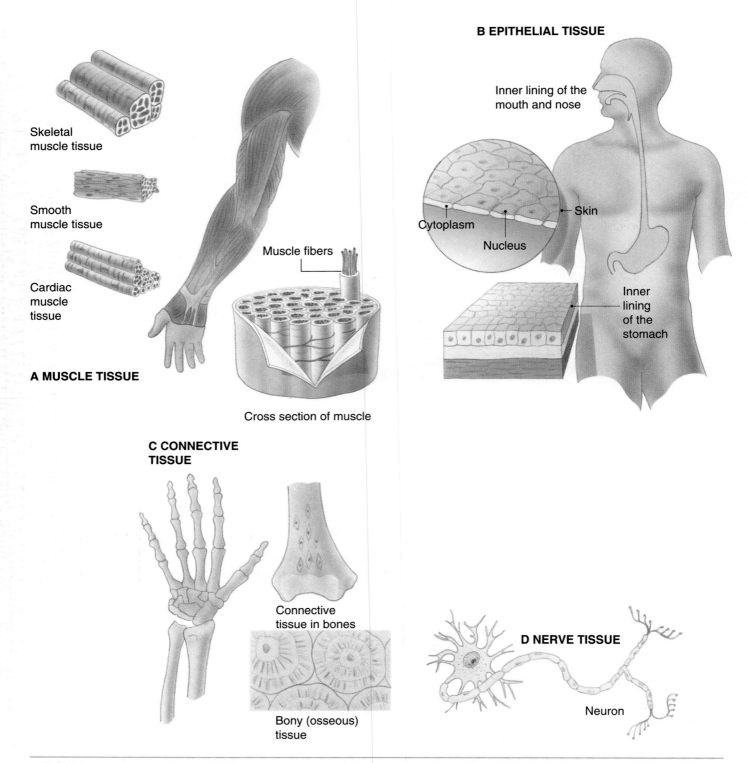

**Skeletal muscle tissue**

**Smooth muscle tissue**

**Cardiac muscle tissue**

**A MUSCLE TISSUE**

Muscle fibers

Cross section of muscle

**B EPITHELIAL TISSUE**

Inner lining of the mouth and nose

Cytoplasm

Nucleus

Skin

Inner lining of the stomach

**C CONNECTIVE TISSUE**

Connective tissue in bones

Bony (osseous) tissue

**D NERVE TISSUE**

Neuron

■ **FIGURE 2.2**   Types of tissue. (A) Muscle tissue makes all body movement possible. (B) Epithelial tissue forms the outer skin and lines the internal organs of the body. (C) Connective tissue supports and protects body structures. (D) Nerve tissue receives stimuli and responds to stimuli.

The body has four types of tissue:

1. **Muscle tissue** produces movement in the body through contraction, or shortening in length. Muscle tissue forms one of three basic types of muscles: **skeletal (SKELL** eh tal) **muscle, smooth muscle,** or **cardiac (CAR** dee ak) **muscle.** Skeletal muscles are the voluntary muscles attached to bones. Smooth muscle is found in internal organs such as the intestines, uterus, and blood vessels. Cardiac muscle is found only in the heart. Smooth muscle and cardiac muscle are involuntary muscles, meaning we have no conscious control over their activity (see ■ Figure 2.2A).

2. **Epithelial** (ep ih **THEE** lee al) **tissue** is found throughout the body as lining for internal organs and also forms the outer **skin.** The stomach is mainly epithelial and muscle tissue. The epithelial tissue secretes gastric juices that aid in digestion. The muscular tissue's movement allows food to come into contact with gastric juices, causing digestion to occur. **Mucous (MYOO** kus) **membranes** are another type of epithelial tissue that lines body passageways and excretes a thick substance (see ■ Figure 2.2B).

3. **Connective tissue** is the supporting and protecting tissue in body structures. **Adipose (ADD** ih pohs) **tissue** or fat, **bone,** and **cartilage (CAR** tih lij) are examples of connective tissue (see ■ Figure 2.2C).

4. **Nervous tissue** forms a network of **nerves** throughout the entire body. This allows for the conduction of electrical impulses to send information between the **brain** and the rest of the body (see ■ Figure 2.2D).

## Organs and Systems

| | | |
|---|---|---|
| **cardiovascular system** | **integumentary system** | **respiratory system** |
| **digestive system** | **lymphatic system** | **special senses** |
| **endocrine system** | **male reproductive system** | **urinary system** |
| **female reproductive system** | **musculoskeletal system** | |
| **hematic system** | **nervous system** | |

Organs are composed of several different types of tissue that work as a unit to perform special functions. For example, the stomach contains muscle fibers, nervous tissue, and epithelial tissue that allows it to contract to mix food with digestive juices.

A system is composed of several organs working in a coordinated manner to perform a complex function or functions. To continue our example, the stomach plus the other digestive system organs—the mouth, esophagus, liver, pancreas, small intestines, and colon—work together to ingest, digest, and absorb our food.

■ Figures 2.3 through 2.14 illustrate the major organs found in each organ system and the special senses. Table 2.1 presents the organ systems that will be studied in this textbook, along with their functions and the medical specialties associated with that system.

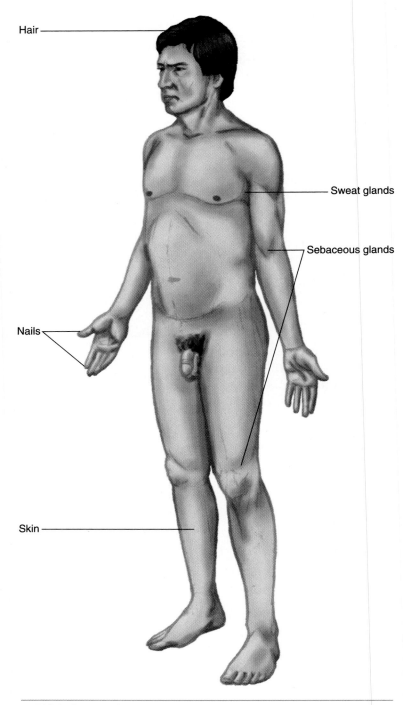

Hair

Sweat glands

Sebaceous glands

Nails

Skin

**FIGURE 2.3** Organs of integumentary system.

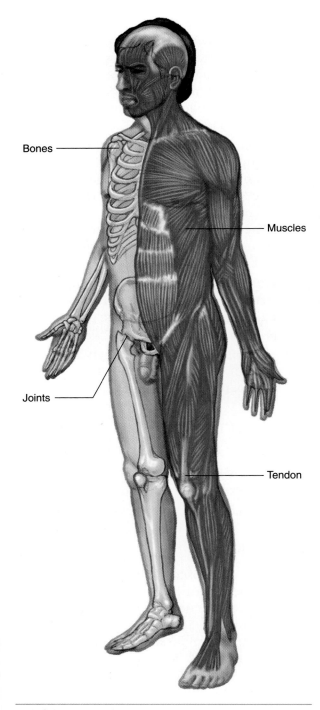

Bones

Muscles

Joints

Tendon

**FIGURE 2.4** Organs of musculoskeletal system.

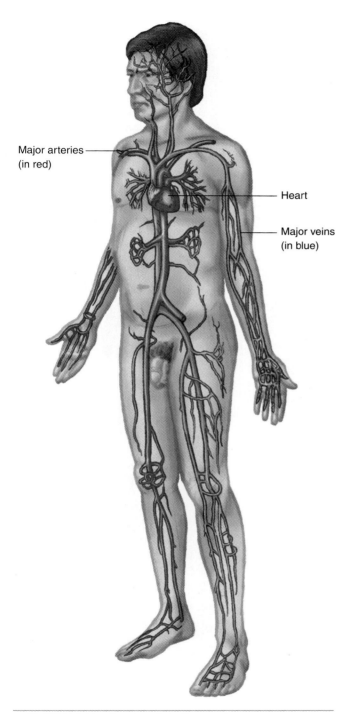

Major arteries
(in red)

Heart

Major veins
(in blue)

**■ FIGURE 2.5**  Organs of cardiovascular system.

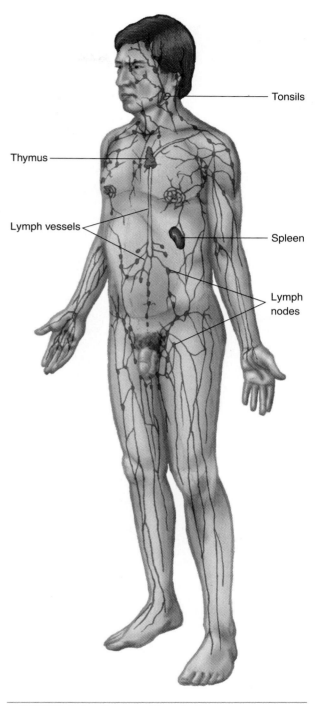

Tonsils

Thymus

Lymph vessels

Spleen

Lymph
nodes

**■ FIGURE 2.6**  Organs of lymphatic system.

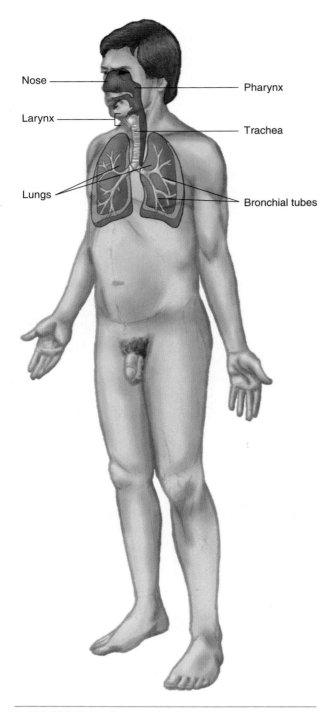

Nose

Larynx

Lungs

Pharynx

Trachea

Bronchial tubes

■ **FIGURE 2.7** Organs of respiratory system.

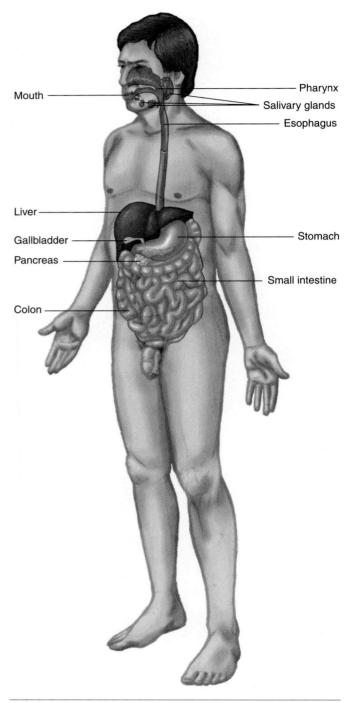

Mouth

Liver

Gallbladder

Pancreas

Colon

Pharynx

Salivary glands

Esophagus

Stomach

Small intestine

■ **FIGURE 2.8** Organs of digestive system.

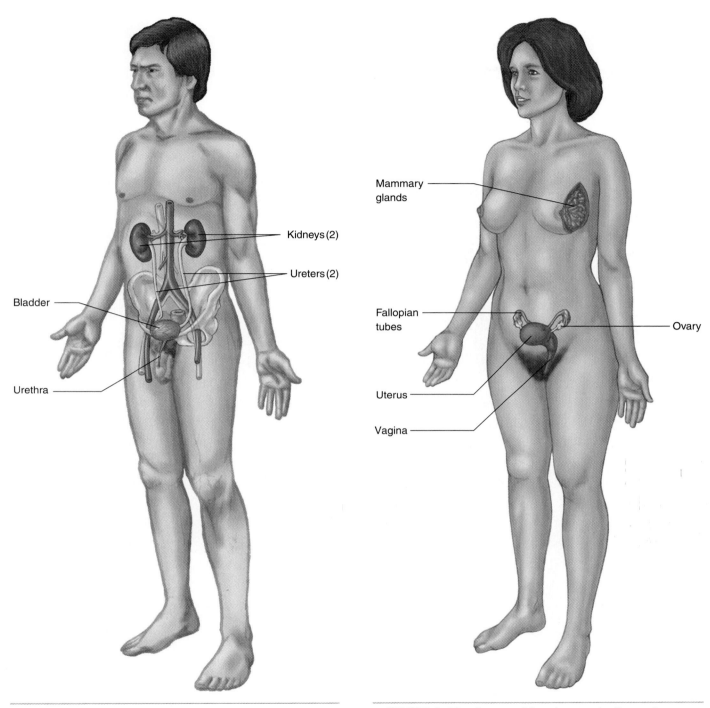

Kidneys(2)

Ureters(2)

Bladder

Urethra

Mammary
glands

Fallopian
tubes

Ovary

Uterus

Vagina

■ **FIGURE 2.9**   Organs of urinary system.

■ **FIGURE 2.10**   Organs of female reproductive system.

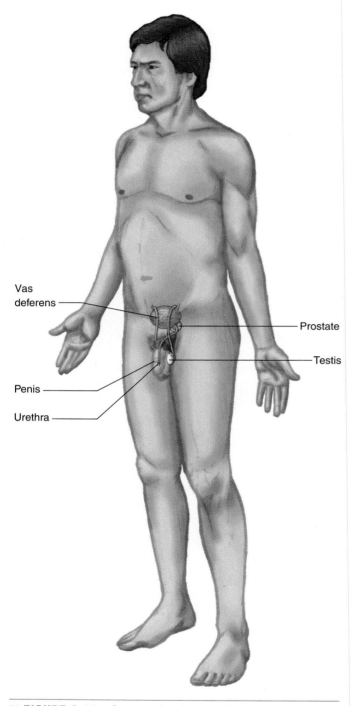

Vas
deferens

Prostate

Penis

Testis

Urethra

**■ FIGURE 2.11**   Organs of male reproductive system.

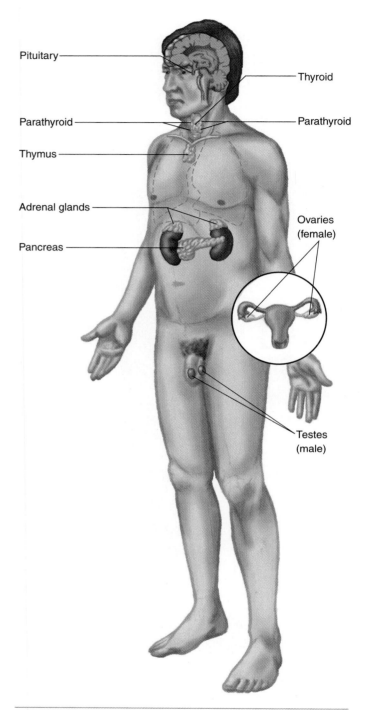

Pituitary

Thyroid

Parathyroid

Parathyroid

Thymus

Adrenal glands

Ovaries
(female)

Pancreas

Testes
(male)

**■ FIGURE 2.12**   Organs of endocrine system.

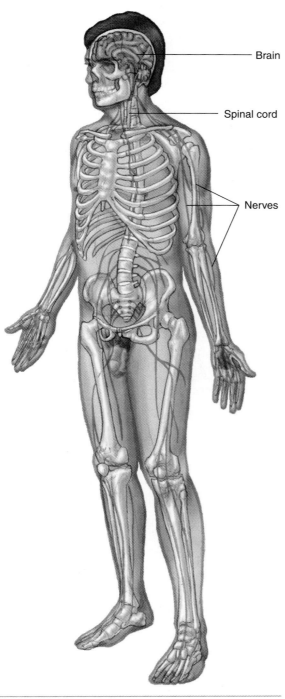

Brain

Spinal cord

Nerves

**FIGURE 2.13**   Organs of nervous system.

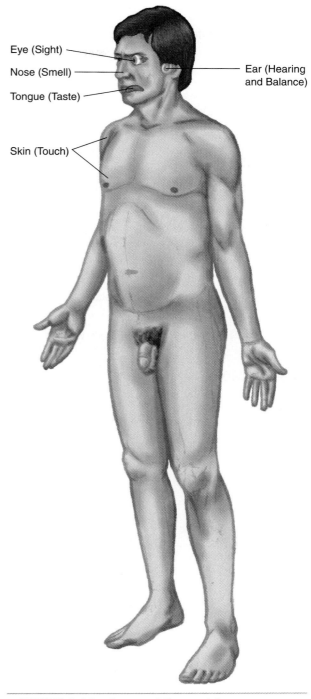

Eye (Sight)

Nose (Smell)

Tongue (Taste)

Ear (Hearing and Balance)

Skin (Touch)

**FIGURE 2.14**   Organs of the special senses.

## Table 2.1 — Organ Systems of the Human Body

| System | Functions | Medical Specialty |
|---|---|---|
| Integumentary (in teg you **MEN** tah ree) | Forms protective two-way barrier and aids in temperature regulation. | dermatology (der mah **TALL** oh jee) |
| Musculoskeletal (mus qu low **SKEL** et all) | Skeleton supports and protects the body, forms blood cells, and stores minerals. Muscles produce movement. | orthopedics (or thoh **PEE** diks) orthopedic (or the **PEE** dik) surgery |
| Cardiovascular (CV) (car dee oh **VAS** kew lar) | Pumps blood throughout the entire body to transport nutrients, oxygen, and wastes. | cardiology (car dee **ALL** oh jee) |
| Blood (Hematic System) (he **MAT** tik) | Transports oxygen, protects against pathogens, and controls bleeding. | hematology (hee mah **TALL** oh jee) |
| Lymphatic (lim **FAT** ik) | Protects the body from disease and invasion from pathogens. | immunology (im yoo **NALL** oh jee) |
| Respiratory | Obtains oxygen and removes carbon dioxide from the body. | otorhinolaryngology (oh toh rye noh lair ing **GALL** oh jee) pulmonology (pull mon **ALL** oh jee) thoracic (tho **RASS** ik) surgery |
| Digestive | Obtains nutrients for the body. | gastroenterology (gas troh en ter **ALL** oh jee) proctology (prok **TOL** oh jee) |
| Urinary (**YOO** rih nair ee) | Filters waste products out of the blood and removes them from the body. | nephrology (neh **FROL** oh jee) urology (yoo **RALL** oh jee) |
| Female reproductive | Produces eggs for reproduction and provides place for growing baby. | gynecology (gigh neh **KOL** oh jee) obstetrics (ob **STET** riks) |
| Male reproductive | Produces sperm for reproduction. | urology (yoo **RALL** oh jee) |
| Endocrine (**EN** doh krin) | Regulates metabolic activities of the body. | endocrinology (en doh krin **ALL** oh jee) |
| Nervous | Receives sensory information and coordinates the body's response. | neurology (noo **RAL** oh jee) neurosurgery (noo roh **SIR** jer ee) |
| Special senses – Eye | Vision | ophthalmology (off thal **MALL** oh jee) |
| Special senses – Ear | Hearing and balance | otorhinolaryngology (oh toh rye noh lair ing **GALL** oh jee) |

## Anatomical Position

The anatomical position is used when describing the positions and relationships of a structure in the human body. A body in the anatomical position is standing erect with the arms at the side of the body, the palms of the hands facing forward, and the eyes looking straight ahead. In addition, the legs are parallel with the feet and the toes pointing forward. For descriptive purposes the assumption is always that the person is in the anatomical position even if the body or parts of the body are in any other position (see ■ Figure 2.15).

## Body Planes

**coronal plane**

**frontal plane**

**horizontal plane**

**median plane**

**sagittal plane**

**transverse plane**

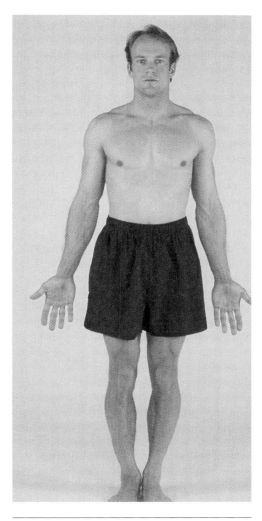

**FIGURE 2.15** In the anatomical position, standing with hands at sides and palms facing forward.

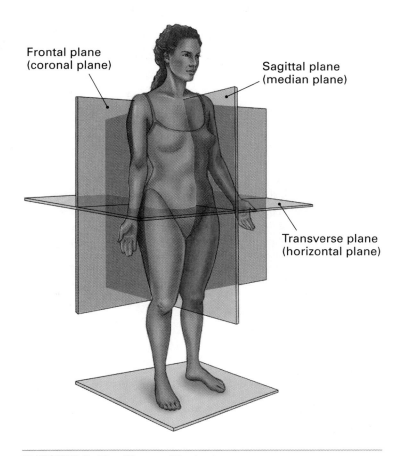

Frontal plane
(coronal plane)

Sagittal plane
(median plane)

Transverse plane
(horizontal plane)

**FIGURE 2.16** Planes of the body.

The terminology for body planes is used to assist medical personnel in describing the body and its parts. To understand body planes, you must imagine cuts slicing through the body at various angles. This imaginary slicing allows us to use more specific language when describing parts of the body. These body planes, illustrated in Figure 2.16, include the following:

1. **Sagittal** (**SAJ** ih tal) **plane:** This vertical plane, also called the **median** (**MEE** dee an) **plane,** runs lengthwise from front to back and divides the body or any of its parts into right and left portions. The right and left sides do not have to be equal.

2. **Frontal plane:** The frontal, or **coronal** (kor **RONE** al), **plane** divides the body into front and back portions. In other words, this is a vertical lengthwise plane running from side to side.

3. **Transverse** (trans **VERS**) **plane:** The transverse, or **horizontal plane** is a crosswise plane that runs parallel to the ground. This imaginary cut would divide the body or its parts into upper and lower portions.

# Directional and Positional Terms

Directional terms assist medical personnel in discussing the position or location of a patient's complaint. Directional or positional terms also help to describe one process, organ, or system as it relates to another. Table 2.2 presents commonly used terms for describing the position of the body or its parts. They are listed in pairs that have opposite meanings: for example, superior versus inferior, anterior versus posterior, medial versus lateral, proximal versus distal, superficial versus deep, and supine versus prone. Directional terms are illustrated in ■ Figure 2.17.

| Table 2.2 | Terms for Describing Body Position |
|---|---|
| **superior** (soo **PEE** ree or) or **cephalic** (seh **FAL** ik) | More toward the head, or above another structure.<br>*Example:* The adrenal glands are superior to the kidneys. |
| **inferior** (in **FEE** ree or) or **caudal** (**KAWD** al) | More toward the feet or tail, or below another structure.<br>*Example:* The intestine is inferior to the heart. |
| **anterior** (an **TEE** ree or) or **ventral** (**VEN** tral) | More toward the front or belly-side of the body.<br>*Example:* The navel is located on the anterior surface of the body. |
| **posterior** (poss **TEE** ree or) or **dorsal** (**DOR** sal) | More toward the back or spinal cord side of the body.<br>*Example:* The posterior wall of the right kidney was excised. |
| **medial** (**MEE** dee al) | Refers to the middle or near the middle of the body or the structure.<br>*Example:* The heart is medially located in the chest cavity. |
| **lateral** (lat) (**LAT** er al) | Refers to the side.<br>*Example:* The ovaries are located lateral to the uterus. |
| **apex** (**AY** peks) | Tip or summit of an organ.<br>*Example:* We hear the heart beat by listening over the apex of the heart. |
| **base** | Bottom or lower part of an organ.<br>*Example:* On the X-ray, a fracture was noted at the base of the skull. |
| **proximal** (**PROK** sim al) | Located nearer to the point of attachment to the body.<br>*Example:* In the anatomical position, the elbow is proximal to the hand. |
| **distal** (**DISS** tal) | Located farther away from the point of attachment to the body.<br>*Example:* The hand is distal to the elbow. |
| **superficial** | More toward the surface of the body.<br>*Example:* The cut was superficial. |
| **deep** | Further away from the surface of the body.<br>*Example:* An incision into an abdominal organ is a deep incision. |
| **supine** (soo **PINE**) | The body lying horizontally and facing upward (see ■ Figure 2.18).<br>*Example:* The patient is in the supine position for abdominal surgery. |
| **prone** (**PROHN**) | The body lying horizontally and facing downward (see ■ Figure 2.19).<br>*Example:* The patient is placed in the prone position for spinal surgery. |

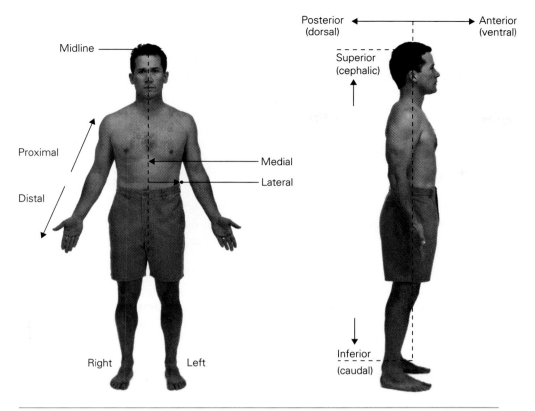

**FIGURE 2.17** Directional terms.

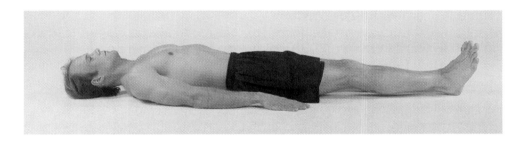

**FIGURE 2.18** The supine position.

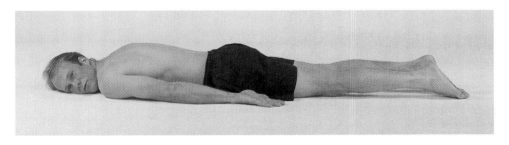

**FIGURE 2.19** The prone position.

# Body Cavities

| | | |
|---|---|---|
| abdominal cavity | parietal pleura | serous membrane |
| abdominopelvic cavity | pelvic cavity | spinal cavity |
| cranial cavity | pericardial cavity | thoracic cavity |
| diaphragm | peritoneum | viscera |
| mediastinum | pleura | visceral layer |
| parietal layer | pleural cavity | visceral peritoneum |
| parietal peritoneum | retroperitoneal | visceral pleura |

The body is not a solid structure; it has many open spaces or cavities. The cavities are part of the normal body structure and are illustrated in ▥ Figure 2.20. We can divide the body into four major cavities using the frontal plane to make two dorsal cavities and two ventral cavities.

The dorsal cavities include the **cranial cavity** (**KRAY** nee al **CAV** ih tee), containing the brain, and the **spinal cavity,** containing the spinal cord.

The ventral cavities include the **thoracic cavity** (tho **RASS** ik **CAV** ih tee) and the **abdominopelvic cavity** (ab dom ih noh **PELL** vik **CAV** ih tee). The thoracic cavity contains the two lungs and a central region between them called the **mediastinum** (mee dee ass **TYE** num). The heart, aorta, esophagus, trachea, and thymus gland are located in the mediastinum. There is an actual physical wall between the thoracic cavity and the abdominopelvic cavity called the **diaphragm** (**DYE** ah fram). The diaphragm is a muscle used for respiration or breathing. The abdominopelvic cavity is generally subdivided into a superior **abdominal cavity** (ab **DOM** ih nal **CAV** ih tee) and an inferior **pelvic cavity** (**PELL** vik **CAV** ih tee). The organs of the digestive, excretory, and reproductive systems are located in these cavities.

The organs within the ventral cavities are referred to as a group as the internal organs or **viscera** (**VISS** er ah). All of the cavities are lined by, and the viscera are encased in, a two-layer **serous** (**SEER** us) **membrane.** These membranes are called the **pleura** (**PLOO** rah) in the thoracic cavity and the **peritoneum** (pair ih toh **NEE** um) in the abdominopelvic cavity. The outer

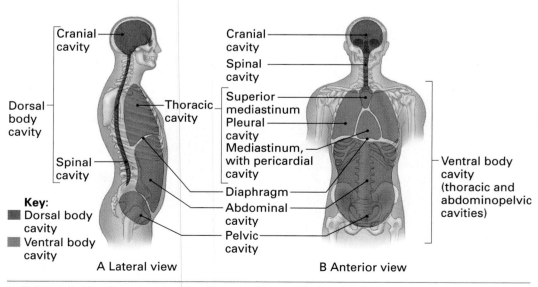

▥ **FIGURE 2.20**   Dorsal and ventral body cavities and their subdivisions.

| Table 2.3 | Body Cavities and Their Major Organs |
|---|---|
| **Cavity** | **Major Organs** |
| Dorsal cavities | |
| Cranial cavity | Brain |
| Spinal cavity | Spinal cord |
| Ventral cavities | |
| Thoracic cavity | Pleural cavity: lungs<br>Pericardial cavity: heart<br>Mediastinum: heart, esophagus, trachea, thymus gland, aorta |
| Abdominopelvic cavity | |
| Abdominal cavity | Stomach, spleen, liver, gallbladder, pancreas, and portions of the small intestines and colon |
| Pelvic cavity | Urinary bladder, ureters, urethra, and portions of the small intestines and colon |
| | *Female:* uterus, ovaries, fallopian tubes, vagina |
| | *Male:* prostate gland, seminal vesicles, portion of the vas deferens |

layer that lines the cavities is called the **parietal** (pah **RYE** eh tal) **layer** (i.e., **parietal pleura** [pah **RYE** eh tal **PLOO** rah] and **parietal peritoneum** [pah **RYE** eh tal pair ih toh **NEE** um], and the inner layer that encases the viscera is called the **visceral** (**VISS** er al) **layer** (i.e., **visceral pleura** [**VISS** er al **PLOO** rah] and **visceral peritoneum** [**VISS** er al pair ih toh **NEE** um]).

Within the thoracic cavity, the pleura is subdivided, forming the **pleural cavity** (**PLOO** ral **CAV** ih tee), containing the lungs, and the **pericardial cavity** (pair ih **CAR** dee al **CAV** ih tee), containing the heart. The larger abdominopelvic cavity is usually subdivided into regions so different areas can be precisely referred to. Two different methods of subdividing this cavity are used: the anatomical divisions and the clinical divisions. Which method a person chooses to use depends partly on personal preference and partly on which system best describes the patient's condition. Table 2.3 describes the body cavities and their major organs.

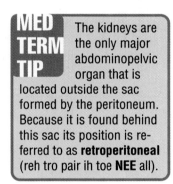

**MED TERM TIP** The kidneys are the only major abdominopelvic organ that is located outside the sac formed by the peritoneum. Because it is found behind this sac its position is referred to as **retroperitoneal** (reh tro pair ih toe **NEE** all).

## Anatomical Divisions of the Abdomen

| | | |
|---|---|---|
| **epigastric** | **left iliac** | **right iliac** |
| **hypogastric** | **left lumbar** | **right lumbar** |
| **left hypochondriac** | **right hypochondriac** | **umbilical** |

The anatomical divisions method divides the abdomen into nine sections or regions, which are frequently referred to in operative reports. The nine regions are as follows (see ■ Figure 2.21):

1. **Right hypochondriac** (high poh **KON** dree ak): Right lateral region of upper row beneath the lower ribs.
2. **Epigastric** (ep ih **GAS** trik): Middle area of upper row above the stomach.
3. **Left hypochondriac:** Left lateral region of the upper row beneath the lower ribs.
4. **Right lumbar:** Right lateral region of the middle row at the waist.

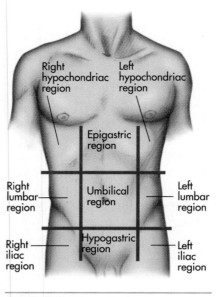

**FIGURE 2.21** Anatomical divisions of the abdomen.

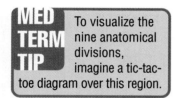

To visualize the nine anatomical divisions, imagine a tic-tac-toe diagram over this region.

5. **Umbilical** (um **BILL** ih kal): Central area over the navel.
6. **Left lumbar:** Left lateral region of the middle row at the waist.
7. **Right iliac** (**ILL** ee ak): Right lateral region of the lower row at the groin.
8. **Hypogastric** (high poh **GAS** trik): Middle region of the lower row beneath the navel.
9. **Left iliac:** Left lateral region of the lower row at the groin.

## Clinical Divisions of the Abdomen

| | |
|---|---|
| **left lower quadrant (LLQ)** | **right lower quadrant (RLQ)** |
| **left upper quadrant (LUQ)** | **right upper quadrant (RUQ)** |

The abdominopelvic region can also be divided into four equal areas or quadrants by visualizing two imaginary lines. One line is horizontal and the other one is vertical, crossing at the navel. These four quadrants are referred to as the clinical divisions of the abdomen. These terms and their abbreviations (for example, right upper quadrant or RUQ) are useful when charting patient assessments and writing operative reports. These quadrants are as follows (see ▓ Figure 2.22):

1. **Right upper quadrant (RUQ):** Contains majority of liver, gallbladder, small portion of pancreas, right kidney, small intestines, and colon.
2. **Right lower quadrant (RLQ):** Contains small intestines and colon, right ovary and fallopian tube, appendix, and right ureter.
3. **Left upper quadrant (LUQ):** Contains small portion of liver, spleen, stomach, majority of pancreas, left kidney, small intestines, and colon.
4. **Left lower quadrant (LLQ):** Contains small intestines and colon, left ovary and fallopian tube, and left ureter.

Some organs, such as the uterus and urinary bladder, fall half in the right quadrant and half in the left quadrant. Therefore, some organs are referred to as *midline organs*.

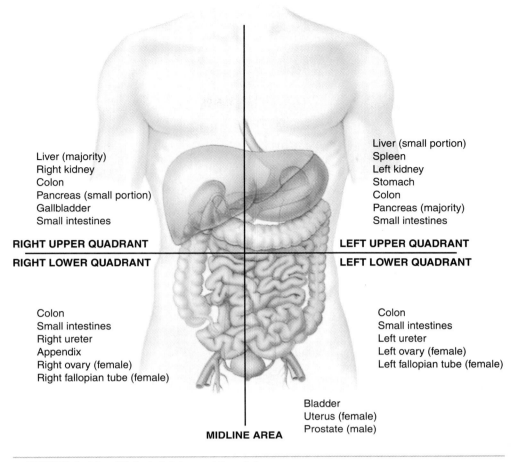

Liver (majority)
Right kidney
Colon
Pancreas (small portion)
Gallbladder
Small intestines

Liver (small portion)
Spleen
Left kidney
Stomach
Colon
Pancreas (majority)
Small intestines

**RIGHT UPPER QUADRANT**

**LEFT UPPER QUADRANT**

**RIGHT LOWER QUADRANT**

**LEFT LOWER QUADRANT**

Colon
Small intestines
Right ureter
Appendix
Right ovary (female)
Right fallopian tube (female)

Colon
Small intestines
Left ureter
Left ovary (female)
Left fallopian tube (female)

Bladder
Uterus (female)
Prostate (male)

**MIDLINE AREA**

■ **FIGURE 2.22**   Clinical divisions of the abdomen.

## Word Building Relating to Body Structure

When using medical terms to indicate different areas of the body or organs, it is usually necessary to turn the combining form into an adjective. For example, *gastr/o* becomes *gastric* or *ventr/o* becomes *ventral*. This is done by adding a suffix to the combining form that translates as *pertaining to*. The following list contains examples of frequently used medical terms relating to body structure that are built directly from word parts. It is important to study this list because there are no rules about which of the several *pertaining to* suffixes to use.

| Combining Form | Suffix | Medical Term | Definition |
|---|---|---|---|
| abdomin/o | -al | abdominal (ab **DOM** ih nal) | pertaining to the abdomen |
| anter/o | -ior | anterior (an **TEE** ree or) | pertaining to the front |
| caud/o | -al | caudal (**KAWD** al) | pertaining to the tail |
| cephal/o | -ic | cephalic (seh **FAL** ik) | pertaining to the head |
| cervic/o | -al | cervical (**SER** vih kal) | pertaining to the neck |
| crani/o | -al | cranial (**KRAY** nee al) | pertaining to the skull |
| dist/o | -al | distal (**DISS** tal) | pertaining to away |

*continued...*

| Combining Form | Suffix | Medical Term | Definition |
|---|---|---|---|
| dors/o | -al | dorsal (**DOR** sal) | pertaining to the spinal cord side |
| epitheli/o | -al | epithelial (ep ih **THEE** lee al) | pertaining to the epithelium |
| infer/o | -ior | inferior (in **FEE** ree or) | pertaining to below |
| later/o | -al | lateral (**LAT** er al) | pertaining to the side |
| medi/o | -al | medial (**MEE** dee al) | pertaining to the middle |
| muscul/o | -ar | muscular (**MUSS** kew lar) | pertaining to muscles |
| neur/o | -al | neural (**NOO** ral) | pertaining to nerves |
| pelv/o | -ic | pelvic (**PELL** vik) | pertaining to the pelvis |
| poster/o | -ior | posterior (poss **TEE** ree or) | pertaining to the back |
| proxim/o | -al | proximal (**PROK** sim al) | pertaining to near |
| somat/o | -ic | somatic (so **MAT** ik) | pertaining to the body |
| spin/o | -al | spinal | pertaining to the spine |
| super/o | -ior | superior (soo **PEE** ree or) | pertaining to above |
| system/o | -ic | systemic (sis **TEM** ik) | pertaining to systems |
| thorac/o | -ic | thoracic (tho **RASS** ik) | pertaining to the chest |
| ventr/o | -al | ventral (**VEN** tral) | pertaining to the belly side |
| viscer/o | -al | visceral (**VISS** er al) | pertaining to internal organs |

# Abbreviations Relating to Body Structure

| | | | | |
|---|---|---|---|---|
| **AP** | anteroposterior | | **LUQ** | left upper quadrant |
| **CV** | cardiovascular | | **MS** | musculoskeletal |
| **GI** | gastrointestinal | | **PA** | posteroanterior |
| **GU** | genitourinary | | **RLQ** | right lower quadrant |
| **lat** | lateral | | **RUQ** | right upper quadrant |
| **LLQ** | left lower quadrant | | **UGI** | upper gastrointestinal |

# Chapter Review

## Pronunciation Practice

You will find the pronunciation for each term on the enclosed CD-ROM.
Check each one off as you master it.

- [ ] abdominal (ab **DOM** ih nal)
- [ ] abdominal cavity (ab **DOM** ih nal **CAV** ih tee)
- [ ] abdominopelvic cavity (ab dom ih noh **PELL** vik **CAV** ih tee)
- [ ] adipose tissue (**ADD** ih pohs)
- [ ] anterior (an **TEE** ree or)
- [ ] apex (**AY** peks)
- [ ] base
- [ ] blood
- [ ] bone
- [ ] brain
- [ ] cardiac (**CAR** dee ak) muscle
- [ ] cardiology (car dee **ALL** oh jee)
- [ ] cardiovascular (car dee oh **VAS** kew lar) system
- [ ] cartilage (**CAR** tih lij)
- [ ] caudal (**KAWD** al)
- [ ] cell (**SELL**)
- [ ] cephalic (seh **FAL** ik)
- [ ] cervical (**SER** vih kal)
- [ ] connective tissue
- [ ] coronal (kor **RONE** al) plane
- [ ] cranial (**KRAY** nee al)
- [ ] cranial cavity (**KRAY** nee al **CAV** ih tee)
- [ ] cytology (sigh **TALL** oh jee)
- [ ] deep
- [ ] dermatology (der mah **TALL** oh jee)
- [ ] diaphragm (**DYE** ah fram)
- [ ] digestive system
- [ ] distal (**DISS** tal)
- [ ] dorsal (**DOR** sal)
- [ ] ear
- [ ] endocrine (**EN** doh krin) system
- [ ] endocrinology (en doh krin **ALL** oh jee)
- [ ] epigastric (ep ih **GAS** trik)
- [ ] epithelial (ep ih **THEE** lee al)

- [ ] epithelial (ep ih **THEE** lee al) tissue
- [ ] eye
- [ ] female reproductive system
- [ ] frontal plane
- [ ] gastroenterology (gas troh en ter **ALL** oh jee)
- [ ] gynecology (gigh neh **KOL** oh jee)
- [ ] hematic system
- [ ] hematology (hee mah **TALL** oh jee)
- [ ] histology (hiss **TALL** oh jee)
- [ ] horizontal plane
- [ ] hypogastric (high poh **GAS** trik)
- [ ] immunology (im yoo **NALL** oh jee)
- [ ] inferior (in **FEE** ree or)
- [ ] integumentary (in teg you **MEN** tah ree) system
- [ ] lateral (**LAT** er al)
- [ ] left hypochondriac (high poh **KON** dree ak)
- [ ] left iliac (**ILL** ee ak)
- [ ] left lower quadrant
- [ ] left lumbar (**LUM** bar)
- [ ] left upper quadrant
- [ ] lymphatic (lim **FAT** ik) system
- [ ] male reproductive system
- [ ] medial (**MEE** dee al)
- [ ] median (**MEE** dee an) plane
- [ ] mediastinum (mee dee ass **TYE** num)
- [ ] mucous (**MYOO** kus) membranes
- [ ] muscle tissue
- [ ] muscular (**MUSS** kyoo lar)
- [ ] musculoskeletal system
- [ ] nephrology (neh **FROL** oh jee)
- [ ] nerves
- [ ] nervous system
- [ ] nervous tissue
- [ ] neural (**NOO** ral)
- [ ] neurology (noo **RAL** oh jee)

- neurons (**NOO** rons)
- neurosurgery (noo roh **SIR** jer ee)
- obstetrics (ob **STET** riks)
- ophthalmology (off thal **MALL** oh jee)
- organism
- organs
- orthopedic (or tho **PEE** dik) surgery
- orthopedics (or tho **PEE** diks)
- otorhinolaryngology (oh toh rye noh lair ing **GALL** oh jee)
- parietal (pah **RYE** eh tal) layer
- parietal peritoneum (pah **RYE** eh tal pair ih toh **NEE** um)
- parietal pleura (pah **RYE** eh tal **PLOO** rah)
- pelvic (**PELL** vik)
- pelvic cavity (**PELL** vik **CAV** ih tee)
- pericardial cavity (pair ih **CAR** dee al **CAV** ih tee)
- peritoneum (pair ih toh **NEE** um)
- pleura (**PLOO** rah)
- pleural cavity (**PLOO** ral **CAV** ih tee)
- posterior (poss **TEE** ree or)
- proctology (prok **TALL** oh jee)
- prone (**PROHN**)
- proximal (**PROK** sim al)
- pulmonology (pull mon **ALL** oh jee)
- respiratory (**RES** pih rah tor ee) system
- retroperitoneal (reh tro pair ih toe **NEE** all)
- right hypochondriac (high poh **KON** dree ak)
- right iliac (**ILL** ee ak)
- right lower quadrant
- right lumbar (**LUM** bar)
- right upper quadrant
- sagittal (**SAJ** ih tal) plane
- serous (**SEER** us) membrane
- skeletal (**SKELL** eh tal) muscle
- skin
- smooth muscle
- somatic (so **MAT** ik)
- special senses
- spinal
- spinal cavity
- superficial
- superior (soo **PEE** ree or)
- supine (soo **PINE**)
- systemic (sis **TEM** ik)
- systems
- thoracic (tho **RASS** ik)
- thoracic cavity (tho **RASS** ik **CAV** ih tee)
- thoracic (tho **RASS** ik) surgery
- tissues
- transverse (trans **VERS**) plane
- umbilical (um **BILL** ih kal)
- urinary (**YOO** rih nair ee) system
- urology (yoo **RALL** oh jee)
- ventral (**VEN** tral)
- viscera (**VISS** er ah)
- visceral (**VISS** er al)
- visceral (**VISS** er al) layer
- visceral peritoneum (**VISS** er al pair ih toh **NEE** um)
- visceral pleura (**VISS** er al **PLOO** rah)

# Practice Exercises

## A. Complete the following statements.

1. The study of tissue is called _____ .

2. The tissue that lines internal organs and serves as a covering for the skin is _____ tissue.

3. The position that describes the body standing erect with arms at the sides and the palms of the hands facing forward is the _____ .

4. The _____ plane of the body is an imaginary line running lengthwise and dividing the body into right and left components.

5. The _____ quadrant of the abdomen contains the appendix.

6. The dorsal cavity contains the _____ cavity and the _____ cavity.

7. There are _____ anatomical divisions in the abdominal cavity.

8. The _____ region of the abdominal cavity is located in the right lower lateral region near the groin.

9. The upper left region located just beneath the ribs is called the _____ region.

## B. Match the planes of the body in column A with the definitions in column B.

**A**

1. _____ frontal plane
2. _____ sagittal plane
3. _____ transverse plane

**B**

a. divides the body into right and left
b. divides the body into upper and lower
c. divides the body into anterior and posterior

## C. Match the terms in column A with the definitions in column B.

**A**

1. _____ distal
2. _____ prone
3. _____ lateral
4. _____ inferior
5. _____ deep
6. _____ apex
7. _____ base
8. _____ posterior
9. _____ superficial
10. _____ supine
11. _____ anterior
12. _____ medial
13. _____ proximal
14. _____ superior

**B**

a. away from the surface
b. toward the surface
c. located closer to point of attachment to the body
d. caudal
e. tip or summit of an organ
f. lying face down
g. cephalic
h. ventral
i. dorsal
j. lying face up
k. to the side
l. middle
m. bottom or lower part of an organ
n. located further away from point of attachment to the body

**D. Circle the prefixes in the following terms and define.**

1. epigastric _____

2. intervertebral _____

3. intramuscular _____

4. pericardium _____

5. postnasal _____

6. retrosternal _____

7. substernal _____

8. transurethral _____

**E. Build terms for the following expressions using the correct prefixes, suffixes, and combining forms.**

1. pertaining to spinal cord side _____

2. pertaining to the chest _____

3. pertaining to above _____

4. pertaining to the tail _____

5. pertaining to internal organs _____

6. pertaining to the side _____

7. pertaining to away from _____

8. pertaining to nerves _____

9. pertaining to systems _____

10. pertaining to the muscles _____

11. pertaining to the belly side _____

12. pertaining to the front _____

13. pertaining to the head _____

14. pertaining to middle _____

**F. Write the abbreviations for the following terms.**

1. musculoskeletal _____

2. lateral _____

3. right upper quadrant _____

4. cardiovascular _____

5. gastrointestinal _____

6. anteroposterior _____

7. genitourinary _____

8. left lower quadrant _____

**G. Define the following combining forms.**

1. viscer/o _____

2. poster/o _____

3. abdomin/o _____

4. thorac/o _____

5. medi/o _____

6. ventr/o _____

7. anter/o _____

8. hist/o _____

9. epitheli/o _____

10. crani/o _____

11. somat/o _____

12. proxim/o _____

13. cephal/o _____

## H. Use the following terms in the sentences that follow.

cardiology          endocrinology        gastroenterology     gynecology

ophthalmology       urology              orthopedics          immunology

otorhinolaryngology proctology           obstetrics

1. John is a musician who plays an electric bass guitar and is experiencing difficulty in hearing soft voices. He would consult a physician in _____ .

2. Ruth is a stock trader with the Chicago Board of Trade. She has had a pounding and racing heartbeat. She would consult a physician specializing in _____ .

3. Mary Ann is experiencing excessive bleeding from fibroid tumors. She would consult a specialist in _____ .

4. Jose has persistent pain in his lower back. He would be seen for an examination by a physician in _____ .

5. A physician who performs eye exams is specializing in the field of _____ .

# Professional Journal

In this exercise you will now have an opportunity to put the words you have learned into practice. Imagine yourself in the role of a physician assistant. If you refer back to the Professional Profile at the beginning of this chapter, you will see that this health care professional is responsible for conducting physical examinations, ordering tests and treatments, and making diagnoses. Use the 10 words listed below to write sentences to describe the patients you saw today. An example of a sentence is *Mr. Jones stepped off a curb wrong today and tore a muscle in his distal leg.*

1.  abdominal cavity _____

2.  dermatology _____

3.  gastroenterology _____

4.  female reproductive system _____

5.  right lower quadrant _____

6.  superior _____

7.  dorsal _____

8.  nerves _____

9.  prone _____

10. lateral _____

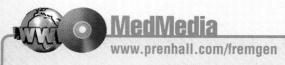

**MedMedia**
www.prenhall.com/fremgen

Use the CD-ROM enclosed with your textbook to gain additional reinforcement through interactive word building exercises, spelling games, labeling activities, and additional quizzes.

Use the above address to access the free, interactive Companion Website created for this textbook. Get hints, instant feedback, and textbook references to chapter-related multiple-choice questions, as well as labeling and matching exercises. In addition, you will find an audio glossary, case studies, and Internet exploration exercises.

# Chapter 3
# Integumentary System

## Learning Objectives

***Upon completion of this chapter, you will be able to:***

- Recognize the combining forms and suffixes introduced in this chapter.

- Gain the ability to pronounce medical terms and major anatomical structures.

- List and describe the three layers of skin and their functions.

- Describe the four purposes of the skin.

- Name and describe the body membranes.

- List and describe the accessory organs of the skin.

- Build integumentary system medical terms from word parts.

- Define vocabulary, pathology, diagnostic, and therapeutic medical terms relating to the integumentary system.

- Interpret abbreviations associated with the integumentary system.

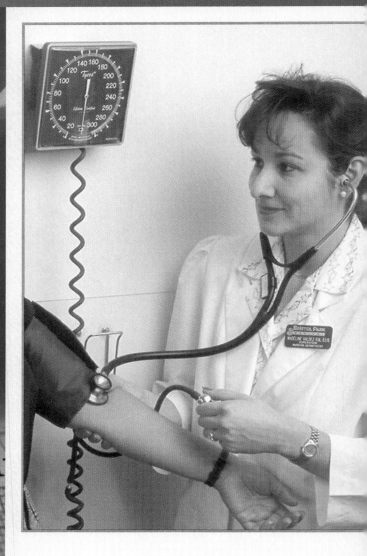

## Professional Profile

### Nursing Service

Nursing service workers assess patients, plan and carry out patient treatments, and evaluate the patient's response to treatment. Skilled nursing care includes intravenous therapy, administering medication and anesthesia, wound care, and patient education. Nursing service personnel are found in acute and long-term care facilities, clinics, physicians' offices, health maintenance organizations, home health agencies, public health agencies, and schools.

### Nurse Practitioner (NP)

- A registered nurse who receives advanced training in a specialized area of nursing such as family health, women's health, pediatric health, gerontological health, or acute care
- Meets all the requirements for becoming a registered nurse
- Completes advanced training and clinical experience in an accredited nurse practitioner program
- Passes national certification examination

### Registered Nurse (RN, BSN, MSN)

- Assesses patient status and progress, provides patient care, administers medications, and provides patient education
- Graduates from an accredited 2-year associate, 4-year bachelor's, or 5-year master's degree nursing program
- Passes national licensing examination

### Licensed Practical/Vocational Nurse (LPN or LVN)

- Trained in basic nursing techniques such as administering medications, dressing wounds, and collecting specimens for laboratory tests
- Works under the supervision of a physician or registered nurse
- Passes national licensing examination

### Certified Nurse Aide (CNA)

- Trained in basic patient care such as taking vital signs, bathing, and feeding
- Works under supervision of RN or LPN
- Completes approved on-the-job certification program

***For more information regarding these health careers, visit the following websites:***
American Nurses Association at **www.nursingworld.org**
National Federation of Licensed Practical Nurses at **www.nflpn.org**
National League for Nursing at **www.nln.org**

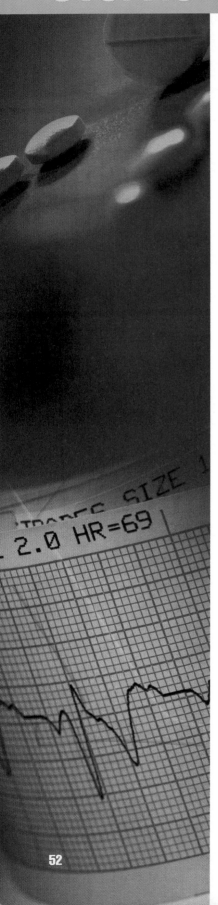

### Organs of the Integumentary System

skin
    dermis
    epidermis
    subcutaneous layer
accessory organs
    hair
    nails
    sebaceous (see **BAY** shus) glands
    sweat glands

### Combining Forms Relating to the Integumentary System

| | | | |
|---|---|---|---|
| adip/o | fat | melan/o | black |
| albin/o | white | myc/o | fungus |
| bi/o | life | necr/o | death |
| cry/o | cold | onych/o | nail |
| cutane/o | skin | pachy/o | thick |
| cyan/o | blue | pil/o | hair |
| derm/o | skin | py/o | pus |
| dermat/o | skin | rhytid/o | wrinkle |
| diaphor/o | profuse sweating | scler/o | hard |
| hidr/o | sweat | seb/o | oil |
| ichthy/o | scaly, dry | trich/o | hair |
| kerat/o | hard, horny | ungu/o | nail |
| leuk/o | white | xanth/o | yellow |
| lip/o | fat | xer/o | dry |

### Suffixes Relating to the Integumentary System

| Suffix | Meaning | Example |
|---|---|---|
| -derma | skin | scleroderma |
| -opsy | view of | biopsy |
| -plakia | a plate | leukoplakia |
| -tome | instrument used to cut | dermatome |

## Anatomy and Physiology of the Integumentary System

| | | |
|---|---|---|
| **hair** | **nails** | **sebum** |
| **integument** | **pathogens** | **sensory receptors** |
| **integumentary system** | **sebaceous glands** | **sweat glands** |

The skin and its accessory organs—**sweat glands, sebaceous** (see **BAY** shus) **glands, hair,** and **nails**—are known as the **integumentary** (in teg you **MEN** tah ree) **system** and **integument** (in **TEG** you mint) is another term for skin. In fact, the skin is the largest organ of the body. It can weigh more than 20 pounds in an adult. The skin serves many purposes for the body: protecting, housing nerve receptors, secreting fluids, and regulating temperature.

The primary function of the skin is protection. It forms a two-way barrier that is capable of keeping **pathogens** (**PATH** oh jenz) (disease-causing organisms) and harmful chemicals from entering the body. It also stops critical body fluids from escaping the body and prevents injury to the internal organs lying underneath the skin.

**Sensory receptors** that detect temperature, pain, touch, and pressure are located in the skin. The messages for these sensations are conveyed to the spinal cord and brain from the nerve endings in the middle layer of the skin.

Fluids are produced in two types of skin glands: sweat and sebaceous. Sweat glands assist the body in maintaining its internal temperature by creating a cooling effect when sweat evaporates. The sebaceous glands, or oil glands, produce a substance called **sebum** (SEE bum). This oily substance lubricates the skin surface.

The structure of skin aids in the regulation of body temperature through a variety of means. As noted previously, the evaporation of sweat cools the body. The body also lowers its internal temperature by dilating superficial blood vessels in the skin. This brings more blood to the surface of the skin, which allows the release of heat. If the body needs to conserve heat, it constricts superficial blood vessels, keeping warm blood away from the surface of the body. Finally, the continuous fat layer of the subcutaneous layer of the skin acts as insulation.

> **MED TERM TIP** Flushing of the skin is a normal response to an increase in temperature in the environment or to a fever. However, in some people, it is also a response to embarrassment. This is called *blushing* and is not easily controlled.

## Body Membranes

connective tissue membranes

cutaneous membrane

epithelial membranes

mucous membranes

mucus

serous membranes

synovial membranes

Several different types of membranes are found in the body. The skin is an example of one of these. Membranes are layers of tissue that cover and protect body surfaces, line body cavities, and line some internal organs, such as the digestive and respiratory passages. Membranes also secrete lubricating fluids to reduce friction during some processes, such as respiration, and serve to anchor organs and bones.

The two major types of membranes are **epithelial** (ep ih **THEE** lee al) **membranes** and **connective tissue membranes.** Epithelial membranes contain two layers of tissue: a superficial layer of epithelial tissue and an underlying layer of connective tissue. In contrast, connective tissue membranes contain only connective tissue and no epithelial cells.

There are three types of epithelial membranes:

1. **Cutaneous** (kew **TAY** nee us) **membrane** is another term for the skin.

2. **Serous** (**SEER** us) **membranes** line body cavities. They secrete a thin, watery fluid that acts as a lubricant to reduce friction when organs rub against each other.

3. **Mucous** (**MYOO** kus) **membranes** line body passages that open directly to the exterior of the body, such as the mouth and reproductive tract. They secrete a sticky fluid, **mucus** (**MYOO** kus), to trap pathogens.

**Synovial** (sin **OH** vee al) **membranes** are the most common connective tissue membrane. They form the lining found in joint capsules and secrete a lubricating fluid for joints.

## The Skin

| | | |
|---|---|---|
| **basal layer** | **epidermis** | **melanocytes** |
| **collagen fibers** | **keratin** | **stratified squamous** |
| **corium** | **lipocytes** | **epithelium** |
| **dermis** | **melanin** | **subcutaneous layer** |

Moving from the outer surface of the skin inward, the three layers are as follows (see ■ Figure 3.1):

1. **Epidermis** (ep ih **DER** mis) is the thin, outer membrane layer.
2. **Dermis** (**DER** mis) or **corium** (**KOH** ree um) is the middle, fibrous connective tissue layer.
3. The **subcutaneous** (sub kyoo **TAY** nee us) (Subcu, Subq) **layer** is the innermost layer, containing fatty tissue.

### Epidermis

The epidermis is composed of squamous epithelial cells (see ■ Figure 3.2). These flat scale-like cells are arranged in overlapping layers or strata referred to as **stratified squamous epithelium** (**STRAT** ih fyde **SKWAY** mus ep ih **THEE** lee um). The epidermis does not have a blood supply or any connective tissue, so it is dependent for nourishment on the deeper layers of skin.

The deepest layer within the epidermis is called the **basal** (BAY sal) **layer.** Cells in this layer continually grow and multiply. New cells that are forming push the old cells toward the outer layer of the epidermis. During this process

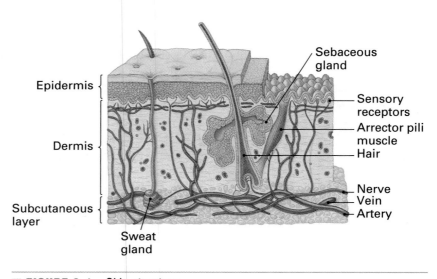

■ **FIGURE 3.1** Skin structure.

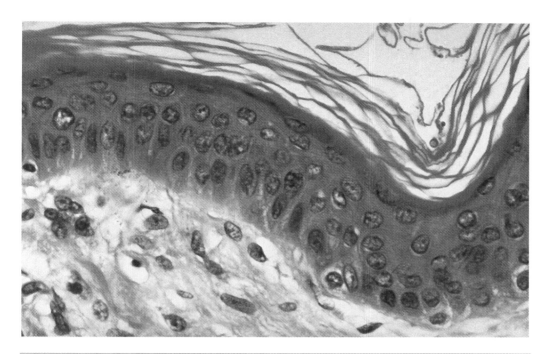

 **FIGURE 3.2** Epidermis.

the cells shrink and die and become filled with a hard protein called **keratin** (**KAIR** ah tin). These dead, keratinized cells allow the skin to act as a barrier to infection and make it waterproof.

The basal layer also contains special cells called **melanocytes** (mel **AN** oh sights), which produce the black pigment **melanin** (**MEL** ah nin). Not only is this pigment responsible for the color of one's skin, but it also protects against damage from the ultraviolet rays of the sun. This damage may be in the form of leather-like skin and wrinkles, which are unwelcomed, but not dangerous. Or it may be one of several forms of skin cancer. Dark-skinned people have more melanin and are generally less likely to have wrinkles or skin cancer.

**MED TERM TIP** We are constantly losing old dead skin cells and replacing them with new younger cells. In fact, because of this process, our skin is replaced entirely about every seven years.

## Dermis

The dermis, also referred to as the corium, is the middle layer of skin, located between the epidermis and the subcutaneous layer. Its name means "true skin." Unlike the thinner epidermis, the dermis is living tissue with a very good blood supply. The dermis itself is composed of connective tissue and **collagen** (**KOL** ah jen) **fibers.** Collagen fibers are made from a strong fibrous protein present in connective tissue, forming a flexible "glue" that gives connective tissue its strength. The dermis houses hair follicles, sweat glands, sebaceous glands, blood vessels, lymph vessels, sensory receptors, nerve fibers, and muscle fibers.

 **MED TERM TIP** Ridges formed in the dermis of our fingertips are what gives each of us unique fingerprints (see Figure 3.3). These do not change during a person's lifetime and are thus a reliable means of identification.

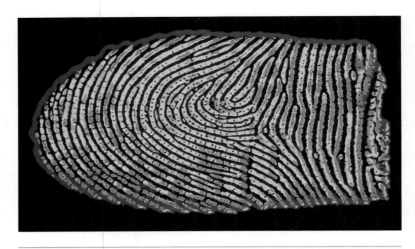

**FIGURE 3.3** Enhanced color fingerprint.
(Scott Camazine/Photo Researchers, Inc.)

### Subcutaneous Layer

This third and deepest layer of the skin is formed of fat. This layer of tissue, composed of fat cells called **lipocytes** (**LIP** oh sights), protects the deeper tissues of the body and acts as insulation for heat and cold.

> **MED TERM TIP**
> A suntan can be thought of as a protective response to the rays of the sun. However, when the melanin in the skin is not able to absorb all the rays of the sun, the skin burns.

## Accessory Organs

The accessory organs of the skin are the anatomical structures located within the dermis. This includes hair, nails, sweat glands, and sebaceous glands.

### Hair

**hair follicle**          **hair root**          **hair shaft**

> **MED TERM TIP**
> Our hair turns gray when we no longer produce melanin. This is a normal part of the aging process.

The fibers that make up our hair are composed of the protein keratin, the same hard protein material that fills the cells of the epidermis. The process of hair formation is much like the process of growth in the epidermal layer of the skin. The deeper cells in the **hair root** (see ▪ Figure 3.4) force older keratinized cells to move upward, forming the **hair shaft.** The hair shaft grows toward the skin surface within the **hair follicle** (**FALL** ikl). Melanin gives hair its color. Sebaceous glands release sebum directly into the hair follicle.

### Nails

| | | |
|---|---|---|
| **cuticle** | **lunula** | **nail body** |
| **cyanosis** | **nail bed** | **nail root** |
| **free edge** | | |

Nails are a flat plate of keratin called the **nail body** that covers the ends of fingers and toes. The nail body is connected to the tissue underneath by the **nail bed** (see ▪ Figure 3.5). Nails grow longer from the **nail root,** which is found at the base of the nail and is covered and protected by the soft tissue **cuticle** (**KEW**

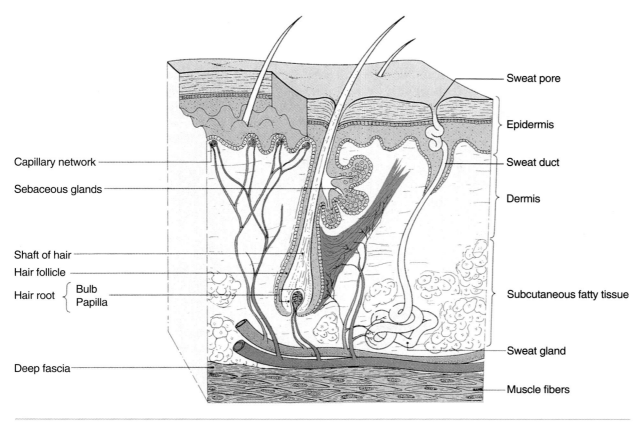

**FIGURE 3.4** Hair follicle/skin structures.

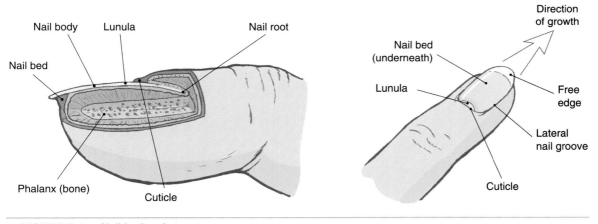

**FIGURE 3.5** Nail bed and structure.

tikl). The **free edge** is the exposed edge that is trimmed when nails become too long. The light-colored half-moon area at the base of the nail is the **lunula** (**LOO** nyoo lah).

**MED TERM TIP**

Because of its rich blood supply and light color, the nail bed is an excellent place to check patients for low oxygen levels in their blood. Deoxygenated blood is a very dark purple-red and gives skin a bluish tinge called **cyanosis** (sigh ah **NOH** sis).

### Sebaceous Glands

Sebaceous glands, found in the dermis, secrete the oil sebum. These oil ducts open into hair follicles and lubricate the hair and skin, thereby helping to prevent drying of the skin (refer to Figure 3.4). Secretion from the sebaceous glands increases during adolescence and begins to diminish as age increases. A loss of sebum in old age, along with sun exposure, can account for wrinkles and dry skin.

### Sweat Glands

**apocrine glands**      **sweat duct**      **sweat pore**
**perspiration**

About two million sweat glands are found throughout the body. The highly coiled gland is located in the dermis. Sweat travels to the surface of the skin in a **sweat duct.** The surface opening of a sweat duct is called a **sweat pore** (refer to Figure 3.4).

Sweat glands function in cooling the body as sweat evaporates. Sweat or **perspiration** contains a small amount of waste products but is normally colorless and odorless. However, there are sweat glands called **apocrine** (**APP** oh krin) **glands** in the pubic and underarm areas. These glands secrete a thicker sweat that can produce an odor when it comes into contact with bacteria on the skin. This is what we recognize as body odor.

## Word Building Relating to the Integumentary System

The following list contains examples of medical terms built directly from word parts. The definition for these terms can be determined by a straightforward translation of the word parts.

| Combining Form | Combined With | Medical Term | Definition |
|---|---|---|---|
| cutane/o | sub- -ous | subcutaneous (sub kyoo **TAY** nee us) | pertaining to under the skin |
| derm/o | epi- -al | epidermal (ep ih **DER** mal) | pertaining to upon the skin |
| | hypo- -ic | hypodermic (high poh **DER** mik) | pertaining to under the skin |
| | intra- -al | intradermal (in trah **DER** mal) | pertaining to within the skin |
| | -tome | dermatome (**DER** mah tohm) | instrument to cut the skin |
| dermat/o | -itis | dermatitis (der mah **TYE** tis) | inflammation of the skin |
| | -logist | dermatologist (der mah **TALL** oh jist) | specialist in skin |
| | -logy | dermatology (der mah **TALL** oh jee) | study of the skin |
| | -pathy | dermatopathy (der mah **TOP** ah thee) | skin disease |
| | -plasty | dermatoplasty (**DER** mah toh plas tee) | surgical repair of the skin |
| hidr/o | an- -osis | anhidrosis (an hi **DROH** sis) | abnormal condition of no sweat |
| | hyper- -osis | hyperhidrosis (high per hi **DROH** sis) | abnormal condition of excessive sweat |

| Combining Form | Combined With | Medical Term | Definition |
|---|---|---|---|
| lip/o | -ectomy | lipectomy (lih **PECK** toh mee) | excision of fat |
| | -oma | lipoma (lip **OH** mah) | fatty growth |
| melan/o | -oma | melanoma (mel ah **NOH** mah) | black tumor |
| necr/o | -osis | necrosis (neh **KROH** sis) | abnormal condition of death |
| onych/o | -ectomy | onychectomy (on ee **KECK** toh mee) | excision of a nail |
| | -malacia | onychomalacia (on ih koh mah **LAY** she ah) | softening of nails |
| | myc/o -osis | onychomycosis (on ih koh my **KOH** sis) | abnormal condition of nail fungus |
| | -phagia | onychophagia (on ih koh **FAY** jee ah) | nail eating (nail biting) |
| py/o | -genic | pyogenic (pye oh **JEN** ik) | pus forming |
| rhytid/o | -ectomy | rhytidectomy (rit ih **DECK** toh mee) | excision of wrinkles |
| | -plasty | rhytidoplasty (**RIT** ih doh plas tee) | surgical repair of wrinkles |
| seb/o | -rrhea | seborrhea (seb or **EE** ah) | oily discharge |
| trich/o | myc/o -osis | trichomycosis (trik oh my **KOH** sis) | abnormal condition of hair fungus |
| ungu/o | -al | ungual (**UNG** gwal) | pertaining to the nails |

| Suffix | Combined With | Medical Term | Meaning |
|---|---|---|---|
| -derma | erythr/o | erythroderma (eh rith roh **DER** mah) | red skin |
| | ichthy/o | ichthyoderma (ick thee oh **DER** mah) | scaly and dry skin |
| | leuk/o | leukoderma (loo koh **DER** mah) | white skin |
| | pachy/o | pachyderma (pak ee **DER** mah) | thick skin |
| | scler/o | scleroderma (sklair ah **DER** mah) | hard skin |
| | xanth/o | xanthoderma (zan thoh **DER** mah) | yellow skin |
| | xer/o | xeroderma (zee roh **DER** mah) | dry skin |

| **Table 3.1** | **Skin Lesions** |

**Primary Skin Lesions**

**Macule**

Flat, nonpalpable change in skin color. Macules are smaller than 1 cm, with a circumscribed border.
*Examples:* freckles, measles, and petechiae.

**Wheal**

Elevated, often reddish area with irregular border caused by diffuse fluid in tissues rather than free fluid in a cavity, as in vesicles. Size varies.
*Examples:* insect bites and hives (extensive wheals).

**Papule**

Elevated, solid, palpable mass with circumscribed border. Papules are smaller than 0.5 cm.
*Examples:* elevated moles, and warts.

**Pustule**

Elevated, pus-filled vesicle or bulla with circumscribed border. Size varies.
*Examples:* acne, impetigo, and carbuncles (large boils).

**Nodule**

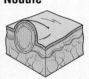

Elevated, solid, hard or soft palpable mass extending deeper into the dermis than a papule. Nodules have circumscribed borders and are 0.5 to 2 cm.
*Examples:* small lipoma, squamous cell carcinoma, fibroma, and intradermal.

**Cyst**

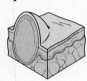

Elevated, encapsulated, fluid-filled or semisolid mass originating in the subcutaneous tissue or dermis, usually 1 cm or larger.
*Examples:* varieties include sebaceous cysts and epidermoid cysts.

**Vesicle**

Elevated, fluid-filled, round or oval shaped palpable mass with thin, translucent walls and circumscribed borders. Vesicles are smaller than 0.5 cm.
*Examples:* herpes simplex/zoster, early chickenpox, poison ivy, and small burn blisters.

**Secondary Skin Lesions**

**Ulcer**

Deep, irregularly shaped area of skin loss extending into the dermis or subcutaneous tissue. May bleed. May leave scar.
*Examples:* decubitus ulcers (pressure sores), stasis ulcers, chancres.

**Cicatrix**

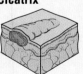

Flat, irregular area of connective tissue left after a lesion or wound has healed. New scars may be red or purple; older scars may be silvery or white.
*Examples:* healed surgical wound or injury, healed acne.

**Fissure**

Linear crack with sharp edges, extending into the dermis.
*Examples:* cracks at the corners of the mouth or in the hands, athlete's foot.

**Keloid**

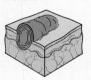

Elevated, irregular, darkened area of excess scar tissue caused by excessive collagen formation during healing. Extends beyond the site of the original injury. Higher incidence in people of African descent.
*Examples:* keloid from ear piercing, surgery, or burn.

NOTE. From *Health Assessment in Nursing* (table 8.4, p.147) by L. Sims, D. D'Amico, J. Stiesmeyer, & J. Webster, 1995. Redwood City, CA: Addison-Wesley. Reprinted by permission.

# Vocabulary Relating to the Integumentary System

| | |
|---|---|
| abrasion (ah BRAY zhun) | A scraping away of the skin surface by friction. |
| abscess (AB sess) | A collection of pus in the skin. |
| albino (al BYE noh) | A genetic condition in which the person is unable to make melanin. Characterized by white hair and skin, and red pupils due to the lack of pigment. |
| alopecia (al oh PEE she ah) | Absence or loss of hair, especially of the head. Commonly called *baldness.* |
| cicatrix (SICK ah trix) | A scar (see Table 3.1). |
| comedo (KOM ee do) | Collection of hardened sebum in hair follicle. Also called a *blackhead.* |
| contusion | Injury caused by a blow to the body; causes swelling, pain, and bruising. The skin is not broken. |
| cyanosis (sigh ah NOH sis) | Bluish tint to the skin caused by deoxygenated blood. |
| cyst (SIST) | Fluid-filled sac under the skin (see Table 3.1). |
| decubitus (dee KYOO bih tus) ulcer (decub) | Open sore caused by pressure over bony prominences cutting off the blood flow to the overlying skin. These can appear in bedridden patients who lie in one position too long and can be difficult to heal. Also called *bedsore* or *pressure sore.* |
| depigmentation (dee pig men TAY shun) | Loss of normal skin color or pigment. |
| dermatologist (der mah TALL oh jist) | Physician who specializes in the treatment of diseases and conditions of the integumentary system. |
| dermatology (der mah TALL oh jee) (Derm, derm) | Study of diseases and conditions of the integumentary system. |
| diaphoresis (dye ah for REE sis) | Profuse sweating. |
| ecchymosis (ek ih MOH sis) | Skin discoloration caused by blood collecting under the skin following blunt trauma to the skin. A bruise (see ▨ Figure 3.6). |
| erythema (er ih THEE mah) | Redness or flushing of the skin. |
| fissure (FISH er) | Crack-like lesion or groove on the skin (see Table 3.1). |
| frostbite | Freezing or the effect of freezing on a part of the body. Exposed areas such as ears, nose, cheeks, fingers, and toes are generally affected (see ▨ Figure 3.7). |
| hemangioma (hee man jee OH ma) | Benign tumor of dilated blood vessels (see ▨ Figure 3.8). |
| hirsutism (HER soot izm) | Excessive hair growth over the body. |
| hyperemia (high per EE mee ah) | Redness of the skin due to increased blood flow. |
| hyperpigmentation (high per pig men TAY shun) | Abnormal amount of pigmentation in the skin. |
| keloid (KEE loyd) | Formation of a raised and thickened hypertrophic scar after an injury or surgery (see Table 3.1 and ▨ Figure 3.9). |
| keratosis (kair ah TOH sis) | Skin condition with an overgrowth and thickening of the epidermis. |
| macule (MACK yool) | Flat, discolored area that is flush with the skin surface. An example would be a freckle or a birthmark (see Table 3.1). |

*continued...*

| | |
|---|---|
| **male pattern baldness** | Pattern of baldness most commonly seen in men. Begins as a receding hairline and progresses to full baldness on top of the head and a fringe of hair around the edges. |
| **nevus (NEV us)** | Pigmented congenital skin blemish, birthmark, or mole. Usually benign but may become cancerous. |
| **nodule (NOD yool)** | Firm, solid mass of cells in the skin (see Table 3.1). |
| **papule (PAP yool)** | Small, solid, circular raised spot on the surface of the skin. Less than 1 cm in diameter (see Table 3.1). |
| **pediculosis (peh dik you LOH sis)** | Infestation with lice. The eggs laid by the lice are called nits and cling tightly to hair. |
| **petechiae (peh TEE kee eye)** | Pinpoint purple or red spots from minute hemorrhages under the skin (see ▧ Figure 3.10). |
| **photosensitivity (foh toh sen sih TIH vih tee)** | Condition in which the skin reacts abnormally when exposed to light, such as the ultraviolet (UV) rays of the sun. |
| **polyp (POLL ip)** | Small tumor with a pedicle or stem attachment. They are commonly found in mucous membranes such as the nasal cavity. |
| **pruritus (proo RIGH tus)** | Severe itching. |
| **purpura (PER pew rah)** | Hemorrhages into the skin due to fragile blood vessels. Commonly seen in elderly people (see ▧ Figure 3.11). |
| **purulent (PYUR yoo lent)** | Containing or producing pus. |
| **pustule (PUS tyool)** | Raised spot on the skin containing pus (see Table 3.1 and ▧ Figure 3.12). |
| **scabies (SKAY bees)** | Contagious skin disease caused by an egg-laying mite that burrows through the skin and causes redness and intense itching; often seen in children. |
| **suppurative (SUP pure a tiv)** | Containing or producing pus. |
| **ulcer (ULL ser)** | Open sore or lesion in skin or mucous membrane (see Table 3.1). |
| **urticaria (er tih KAY ree ah)** | Also called *hives;* a skin eruption of pale reddish wheals with severe itching. Usually associated with food allergy, stress, or drug reactions. |
| **verruca (ver ROO kah)** | Commonly called *warts;* a benign growth caused by a virus. Has a rough surface that is removed by chemicals and/or laser therapy. |
| **vesicle (VESS ikl)** | A blister; small, fluid-filled raised spot on the skin (see Table 3.1 and ▧ Figure 3.13). |
| **vitiligo (vit ill EYE go)** | Disappearance of pigment from the skin in patches, causing a milk-white appearance. Also called *leukoderma.* |
| **wheal (WEEL)** | Small, round, raised area on the skin that may be accompanied by itching (see Table 3.1 and ▧ Figure 3.14). |

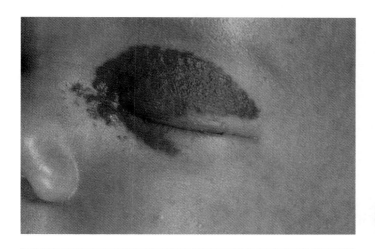

**■ FIGURE 3.6** Ecchymosis.
(NMSB/Custom Medical Stock)

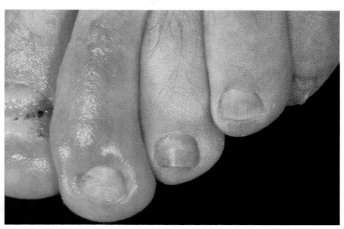

**■ FIGURE 3.7** Frostbite of toes.
(BioPhoto Associates/Photo Researchers, Inc.)

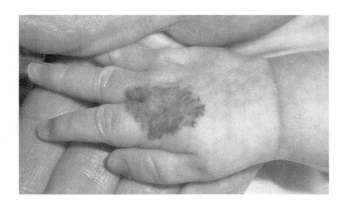

**■ FIGURE 3.8** Hemangioma (birthmark) on baby's hand.
(Dr. H. C. Robinson/Science Photo Library/Photo Researchers, Inc.)

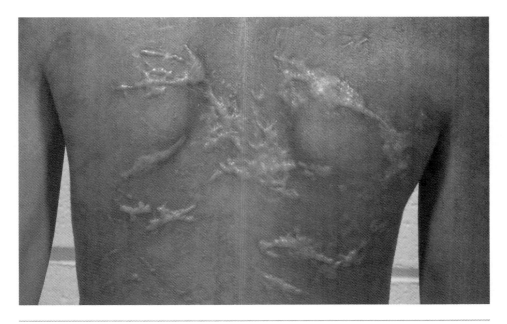

**■ FIGURE 3.9** Keloids on back.
(Martin Rotker/Phototake NYC)

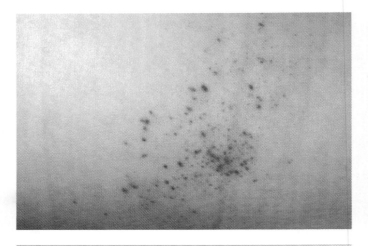

■ **FIGURE 3.10**   Petechiae.
(Custom Medical Stock)

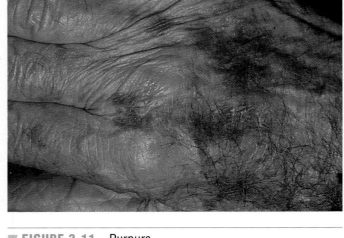

■ **FIGURE 3.11**   Purpura.
(Copyright © Carroll H. Weiss. All rights reserved.)

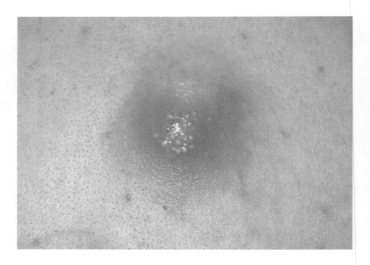

■ **FIGURE 3.12**   Pustule.
(Charles Stewart And Associates)

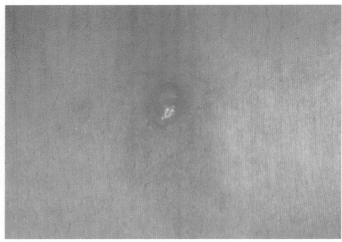

■ **FIGURE 3.13**   Vesicle associated with chicken pox.
(Charles Stewart and Associates)

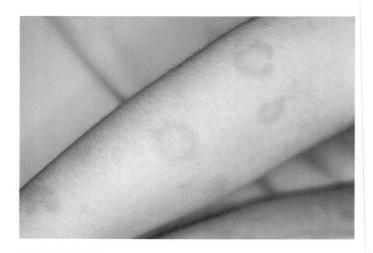

■ **FIGURE 3.14**   Wheals.
(CNRI/Phototake NYC)

# Pathology Relating to the Integumentary System

| | |
|---|---|
| **acne (ACK nee)** | Inflammatory disease of the sebaceous glands and hair follicles that results in papules and pustules. |
| **acne rosacea (ACK nee roh ZAY she ah)** | Form of acne seen in adults, especially on the nose and cheeks. |
| **acne vulgaris (ACK nee vul GAY ris)** | Common form of acne seen in teenagers. Characterized by comedo, papules, and pustules. |
| **basal cell carcinoma (BAY sal sell kar sin NOH ma) (BCC)** | Cancerous tumor of the basal cell layer of the epidermis. A frequent type of skin cancer that rarely metastasizes or spreads. These cancers can arise on sun-exposed skin. |
| **burn** | Damage to the skin that can result from exposure to open fire, electricity, ultraviolet light from the sun, or caustic chemicals. Seriousness depends on the amount of body surface involved and the depth of the burn. Extent of a burn is estimated using the Rule of Nines (see ▨ Figure 3.15). Depth is determined by the number of layers of skin involved (see ▨ Figure 3.16). |
| **burn, 1st degree** | Damage to the epidermis layer of the skin. Characterized by hyperemia, but no blisters or scars (see ▨ Figures 3.16 and 3.17). |
| **burn, 2nd degree** | Damage extends through the epidermis and into the dermis, causing vesicles to form. Scarring may occur. Also called *partial thickness burn* (see ▨ Figures 3.16 and 3.18). |
| **burn, 3rd degree** | Damage to full thickness of skin and into underlying tissues. Infection is a major concern with 3rd degree burns, and fluid loss can be life threatening. Grafts are usually required and scarring will occur. Also called *full-thickness burn* (see ▨ Figures 3.16 and 3.19). |
| **carbuncle (CAR bung kl)** | Furuncle involving several hair follicles. |
| **cellulitis (sell you LYE tis)** | A diffuse, acute infection and inflammation of the skin (see ▨ Figure 3.20). |
| **dry gangrene (GANG green)** | Late stages of gangrene characterized by the affected area becoming black and leathery. |
| **eczema (EK zeh mah)** | Superficial dermatitis of unknown cause accompanied by papules, vesicles, and crusting. |
| **furuncle (FOO rung kl)** | Bacterial infection of a hair follicle. Characterized by redness, pain, and swelling. Also called a *boil.* |
| **gangrene (GANG green)** | Tissue necrosis usually due to deficient blood supply. |
| **ichthyosis (ick thee OH sis)** | Condition in which the skin becomes dry, scaly, and keratinized. |
| **impetigo (im peh TYE goh)** | A bacterial infection of the skin with pustules that rupture and become crusted over (see ▨ Figure 3.21). |
| **Kaposi's sarcoma (KAP oh seez sar KOH mah)** | Form of skin cancer frequently seen in acquired immunodeficiency syndrome (AIDS) patients. Consists of brownish-purple papules that spread from the skin and metastasize to internal organs (see ▨ Figure 3.22). Named for Moritz Kaposi, an Austrian dermatologist. |
| **leukoplakia (loo koh PLAY kee ah)** | Change in mucous membrane that results in thick, white plate-like patches on the mucous membrane of the tongue and cheek. Considered precancerous, it is associated with smoking. |

*continued...*

| | |
|---|---|
| **malignant melanoma (mah LIG nant mel a NOH ma) (MM)** | Dangerous form of skin cancer caused by an uncontrolled growth of melanocytes. May quickly metastasize or spread to internal organs (see ▦ Figure 3.23). |
| **onychia (oh NICK ee ah)** | Infected nail bed. |
| **paronychia (pair oh NICK ee ah)** | Infection around a nail. |
| **pemphigus vulgaris (PEM fih gus vul GAY ris)** | Skin condition in which blisters form in the skin and mucous membranes. |
| **psoriasis (soh RYE ah sis)** | Chronic inflammatory condition consisting of crusty papules forming patches with circular borders (see ▦ Figure 3.24). |
| **rubella (roo BELL ah)** | Contagious viral skin infection. Commonly called *German measles.* |
| **sebaceous cyst (see BAY shus SIST)** | Sac under the skin filled with sebum or oil from a sebaceous gland. This can grow to a large size and may need to be excised. |
| **shingles (SHING lz)** | Eruption of vesicles along a nerve path, causing a rash and pain. Caused by the same virus as chicken pox. |
| **squamous cell carcinoma (SKWAY mus sell kar sih NOH mah) (SCC)** | Epidermal cancer that may go into deeper tissue but does not generally metastasize. |
| **systemic lupus erythematosus (sis TEM ik LOO pus air ih them ah TOH sis) (SLE)** | Chronic disease of the connective tissue that injures the skin, joints, kidneys, nervous system, and mucous membranes. May produce a characteristic butterfly rash across the cheeks and nose. |
| **tinea (TIN ee ah)** | Fungal skin disease resulting in itching, scaling lesions. |
| **tinea capitis (TIN ee ah CAP it is)** | Fungal infection of the scalp. Commonly called *ringworm.* |
| **tinea pedis (TIN ee ah PED is)** | Fungal infection of the foot. Commonly called *athlete's foot.* |
| **varicella (VAIR ih chell a)** | Contagious viral skin infection. Commonly called *chicken pox* (see ▦ Figure 3.25). |
| **wet gangrene (GANG green)** | Area of gangrene becoming infected by pus-producing bacteria. |

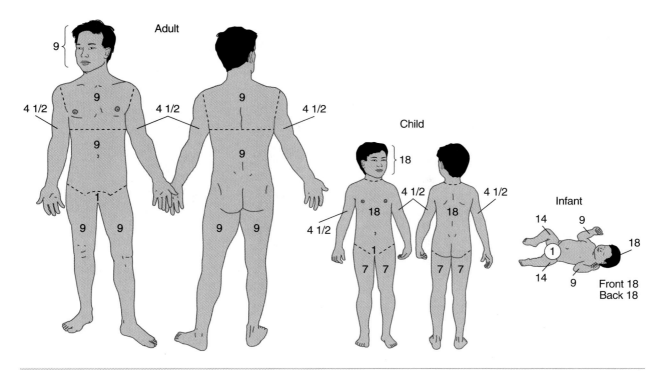

**FIGURE 3.15** Rule of Nines for burns (all numbers are % of body surface).
(Dr. P. Marazzi/Science Photo Library/Photo Researchers, Inc.)

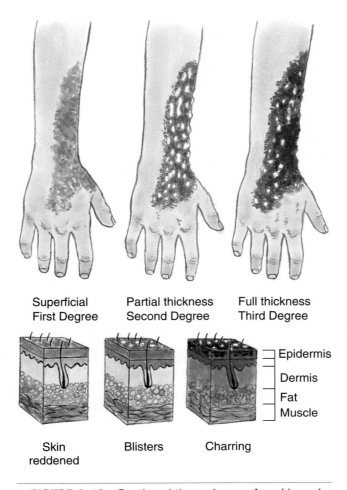

| Superficial First Degree | Partial thickness Second Degree | Full thickness Third Degree |
|---|---|---|

Epidermis
Dermis
Fat
Muscle

| Skin reddened | Blisters | Charring |
|---|---|---|

**FIGURE 3.16** Depth and tissue damage found in each degree of burn.

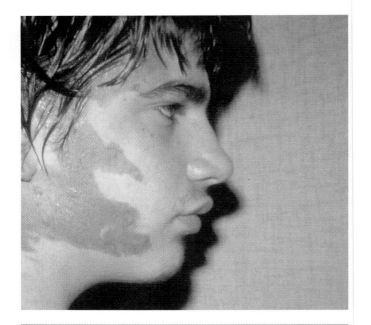

**FIGURE 3.17** First-degree burns on face.

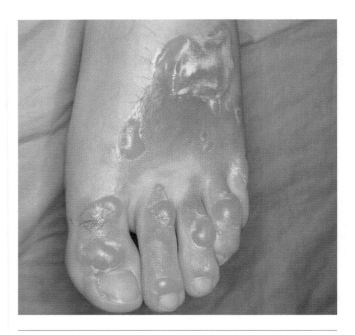

**FIGURE 3.18** Second-degree burns on feet.
(Moynahan Medical Center)

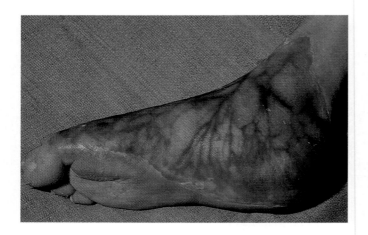

**FIGURE 3.19** Third-degree burn on right foot.
(Courtesy of Dr. William Dominic, Valley Medical Center)

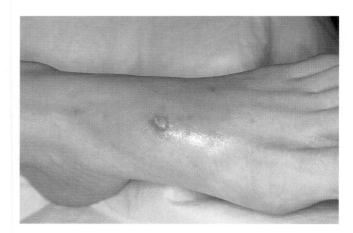

**FIGURE 3.20** Cellulitis on foot.
(Barts Medical Library/Phototake NYC)

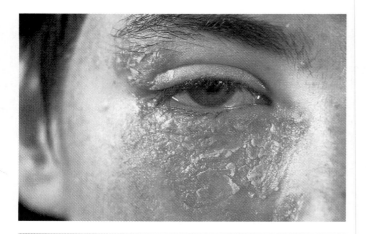

**FIGURE 3.21** Impetigo.
(Charles Stewart and Associates)

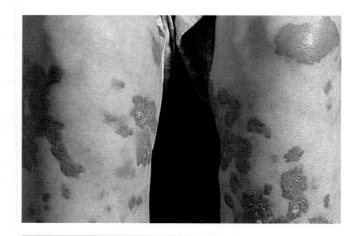

**FIGURE 3.22** Kaposi's sarcoma lesions.
(Zeva Oelbaum/Peter Arnold, Inc.)

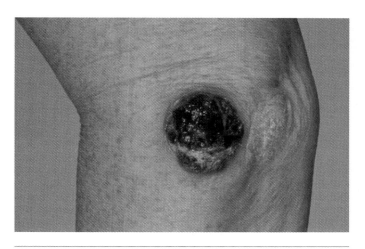

■ **FIGURE 3.23**  Malignant melanoma.
(BioPhoto Associates/Science Source/Photo Researchers, Inc.)

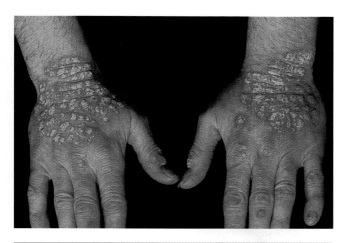

■ **FIGURE 3.24**  Psoriasis lesions.

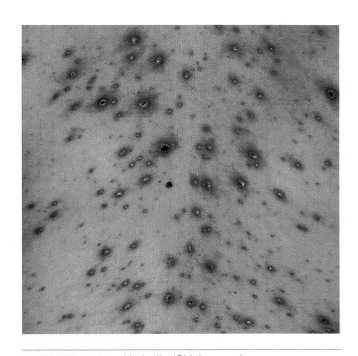

■ **FIGURE 3.25**  Varicella (Chicken pox).

## Diagnostic Procedures Relating to the Integumentary System

| | |
|---|---|
| **biopsy (BYE op see) (BX, bx)** | A piece of tissue is removed by syringe and needle, knife, punch, or brush to examine under a microscope. Used to aid in diagnosis. |
| **culture and sensitivity (C&S)** | A laboratory test that grows a colony of bacteria removed from an infected area in order to identify the specific infecting bacteria and then determine its sensitivity to a variety of antibiotics. |
| **exfoliative cytology (ex FOH lee ah tiv sigh TALL oh jee)** | Scraping cells from tissue and then examining them under a microscope. |

*continued...*

| | |
|---|---|
| frozen section (FS) | A thin piece of tissue is cut from a frozen specimen for rapid examination under a microscope. |
| fungal scrapings | Scrapings, taken with a curette or scraper, of tissue from lesions are placed on a growth medium and examined under a microscope to identify fungal growth. |
| needle biopsy | Using a sterile needle to remove tissue for examination under a microscope. |
| skin tests (ST) | Test to determine the patient's reaction to a suspected allergen by injecting a small amount under the skin (intradermal) with a needle. The reaction of the patient to this material is then read to indicate any allergy. Examples of such tests are the tuberculin (TB) test, Mantoux (PPD) test, patch test, and Schick test. |
| sweat test | Test performed on sweat to determine the level of chloride. An increase in skin chloride is seen with the disease cystic fibrosis. |

# Therapeutic Procedures Relating to the Integumentary System

| | |
|---|---|
| adipectomy (add ih PECK toh mee) | Surgical removal of fat. |
| allograft (AL oh graft) | Skin graft from one person to another; donor is usually a cadaver. |
| autograft (AW toh graft) | Skin graft from a person's own body (see Figure 3.26). |
| cauterization (kaw ter ih ZAY shun) | Destruction of tissue with a caustic chemical, electric current, freezing, or hot iron. |
| chemabrasion (kee moh BRAY zhun) | Abrasion using chemicals. Also called a *chemical peel.* |
| cryosurgery (cry oh SER jer ee) | The use of extreme cold to freeze and destroy tissue. |
| curettage (koo REH tahz) | Removal of superficial skin lesions with a curette (surgical instrument shaped like a spoon) or scraper. |
| debridement (de BREED mint) | Removal of foreign material and dead or damaged tissue from a wound. |
| dermabrasion (DERM ah bray shun) | Abrasion or rubbing using wire brushes or sandpaper. Performed to remove acne scars, tattoos, and scar tissue. |
| dermatome (DER mah tohm) | Instrument for cutting the skin or thin transplants of skin. |
| dermatoplasty (DER mah toh plas tee) | Skin grafting; transplantation of skin. |
| electrocautery (ee leck troh KAW teh ree) | To destroy tissue with an electric current. |
| heterograft (HET ur oh graft) | Skin graft from an animal of another species (usually a pig) to a human. Also called *xenograft.* |
| incision and drainage (I&D) | Making an incision to create an opening for the drainage of material such as pus. |
| laser therapy | Removal of skin lesions and birthmarks using a laser beam that emits intense heat and power at a close range. The laser converts frequencies of light into one small, powerful beam. |
| liposuction (LIP oh suck shun) | Removal of fat beneath the skin by means of suction. |

| plication (plye KAY shun) | Taking tucks surgically in a structure to shorten it. |
| --- | --- |
| rhytidectomy (rit ih DECK toh mee) | Surgical removal of excess skin to eliminate wrinkles. Commonly referred to as a *face lift*. |
| skin graft (SG) | The transfer of skin from a normal area to cover another site. Used to treat burn victims and after some surgical procedures. |
| xenograft (ZEN oh graft) | Skin graft from an animal of another species (usually a pig) to a human. Also called *heterograft*. |

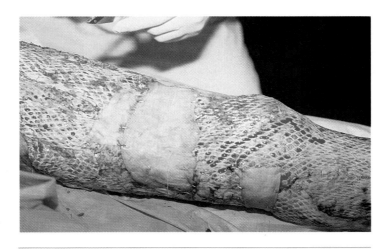

**■ FIGURE 3.26** Autograft.
(Courtesy of Dr. William Dominic, Valley Medical Center)

# Pharmacology Relating to the Integumentary System

| anesthetics (an es THET tics) | Applied to the skin to deaden pain. |
| --- | --- |
| antibiotics (an tye bye AW tics) | Kill bacteria causing skin infections. |
| antifungals (an tye FUNG alls) | Kill fungi infecting the skin. |
| anti-inflammatory drugs | Reduce skin inflammation or itching. |
| antiparasitics (an tye pair ah SIT tics) | Kill mites or lice. |
| antipruritics (an tye proo RIGH tiks) | Reduce severe itching. |
| antiseptics (an tye SEP tics) | Used to kill bacteria in skin cuts and wounds or at a surgical site. |
| corticosteroid cream | Specific type of powerful anti-inflammatory cream. |

NOTE. From *Health Assessment in Nursing* (table 8.4, p.147) by L. Sims, D. D'Amico, J. Stiesmeyer, & J. Webster, 1995. Redwood City, CA: Addison-Wesley. Reprinted by permission.

## Abbreviations Relating to the Integumentary System

| | | | |
|---|---|---|---|
| **BCC** | basal cell carcinoma | **SCC** | squamous cell carcinoma |
| **BX, bx** | biopsy | **SG** | skin graft |
| **C&S** | culture and sensitivity | **SLE** | systemic lupus erythematosus |
| **decub** | decubitus ulcer | **ST** | skin test |
| **Derm, derm** | dermatology | **STSG** | split-thickness skin graft |
| **FS** | frozen section | **subcu, SC,** | subcutaneous |
| **I&D** | incision and drainage | **sc, subq** | |
| **ID** | intradermal | **ung** | ointment |
| **MM** | malignant melanoma | **UV** | ultraviolet |

# Chapter Review

## Pronunciation Practice

 *You will find the pronunciation for each term on the enclosed CD-ROM. Check each one off as you master it.*

- ☐ abrasion (ah **BRAY** zhun)
- ☐ abscess (**AB** sess)
- ☐ acne (**ACK** knee)
- ☐ acne rosacea (**ACK** knee roh **ZAY** she ah)
- ☐ acne vulgaris (**ACK** nee vul **GAY** ris)
- ☐ adipectomy (add ih **PECK** toh mee)
- ☐ albino (al **BYE** noh)
- ☐ allograft (**AL** oh graft)
- ☐ alopecia (al oh **PEE** she ah)
- ☐ anesthetics (an es **THET** tics)
- ☐ anhidrosis (an hi **DROH** sis)
- ☐ antibiotics (an tye bye **AW** tics)
- ☐ antifungals (an tye **FUNG** alls)
- ☐ anti-inflammatory drugs
- ☐ antiparasitics (an tye pair ah **SIT** tics)
- ☐ antipruritics (an tye proo **RIGH** tiks)
- ☐ antiseptics (an tye **SEP** tics)
- ☐ apocrine (**APP** oh krin) glands
- ☐ autograft (**AW** toh graft)
- ☐ basal cell carcinoma (**BAY** sal sell kar sin **NOH** mah)
- ☐ basal (**BAY** sal) layer
- ☐ biopsy (**BYE** op see)
- ☐ burn
- ☐ burn, 1st degree
- ☐ burn, 2nd degree
- ☐ burn, 3rd degree
- ☐ carbuncle (**CAR** bung kl)
- ☐ cauterization (kaw ter ih **ZAY** shun)
- ☐ cellulitis (sell you **LYE** tis)
- ☐ chemabrasion (kee mah **BRAY** zhun)
- ☐ cicatrix (**SIK** ah trix)
- ☐ collagen (**KOL** ah jen) fibers
- ☐ comedo (**KOM** ee doh)
- ☐ connective tissue membranes
- ☐ contusion

- ☐ corium (**KOH** ree um)
- ☐ corticosteroid cream
- ☐ cryosurgery (cry oh **SER** jer ee)
- ☐ culture and sensitivity
- ☐ curettage (koo **REH** tahz)
- ☐ cutaneous (kew **TAY** nee us) membrane
- ☐ cuticle (**KEW** tikl)
- ☐ cyanosis (sigh ah **NOH** sis)
- ☐ cyst (**SIST**)
- ☐ debridement (day breed **MON**)
- ☐ decubitus ulcer (dee **KYOO** bih tus **ULL** ser)
- ☐ depigmentation (dee pig men **TAY** shun)
- ☐ dermabrasion (**DERM** ah bray shun)
- ☐ dermatitis (der mah **TYE** tis)
- ☐ dermatologist (der mah **TALL** oh jist)
- ☐ dermatology (der mah **TALL** oh jee)
- ☐ dermatome (**DER** mah tohm)
- ☐ dermatopathy (der mah **TOP** ah thee)
- ☐ dermatoplasty (**DER** mah toh plas tee)
- ☐ dermis (**DER** mis)
- ☐ diaphoresis (dye ah for **REE** sis)
- ☐ dry gangrene (**GANG** green)
- ☐ ecchymosis (ek ih **MOH** sis)
- ☐ eczema (**EK** zeh mah)
- ☐ electrocautery (ee leck troh **KAW** teh ree)
- ☐ epidermal (ep ih **DER** mal)
- ☐ epidermis (ep ih **DER** mis)
- ☐ epithelial (ep ih **THEE** lee al) membranes
- ☐ erythema (er ih **THEE** mah)
- ☐ erythroderma (eh rith roh **DER** ma)
- ☐ exfoliative cytology (ex **FOH** lee ah tiv sigh **TALL** oh jee)
- ☐ fissure (**FISH** er)
- ☐ free edge
- ☐ frostbite
- ☐ frozen section

- ❏ fungal scrapings (**FUN** gal)
- ❏ furuncle (**FOO** rung kl)
- ❏ gangrene (**GANG** green)
- ❏ hair
- ❏ hair follicle (**FALL** ikl)
- ❏ hair root
- ❏ hair shaft
- ❏ hemangioma (hee man jee **OH** mah)
- ❏ heterograft (**HET** ur oh graft)
- ❏ hirsutism (**HER** soot izm)
- ❏ hyperemia (high per **EE** mee ah)
- ❏ hyperhidrosis (high per hi **DROH** sis)
- ❏ hyperpigmentation (high per pig men **TAY** shun)
- ❏ hypodermic (high poh **DERM** ik)
- ❏ ichthyoderma (ick thee oh **DER** mah)
- ❏ ichthyosis (ick thee **OH** sis)
- ❏ impetigo (im peh **TYE** goh)
- ❏ incision and drainage
- ❏ integument (in **TEG** you mint)
- ❏ integumentary (in teg you **MEN** tah ree) system
- ❏ intradermal (in trah **DER** mal)
- ❏ Kaposi's sarcoma (**KAP** oh seez sar **KOH** mah)
- ❏ keloid (**KEE** loyd)
- ❏ keratin (**KAIR** ah tin)
- ❏ keratosis (kair ah **TOH** sis)
- ❏ laser therapy
- ❏ leukoderma (loo koh **DER** mah)
- ❏ leukoplakia (loo koh **PLAY** kee ah)
- ❏ lipectomy (lih **PECK** toh mee)
- ❏ lipocytes (**LIP** oh sights)
- ❏ lipoma (lip **OH** mah)
- ❏ liposuction (**LIP** oh suck shun)
- ❏ lunula (**LOO** nyoo lah)
- ❏ macule (**MACK** yool)
- ❏ male pattern baldness
- ❏ malignant melanoma (mah **LIG** nant mel ah **NOH** mah)
- ❏ melanin (**MEL** an in)
- ❏ melanocytes (mel **AN** oh sights)
- ❏ melanoma (mel ah **NOH** ma)
- ❏ mucous (**MYOO** kus) membrane
- ❏ mucus (**MYOO** kus)
- ❏ nail bed
- ❏ nail body
- ❏ nail root
- ❏ nails
- ❏ necrosis (neh **KROH** sis)
- ❏ needle biopsy
- ❏ nevus (**NEV** us)
- ❏ nodule (**NOD** yool)
- ❏ onychectomy (on ee **KECK** toh me)
- ❏ onychia (oh **NICK** ee ah)
- ❏ onychomalacia (on ih koh mah **LAY** she ah)
- ❏ onychomycosis (on ih koh my **KOH** sis)
- ❏ onychophagia (on ih koh **FAY** jee ah)
- ❏ pachyderma (pak ee **DER** mah)
- ❏ papule (**PAP** yool)
- ❏ paronychia (pair oh **NICK** ee ah)
- ❏ pathogens (**PATH** oh jenz)
- ❏ pediculosis (peh dik you **LOH** sis)
- ❏ pemphigus vulgaris (**PEM** fih gus vul **GAY** ris)
- ❏ perspiration
- ❏ petechiae (peh **TEE** kee eye)
- ❏ photosensitivity (foh toh sen sih **TIH** vih tee)
- ❏ plication (plye **KAY** shun)
- ❏ polyp (**POLL** ip)
- ❏ pruritus (proo **RIGH** tus)
- ❏ psoriasis (soh **RYE** ah sis)
- ❏ purpura (**PER** pew rah)
- ❏ purulent (**PYUR** yoo lent)
- ❏ pustule (**PUS** tyool)
- ❏ pyogenic (pye oh **JEN** ik)
- ❏ rhytidectomy (rit ih **DECK** toh mee)
- ❏ rhytidoplasty (**RIT** ih doh plas tee)
- ❏ rubella (roo **BELL** ah)
- ❏ scabies (**SKAY** bees)
- ❏ scleroderma (sklair ah **DER** mah)
- ❏ sebaceous cyst (see **BAY** shus **SIST**)
- ❏ sebaceous (see **BAY** shus) gland
- ❏ seborrhea (seb or **EE** ah)
- ❏ sebum (**SEE** bum)
- ❏ sensory (**SEN** soh ree) receptors
- ❏ serous (**SEER** us) membrane
- ❏ shingles (**SHING** lz)
- ❏ skin graft

- [ ] skin tests
- [ ] squamous cell carcinoma (**SKWAY** mus sell kar sih **NOH** mah)
- [ ] stratified squamous epithelium (**STRAT** ih fyde **SKWAY** mus ep ih **THEE** lee um)
- [ ] subcutaneous (sub kyoo **TAY** nee us)
- [ ] subcutaneous (sub kyoo **TAY** nee us) layer
- [ ] suppurative (**SUP** pure a tiv)
- [ ] sweat duct
- [ ] sweat glands
- [ ] sweat pore
- [ ] sweat test
- [ ] synovial (sin **OH** vee al) membrane
- [ ] systemic lupus erythematosus (sis **TEM** ik **LOO** pus air ih them ah **TOH** sis)
- [ ] tinea (**TIN** ee ah)
- [ ] tinea capitis (**TIN** ee ah **CAP** it is)
- [ ] tinea pedis (**TIN** ee ah **PED** is)
- [ ] trichomycosis (trik oh my **KOH** sis)
- [ ] ulcer (**ULL** ser)
- [ ] ungual (**UNG** gwal)
- [ ] urticaria (er tih **KAY** ree ah)
- [ ] varicella (**VAIR** ih chell a)
- [ ] verruca (ver **ROO** kah)
- [ ] vesicle (**VESS** ikl)
- [ ] vitiligo (vit ill **EYE** go)
- [ ] wet gangrene (**GANG** green)
- [ ] wheal (**WEEL**)
- [ ] xanthoderma (zan thoh **DER** mah)
- [ ] xenograft (**ZEN** oh graft)
- [ ] xeroderma (zee roh **DER** ma)

# Case Study

## Dermatology Consultation Report

**Reason for Consultation:** Evaluate patient for excision of recurrent basal cell carcinoma, left cheek.

**History of Present Illness:** Patient is a 74-year-old male first seen by his regular physician 5 years ago for persistent facial lesions. Biopsies revealed basal cell carcinoma in two lesions, one on the nasal tip and the other on the left cheek. These were excised and healed with a normal cicatrix. The patient noted that the left cheek lesion returned approximately 1 year ago. Patient admits to not following his physician's advice to use sunscreen and a hat. Patient reports pruritus and states the lesion is growing larger. Patient has been referred for dermatology evaluation regarding deep excision of the lesion and dermatoplasty.

**Past Medical History:** Patient's activity level is severely restricted due to congestive heart failure (CHF) with dyspnea, lower extremity edema, and cyanosis. He takes several cardiac medications daily and occasionally requires oxygen by nasal canula. History is negative for other types of cancer.

**Results of Physical Exam:** Examination revealed a 10- × 14-mm lesion on left cheek 20 mm anterior to the ear. The lesion displays marked erythema and poorly defined borders. The area immediately around the lesion shows depigmentation with vesicles. There is a well-healed cicatrix on the nasal tip with no evidence of the neoplasm returning.

**Assessment:** Even without a biopsy, this is most likely a recurrence of this patient's basal cell carcinoma.

**Recommendations:** Due to the lesion's size, shape, and reoccurrence, recommend deep excision of the neoplasm through the epidermis and dermis layers. The patient will then require dermatoplasty. The most likely donor site will be the proximal-medial thigh. This patient is at high risk for basal cell carcinoma and should never go outside without sunscreen and a hat. I have discussed the surgical procedure with the patient and he fully understands the procedure, risks, and alternate treatment choices. In light of his cardiac status, if he decides to proceed with the surgery, he will need a thorough workup by his cardiologist.

## Critical Thinking Questions

1. Which of the following symptoms was reported by the patient?
   a. easy bruising
   b. excessive scarring
   c. intense itching
   d. yellow skin

2. In your own words, describe the lesion on the patient's face.

3. What advice did this patient fail to follow? What happened, in part, because he did not follow instructions?

4. This patient has a serious health condition other than his facial lesion. Name that condition and describe it in your own words. What is the abbreviation for this condition? This patient has three symptoms of this condition. List the three symptoms and describe each in your own words. This condition and its symptoms use terminology that has not been introduced yet. You will need to use your text as a reference to answer this question.

   The condition is: _____ .

   The abbreviation for this condition is: _____ .

   The three symptoms are: _____ .

5. What procedure was performed on the original lesion that confirmed the diagnosis? Explain, in your own words, what this procedure involves.

6. Briefly describe, in your own words, the two stages of the surgical procedure the physician recommends.

# Chart Note Transcription

## Chart Note

The chart note below contains 10 phrases that can be re-worded with a medical term that you learned in this chapter. Each phrase is identified with an underline. Determine the medical term and write your answers in the space provided.

**Current Complaint:** A 64-year-old female with an <u>open sore</u> ① on her right leg is seen by the <u>specialist in treating diseases of the skin</u>. ②

**Past History:** Patient states she first noticed an area of pain, <u>severe itching</u>, ③ and <u>redness of the skin</u> ④ just below her right knee about 6 weeks ago. One week later <u>raised spots containing pus</u> ⑤ appeared. Patient states the raised spots containing pus ruptured and the open sore appeared.

**Signs and Symptoms:** Patient has a deep open sore $5 \times 3$ cm: It is 4 cm distal to the knee on the lateral aspect of the right leg. It appears to extend into the <u>middle skin layer</u>, ⑥ and the edges show signs of <u>tissue death</u>. ⑦ The open sore has a small amount of drainage but there is no odor. A <u>sample of the drainage that was grown in the lab to identify the microorganism and determine the best antibiotic</u> ⑧ of the drainage revealed *Staphylococcus* bacteria in the open sore.

**Diagnosis:** <u>Inflammation of skin cells and tissues.</u> ⑨

**Treatment:** <u>Removal of damaged tissue</u> ⑩ of the open sore followed by application of an antibiotic cream. Patient was instructed to return to the specialist in treating diseases of the skin's office in 2 weeks, or sooner if the open sore does not heal, or if it begins draining pus.

1. _____

2. _____

3. _____

4. _____

5. _____

6. _____

7. _____

8. _____

9. _____

10. _____

# Practice Exercises

**A. State the terms described using the combining forms provided.**

The combining form *dermat/o* refers to the skin. Use it to write a term that means

1. inflammation of the skin _____
2. any abnormal skin condition _____
3. an instrument for cutting the skin _____
4. specialist in skin _____
5. surgical repair of the skin _____
6. study of the skin _____

The combining form *melan/o* means black. Use it to write a term that means

7. a black tumor _____
8. a black cell _____

The combining form *rhytid/o* means wrinkles. Use it to write a term that means

9. wrinkle excision _____
10. wrinkle surgical repair _____

The combining form *trich/o* refers to the hair. Use it to write a term that means

11. an abnormal condition of the hair caused by a fungus _____

The combining form *onych/o* refers to the nail. Use it to write a term that means

12. softening of the nails _____
13. infection around the nail _____
14. nail eating (biting) _____
15. excision of the nail _____

**B. Define the following combining forms.**

1. cry/o _____
2. cutane/o _____
3. diaphor/o _____
4. py/o _____
5. cyan/o _____
6. onych/o _____
7. lip/o _____
8. kerat/o _____

**C. Define the following terms.**

1. integumentary _____
2. melanin _____
3. sebum _____

4. cutaneous membrane _____

5. epidermis _____

6. keratin _____

7. cuticle _____

8. hair follicle _____

## D. Describe the following types of burns.

1. first degree _____

2. second degree _____

3. third degree _____

## E. Match the terms in column A with the definitions in column B.

| A | | B |
|---|---|---|
| 1. _____ eczema | | a. decubitus ulcer |
| 2. _____ nevus | | b. lack of skin pigment |
| 3. _____ lipoma | | c. acne commonly seen in adults |
| 4. _____ urticaria | | d. hardened skin |
| 5. _____ bedsore | | e. papules, vesicles, crusts |
| 6. _____ acne rosacea | | f. white patches |
| 7. _____ acne vulgaris | | g. birthmark |
| 8. _____ leukoplakia | | h. excessive hair growth |
| 9. _____ hirsutism | | i. death of tissue |
| 10. _____ alopecia | | j. fatty tumor |
| 11. _____ gangrene | | k. hives |
| 12. _____ scleroderma | | l. baldness |
| 13. _____ albino | | m. acne of adolescence |

## F. Match the terms in column A with the procedures in column B.

| A | | B |
|---|---|---|
| 1. _____ debridement | | a. surgical removal of wrinkled skin |
| 2. _____ cauterization | | b. instrument to cut thin slices of skin |
| 3. _____ lipectomy | | c. removal of fat with suction |
| 4. _____ dermatoplasty | | d. surgical removal of fat |
| 5. _____ liposuction | | e. skin grafting |
| 6. _____ rhytidectomy | | f. removal of lesions with scraper |
| 7. _____ curettage | | g. remove skin with brushes |
| 8. _____ dermabrasion | | h. remove damaged skin |
| 9. _____ dermatome | | i. destruction of tissue with electric current |

## G. Write the abbreviations for the following terms.

1. frozen section _____

2. incision and drainage _____

3. intradermal _____

4. subcutaneous _____

5. ultraviolet _____

6. ointment _____

7. biopsy _____

## H. Use the following terms in the sentences that follow.

| | | | |
|---|---|---|---|
| cyst | impetigo | malignant melanoma | pustule |
| fissure | furuncle | petechiae | vesicle |
| macule | carbuncle | dermis | keloid |
| nodule | scabies | epidermis | Kaposi's sarcoma |
| papule | tinea | paronychia | xeroderma |
| polyp | verruca | pachyderma | shingles |

1. The middle layer of the skin is called the _____ .

2. Meyer has a painful eruption of vesicles along a nerve. This condition is called _____ .

3. The winter climates can cause dry skin. The medical term for this is _____ .

4. Kim has experienced small pinpoint purplish spots caused by bleeding under the skin. This is called _____ .

5. Janet has a fungal skin disease. This is called _____ .

6. A contagious skin disease caused by a mite is _____ .

7. An infection around the entire nail is called _____ .

8. A form of skin cancer affecting AIDS patients is called _____ .

9. An especially dangerous type of skin cancer caused by an overproduction of melanin is called _____ .

10. Latrivia has a bacterial skin infection that results in pustules crusting and rupturing. It is called _____ .

11. A pus-containing raised spot on the skin is called a _____ .

12. A small, flat, discolored area, such as a freckle, is called a _____ .

13. A small tumor with a pedicle or stem is called a _____ .

14. A solid raised group of cells is called a _____ .

15. A crack or groove in the skin is referred to as a _____ .

## I. Use the following prefixes to write a word that means

epi-            sub-

intra-           hypo-

1. under the skin _____ or _____

2. within the skin _____

3. on the skin _____

# Professional Journal

In this exercise you will now have an opportunity to put the words you have learned into practice. Imagine yourself in the role of a registered nurse. If you refer back to the Professional Profile at the beginning of this chapter, you will see that this health care professional is responsible for assessing patient status and progress, providing patient care, administering medications, and providing patient education. Use the 10 words listed below to write sentences to describe the patients you saw today.

An example of a sentence is *The young lady had recently developed* **photosensitivity** *and needed education regarding ways to avoid the sun.*

1. abrasion _____

2. antibiotic _____

3. autograft _____

4. culture and sensitivity _____

5. wheal _____

6. ulcer _____

7. malignant melanoma _____

8. pediculosis _____

9. rubella _____

10. second-degree burn _____

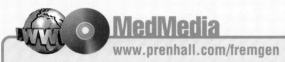

## MedMedia
### www.prenhall.com/fremgen

Use the CD-ROM enclosed with your textbook to gain additional reinforcement through interactive word building exercises, spelling games, labeling activities, and additional quizzes.

Use the above address to access the free, interactive Companion Website created for this textbook. Get hints, instant feedback, and textbook references to chapter-related multiple-choice questions, as well as labeling and matching exercises. In addition, you will find an audio glossary, case studies, and Internet exploration exercises.

***For more information regarding dermatology and skin diseases visit the following websites:***

National Library of Medicine at **www.nlm.nih.gov/medlineplus/skindiseasesgeneral.html**

National Institute of Arthritis and Musculoskeletal and Skin Diseases at
   **www.niams.nih.gov/hi/index/htm**

New Zealand Dermatology Society at **www.dermnetnz.org/index/html**

# Chapter 4
# Musculoskeletal System

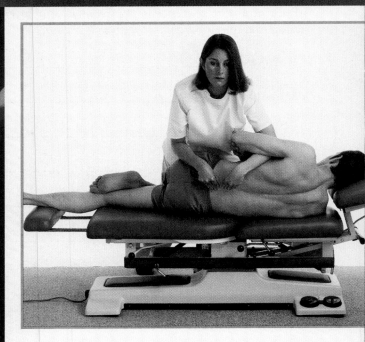

## Learning Objectives

*Upon completion of this chapter, you will be able to:*

- Recognize the combining forms and suffixes introduced in this chapter.
- Gain the ability to pronounce medical terms and major anatomical structures.
- List the major organs of the musculoskeletal system and describe their functions.
- Correctly place bones in either the axial or the appendicular skeleton.
- Recognize the components of a long bone.
- Identify bony projections and depressions.
- Identify the parts of a synovial joint.
- Describe the characteristics of the three types of muscle tissue.
- Distinguish the major muscles of the body.
- Use movement terminology correctly.
- Build musculoskeletal system medical terms from word parts.
- Define vocabulary, pathology, diagnostic, and therapeutic medical terms relating to the musculoskeletal system.
- Recognize types of medication associated with the musculoskeletal system.
- Interpret abbreviations associated with the musculoskeletal system.

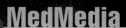

## MedMedia

## Professional Profile

### Chiropractic Medicine

Chiropractic medicine is based on the philosophy that many health problems are directly linked to problems of the muscular, nervous, and skeletal systems. Chiropractors utilize manipulation, especially of the spinal column, to correct skeletal alignment problems in order to alleviate stresses that may be affecting other body systems. In addition to manipulation, chiropractors also utilize massage, exercise, and nutritional means to treat their patients. Chiropractors also educate patients on ways to improve their lifestyles especially through improved nutrition and exercise.

### Doctor of Chiropractic (DC)

- Enters a chiropractic program after completing 90 hours of undergraduate work
- Graduates from an accredited 4-year chiropractic program
- Passes a licensing examination

*For more information regarding these health careers, visit the following websites:*
American Chiropractic Association at **www.amerchiro.org**
Council on Chiropractic Education at **www.cce-usa.org**

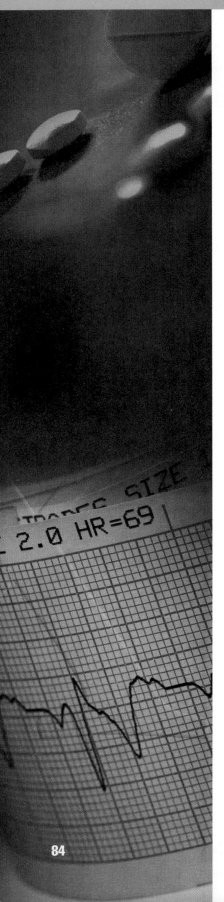

## Part I: Skeletal System

**Organs of the Skeletal System**

bones
joints

**Combining Forms Relating to the Skeletal System**

| | | | |
|---|---|---|---|
| ankyl/o | stiff joint | metacarp/o | metacarpals, hand bones |
| arthr/o | joint | metatars/o | metatarsals, foot bones |
| articul/o | joint | myel/o | bone marrow |
| burs/o | sac | orth/o | straight |
| carp/o | wrist | oste/o | bone |
| cervic/o | neck | patell/o | patella, knee cap |
| chondr/o | cartilage | ped/o | foot |
| clavicul/o | clavicle, collarbone | pelv/o | pelvis |
| coccyg/o | coccyx, tailbone | phalang/o | phalanges, bones of fingers and toes |
| cost/o | rib | | |
| crani/o | skull, head | pub/o | pubis, part of hipbone |
| femor/o | femur, thigh bone | radi/o | radius, lower arm bone |
| fibul/o | fibula, smaller outer bone of lower leg | sacr/o | sacrum |
| | | scapul/o | scapula, shoulder blade |
| humer/o | humerus, upper arm bone | scoli/o | crooked, bent |
| ili/o | ilium, part of hipbone | spondyl/o | vertebrae, backbone |
| ischi/o | ischium, part of hipbone | stern/o | sternum, breastbone |
| kyph/o | hump | synovi/o | synovial membrane |
| lamin/o | lamina, part of vertebra | tars/o | ankle |
| lord/o | swayback, curve | thorac/o | chest |
| lumb/o | loin, lower back | tibi/o | tibia, inner bone of lower leg |
| mandibul/o | mandible, jawbone | uln/o | ulna, lower arm bone |
| maxill/o | maxilla, upper jawbone | vertebr/o | vertebra, backbone |

**Suffixes Relating to the Skeletal System**

| Suffix | Meaning | Example |
|---|---|---|
| -blast | immature, embryonic | osteoblast |
| -clasia | to surgically break | osteoclasia |
| -desis | stabilize, fuse | arthrodesis |
| -listhesis | slipping | spondylolisthesis |
| -malacia | softening | osteomalacia |
| -porosis | porous | osteoporosis |
| -scopy | procedure to visually examine | arthroscopy |
| -tome | instrument to cut | osteotome |

# Anatomy and Physiology of the Skeletal System

| | |
|---|---|
| **bone marrow** | **joints** |
| **bones** | **muscles** |

The **bones** of the skeleton serve as the body's frame, protect vital organs, and store minerals. **Bone marrow** is the site of blood cell production. A **joint** is the place where two bones meet. This gives flexibility to the skeleton. The skeleton, joints, and **muscles** work together to produce movement.

## Bones

| | | |
|---|---|---|
| **appendicular skeleton** | **osseous tissue** | **osteoblasts** |
| **axial skeleton** | **ossification** | **osteocytes** |
| **cartilage** | | |

Bone, also called **osseous** (**OSS** ee us) **tissue**, is one of the hardest materials in the body. Bones are formed from a gradual process beginning before birth called **ossification** (oss sih fih **KAY** shun). The fetal skeleton is formed from a **cartilage** (**CAR** tih lij) model. This flexible tissue is gradually replaced by **osteoblasts** (**OSS** tee oh blasts), immature bone cells. In adult bone, the osteoblasts have matured into **osteocytes** (**OSS** tee oh sights). The formation of strong bones is greatly dependent on an adequate supply of minerals such as calcium and phosphorus.

The human body contains 206 bones (see ▧ Figure 4.1). Each bone is a unique organ that carries its own blood supply, nerves, and lymphatic vessels. The human skeleton has two divisions: the **axial** (**AK** see al) **skeleton** and the **appendicular** (app en **DIK** yoo lar) **skeleton**. Figures 4.2 and 4.6 illustrate the axial and appendicular skeletons.

## Axial Skeleton

| | | |
|---|---|---|
| **cervical vertebrae** | **lumbar vertebrae** | **sacrum** |
| **coccyx** | **mandible** | **sphenoid bone** |
| **cranium** | **maxilla** | **sternum** |
| **ethmoid bone** | **nasal bone** | **temporal bone** |
| **facial bones** | **occipital bone** | **thoracic vertebrae** |
| **frontal bone** | **palatine bone** | **vertebral column** |
| **hyoid bone** | **parietal bone** | **vomer bone** |
| **lacrimal bone** | **rib cage** | **zygomatic bone** |

The axial skeleton includes the bones in the head, neck, spine, chest, and trunk of the body (see ▧ Figure 4.2). These bones form the central axis for the whole body and protect many of the internal organs such as the brain, lungs, and heart.

The head or skull is divided into two parts consisting of the **cranium** (**KRAY** nee um) and **facial bones.** These bones protect the brain and special sense organs from injury. The cranium covers the brain and the facial bones surround the mouth, nose, and eyes. Muscles for chewing and head movements are attached to the cranial bones. The cranium consists of the **frontal, parietal** (pah **RYE** eh tal), **temporal** (**TEM** por al), **ethmoid** (**ETH** moyd), **sphenoid** (**SFEE** noyd), and **occipital** (ock **SIP** eh tal) **bones.** The facial bones are

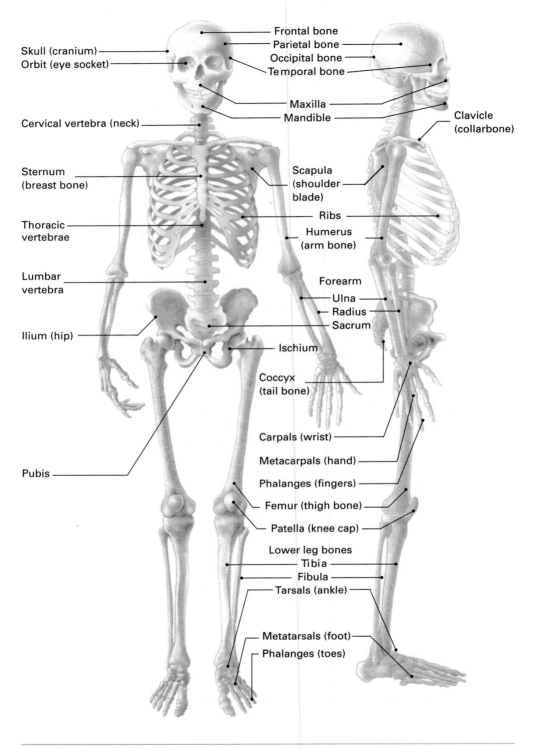

Frontal bone

Skull (cranium)
Orbit (eye socket)

Parietal bone
Occipital bone
Temporal bone

Maxilla
Mandible

Cervical vertebra (neck)

Clavicle
(collarbone)

Sternum
(breast bone)

Scapula
(shoulder
blade)

Ribs

Thoracic
vertebrae

Humerus
(arm bone)

Lumbar
vertebra

Forearm
Ulna
Radius
Sacrum

Ilium (hip)

Ischium

Coccyx
(tail bone)

Carpals (wrist)

Metacarpals (hand)

Pubis

Phalanges (fingers)

Femur (thigh bone)

Patella (knee cap)

Lower leg bones
Tibia
Fibula
Tarsals (ankle)

Metatarsals (foot)
Phalanges (toes)

**■ FIGURE 4.1**  The human skeleton.

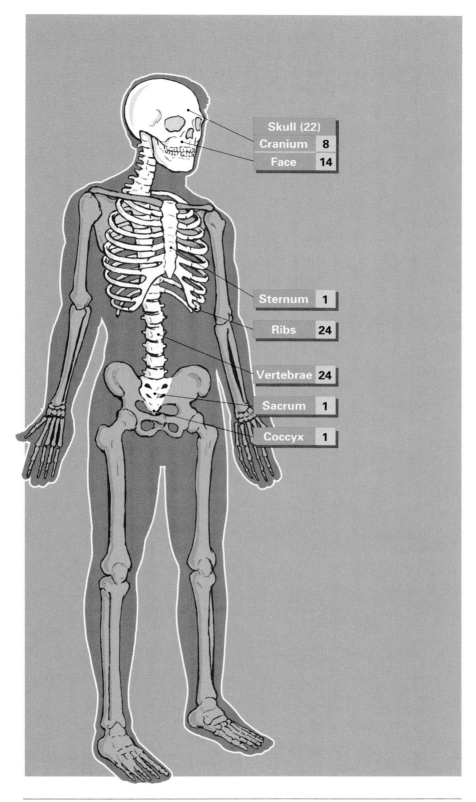

Skull (22)
Cranium 8
Face 14

Sternum 1

Ribs 24

Vertebrae 24

Sacrum 1

Coccyx 1

**■ FIGURE 4.2** The axial skeleton.

the **mandible** (**MAN** dih bl), **maxilla** (mack **SIH** lah), **zygomatic** (zeye go **MAT** ik), **vomer** (**VOH** mer), **palatine** (**PAL** ah tine), **nasal** (**NAY** zl), and **lacrimal** (**LACK** rim al) **bones.** The cranial and facial bones are illustrated in ▓ Figure 4.3 and described in Table 4.1.

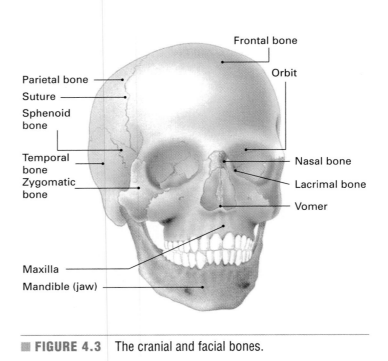

▓ **FIGURE 4.3** The cranial and facial bones.

| Table 4.1 | Bones of the Skull | |
|---|---|---|
| **Name** | **Number** | **Description** |
| ***Cranial Bones*** | | |
| Frontal bone | 1 | Forehead |
| Parietal bone | 2 | Upper sides of cranium and roof of skull |
| Occipital bone | 1 | Back and base of skull |
| Temporal bone | 2 | Sides and base of cranium |
| Sphenoid bone | 1 | Bat-shaped bone that forms part of the base of the skull, floor, and sides of eye orbit |
| Ethmoid bone | 1 | Forms part of eye orbit, nose, and floor of cranium |
| ***Facial Bones*** | | |
| Lacrimal bone | 2 | Inner corner of each eye |
| Nasal bone | 2 | Form part of nasal septum and support bridge of nose |
| Maxilla | 1 | Upper jaw |
| Mandible | 1 | Lower jawbone; only movable bone of the skull |
| Zygomatic bone | 2 | Cheekbones |
| Vomer bone | 1 | Base of nasal septum |
| Palatine bone | 1 | Hard palate (**PAH** lat) of mouth and floor of the nose |

The **hyoid** (**HIGH** oyd) **bone** is a single U-shaped bone suspended in the neck between the mandible and larynx. It is a point of attachment for swallowing and speech muscles.

The trunk of the body consists of the **vertebral** (**VER** teh bral) **column, sternum** (**STER** num), and **rib cage.** The vertebral or spinal column can be divided into five sections: **cervical vertebrae** (**SER** vih kal **VER** teh bray), **thoracic vertebrae** (tho **RASS** ik **VER** teh bray), **lumbar vertebrae** (**LUM** bar **VER** teh bray), **sacrum** (**SAY** crum), and **coccyx** (**COCK** six) (see Table 4.2 and ▦ Figure 4.4). The rib cage has 12 pairs of ribs attached at the back to the vertebral or spinal column. Ten of the pairs are also attached to the breastbone or sternum in the front (see ▦ Figure 4.5). The remaining two pairs are called *floating ribs* and are attached only to the vertebral column. The rib cage serves to provide support for other organs, such as the heart and lungs.

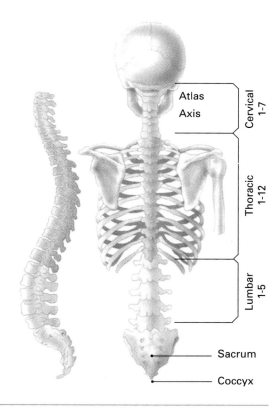

Atlas
Axis
Cervical 1-7
Thoracic 1-12
Lumbar 1-5
Sacrum
Coccyx

▦ **FIGURE 4.4** The spinal column.

| Table 4.2 | Bones of the Vertebral/Spinal Column | |
|---|---|---|
| **Name** | **Number** | **Description** |
| Cervical vertebra | 7 | Vertebrae in the neck region |
| Thoracic vertebra | 12 | Vertebrae in the chest region with ribs attached |
| Lumbar vertebra | 5 | Vertebrae in the small of the back, about waist level |
| Sacrum | 1 | Five vertebrae that become fused into one triangular-shaped flat bone at the base of the vertebral column |
| Coccyx | 1 | Three to five very small vertebrae attached to the sacrum, often become fused |

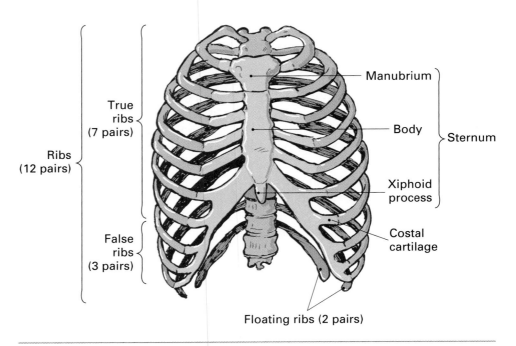

Manubrium

True ribs (7 pairs)

Ribs (12 pairs)

Body

Sternum

Xiphoid process

False ribs (3 pairs)

Costal cartilage

Floating ribs (2 pairs)

**■ FIGURE 4.5** The rib cage.

## Appendicular Skeleton

| | | |
|---|---|---|
| **carpals** | **lower extremities** | **pubis** |
| **clavicle** | **metacarpals** | **radius** |
| **femur** | **metatarsals** | **scapula** |
| **fibula** | **os coxae** | **tarsals** |
| **humerus** | **patella** | **tibia** |
| **ilium** | **pectoral girdle** | **ulna** |
| **innominate bone** | **pelvic girdle** | **upper extremities** |
| **ischium** | **phalanges** | |

**MED TERM TIP** The elbow is commonly referred to as the *funny bone.* It is actually a projection of the ulna called the olecranon process.

The appendicular skeleton consists of the **upper extremities, lower extremities, pectoral girdle,** and **pelvic girdle** (see ■ Figure 4.6). These are the bones for our appendages or limbs and, along with the muscles attached to them, they are responsible for body movement.

The pelvic girdle consists of the **clavicle** (**CLAV** ih kl) and **scapula** (**SKAP** yoo lah) bones. It functions to attach the upper extremity, or arm, to the axial skeleton by articulating with the sternum anteriorly and the vertebral column posteriorly. The bones of the upper extremity include the **humerus** (**HYOO** mer us), **ulna** (**UHL** nah), **radius** (**RAY** dee us), **carpals** (**CAR** pals), **metacarpals** (met ah **CAR** pals), and **phalanges** (fah **LAN** jeez). These bones are illustrated in ■ Figure 4.7.

The pelvic girdle is called the **os coxae** (**OSS KOK** sigh) or the **innominate** (ih **NOM** ih nayt) **bone** or hipbone. It contains the **ilium** (**ILL** ee um), **ischium** (**ISS** kee um), and **pubis** (**PYOO** bis). It articulates with the sacrum posteriorly to attach the lower extremity, or leg, to the axial skeleton. The lower extremity bones include the **femur** (**FEE** mer), **patella** (pah **TELL** ah), **tibia** (**TIB** ee ah), **fibula** (**FIB** yoo lah), **tarsals** (**TAHR** sals), **metatarsals** (met ah **TAHR** sals), and phalanges. These bones are illustrated in ■ Figure 4.8.

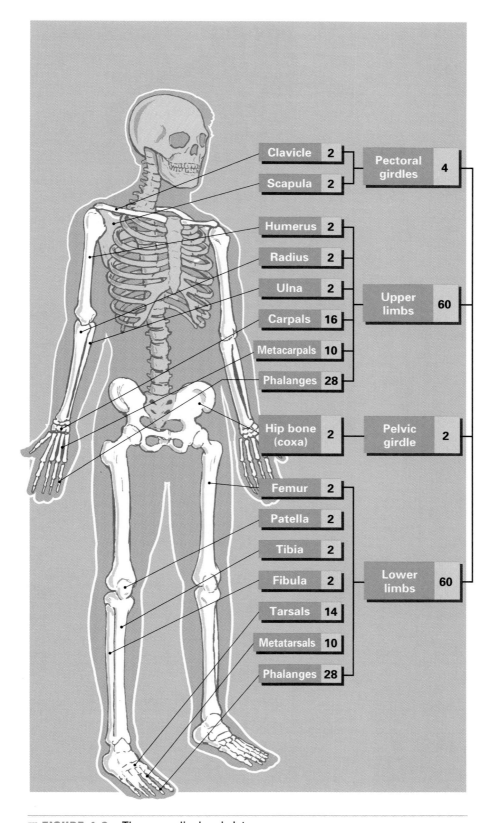

**FIGURE 4.6** The appendicular skeleton.

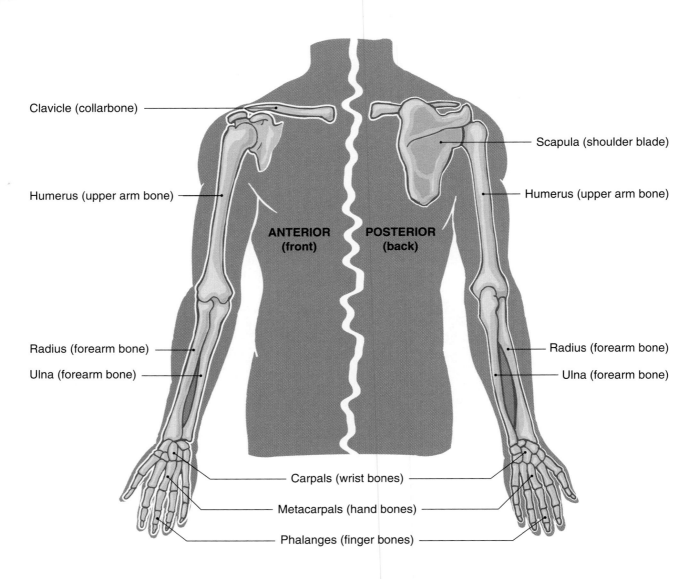

Clavicle (collarbone)

Scapula (shoulder blade)

Humerus (upper arm bone)

Humerus (upper arm bone)

ANTERIOR (front)

POSTERIOR (back)

Radius (forearm bone)

Ulna (forearm bone)

Radius (forearm bone)

Ulna (forearm bone)

Carpals (wrist bones)

Metacarpals (hand bones)

Phalanges (finger bones)

### Bones in the Upper Extremities

| Name | Number | Description |
|------|--------|-------------|
| Clavicle | 2 | Collar bone |
| Scapula | 2 | Shoulder blade |
| Humerus | 2 | Upper arm bone |
| Radius | 2 | Forearm bone on thumb side of lower arm |
| Ulna | 2 | Forearm bone on little finger side of lower arm |
| Carpal | 16 | Bones of wrist |
| Metacarpals | 10 | Bones in palm of hand |
| Phalanges | 28 | Finger bones; three in each finger and two in each thumb |

■ **FIGURE 4.7** Bones of the upper extremities.

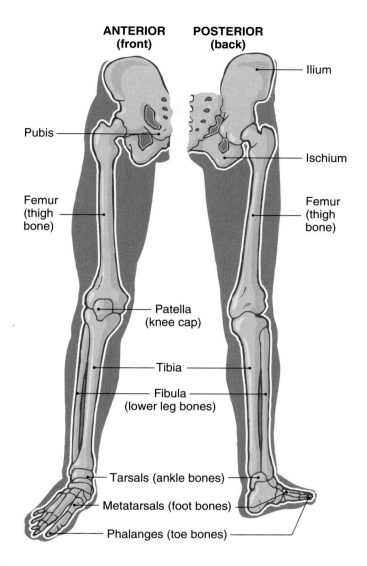

ANTERIOR (front)    POSTERIOR (back)

Ilium

Pubis

Ischium

Femur (thigh bone)

Femur (thigh bone)

Patella (knee cap)

Tibia

Fibula (lower leg bones)

Tarsals (ankle bones)

Metatarsals (foot bones)

Phalanges (toe bones)

### Bones in the Lower Extremities

| Name | Number | Description |
|---|---|---|
| Os coxae | 2 | Hipbone (ilium, ischium, pubis) |
| Femur | 2 | Upper leg bone; thigh bone |
| Patella | 2 | Knee cap |
| Tibia | 2 | Shin bone; thicker lower leg bone |
| Fibula | 2 | Thinner, long bone in lateral side of lower leg |
| Tarsals | 14 | Ankle and heel bones |
| Metatarsals | 10 | Fore foot bones |
| Phalanges | 28 | Toe bones; three in each toe and two in each great toe |

**FIGURE 4.8** Bones of the lower extremities.

**MED TERM TIP** The term *girdle*, meaning something that encircles or confines, refers to the entire bony structure of the shoulder and the pelvis. Therefore, if just one bone from these two areas is being discussed, such as the ilium of the pelvis, it would be named as such. If, however, the entire pelvis is being discussed, it would be called the pelvic girdle.

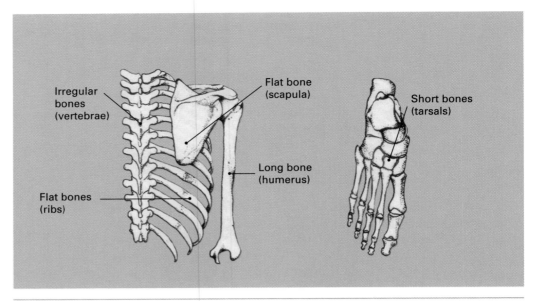

**FIGURE 4.9** Classification of bones.

## Bone Structure

cancellous bone

compact bone

cortical bone

diaphysis

epiphysis

flat bones

irregular bones

long bones

medullary cavity

periosteum

red bone marrow

short bones

spongy bone

yellow bone marrow

**MED TERM TIP** Do not confuse a long bone with a large bone. A long bone is not necessarily a large bone. The bones of your fingers are short in length, but since they are longer than they are wide, they are classified as long bones.

Several different types of bones are found throughout the body. They basically fall into four categories: **long bones, short bones, flat bones,** and **irregular bones** (see Figure 4.9). Long bones are longer than they are wide. Examples are the femur and humerus. Short bones are roughly as long as they are wide. The carpals and tarsals are short bones. Irregular bones received their name because the shapes of the bones are very irregular. The vertebrae are irregular bones. Flat bones are usually plate-shaped bones such as the sternum, scapulae, and pelvis.

The majority of bones in the human body are long bones. These bones have similar structure with a central shaft or **diaphysis** (dye **AFF** ih sis) that widens at each end, which is called an **epiphysis** (eh **PIFF** ih sis). Most bones are covered with a thin connective tissue membrane called the **periosteum** (pair ee **AH** stee um), which contains numerous blood vessels, nerves, and lymphatic vessels. The dense and hard exterior surface bone is called **cortical** (**KOR** ti kal) or **compact bone. Cancellous** (**CAN** sell us) or **spongy bone** is found inside the bone. As its name indicates, spongy bone has spaces in it, giving it a sponge-like appearance. These spaces contain **red bone marrow.** Red bone marrow manufactures most of the blood cells and is found in some parts of all bones. The center of the diaphysis is a single open space called the **medullary** (**MED** you lair ee) **cavity.** This cavity contains **yellow bone marrow,** which is mainly fat cells. Figure 4.10 contains an illustration of the structure of long bones.

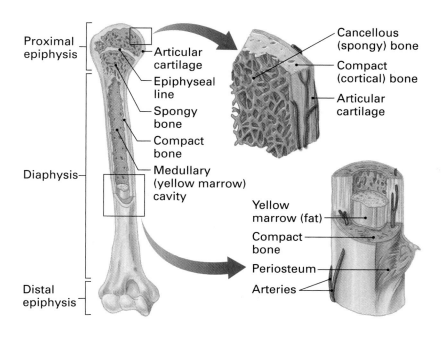

**■ FIGURE 4.10**   Composition of bone.

## Bone Projections and Depressions

| | | |
|---|---|---|
| **condyle** | **fossa** | **sinus** |
| **epicondyle** | **head** | **trochanter** |
| **fissure** | **neck** | **tubercle** |
| **foramen** | **process** | **tuberosity** |

Bones have many projections and depressions. Some are rounded and smooth in order to articulate with another bone in a joint. Others are rough to provide muscles with attachment points. Generally, the term **process** is used when discussing bony projections. These terms are commonly used on operative reports and in physicians' records for clear identification of areas on the individual bones. Some of the common bony processes include the following:

1. The **head** is a large ball-shaped end on a long bone. It may be separated from the body or shaft of the bone by a narrow area called the **neck.**

2. A **condyle** (**KON** dile) refers to a smooth rounded portion at the end of a bone.

3. The **epicondyle** (ep ih **KON** dile) is a projection located above or on a condyle.

4. The **trochanter** (tro **KAN** ter) refers to the large rough process on the femur for the attachment of a muscle.

5. A **tubercle** (**TOO** ber kl) is a rough process that provides the attachment for tendons and muscles.

6. The **tuberosity** (too ber **OSS** ih tee) is a rough process that provides the attachment of tendons and muscles.

See ■ Figure 4.11 for an illustration of the processes found on the femur.

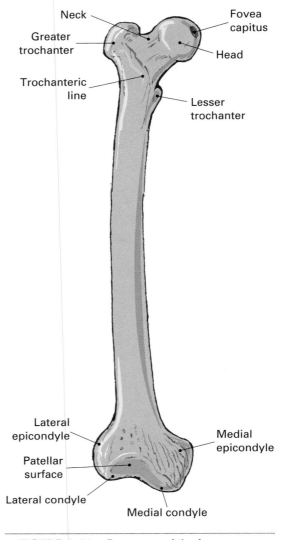

**Neck**

**Fovea capitus**

**Greater trochanter**

**Head**

**Trochanteric line**

**Lesser trochanter**

**Lateral epicondyle**

**Medial epicondyle**

**Patellar surface**

**Lateral condyle**

**Medial condyle**

■ **FIGURE 4.11** Processes of the femur.

In addition, bones have hollow regions or depressions. The most common depressions are as follows:

1. A **sinus** (**SIGH** nus), which is a hollow cavity within a bone.
2. A **foramen** (for **AY** men), which is a smooth round opening for nerves and blood vessels.
3. A **fossa** (**FOSS** ah), which consists of a shallow cavity or depression on the surface of a bone.
4. A **fissure** (**FISH** er), which is a slit-type opening.

## Joints

| | | |
|---|---|---|
| **articular cartilage** | **fibrous joints** | **sutures** |
| **articulation** | **joint capsule** | **synovial fluid** |
| **ball-and-socket joint** | **ligaments** | **synovial joint** |
| **bursa** | **pubic symphysis** | **synovial membrane** |
| **cartilaginous joints** | | |

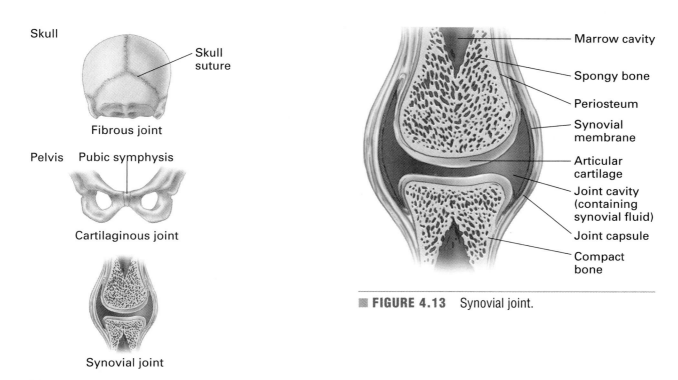

**FIGURE 4.12** Types of joints found in the body.

**FIGURE 4.13** Synovial joint.

Joints are formed when two or more bones meet. This is also referred to as an **articulation** (ar tik yoo **LAY** shun). There are three types of joints based on the amount of movement allowed between the two bones. The types are **synovial** (sin **OH** vee al) **joints, cartilaginous** (car tih **LAJ** ih nus) **joints,** and **fibrous** (**FYE** bruss) **joints** (see ▓ Figure 4.12).

Most joints are freely moving synovial joints (see ▓ Figure 4.13). These joints are enclosed by an elastic **joint capsule** and contain a lubricating fluid called **synovial fluid** secreted by the **synovial membrane.** The ends of bones in a synovial joint are covered by a layer of **articular** (ar **TIK** yoo lar) **cartilage.** Cartilage is very tough, but still flexible. It withstands high levels of stress to act as a shock absorber for the joint and prevents bone from rubbing against bone. Cartilage is found in several other areas of the body, such as the nasal septum, external ear, eustachian tube, larynx, trachea, bronchi, and intervertebral disks. One example of a synovial joint is the **ball-and-socket joint,** which is found at the shoulder and hip. The ball rotating in the socket allows for a wide range of motion. Bands of strong connective tissue called **ligaments** (**LIG** ah ments) bind bones together at the joint.

Some synovial joints contain a **bursa** (**BER** sah), which is a sac-like structure composed of connective tissue and lined with synovial membrane. They are most commonly found between bones and ligaments or tendons and function to reduce friction. Some common bursa locations are the elbow, knee, and shoulder joints.

Not all joints are freely moving. Fibrous joints allow almost no movement since the ends of the bones are joined by thick fibrous tissue, which may even fuse into solid bone. The **sutures** (**SOO** chers) of the skull are an example of a fibrous joint. Cartilaginous joints allow for slight movement but hold bones firmly in place by a solid piece of cartilage. An example of this type of joint is the **pubic symphysis** (**PYOO** bik **SIM** fih sis), the point at which the left and right pubic bones meet in the front of the lower abdomen.

> **MED TERM TIP**
>
> *Bursitis* (bur **SIGH** tis) is an inflammation of the bursa located between bony prominences such as at the shoulder. Housemaid's knee is a form of bursitis and carries the medical name *prepatellar bursitis* (pre pah **TELL** er bur **SIGH** tis). The term is thought to have originated from the damage to the knees that occurred when maids knelt to scrub floors.

# Word Building Relating to the Skeletal System

The following list contains examples of medical terms built directly from word parts. The definition for these terms can be determined by a straightforward translation of the word parts.

| Combining Form | Combined With | Medical Term | Definition |
|---|---|---|---|
| arthr/o | -algia | arthralgia (ar **THRAL** jee ah) | joint pain |
| | -centesis | arthrocentesis (ar thro sen **TEE** sis) | puncture to withdraw fluid from a joint |
| | -clasia | arthroclasia (ar throh **KLAY** see ah) | surgically breaking a joint |
| | -desis | arthrodesis (ar throh **DEE** sis) | fusion of a joint |
| | -itis | arthritis (ar **THRY** tis) | joint inflammation |
| | -otomy | arthrotomy (ar **THROT** oh mee) | incision into a joint |
| | -scopy | arthroscopy (ar **THROS** koh pee) | visual examination of inside a joint |
| burs/o | -ectomy | bursectomy (ber **SEK** toh mee) | excision of a bursa |
| | -itis | bursitis (ber **SIGH** tis) | inflammation of a bursa |
| | -lith | bursolith (**BER** soh lith) | stone in a bursa |
| chondr/o | -ectomy | chondrectomy (kon **DREK** toh mee) | excision of cartilage |
| | -malacia | chondromalacia (kon droh mah **LAY** she ah) | cartilage softening |
| | -plasty | chondroplasty (**KON** droh plas tee) | surgical repair of cartilage |
| crani/o | intra- -al | intracranial (in trah **KRAY** nee al) | pertaining to inside the skull |
| | -otomy | craniotomy (kray nee **OTT** oh mee) | incision into the skull |
| myel/o | -oma | myeloma (my ah **LOH** mah) | bone marrow tumor |
| oste/o | carcin/o -oma | osteocarcinoma (oss tee oh kar sin **OH** mah) | cancerous bone tumor |
| | chondr/o -oma | osteochondroma (oss tee oh kon **DROH** mah) | bone and cartilage tumor |
| | -clasia | osteoclasia (oss tee oh **KLAY** see ah) | to surgically break a bone |
| | -malacia | osteomalacia (oss tee oh mah **LAY** she ah) | bone softening |
| | myel/o -itis | osteomyelitis (oss tee oh mi ell **EYE** tis) | inflammation of bone and bone marrow |

| | -otomy | osteotomy (oss tee **OTT** ah me) | incision into a bone |
|---|---|---|---|
| | -pathy | osteopathy (oss tee **OPP** ah thee) | bone disease |
| | -porosis | osteoporosis (oss tee oh por **ROH** sis) | abnormal condition of porous bones |
| | -tome | osteotome (**OSS** tee oh tohm) | instrument to cut bone |
| vertebr/o | inter- -al | intervertebral (in ter **VER** teh bral) | pertaining to between vertebrae |

## Building Adjective Forms of Bone Names

It is important to learn the names and combining forms of all the bones in medical terminology because they are so frequently used as adjectives to indicate location.

| Adjective Suffix | Combined With | Adjective Form | Noun Form |
|---|---|---|---|
| -ac | ili/o | iliac | ilium |
| -al | cervic/o | cervical | neck |
| | cost/o | costal | rib |
| | femor/o | femoral | femur |
| | humer/o | humeral | humerus |
| | ischi/o | ischial | ischium |
| | radi/o | radial | radius |
| | sacr/o | sacral | sacrum |
| | stern/o | sternal | sternum |
| | tibi/o | tibial | tibia |
| -ar | clavicul/o | clavicular | clavicle |
| | fibul/o | fibular | fibula |
| | lumb/o | lumbar | low back |
| | mandibul/o | mandibular | mandible |
| | patell/o | patellar | patella |
| | scapul/o | scapular | scapula |
| | uln/o | ulnar | ulna |
| -ary | maxill/o | maxillary | maxilla |
| -eal | coccyg/o | coccygeal | coccyx |
| | phalang/o | phalangeal | phalanges |
| -ic | pub/o | pubic | pubis |
| | thorac/o | thoracic | thorax |

# Vocabulary Relating to the Skeletal System

| | |
|---|---|
| **callus (KAL us)** | The mass of bone tissue that forms at a fracture site during its healing. |
| **crepitation (krep ih TAY shun)** | The noise produced by bones or cartilage rubbing together in conditions such as arthritis. |
| **exostosis (eck sos TOH sis)** | A bone spur. |
| **kyphosis (ki FOH sis)** | Abnormal increase in the outward curvature of the thoracic spine. Also known as *hunchback* or *humpback*. See ▓ Figure 4.14 for an illustration of abnormal spine curvatures. |
| **lordosis (lor DOH sis)** | Abnormal increase in the forward curvature of the lumbar spine. Also known as *swayback*. See Figure 4.14 for an illustration of abnormal spine curvatures. |
| **orthopedics (or thoh PEE diks)** | Branch of medicine specializing in the diagnosis and treatment of conditions of the musculoskeletal system. |
| **orthopedist (or thoh PEE dist)** | Physician who specializes in treatment of conditions of the musculoskeletal system. |
| **orthotics (or THOT iks)** | A brace or splint used to prevent or correct deformities. |
| **orthotist (or THOT ist)** | Person skilled in making and fitting orthotics. |
| **podiatrist (po DYE ah trist)** | Specialist in treating disorders of the feet. |
| **prosthesis (pross THEE sis)** | Artificial device that is used as a substitute for a body part that is either congenitally missing or is absent as a result of accident or disease (for instance, an artificial leg or hip). |
| **prosthetist (PROSS thah tist)** | Person who fabricates and fits prostheses. |

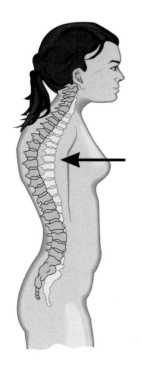
Excessive kyphosis (slouch)

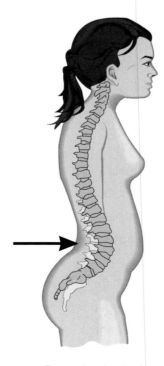
Excessive lordosis (swayback)

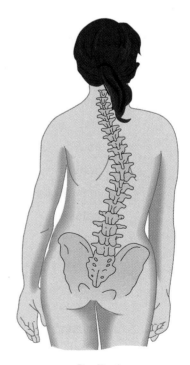
Scoliosis

▓ **FIGURE 4.14**  Abnormal spinal curvatures.

# Pathology Relating to the Skeletal System

| | |
|---|---|
| **ankylosing spondylitis (ang kih LOH sing spon dih LYE tis)** | Inflammatory spinal condition that resembles rheumatoid arthritis. Results in gradual stiffening and fusion of the vertebrae. More common in men than women. |
| **bunion (BUN yun)** | Inflammation of the bursa of the great toe. |
| **carpal tunnel syndrome (CTS) (CAR pal TUN el SIN drohm)** | Pain caused by compression of the nerve as it passes between the bones and ligaments of the wrist. |
| **closed fracture** | A fracture in which there is no open skin wound. Also called a *simple fracture* (see ▉ Figure 4.15). |
| **Colles' (COL eez) fracture** | A common type of wrist fracture (see ▉ Figure 4.16). |
| **comminuted fracture (kom ih NYOOT ed)** | Fracture in which the bone is shattered, splintered, or crushed into many small pieces or fragments. |
| **compound fracture** | Fracture in which the skin has been broken through to the fracture. Also called an *open fracture* (see also Figure 4.15). |
| **dislocation** | Occurs when the bones in a joint are displaced from their normal alignment. |
| **Ewing's sarcoma (YOO wings sar KOH mah)** | Malignant growth found in the shaft of long bones that spreads through the periosteum. Removal is treatment of choice, because this tumor will metastasize or spread to other organs. Named for James Ewing, an American pathologist. |
| **fracture (FX, Fx)** | A broken bone. |
| **gout (GOWT)** | Inflammation of the joints caused by excessive uric acid. |
| **greenstick fracture** | Fracture in which there is an incomplete break; one side of bone is broken and the other side is bent. This type of fracture is commonly found in children due to their softer and more pliable bone structure. |
| **herniated nucleus pulposus (HER nee ated NOO klee us pull POH sus) (HNP)** | Herniation or protrusion of an intervertebral disk; also called *herniated disk*. May require surgery. |
| **impacted fracture** | Fracture in which bone fragments are pushed into each other. |
| **myeloma (my ah LOH mah)** | Malignant tumor originating in the bone marrow. |
| **oblique (oh BLEEK) fracture** | Fracture at an angle to the bone (see ▉ Figure 4.17). |
| **open fracture** | Fracture in which the skin has been broken through to the fracture. Also called a *compound fracture* (see also Figure 4.15). |
| **osteoarthritis (oss tee oh ar THRY tis) (OA)** | Arthritis resulting in degeneration of the bones and joints, especially those bearing weight. Results in bone rubbing against bone. |
| **osteogenic sarcoma (oss tee oh GIN ik sark OH mah)** | The most common type of bone cancer. Usually begins in osteocytes found at the ends of long bones. |
| **osteomalacia (oss tee oh mah LAY she ah)** | Softening of the bones caused by a deficiency of calcium. It is thought that in children the cause is insufficient sunlight and vitamin D. |
| **osteoporosis (oss tee oh por ROH sis)** | Decrease in bone mass that results in a thinning and weakening of the bone with resulting fractures. The bone becomes more porous, especially in the spine and pelvis. |
| **Paget's (PAH jets) disease** | A fairly common metabolic disease of the bone from unknown causes. It usually attacks middle-aged and elderly people and is characterized by bone destruction and deformity. Named for Sir James Paget, a British surgeon. |

*continued...*

| Pathology Relating to the Skeletal System (continued) | |
|---|---|
| **pathologic (path a LOJ ik) fracture** | Fracture caused by diseased or weakened bone. |
| **rheumatoid arthritis (ROO mah toyd ar THRY tis) (RA)** | Chronic form of arthritis with inflammation of the joints, swelling, stiffness, pain, and changes in the cartilage that can result in crippling deformities (see Figure 4.18). |
| **rickets (RIK ets)** | Deficiency in calcium and vitamin D found in early childhood that results in bone deformities, especially bowed legs. |
| **scoliosis (skoh lee OH sis)** | Abnormal lateral curvature of the spine. See Figure 4.14 for an illustration of abnormal spine curvatures. |
| **simple fracture** | A fracture in which there is no open skin wound. Also called a *closed fracture* (see Figure 4.15). |
| **spina bifida (SPY nah BIF ih dah)** | A congenital anomaly that occurs when a vertebra fails to fully form around the spinal cord. |
| **spinal stenosis (ste NOH sis)** | Narrowing of the spinal canal causing pressure on the cord and nerves. |
| **spiral fracture** | Fracture in which the fracture line spirals around the shaft of the bone. Can be caused by a twisting injury and is often slower to heal than other types of fractures. |
| **spondylolisthesis (spon dih loh liss THEE sis)** | The forward sliding of a lumbar vertebra over the vertebra below it. |
| **spondylosis (spon dih LOH sis)** | A degenerative condition of the vertebral column. |
| **strain** | Damage to the ligaments surrounding a joint due to overstretching, but no dislocation of the joint. |
| **systemic lupus erythematosus (sis TEM ik LOOP us air ih them ah TOH sis) (SLE)** | Chronic inflammatory disease of connective tissue that causes injury to the joints, skin, kidneys, heart, lungs, and nervous system. A characteristic butterfly rash or erythema may be present. |
| **talipes (TAL ih peez)** | Congenital deformity of the foot. Also referred to as a *clubfoot*. |
| **transverse fracture** | Complete fracture that is straight across the bone at right angles to the long axis of the bone (see Figure 4.19). |
| **whiplash** | Injury to the bones in the cervical spine as a result of a sudden movement forward and backward of the head and neck. Can occur as a result of a rear-end auto collision. |

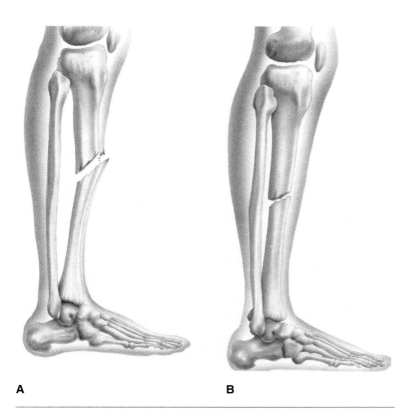

**A**                    **B**

■ **FIGURE 4.15**    (A) Open (or compound) and (B) closed (or simple) fractures.

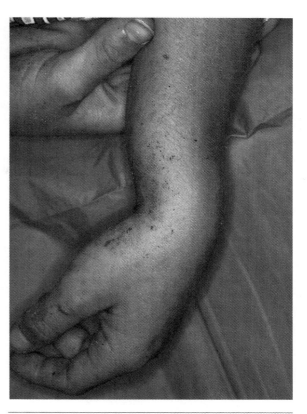

■ **FIGURE 4.16**    Colles' fracture.
(Charles Stewart and Associates)

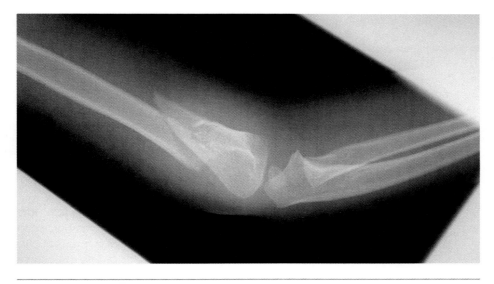

■ **FIGURE 4.17**    Fractured humerus.
(Charles Stewart and Associates)

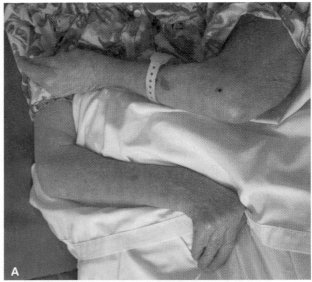

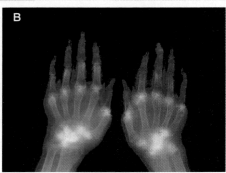

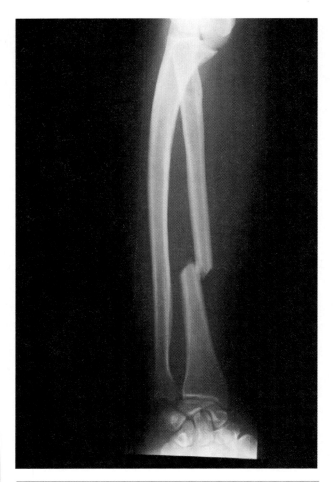

■ **FIGURE 4.18** (A) Contractures of rheumatoid arthritis. (B) Enhanced color X-ray of arthritis in hands and wrists.
(CNRI/Science Photo Library/Photo Researchers, Inc.)

■ **FIGURE 4.19** X-ray of complete fracture of radius.
(James Stevenson/Science Photo Library/Photo Researchers, Inc.)

## Diagnostic Procedures Relating to the Skeletal System

| | |
|---|---|
| **arthrography** (ar THROG rah fee) | Visualization of a joint by radiographic study after injection of a contrast medium into the joint space. |
| **arthroscopy** (ar THROS koh pee) | Examination of the interior of a joint by entering the joint with an arthroscope. Torn ligaments can be repaired while the patient is undergoing arthroscopy. The arthroscope contains a small television camera that allows the physician to view the interior of the joint on a monitor during the procedure (see ■ Figure 4.20). |
| **bone scan** | Patient is given a radioactive dye and then scanning equipment is used to visualize bones. It is especially useful in observing progress of treatment for osteomyelitis and cancer metastases to the bone. |
| **myelography** (my eh LOG rah fee) | Study of the spinal column after injecting opaque contrast material; particularly useful in identifying herniated nucleus pulposus. |
| **photon absorptiometry** (FOH ton ab sorp she AHM eh tree) | Measurement of bone density using an instrument for the purpose of detecting osteoporosis. |

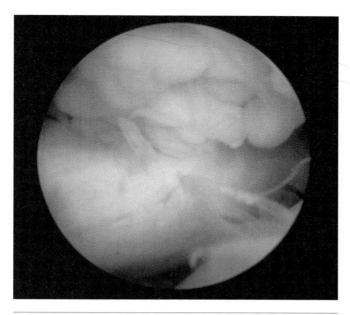

**FIGURE 4.20** Arthroscopy of the knee.
(Southern Illinois University/ Photo Researchers, Inc.)

## Therapeutic Procedures Relating to the Skeletal System

| | |
|---|---|
| **amputation**<br>**(am pew TAY shun)** | Partial or complete removal of a limb for a variety of reasons, including tumors, gangrene, intractable pain, crushing injury, or uncontrollable infection. |
| **arthroscopic**<br>**(ar throh SKOP ic) surgery** | Use of an arthroscope to facilitate performing surgery on a joint (see Figure 4.20). |
| **bone graft** | Piece of bone taken from the patient that is used to take the place of a removed bone or a bony defect at another site. |
| **bunionectomy**<br>**(bun yun ECK toh mee)** | Removal of the bursa at the joint of the great toe. |
| **carpal tunnel**<br>**(CAR pal TUN el) release** | Surgical cutting of the ligament in the wrist to relieve nerve pressure caused by carpal tunnel syndrome, which can result from repetitive motion such as typing. |
| **cast** | Application of a solid material to immobilize an extremity or portion of the body as a result of a fracture, dislocation, or severe injury. It is most often made of plaster of Paris (see Figure 4.21). |
| **diskectomy (disk EK toh mee)** | Removal of a herniated intervertebral disk. |
| **laminectomy**<br>**(lam ih NEK toh mee)** | Removal of the vertebral posterior arch to correct severe back problems and pain caused by compression of a spinal nerve. |
| **reduction** | Correcting a fracture by realigning the bone fragments. Closed reduction is doing this manipulation without entering the body. Open reduction is the process of making a surgical incision at the site of the fracture to do the reduction. This is commonly necessary when bony fragments need to removed. |
| **spinal fusion** | Surgical immobilization of adjacent vertebrae. This may be done for several reasons, including correction for a herniated disk. |
| **total hip replacement (THR)** | Surgical reconstruction of a hip by implanting a prosthetic or artificial hip joint. Also called *total hip arthroplasty (THA)* (see Figure 4.22). |
| **total knee replacement (TKR)** | Surgical reconstruction of a knee joint by implanting a prosthetic knee joint. Also called *total knee arthroplasty (TKA).* |

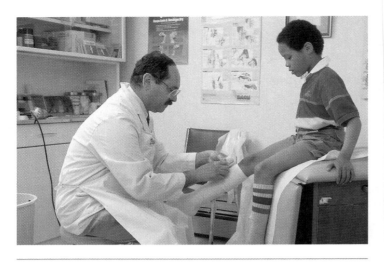

■ **FIGURE 4.21** Physician applying cast to right leg.

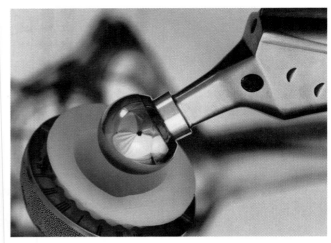

■ **FIGURE 4.22** Prosthetic hip joint.
(Lawrence Livermore National Library/Science Photo Library/Photo Researchers, Inc.)

## Pharmacology Relating to the Skeletal System

| | |
|---|---|
| **bone reabsorption inhibitors** | Conditions that result in weak and fragile bones, such as osteoporosis and Paget's disease, are improved by medications that reduce the reabsorption of bones. |
| **calcium supplements and Vitamin D therapy** | Maintaining high blood levels of calcium in association with vitamin D helps maintain bone density and treats osteomalacia, osteoporosis, and rickets. |
| **corticosteroids** | A hormone produced by the adrenal cortex that has very strong anti-inflammatory properties. It is particularly useful in treating rheumatoid arthritis. |
| **nonsteroidal anti-inflammatory drugs (NSAIDs)** | A large group of drugs including aspirin and ibuprofen that provide mild pain relief and anti-inflammatory benefits for conditions such as arthritis. |

## Abbreviations Relating to the Skeletal System

| | | | |
|---|---|---|---|
| **AE** | above elbow | **LUE** | left upper extremity |
| **AK** | above knee | **NSAID** | nonsteroidal anti-inflammatory drug |
| **BDT** | bone density testing | **OA** | osteoarthritis |
| **BE** | below elbow | **ORIF** | open reduction–internal fixation |
| **BK** | below knee | **Orth, ortho** | orthopedics |
| **C1, C2, etc.** | first cervical vertebra, second cervical vertebra, etc. | **RA** | rheumatoid arthritis |
| | | **RLE** | right lower extremity |
| **CDH** | congenital dislocation of the hip | **RUE** | right upper extremity |
| **CTS** | carpal tunnel syndrome | **SLE** | systemic lupus erythematosus |
| **DJD** | degenerative joint disease | **T1, T2, etc.** | first thoracic vertebra, second thoracic vertebra, etc. |
| **FX, Fx** | fracture | | |
| **HNP** | herniated nucleus pulposus | **THA** | total hip arthroplasty |
| **JRA** | juvenile rheumatoid arthritis | **THR** | total hip replacement |
| **L1, L2, etc.** | first lumbar vertebra, second lumbar vertebra, etc. | **TKA** | total knee arthroplasty |
| | | **TKR** | total knee replacement |
| **LAT, lat** | lateral | **TMJ** | temporomandibular joint |
| **LE** | lower extremity | **TX, Tx** | traction, treatment |
| **LLE** | left lower extremity | **UE** | upper extremity |

# Overview

## Part II: Muscular System

### Organs of the Muscular System

fascia
muscles
tendons

### Combining Forms Relating to the Muscular System

| | |
|---|---|
| fasci/o | fibrous band |
| fibr/o | fibers |
| leiomy/o | smooth muscle |
| muscul/o | muscle |
| my/o | muscle |
| myocardi/o | heart muscle |
| myos/o | muscle |
| plant/o | sole of foot |
| rhabdomy/o | skeletal muscle |
| ten/o | tendon |
| tend/o | tendon |
| tendin/o | tendon |

### Suffixes Relating to the Muscular System

| Suffix | Meaning | Example |
|---|---|---|
| -asthenia | weakness | myasthenia |
| -kinesia | movement | bradykinesia |
| -trophy | development, nourishment | hypertrophy |

### Prefixes Relating to the Muscular System

| Prefix | Meaning | Example |
|---|---|---|
| ab- | away from | abduction |
| ad- | toward | adduction |
| circum- | around | circumduction |

## Anatomy and Physiology of the Muscular System

**muscle tissue fibers**　　　　**myoneural junction**

Muscles are bundles of parallel **muscle tissue fibers.** As these fibers contract (shorten in length) they pull whatever they are attached to closer together. This may move two bones closer together or make an opening narrower. A muscle contraction occurs when a message is transmitted from the brain through the

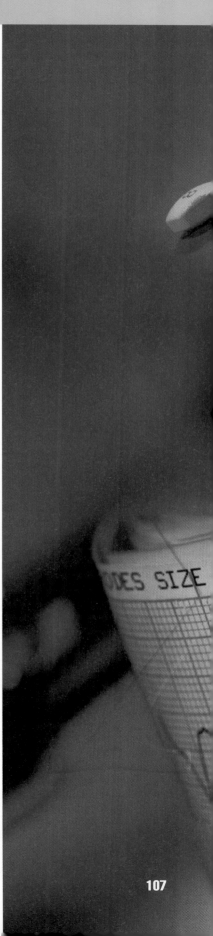

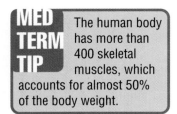
nervous system to the muscles. The point at which a nerve contacts a muscle fiber is called the **myoneural** (**MY** oh **NOO** rall) **junction**.

## Types of Muscles

| | | |
|---|---|---|
| **adductor longus** | **gluteus maximus** | **skeletal muscle** |
| **biceps** | **myocardium** | **smooth muscle** |
| **cardiac muscle** | **rectus abdominis** | **tendon** |
| **fascia** | | |

Three basic types of muscle tissue are **skeletal** (**SKELL** eh tal) **muscle, smooth muscle,** and **cardiac** (**CAR** dee ak) **muscle** (see Figure 4.23). These muscle tissues are either voluntary or involuntary. Voluntary muscle tissue allows the person to dictate the function. The skeletal muscles of the arm and leg are examples of this type of muscle. Involuntary muscles generally act without any conscious direction from the person. The smooth muscles found in internal organs and cardiac muscles are examples of involuntary muscle tissue (see Figure 4.24).

Skeletal muscles are attached to the skeletal bones and allow for voluntary movement. These muscles are wrapped in layers of connective tissue called **fascia** (**FASH** ee ah). The fascia covering tapers at each end of a skeletal mus-

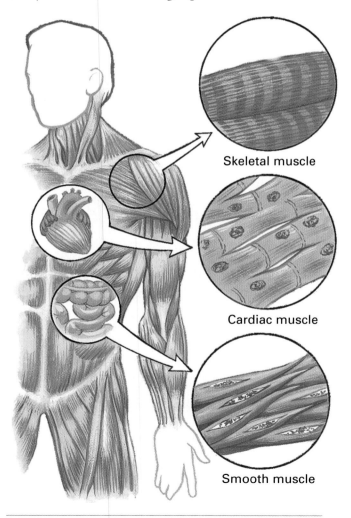

Skeletal muscle

Cardiac muscle

Smooth muscle

**FIGURE 4.23** Types of muscles.

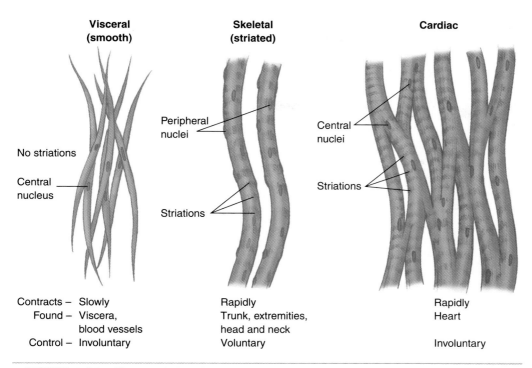

| Visceral (smooth) | Skeletal (striated) | Cardiac |
|---|---|---|

No striations

Peripheral nuclei

Central nucleus

Central nuclei

Striations

Striations

Contracts – Slowly
    Found – Viscera, blood vessels
 Control – Involuntary

Rapidly
Trunk, extremities, head and neck
Voluntary

Rapidly
Heart

Involuntary

**FIGURE 4.24**   *Characteristics of muscle tissue.*

cle to form a very strong **tendon** (**TEN** dun). The tendon then inserts into the periosteum covering a bone to attach the muscle to the bone. Skeletal muscles are stimulated by motor neurons of the nervous system. See Figure ▒ 4.25 for an illustration of the most commonly discussed skeletal muscles.

Smooth muscle tissue is found in the walls of the hollow organs, such as the stomach, and tube-shaped organs, such as the respiratory airways and blood vessels. It is responsible for the involuntary muscle action associated with movement of the internal organs.

Cardiac muscle, or **myocardium** (my oh **CAR** dee um), occurs in the walls of the heart and allows for the heart's involuntary pumping action. This muscle will be more thoroughly described in Chapter 5, Cardiovascular System.

The name of a muscle often reflects its location, size, fiber direction, or number of attachment points, as the following examples illustrate.

- **Location:** The term **rectus abdominis** (**REK** tus ab **DOM** ih nis) means straight (rectus) abdominal muscle.
- **Size:** When gluteus, meaning rump area, is combined with maximus, meaning large, we have the term **gluteus maximus** (**GLOO** tee us **MACKS** ih mus).
- **Fiber direction:** The **adductor** (ad **DUCK** tor) **longus** is the long thigh muscle responsible for adduction.
- **Number of attachment points:** The term *bi*, meaning two, can form the medical term **biceps** (**BYE** seps), which stands for the muscle in the upper arm that has two heads or connecting points.

## Terminology for Muscle Actions

**action**                              **insertion**

**antagonistic pairs**          **origin**

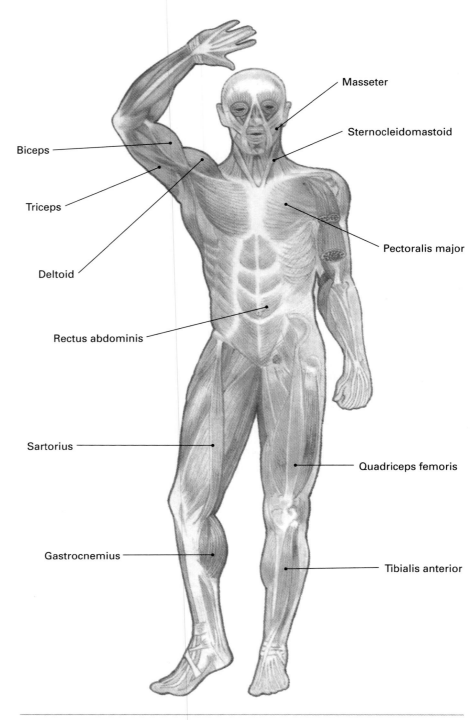

**FIGURE 4.25** Muscles: anterior view.

Skeletal muscles are attached to two different bones and overlap a joint. When a muscle contracts, the two bones move, but not usually equally. The less movable of the two bones is called the **origin** for the muscle, while the more movable bone is the **insertion** for the muscle. The type of movement a muscle produces is called its **action.** The muscles are often arranged around joints in **antagonistic pairs,** meaning they produce opposite actions. For example, one muscle will bend a joint while its antagonist is responsible for straightening the joint. Some common terminology for muscle actions arranged in antagonistic pairs follows:

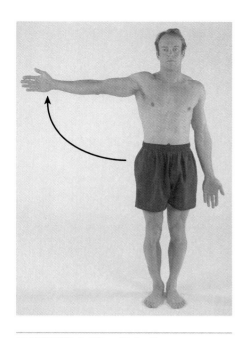

■ FIGURE 4.26   Abduction.

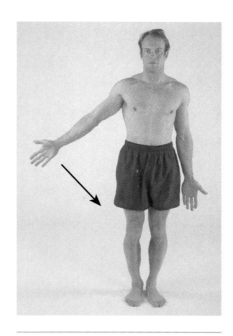

■ FIGURE 4.27   Adduction.

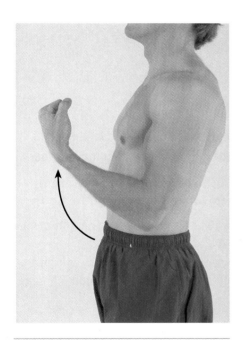

■ FIGURE 4.28   Flexion of left forearm.

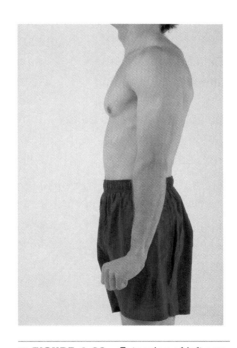

■ FIGURE 4.29   Extension of left arm.

**abduction** (ab **DUCK** shun)    Movement away from midline of the body (see ■ Figure 4.26).

**adduction** (ah **DUCK** shun)    Movement toward midline of the body (see ■ Figure 4.27).

**flexion** (**FLEK** shun)    Act of bending or being bent (see ■ Figure 4.28).

**extension** (eks **TEN** shun)    Movement that brings limb into or toward a straight condition (see ■ Figure 4.29).

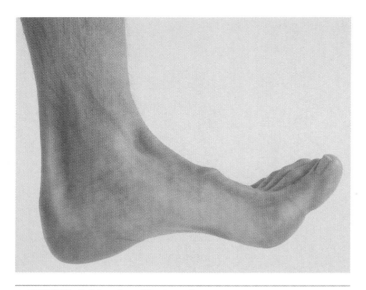

**FIGURE 4.30**  Dorsiflexion of toes.

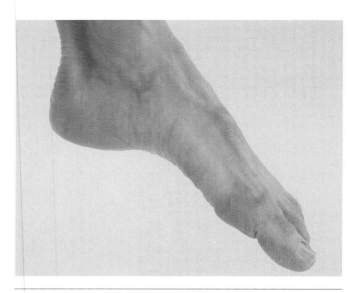

**FIGURE 4.31**  Plantar flexion of foot.

| | |
|---|---|
| **dorsiflexion** (dor see **FLEK** shun) | Backward bending, as of hand or foot (see ▥ Figure 4.30). |
| **plantar flexion** (**PLAN** tar **FLEK** shun) | Bending sole of foot; pointing toes downward (see ▥ Figure 4.31). |
| **eversion** (ee **VER** zhun) | Turning outward. |
| **inversion** (in **VER** zhun) | Turning inward. |
| **pronation** (proh **NAY** shun) | To turn downward or backward as with the hand or foot. |
| **supination** (soo pin **NAY** shun) | Turning the palm or foot upward. |
| **elevation** | To raise a body part, as in shrugging the shoulders. |
| **depression** | A downward movement, as in dropping the shoulders. |

    The following three actions are not antagonistic pairs. Rather they are three terms that describe different types of circular movements made by the body.

| | |
|---|---|
| **circumduction** (sir kum **DUCK** shun) | Movement in a circular direction from a central point. Imagine drawing a large circle in the air. |
| **opposition** | Moving thumb away from palm; the ability to move the thumb into contact with the other fingers. |
| **rotation** | Moving around a central axis. |

## Word Building Relating to the Muscular System

The following list contains examples of medical terms built directly from word parts. The definition for these terms can be determined by a straightforward translation of the word parts.

| Combining Form | Combined With | Medical Term | Definition |
|---|---|---|---|
| fasci/o | -itis | fasciitis (fas ee **EYE** tis) | inflammation of fascia |
| | -rrhaphy | fasciorrhaphy (fas ee **OR** ah fee) | suture fascia |
| | -tomy | fasciotomy (fas ee **OT** oh mee) | incision into fascia |

| leiomy/o | fibr/o -oma | leiomyofibroma (lye oh my oh fye **BRO** mah) | fibrous smooth muscle tumor |
| | -oma | leiomyoma (lye oh my **OH** mah) | smooth muscle tumor |
| my/o | electr/o -gram | electromyogram (ee lek troh **MY** oh gram) (EMG) | record of muscle electricity |
| | -pathy | myopathy (my **OPP** ah thee) | muscle disease |
| | -plasty | myoplasty (**MY** oh plas tee) | surgical repair of muscle |
| | -rrhaphy | myorrhaphy (**MY** or ah fee) | suture a muscle |
| myos/o | poly- -itis | polymyositis (pol ee my oh **SIGH** tis) | inflammation of many muscles |
| rhabdomy/o | -lysis | rhabdomyolysis (rab doh my oh **LYE** sis) | skeletal muscle destruction |
| | -oma | rhabdomyoma (rab doh my **OH** mah) | skeletal muscle tumor |
| ten/o | -dynia | tenodynia (ten oh **DIN** ee ah) | tendon pain |
| | my/o -pathy | tenomyopathy (ten oh my **OP** oh thee) | disease of tendons and muscle |
| | -rrhaphy | tenorrhaphy (tah **NOR** ah fee) | suture a tendon |
| tend/o | -plasty | tendoplasty (**TEN** doh plas tee) | surgical repair of tendon |
| | -tomy | tendotomy (tend **OT** oh mee) | incision into tendon |
| tendin/o | -itis | tendinitis (ten dih **NIGH** tis) | inflammation of tendon |
| | -ous | tendinous (**TEN** din us) | pertaining to tendons |

| Suffix | Combined With Prefix | Medical Term | Definition |
|---|---|---|---|
| -kinesia | brady- | bradykinesia (brad ee kih **NEE** see ah) | slow movement |
| | dys- | dyskinesia (dis kih **NEE** see ah) | difficult or painful movement |
| | hyper- | hyperkinesia (high per kih **NEE** see ah) | excessive movement |
| -trophy | a- | atrophy (**AT** rah fee) | lack of development |
| | dys- | dystrophy (**DIS** troh fee) | difficult (poor) development |
| | hyper- | hypertrophy (high **PER** troh fee) | excessive development |

# Vocabulary Relating to the Muscular System

| **adhesion** | Scar tissue forming in the fascia surrounding a muscle, making it difficult to stretch the muscle. |
|---|---|
| **contracture (kon TRACK chur)** | An abnormal shortening of a muscle, making it difficult to stretch the muscle. |
| **spasm** | A sudden, involuntary, strong muscle contraction. |
| **torticollis (tore tih KOLL iss)** | Severe neck spasms pulling the head to one side. Commonly called *wryneck* or a *crick in the neck*. |

## Pathology Relating to the Muscular System

| | |
|---|---|
| **fibromyalgia**<br>**(figh broh my AL jee ah)** | A condition with widespread aching and pain in the muscles and soft tissue. |
| **ganglion (GANG lee on)** | Cyst that forms on tendon sheath, usually on hand, wrist, or ankle. |
| **lateral epicondylitis**<br>**(ep ih kon dih LYE tis)** | Inflammation of the muscle attachment to the lateral epicondyle of the elbow. Often caused by strongly gripping. Commonly called *tennis elbow*. |
| **muscular dystrophy**<br>**(MUSS kew ler DIS troh fee) (MD)** | Inherited disease causing a progressive muscle degeneration, weakness, and atrophy. |
| **pseudohypertrophic**<br>**(soo doh HIGH per troh fic)**<br>**muscular dystrophy** | One type of inherited muscular dystrophy in which the muscle tissue is gradually replaced by fatty tissue, making the muscle look strong. Also called *Duchenne's muscular dystrophy*. |
| **sprain** | Damage to the muscle and soft tissue due to overuse of overstretching. |

## Diagnostic Procedures Relating to the Muscular System

| | |
|---|---|
| **creatine phosphokinase**<br>**(KREE ah teen foss foe KYE nase) (CPK)** | A muscle enzyme found in skeletal muscle and cardiac muscle. Blood levels become elevated in disorders such as heart attack, muscular dystrophy, and other skeletal muscle pathologies. |
| **deep tendon reflexes** | Muscle contraction in response to a stretch caused by striking the muscle tendon with a reflex hammer. Test used to determine if muscles are responding properly. |
| **electromyography**<br>**(ee lek troh my OG rah fee)** | Study and record of the strength and quality of muscle contractions as a result of electrical stimulation. |
| **muscle biopsy (BYE op see)** | Removal of muscle tissue for pathological examination. |

## Pharmacology Relating to the Muscular System

| | |
|---|---|
| muscle relaxants | Medication to relax skeletal muscles in order to reduce muscle spasms. Also called *antispasmodics*. |

## Abbreviations Relating to the Muscular System

| | | | | |
|---|---|---|---|---|
| **CPK** | creatine phosphokinase | | **IM** | intramuscular |
| **DTR** | deep tendon reflex | | **MD** | muscular dystrophy |
| **EMG** | electromyogram | | **ROM** | range of motion |

# Chapter Review

## Pronunciation Practice

*You will find the pronunciation for each term on the enclosed CD-ROM. Check each one off as you master it.*

- ☐ abduction (ab **DUCK** shun)
- ☐ action
- ☐ adduction (ad **DUCK** shun)
- ☐ adductor (ad **DUCK** tor) longus
- ☐ adhesion
- ☐ amputation (am pew **TAY** shun)
- ☐ ankylosing spondylitis (ang kih **LOH** sing spon dih **LYE** tis)
- ☐ antagonistic pairs
- ☐ appendicular (app en **DIK** yoo lar) skeleton
- ☐ arthralgia (ar **THRAL** jee ah)
- ☐ arthritis (ar **THRY** tis)
- ☐ arthrocentesis (ar throh sen **TEE** sis)
- ☐ arthroclasia (ar throh **KLAY** see ah)
- ☐ arthrodesis (ar throh **DEE** sis)
- ☐ arthrography (ar **THROG** rah fee)
- ☐ arthroscopic (ar throh **SKOP** ik) surgery
- ☐ arthroscopy (ar **THROS** koh pee)
- ☐ arthrotomy (ar **THROT** oh mee)
- ☐ articular (ar **TIK** yoo lar) cartilage
- ☐ articulation (ar tik yoo **LAY** shun)
- ☐ atrophy (**AT** rah fee)
- ☐ axial (**AK** see al) skeleton
- ☐ ball-and-socket joint
- ☐ biceps (**BYE** seps)
- ☐ bone graft
- ☐ bone marrow
- ☐ bone reabsorption inhibitors
- ☐ bone scan
- ☐ bones
- ☐ bradykinesia (brad ee kih **NEE** see ah)
- ☐ bunion (**BUN** yun)
- ☐ bunionectomy (bun yun **ECK** toh mee)
- ☐ bursa (**BER** sah)
- ☐ bursectomy (ber **SEK** toh mee)
- ☐ bursitis (ber **SIGH** tis)

- ☐ bursolith (**BER** soh lith)
- ☐ calcium supplements
- ☐ callus (**KAL** us)
- ☐ cancellous (**CAN** sell us) bone
- ☐ cardiac (**CAR** dee ak) muscle
- ☐ carpal tunnel (**CAR** pal **TUN** el) release
- ☐ carpal tunnel syndrome (**CAR** pal **TUN** el **SIN** drohm)
- ☐ carpals (**CAR** pals)
- ☐ cartilage (**CAR** tih lij)
- ☐ cartilaginous (car tih **LAJ** ih nus) joints
- ☐ cast
- ☐ cervical
- ☐ cervical vertebrae (**SER** vih kal **VER** teh bray)
- ☐ chondrectomy (kon **DREK** toh mee)
- ☐ chondromalacia (kon droh mah **LAY** she ah)
- ☐ chondroplasty (**KON** droh plas tee)
- ☐ circumduction (sir kum **DUCK** shun)
- ☐ clavicle (**CLAV** ih kl)
- ☐ clavicular
- ☐ closed fracture
- ☐ coccygeal
- ☐ coccyx (**COCK** six)
- ☐ Colles' (**COL** eez) fracture
- ☐ comminuted (kom ih **NYOOT** ed) fracture
- ☐ compact bone
- ☐ compound fracture
- ☐ condyle (**CON** dile)
- ☐ contracture (kon **TRACK** chur)
- ☐ cortical bone (**KOR** tih kal)
- ☐ corticosteroids
- ☐ costal
- ☐ craniotomy (kray nee **OTT** oh mee)
- ☐ cranium (**KRAY** nee um)
- ☐ creatine phosphokinase (**KREE** ah teen foss foe **KYE** nase)
- ☐ crepitation (krep ih **TAY** shun)

- ❑ deep tendon reflex
- ❑ depression
- ❑ diaphysis (dye **AFF** ih sis)
- ❑ diskectomy (disk **EK** toh mee)
- ❑ dislocation
- ❑ dorsiflexion (dor see **FLEK** shun)
- ❑ dyskinesia (dis kih **NEE** see ah)
- ❑ dystrophy (**DIS** troh fee)
- ❑ electromyogram (ee lek troh **MY** oh gram)
- ❑ electromyography (ee lek troh my **OG** rah fee)
- ❑ elevation
- ❑ epicondyle (ep ih **KON** dile)
- ❑ epiphysis (eh **PIFF** ih sis)
- ❑ ethmoid (**ETH** moyd) bone
- ❑ eversion (ee **VER** zhun)
- ❑ Ewing's sarcoma (**YOO** wings sar **KOH** ma)
- ❑ exostosis (eck sos **TOH** sis)
- ❑ extension (eks **TEN** shun)
- ❑ facial bones
- ❑ fascia (**FASH** ee ah)
- ❑ fasciitis (fas ee **EYE** tis)
- ❑ fasciorrhaphy (fas ee **OR** ah fee)
- ❑ fasciotomy (fas ee **OT** oh mee)
- ❑ femoral
- ❑ femur (**FEE** mer)
- ❑ fibromyalgia (figh broh my **AL** jee ah)
- ❑ fibrous (**FYE** bruss) joints
- ❑ fibula (**FIB** yoo lah)
- ❑ fibular
- ❑ fissure (**FISH** er)
- ❑ flat bones
- ❑ flexion (**FLEK** shun)
- ❑ foramen (for **AY** men)
- ❑ fossa (**FOSS** ah)
- ❑ fracture
- ❑ frontal bone
- ❑ ganglion (**GANG** lee on)
- ❑ gout (**GOWT**)
- ❑ greenstick fracture
- ❑ head
- ❑ herniated nucleus pulposus (**HER** nee ated **NOO** klee us pull **POH** sus)

- ❑ humeral
- ❑ humerus (**HYOO** mer us)
- ❑ hyoid (**HIGH** oyd) bone
- ❑ hyperkinesia (high per kih **NEE** see ah)
- ❑ hypertrophy (high **PER** troh fee)
- ❑ iliac
- ❑ ilium (**ILL** ee um)
- ❑ impacted fracture
- ❑ innominate (ih **NOM** ih nayt) bone
- ❑ insertion
- ❑ intervertebral (in ter **VER** teh bral)
- ❑ intracranial (in trah **KRAY** nee al)
- ❑ inversion (in **VER** zhun)
- ❑ irregular bones
- ❑ ischial
- ❑ ischium (**ISS** kee um)
- ❑ joint capsule
- ❑ joints
- ❑ kyphosis (ki **FOH** sis)
- ❑ lacrimal (**LACK** rim al) bone
- ❑ laminectomy (lam ih **NEK** toh mee)
- ❑ lateral epicondylitis (ep ih kon dih **LYE** tis)
- ❑ leiomyofibroma (lye oh my oh fye **BRO** mah)
- ❑ leiomyoma (lye oh my **OH** mah)
- ❑ ligaments (**LIG** ah ments)
- ❑ long bones
- ❑ lordosis (lor **DOH** sis)
- ❑ lower extremities
- ❑ lumbar (**LUM** bar)
- ❑ lumbar vertebrae (**LUM** bar **VER** teh bray)
- ❑ mandible (**MAN** dih bl)
- ❑ mandibular
- ❑ maxilla (mack **SIH** lah)
- ❑ maxillary
- ❑ medullary (**MED** you lair ee) cavity
- ❑ metacarpals (met ah **CAR** pals)
- ❑ metatarsals (met ah **TAHR** sals)
- ❑ muscle biopsy (**BYE** op see)
- ❑ muscle relaxants
- ❑ muscle tissue fibers
- ❑ muscles
- ❑ muscular dystrophy (**MUSS** kew ler **DIS** troh fee)

- myelography (my eh **LOG** rah fee)
- myeloma (my ah **LOH** mah)
- myocardium (my oh **CAR** dee um)
- myoneural (**MY** oh **NOO** rall) junction
- myopathy (my **OPP** ah thee)
- myoplasty (**MY** oh plas tee)
- myorrhaphy (my **OR** ah fee)
- nasal (**NAY** zl) bone
- neck
- nonsteroidal anti-inflammatory drugs
- oblique (oh **BLEEK**) fracture
- occipital (ock **SIP** eh tal) bone
- open fracture
- opposition
- origin
- orthopedics (or thoh **PEE** diks)
- orthopedist (or thoh **PEE** dist)
- orthotics (or **THOT** iks)
- orthotist (or **THOT** ist)
- os coxae (**OSS KOK** sigh)
- osseous (**OSS** ee us) tissue
- ossification (oss sih fih **KAY** shun)
- osteoarthritis (oss tee oh ar **THRY** tis)
- osteoblast (**OSS** tee oh blast)
- osteocarcinoma (oss tee oh kar sin **OH** ma)
- osteochondroma (oss tee oh kon **DROH** mah)
- osteoclasia (oss tee oh **KLAY** see ah)
- osteocytes (**OSS** tee oh sights)
- osteogenic sarcoma (oss tee oh **GIN** ik sark OH mah)
- osteomalacia (oss tee oh mah **LAY** she ah)
- osteomyelitis (oss tee oh my ell **EYE** tis)
- osteopathy (oss tee **OPP** ah thee)
- osteoporosis (oss tee oh por **ROH** sis)
- osteotome (**OSS** tee oh tohm)
- osteotomy (oss tee **OTT** ah mee)
- Paget's (**PAH** jets) disease
- palatine (**PAL** ah tine) bone
- parietal (pah **RYE** eh tal) bone
- patella (pah **TELL** ah)
- patellar
- pathologic (path ah **LOJ** ik) fracture
- pectoral girdle
- pelvic girdle
- periosteum (pair ee **AH** stee um)
- phalangeal
- phalanges (fah **LAN** jeez)
- photon absorptiometry (**FOH** ton ab sorp she **AHM** eh tree)
- plantar flexion (**PLAN** tar **FLEK** shun)
- podiatrist (po **DYE** ah trist)
- polymyositis (pol ee my oh **SIGH** tis)
- process
- pronation (proh **NAY** shun)
- prosthesis (pross **THEE** sis)
- prosthetist (**PROSS** thah tist)
- pseudohypertrophic (soo doh **HIGH** per troh fic) muscular dystrophy
- pubic
- pubic symphysis (**PYOO** bik **SIM** fih sis)
- pubis (**PYOO** bis)
- radial
- radius (**RAY** dee us)
- rectus abdominis (**REK** tus ab **DOM** ih nis)
- red bone marrow
- reduction
- rhabdomyolysis (rab doh my oh **LYE** sis)
- rhabdomyoma (rab doh my **OH** mah)
- rheumatoid arthritis (**ROO** mah toyd ar **THRY** tis)
- rib cage
- rickets (**RIK** ets)
- rotation (roh **TAY** shun)
- sacral
- sacrum (**SAY** crum)
- scapula (**SKAP** yoo lah)
- scapular
- scoliosis (skoh lee **OH** sis)
- short bones
- simple fracture
- sinus (**SIGH** nus)
- skeletal (**SKELL** eh tal) muscle
- smooth muscle
- spasm
- sphenoid (**SFEE** noyd) bone
- spina bifida (**SPY** nah **BIF** ih dah)
- spinal fusion
- spinal stenosis (ste **NOH** sis)

- spiral fracture
- spondylolisthesis (spon dih loh liss **THEE** sis)
- spondylosis (spon dih **LOH** sis)
- spongy bone
- sprain
- sternal
- sternum (**STER** num)
- strain
- supination (soo pin **NAY** shun)
- sutures (**SOO** chers)
- synovial (sin **OH** vee al) fluid
- synovial (sin **OH** vee al) joint
- synovial membrane (sin **OH** vee al **MEM** brayn)
- systemic lupus erythematosus
  (sis **TEM** ik **LOO** pus air ih them ah **TOH** sis)
- talipes (**TAL** ih peez)
- tarsals (**TAHR** sals)
- temporal (**TEM** por al) bone
- tendinitis (ten dih **NIGH** tis)
- tendinous (**TEN** din us)
- tendon (**TEN** dun)
- tendoplasty (**TEN** doh plas tee)
- tendotomy (tend **OT** oh mee)
- tenodynia (ten oh **DIN** ee ah)
- tenomyopathy (ten oh my **OP** oh thee)
- tenorrhaphy (tah **NOR** ah fee)
- thoracic (tho **RASS** ik)
- thoracic vertebrae (tho **RASS** ik **VER** teh bray)
- tibia (**TIB** ee ah)
- tibial
- torticollis (tore tih **KOLL** iss)
- total hip replacement
- total knee replacement
- transverse fracture
- trochanter (tro **KAN** ter)
- tubercle (**TOO** ber kl)
- tuberosity (too ber **OSS** ih tee)
- ulna (**UHL** nah)
- ulnar
- upper extremities
- vertebral (**VER** teh bral) column
- Vitamin D therapy
- vomer (**VOH** mer) bone
- whiplash
- yellow bone marrow
- zygomatic (zeye go **MAT** ik) bone

# Case Study

## Discharge Summary

**Admitting Diagnosis:** Osteoarthritis bilateral knees.

**Final Diagnosis:** Osteoarthritis bilateral knees with prosthetic right knee replacement.

**History of Present Illness:** Patient is a 68-year-old male. He reports he has experienced occasional knee pain and swelling since he injured his knees playing football in high school. These symptoms became worse while he was in his 50s and working on a concrete surface. The right knee has always been more painful than the left. Arthroscopy 12 years ago revealed a torn lateral meniscus and chondromalacia of the patella on the right. He had an arthroscopic meniscectomy with a 50% improvement in symptoms at that time. He returned to his orthopedic surgeon 6 months ago because of constant knee pain and swelling severe enough to interfere with sleep and all activities. He required a cane to walk. CT scan indicated severe bilateral osteoarthritis, with complete loss of the joint space on the right. He was referred to a physiatrist who prescribed Motrin; physical therapy for ROM; strengthening exercises; and a low-fat, low-calorie weight loss diet for moderate obesity that greatly added to the strain on his knees. Over the course of the next 2 months, the left knee improved, but the right knee did not. Due to the failure of conservative treatment, he is admitted to the hospital at this time for prosthetic replacement of the right knee. Patient's other medical history is significant for hypertension and coronary artery disease that is controlled with medication. He has lost weight through diet, which has improved his hypertension, if not his knee pain.

**Summary of Hospital Course:** Patient tolerated the surgical procedure well. He began intensive physical therapy for lower extremity ROM and strengthening exercises and gait training with a walker. He received occupational therapy instruction in ADLs, especially dressing and personal care. He was able to transfer himself out of bed by the 3rd post-op day and was able to ambulate 150 ft with a walker and dress himself on the 5th post-op day. His right knee flexion was 90° and he lacked 5° of full extension.

**Discharge Plans:** Patient was discharged home with his wife 1 week post-op. He will continue rehabilitation as an outpatient. Return to office for post-op checkup in 1 week.

## Critical Thinking Questions

1. What is the specialty of a physiatrist? Describe in your own words what the physiatrist ordered for this patient.

2. What surgical procedure did the patient have 12 years ago? What two pathologies were revealed by that procedure? What surgical procedure was performed to correct his problems at that time?

3. The following medical terms are not defined in your text. Based on your reading of this discharge summary, what do you think each term means in general—not the specifics of this patient.

   a. conservative treatment

   b. outpatient

4. What two types of post-op therapy did this patient receive? Describe the treatment each type of therapy provided for this patient.

5. Describe how much the patient could move his right knee when he was discharged from the hospital.

6. The following medical terms are introduced in a later chapter. Use your text as a dictionary to describe, in your own words, what each term means.

   a. coronary artery disease

   b. hypertension

# Chart Note Transcription

## Chart Note

The chart note below contains 11 phrases that can be reworded with a medical term that you learned in this chapter. Each phrase is identified with an underline. Determine the medical term and write your answers in the space provided.

**Current Complaint:** An 82-year-old female was transported to the Emergency Room via ambulance with severe left hip pain following a fall on the ice.

**Past History:** Patient suffered a <u>wrist broken bone</u>.① 2 years earlier that required <u>immobilization by solid material</u>.② Following this <u>broken bone</u>,③ her <u>physician who specializes in treatment of bone conditions</u>④ diagnosed her with moderate <u>porous bones</u>⑤ on the basis of a <u>computer-assisted X-ray</u>.⑥

**Signs and Symptoms:** Patient reported severe left hip pain, rating it as 8 on a scale of 1 to 10. She held her hip <u>in a bent position</u>⑦ and could not tolerate <u>movement toward a straight position</u>.⑧ X-rays of the left hip and leg were taken.

**Diagnosis:** <u>Shattered broken bone</u>⑨ in the neck of the left <u>thigh bone</u>.⑩

**Treatment:** <u>Implantation of an artificial hip joint</u>⑪ on the left.

1. _____

2. _____

3. _____

4. _____

5. _____

6. _____

7. _____

8. _____

9. _____

10. _____

11. _____

# Practice Exercises

## A. Complete the following statements.

1. The two divisions of the human skeleton are the _____ and _____ .

2. The five regions of the spinal column are the _____ , _____ , _____ , _____ , and _____ .

3. The five functions of the skeletal system are to _____ , _____ , _____ , _____ , and _____ .

4. The anatomical name for the thigh bone is _____ .

5. The anatomical term for the knee cap is _____ .

6. The membrane covering bones is called the _____ .

7. A Colles' fracture occurs in the _____ .

8. There are _____ skeletal muscles.

9. There are _____ bones in the human body.

10. The three types of muscle are _____ , _____ , and _____ .

11. A physician specializing in diseases and injuries of the bones and muscles is a(n) _____ .

12. A specialist in treating disorders of the feet is a(n) _____ .

## B. State the terms described using the combining forms provided.

The combining form *oste/o* refers to bone. Use it to write a term that means

1. bone cell _____

2. embryonic bone cell _____

3. porous bone _____

4. surgical repair of the bone _____

5. incision of the bone _____

6. instrument to cut bone _____

7. inflammation of the bone and bone marrow _____

8. softening of the bones _____

9. tumor composed of both bone and cartilage _____

The combining form *my/o* refers to muscle. Use it to write a term that means

10. muscle disease _____

11. surgical repair of muscle _____

12. suture of muscle _____

The combining form *rhabdomy/o* refers to skeletal muscle. Use it to write a term that means

13. skeletal muscle tumor _____

14. skeletal muscle destruction _____

The combining form *ten/o* refers to tendons. Use it to write a term that means

15. tendon pain _____

16. tendon and muscle disease _____

The combining form *arthr/o* refers to the joints. Use it to write a term that means

17.  surgical fusion of a joint _____

18.  surgical repair of a joint _____

19.  incision into a joint _____

20.  inflammation of a joint _____

21.  inflammation of joint and cartilage _____

22.  pain in the joints _____

The combining form *crani/o* refers to the head or skull. Use it to write a term that means

23.  surgical incision into the skull _____

24.  surgical repair of the skull _____

25.  pertaining to inside the skull _____

## C. Write the suffix for each expression and provide an example of its use.

1.  fuse _____

2.  weakness _____

3.  abnormal softening _____

4.  to surgically break _____

5.  movement _____

6.  porous _____

## D. Give the adjective form for the following bones.

1.  femur _____

2.  sternum _____

3.  clavicle _____

4.  coccyx _____

5.  maxilla _____

6.  tibia _____

7.  patella _____

8.  phalanges _____

9.  humerus _____

10.  pubis _____

## E. Define the following word roots/combining forms.

1.  lamin/o _____

2.  ankyl/o _____

3.  chondr/o _____

4.  spondyl/o _____

5.  my/o _____

6.  orth/o _____

7.  kyph/o _____

8.  tend/o _____

9. myel/o _____

10. articul/o _____

## F. Define the following terms.

1. chondroplasty _____

2. bradykinesia _____

3. osteoporosis _____

4. lordosis _____

5. atrophy _____

6. myeloma _____

7. phalanges _____

8. coccyx _____

9. arthrocentesis _____

10. bursolith _____

## G. Name the five regions of the spinal column and indicate the number of bones in each area.

| Name | Number of Bones |
|------|-----------------|
| 1. _____ | _____ |
| 2. _____ | _____ |
| 3. _____ | _____ |
| 4. _____ | _____ |
| 5. _____ | _____ |

## H. Circle the prefix and suffix and place a *P* for prefix or an *S* for suffix over these word parts. In the space provided, define the term.

1. arthroscopy _____

2. intervertebral _____

3. chondromalacia _____

4. diskectomy _____

5. myorrhaphy _____

6. subscapular _____

## I. Match the terms in column A with the definitions in column B.

|  | A | B |
|---|---|---|
| 1. | _____ abduction | a. backward bending of the foot |
| 2. | _____ rotation | b. bending the foot to point toes toward the ground |
| 3. | _____ plantar flexion | c. straightening motion |
| 4. | _____ extension | d. motion around a central axis |
| 5. | _____ dorsiflexion | e. motion away from the body |
| 6. | _____ flexion | f. moving the thumb away from the palm |
| 7. | _____ adduction | g. motion toward the body |
| 8. | _____ opposition | h. bending motion |

**J. Match types of fractures in column A with the definitions in column B.**

|  | A |  | B |
|---|---|---|---|
| 1. | _____ comminuted | a. | fracture line is at an angle |
| 2. | _____ greenstick | b. | fracture line curves around the bone |
| 3. | _____ compound | c. | bone is splintered or crushed |
| 4. | _____ simple | d. | bone is pressed into itself |
| 5. | _____ impacted | e. | fracture line is straight across bone |
| 6. | _____ transverse | f. | skin has been broken |
| 7. | _____ oblique | g. | no open wound |
| 8. | _____ spiral | h. | bone only partially broken |

**K. Define the following medical specialties and specialists.**

1. orthopedics _____

2. chiropractic _____

3. podiatrist _____

4. orthotics _____

5. prosthetics _____

**L. Identify the following abbreviations.**

1. DJD _____

2. EMG _____

3. C1 _____

4. T6 _____

5. IM _____

6. ROM _____

7. JRA _____

8. LLE _____

9. ortho _____

10. CTS _____

**M. Write the abbreviations for the following terms.**

1. congenital dislocation of hip _____

2. total knee replacement _____

3. herniated nucleus pulposus _____

4. deep tendon reflex _____

5. upper extremity _____

6. fifth lumbar vertebra _____

7. bone density testing _____

8. above the knee _____

9. fracture _____

10. nonsteroidal anti-inflammatory drug _____

**N. Use the following terms in the sentences that follow.**

| | | |
|---|---|---|
| talipes | myasthenia gravis | laminectomy |
| osteogenic sarcoma | lateral epicondylitis | scoliosis |
| osteoporosis | rickets | pseudotrophic muscular dystrophy |
| whiplash | ganglion cyst | systemic lupus erythematosus |

1. Mrs. Lewis, age 84, is being treated for a broken hip. Her physician will be running tests for what potential ailment? _____

2. Jamie, age 6 months, is being given orange juice and vitamin supplements to avoid what condition? _____

3. George began to have severe elbow pain after playing tennis several days in a row. He most probably has what condition? _____

4. Marshall was involved in a rear-end collision. He is complaining of severe headaches and neck stiffness. What condition may he have suffered? _____

5. Mr. Jefferson's physician has discovered a tumor at the end of his femur. He has been admitted to the hospital for a biopsy to rule out what type of bone cancer? _____

6. The school nurse has asked Janelle to bend over so that she may examine her back to see if she is developing a lateral curve. What is the nurse looking for? _____

7. Gerald has experienced a gradual loss of muscle strength over the past 5 years even though his muscles look large and healthy. The doctors believe he has an inherited muscle disease. What is that disease? _____

8. Roberta has suddenly developed arthritis in her hands and knees, an aversion to the sun, and a butterfly rash across her nose and cheeks. What is one of the diseases that her physician will wish to rule out? _____

# Professional Journal

In this exercise you will now have an opportunity to put the words you have learned into practice. Imagine yourself in the role of a chiropractor. If you refer back to the Professional Profile at the beginning of this chapter, you will see that this health care professional is responsible for treating disorders involving the skeleton and muscles. Use the 10 words listed below, or any other new terms from this chapter, to write sentences to describe the patients you saw today.

An example of a sentence is *Mrs. Jones'* **whiplash** *was much improved after her treatment.*

1. flexion _____

2. arthritis _____

3. calcium supplements _____

4. femur _____

5. lumbar vertebrae _____

6. deep tendon reflex _____

7. fibromyalgia _____

8. ball-and-socket joint _____

9. atrophy _____

10. kypohsis _____

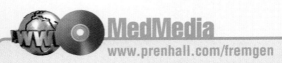

## MedMedia
www.prenhall.com/fremgen

Use the CD-ROM enclosed with your textbook to gain additional reinforcement through interactive word building exercises, spelling games, labeling activities, and additional quizzes.

Use the above address to access the free, interactive Companion Website created for this textbook. Get hints, instant feedback, and textbook references to chapter-related multiple-choice questions, as well as labeling and matching exercises. In addition, you will find an audio glossary, case studies, and Internet exploration exercises.

***For more information regarding orthopedics and musculoskeletal diseases visit the following websites:***

National Institute of Arthritis and Musculoskeletal and Skin Diseases at **www.niams.nih.gov**

Karolinska Institute of Stockholm, Sweden University Library Disease and Disorder Links at **www.mic.ki.se/diseases/c05.html**

American Academy of Orthopedic Surgeons "Your Orthopedic Connection" page at **www.orthoinfo.aaos.org**

DynoMed patient information at **www.dynomed.com/encyclopedia/encyclopedia/cfm**

# Chapter 5
# Cardiovascular System

## Learning Objectives

*Upon completion of this chapter,*
*you will be able to:*

- Recognize the combining forms, prefixes, and suffixes introduced in this chapter.

- Gain the ability to pronounce medical terms and major anatomical structures.

- List the major organs of the cardiovascular system and their functions.

- Describe the flow of blood through the heart and the body.

- Explain how the electrical conduction system controls the heartbeat.

- Build cardiovascular system medical terms from word parts.

- Define vocabulary, pathology, diagnostic, and therapeutic medical terms relating to the cardiovascular system.

- Recognize types of medication associated with the cardiovascular system.

- Interpret abbreviations associated with the cardiovascular system.

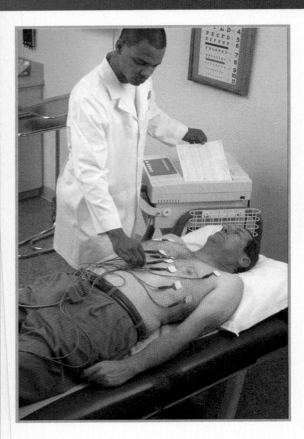

## MedMedia
www.prenhall.com/fremgen
Additional interactive resources and activities for this chapter can be found on the Companion Website. For animations, audio glossary, and review, access the accompanying CD-ROM in this book.

## Professional Profile

### Cardiovascular Professionals

Cardiology technologists, electrocardiogram technicians, and cardiac sonographers are all involved in the diagnosis and treatment of heart and blood vessel disease. The results of the tests and procedures they conduct are vitally important for the diagnosis and treatment of cardiovascular disease. These health care professionals are found wherever procedures to study the functioning of the cardiovascular system are performed. This includes hospitals, physicians' offices, cardiac rehabilitation programs, and diagnostic centers.

### Cardiology Technologist

- Assists with invasive heart procedures
- Includes cardiac catheterizations and angioplasty procedures
- Must complete an accredited 2-to 4-year program

### Electrocardiogram Technician

- Conducts tests to record the electrical activity of the heart
- Includes electrocardiography (EKGs), Holter monitoring, and stress testing
- May complete a 1-year certification program or receive on-the-job training

### Cardiac Sonographer

- Uses ultrasound to produce a moving image of the heart for diagnostic purposes
- Graduates from a 1-year certification, 2-year associate's degree, or 4-year baccalaureate program

*For more information regarding these health careers, visit the following websites:*
Alliance of Cardiovascular Professionals at **www.acp-online.org**
American Society of Echocardiography at **www.asecho.org**

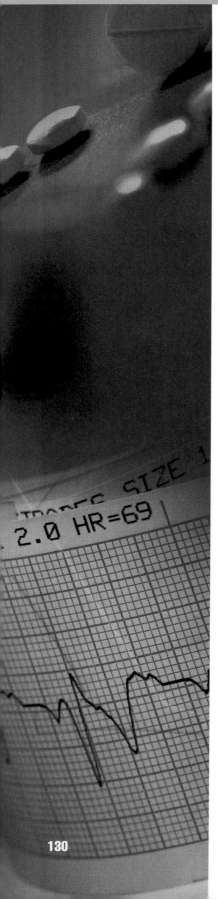

## Overview

### Organs of the Cardiovascular System

blood vessels
   arteries
   capillaries
   veins
heart

### Combining Forms Relating to the Cardiovascular System

| angi/o | vessel | ox/o | oxygen |
|--------|--------|------|--------|
| aort/o | aorta | pericardi/o | pericardium |
| arteri/o | artery | phleb/o | vein |
| ather/o | fatty substance | sphygm/o | pulse |
| atri/o | atrium | steth/o | chest |
| cardi/o | heart | thromb/o | clot |
| coron/o | heart | valv/o | valve |
| cyan/o | blue | valvul/o | valve |
| hemangi/o | blood vessel | ven/o | vein |
| ox/i | oxygen | ventricul/o | ventricle |

### Prefixes Relating to the Cardiovascular System

| Prefix | Meaning | Example |
|--------|---------|---------|
| brady- | slow | bradycardia |
| tachy- | fast | tachycardia |

### Suffixes Relating to the Cardiovascular System

| Suffix | Meaning | Example |
|--------|---------|---------|
| -manometer | instrument to measure pressure | sphygmomanometer |
| -ole | small | arteriole |
| -sclerosis | hardening | arteriosclerosis |
| -stenosis | narrowing | angiostenosis |
| -tension | pressure | hypotension |
| -ule | small | venule |

## Anatomy and Physiology of the Cardiovascular System

| | | |
|--------|--------|--------|
| amino acids | circulatory system | oxygen |
| arteries | deoxygenated | oxygenated |
| blood vessels | glucose | pulmonary circulation |
| capillaries | heart | systemic circulation |
| carbon dioxide | metabolism | veins |

The cardiovascular (CV) system is also called the **circulatory system.** This system, which maintains the distribution of blood throughout the body, is composed of the **heart** and the **blood vessels—arteries, capillaries,** and **veins.**

The circulatory system is composed of two parts: the **pulmonary circulation** (**PULL** mon air ee ser kew **LAY** shun) and the **systemic circulation** (sis **TEM** ik ser kew **LAY** shun). The pulmonary circulation, between the heart and lungs, transports **deoxygenated** (dee **OK** sih jen ay ted) blood to the lungs to get oxygen, and then back to the heart. The systemic circulation carries **oxygenated** (**OK** sih jen ay ted) blood away from the heart to the tissues and cells, and then back to the heart. In this way all the body cells receive blood and oxygen (see ■ Figure 5.1).

In addition to distributing **oxygen** and other nutrients, such as **glucose** (**GLOO** kohs) and **amino acids,** the cardiovascular system collects the waste products from the cells. **Carbon dioxide** and other waste products from **metabolism** (meh **TAB** oh lizm) are transported by the cardiovascular system to the lungs and kidneys, where they are eliminated from the body.

## Heart

**apex**                         **cardiac muscle**

The heart is actually a muscular pump made up of **cardiac** (**CAR** dee ak) **muscle** fibers that could be called a muscle rather than an organ. It has four chambers or cavities and beats an average of 60 to 100 beats per minute (bpm) or about 100,000 times in one day. Each time the cardiac muscle contracts, blood is ejected from the heart and pushed throughout the body within the blood vessels.

The heart is located in the mediastinum in the center of the chest cavity. However, it is not exactly centered; more of the heart is on the left side of the mediastinum than the right. It is about the size of a fist and is shaped like an upside-down pear (see ■ Figure 5.2). The tip of the heart at the lower edge is called the **apex** (**AY** peks). The sternum is located directly in front of the heart.

> **MED TERM TIP** Locating the tip of the sternum, called the *xiphoid process,* is important when administering cardiopulmonary resuscitation (CPR). Chest compressions must be made over the center of the sternum and not over the xiphoid process.

### Heart Layers

**endocardium**          **myocardium**          **pericardium**
**epicardium**            **parietal pericardium**  **visceral pericardium**

The wall of the heart is quite thick and composed of three layers (see ■ Figure 5.3):

1. The **endocardium** (en doh **CAR** dee um) is the inner layer of the heart that lines the heart chambers. It is a very smooth, thin layer that serves to reduce friction as the blood passes through the heart chambers.

2. The **myocardium** (my oh **CAR** dee um) is the thick muscular middle layer of the heart. Contraction of this muscle layer develops the pressure required to pump blood through the blood vessels.

3. The **epicardium** (ep ih **CAR** dee um) is the outer layer of the heart. The heart is enclosed within the double-layered pleural sac, the **pericardium** (pair ih **CAR** dee um). The epicardium is the **visceral pericardium** (**VISS** er al pair ih **CAR** dee um), or inner layer of the sac. The outer layer of the sac is the **parietal pericardium** (pah **RYE** eh tal pair ih **CAR** dee um). Fluid between the two layers of the sac reduces friction as the heart beats.

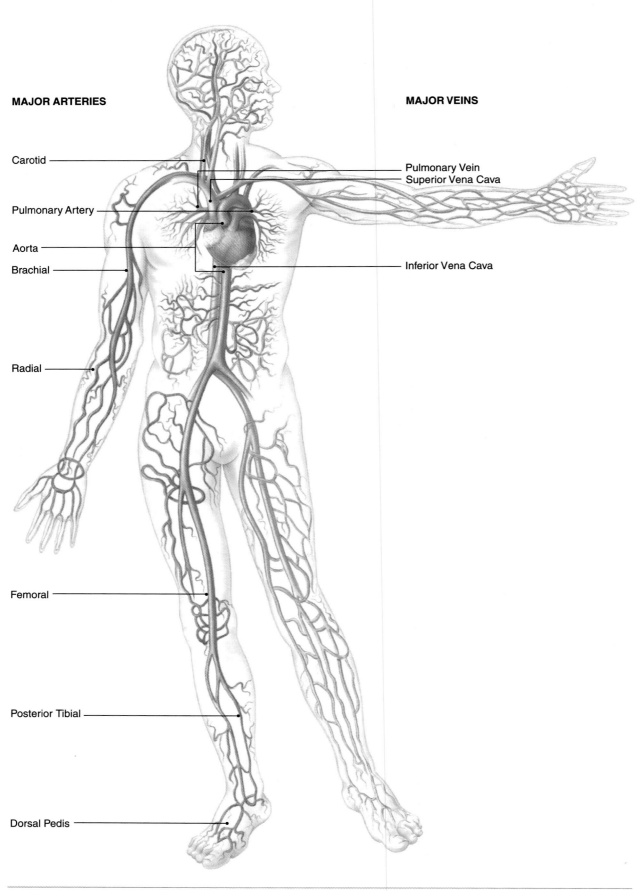

**MAJOR ARTERIES**

Carotid

Pulmonary Artery

Aorta

Brachial

Radial

Femoral

Posterior Tibial

Dorsal Pedis

**MAJOR VEINS**

Pulmonary Vein
Superior Vena Cava

Inferior Vena Cava

**■ FIGURE 5.1** The circulatory system.

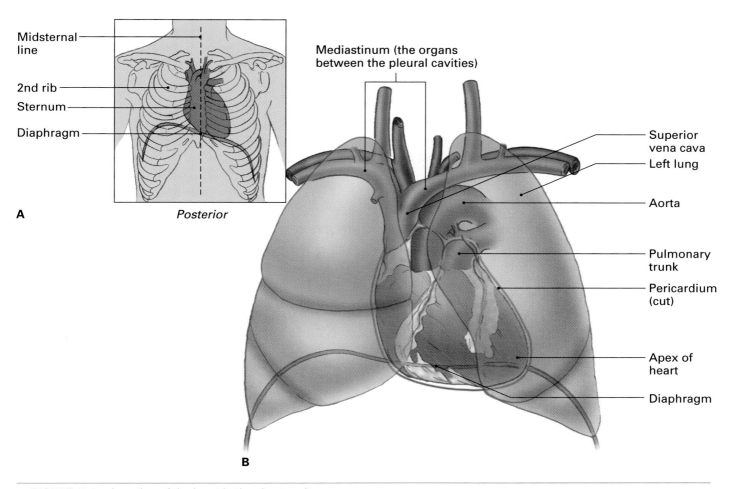

Midsternal line

2nd rib

Sternum

Diaphragm

**A**

*Posterior*

Mediastinum (the organs between the pleural cavities)

Superior vena cava

Left lung

Aorta

Pulmonary trunk

Pericardium (cut)

Apex of heart

Diaphragm

**B**

▓ **FIGURE 5.2**   Location of the heart in the chest cavity.

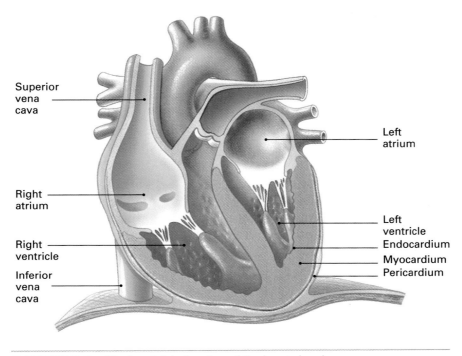

Superior vena cava

Right atrium

Right ventricle

Inferior vena cava

Left atrium

Left ventricle

Endocardium

Myocardium

Pericardium

▓ **FIGURE 5.3**   The heart: interior view of the heart chambers.

## Heart Chambers

| | |
|---|---|
| **atria** | **interventricular septum** |
| **interatrial septum** | **ventricles** |

The heart is divided into four chambers or cavities (see Figure 5.3). There are two **atria** (**AY** tree ah), or upper chambers, and two **ventricles** (**VEN** trik lz), or lower chambers. These are divided into right and left sides by walls called the **interatrial septum** (in ter **AY** tree al **SEP** tum) and the **interventricular septum** (in ter ven **TRIK** yoo lar **SEP** tum). The atria are the receiving chambers of the heart. Blood returning to the heart via veins first collects in the atria. The ventricles are the pumping chambers. They have a much thicker myocardium and its contraction ejects blood out of the heart and into the great arteries.

## Heart Valves

| | | |
|---|---|---|
| **aortic valve** | **cusps** | **semilunar valve** |
| **atrioventricular valve** | **mitral valve** | **tricuspid valve** |
| **bicuspid valve** | **pulmonary valve** | |

Four valves act as restraining gates to control the direction of blood flow. They are situated at the entrances and exits to the ventricles (see ▦ Figures 5.4 and 5.5). Properly functioning valves allow blood to flow only in the forward direction by blocking it from returning to the previous chamber.

The valves are as follows:

1. **Tricuspid** (try **CUSS** pid) **valve**: This is an **atrioventricular** (ay tree oh ven **TRIK** yoo lar) **valve** (AV), meaning that it controls the opening between the right atrium and the right ventricle. Once the blood enters the right ventricle it cannot back up into the atrium again. The prefix *tri-*, meaning three, indicates that this valve has three leaflets or **cusps.**

2. **Pulmonary** (**PULL** mon air ee) **valve**: This is a **semilunar** (sem ih **LOO** nar) **valve**. The prefix *semi-*, meaning half, and the term *lunar*, meaning moon, indicate that this valve looks like a half moon. Located between the right ventricle and the pulmonary artery, this important valve allows blood to flow from the right ventricle into the pulmonary artery.

3. **Mitral** (**MY** tral) **valve**: This is also called the **bicuspid** (bye **CUSS** pid) **valve**, indicating that it has two cusps. Blood flows through this atrioventricular valve to the left ventricle and cannot back up into the left atrium.

4. **Aortic** (ay **OR** tik) **valve**: Blood leaves the left ventricle through this semilunar valve between the left ventricle and into the aorta.

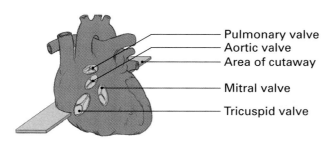

- Pulmonary valve
- Aortic valve
- Area of cutaway
- Mitral valve
- Tricuspid valve

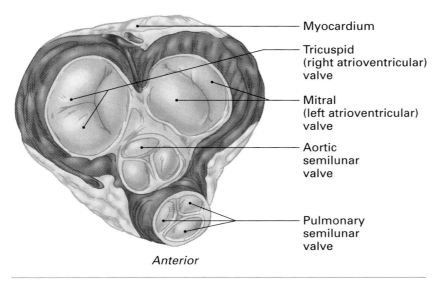

- Myocardium
- Tricuspid (right atrioventricular) valve
- Mitral (left atrioventricular) valve
- Aortic semilunar valve
- Pulmonary semilunar valve

*Anterior*

**FIGURE 5.4**   The valves of the heart.

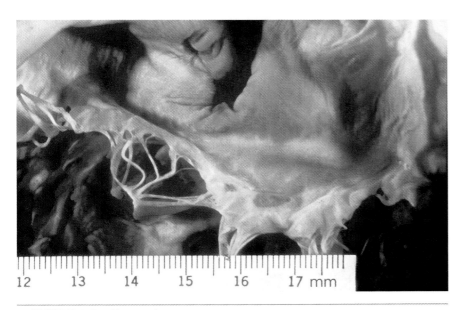

**FIGURE 5.5**   Heart valves.
(Charles Stewart and Associates)

**MED TERM TIP**

The heart makes two distinct sounds referred to as "lub-dupp." These sounds are produced by the forceful snapping shut of the heart valves. *Lub* is the closing of the atrioventricular valves. *Dupp* is the closing of the semilunar valves. Listening to these sounds with a stethoscope is part of determining if the valves are functioning properly.

## Blood Flow Through the Heart

**aorta**                    **pulmonary artery**          **superior vena cava**

**diastole**                 **pulmonary veins**           **systole**

**inferior vena cava**

The flow of blood through the heart is quite orderly (see ■ Figure 5.6). It progresses through the heart to the lungs, where it receives oxygen; back to the heart; and then out to the body tissues and parts. The normal blood flow is as follows:

1. Deoxygenated blood from all the tissues in the body, except lung tissue, enters a relaxed right atrium via two large veins called the **superior vena cava** (soo **PEE** ree or **VEE** nah **KAY** vah) and **inferior vena cava**. (in **FEE** ree or **VEE** nah **KAY** vah).

2. The right atrium contracts and blood flows through the tricuspid valve into the relaxed right ventricle.

3. The right ventricle then contracts and blood is pumped through the pulmonary valve into the **pulmonary** (**PULL** mon air ee) **artery,** which carries it to the lungs.

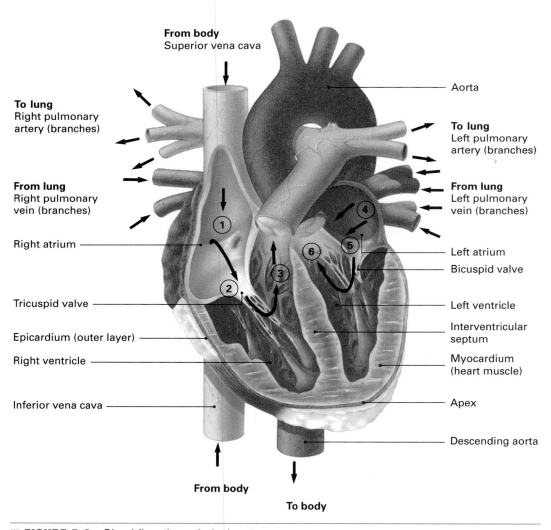

■ **FIGURE 5.6**   Blood flow through the heart.

4. The left atrium receives blood that has been oxygenated by the lungs. This blood enters the relaxed left atrium from the four **pulmonary** (**PULL** mon air ee) **veins**.

5. The left atrium contracts and blood flows through the mitral valve into the relaxed left ventricle.

6. When the left ventricle contracts, the blood is pumped through the aortic valve and into the **aorta** (ay **OR** tah), the largest artery in the body. The aorta carries blood to all parts of the body except the lungs.

It can be seen that the heart chambers alternate between relaxing in order to fill and contracting to push blood forward. The period of time a chamber is relaxed is **diastole** (dye **ASS** toe lee). The contraction phase is **systole** (**SIS** toe lee).

## Conduction System of the Heart

| | | |
|---|---|---|
| **atrioventricular node** | **bundle of His** | **Purkinje fibers** |
| **autonomic nervous system** | **pacemaker** | **sinoatrial node** |
| **bundle branches** | | |

The **autonomic nervous system** (aw toh NOM ik NER vus SIS tem) regulates heart rate; therefore we have no voluntary control over the beating of our heart. Special tissue within the heart is responsible for conducting an electrical impulse that stimulates the different chambers to contract in the correct order.
The path that the impulses travel is as follows (see ■ Figure 5.7):

1. The **sinoatrial** (sigh noh **AY** tree al) (SA) **node,** or **pacemaker,** is where the electrical impulse begins. From the sinoatrial node a wave of electricity travels through the atria, causing them to contract, or go into systole.

2. Next, the **atrioventricular** (ay tree oh ven **TRIK** yoo lar) **node** is stimulated.

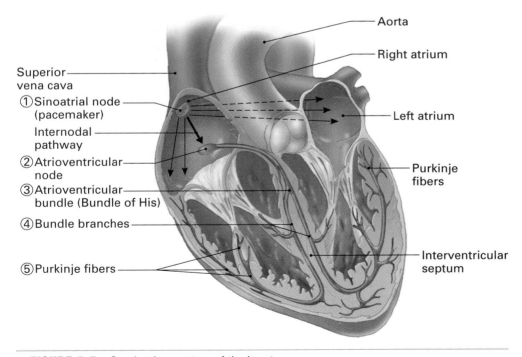

**■ FIGURE 5.7** Conduction system of the heart.

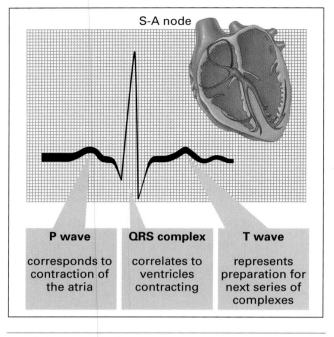

|  P wave | QRS complex | T wave |
| --- | --- | --- |
| corresponds to contraction of the atria | correlates to ventricles contracting | represents preparation for next series of complexes |

**FIGURE 5.8** EKG tracing.

3. This node transfers the stimulation wave to the **bundle of His.**

4. The electrical signal next travels down the **bundle branches** within the interventricular septum.

5. Finally, the **Purkinje** (per KIN gee) **fibers** out in the ventricular myocardium are stimulated, which results in ventricular systole.

> **MED TERM TIP**
>
> The electrocardiogram, which is referred to as an EKG or ECG, is a measurement of the electrical activity of the heart (see ▪ Figure 5.8). This can give the physician information about the health of the heart, especially the myocardium.

## Blood Vessels

| | |
| --- | --- |
| **arterioles** | **coronary arteries** |
| **capillary bed** | **venules** |

There are three types of blood vessels: arteries, capillaries, and veins. The arteries are the large, thick-walled vessels that carry the blood away from the heart (see ▪ Figure 5.9). The pulmonary artery carries deoxygenated blood, or blood without oxygen, from the right ventricle to the lungs. The largest artery, the aorta, begins from the left ventricle of the heart and carries oxygenated blood, or blood with oxygen, to all the body systems. The **coronary arteries** (**KOR** ah nair ee **AR** te reez) then branch from the aorta and provide blood to the myocardium (see ▪ Figure 5.10). As they travel through the body the arteries branch into progressively smaller arteries. The smallest arteries are called **arterioles** (ar **TEE** ree ohlz). Arterioles deliver blood to the capillaries.

Capillaries are a network of tiny blood vessels referred to as a **capillary bed.** Arterial blood flows into a capillary bed and venous blood flows back out. Capillaries are very thin walled, allowing for the diffusion of the oxygen from the

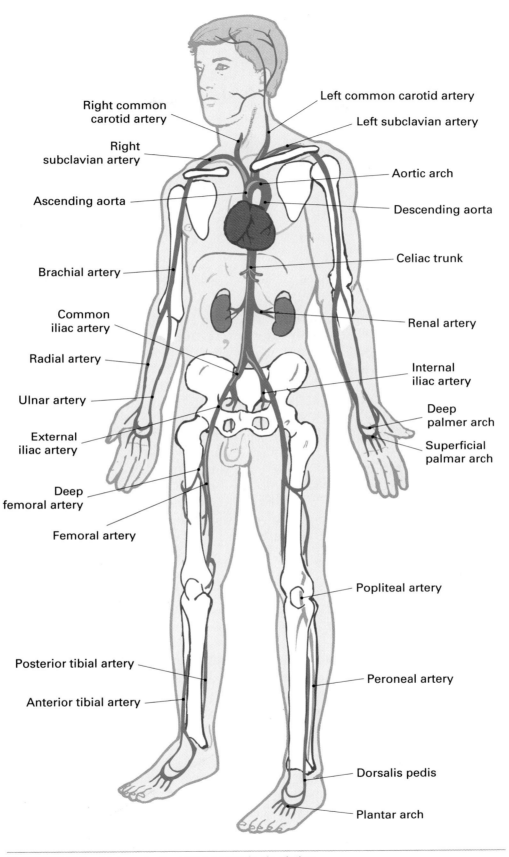

**FIGURE 5.9** Major arteries of the systemic circulation.

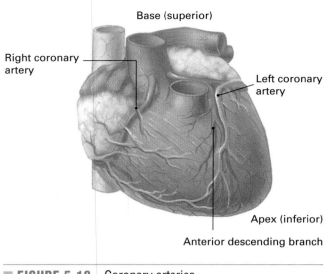

Base (superior)

Right coronary
artery

Left coronary
artery

Apex (inferior)

Anterior descending branch

**FIGURE 5.10** Coronary arteries.

blood and into the body tissues. Likewise, waste products are able to diffuse out of the body tissues and into the bloodstream to be carried away. Since the capillaries are so small in diameter, the blood will not flow as quickly through them as it does through the arteries and veins. This means that the blood has time for an exchange of nutrients, oxygen, and waste material to take place. As blood exits a capillary bed, it returns to the heart in a vein.

The veins carry blood back to the heart (see ▦ Figure 5.11). Blood leaving capillaries first enters small **venules** (**VEN** yools), which then merge into larger veins. Veins have much thinner walls than arteries, causing them to collapse easily. The veins also have valves that allow the blood to move only toward the heart. These valves prevent blood from backing away from the heart. The two large veins that enter the heart are the superior vena cava, which carries blood from the upper body, and the inferior vena cava, which carries blood from the lower body. Blood pressure in the veins is much lower than it is in the arteries. Muscular action against the veins and skeletal muscle contractions help in the movement of blood.

See ▦ Figure 5.12 for an illustration of blood circulation through the cardiovascular system.

## Blood Pressure

| | |
|---|---|
| **blood pressure (BP)** | **sphygmomanometer** |
| **diastolic pressure** | **systolic pressure** |

**Blood pressure** (BP) is a measurement of the force exerted by blood against the wall of a blood vessel. During ventricular systole, blood is under a lot of pressure from the ventricular contraction, giving the highest blood pressure reading—the **systolic** (sis **TOL** ik) **pressure**. During ventricular diastole, blood is not being pushed by the heart at all and the blood pressure reading drops to its lowest point—the **diastolic** (dye ah **STOL** ik) **pressure.** Therefore, to see the full range of what is occurring with blood pressure, both numbers are required. Blood pressure is also affected by several other characteristics of the blood and the blood vessels. These include the elasticity of the arteries, the diameter of the blood vessels, the viscosity of the blood, the volume of blood flowing through the vessels, and the amount of resistance there is to blood flow.

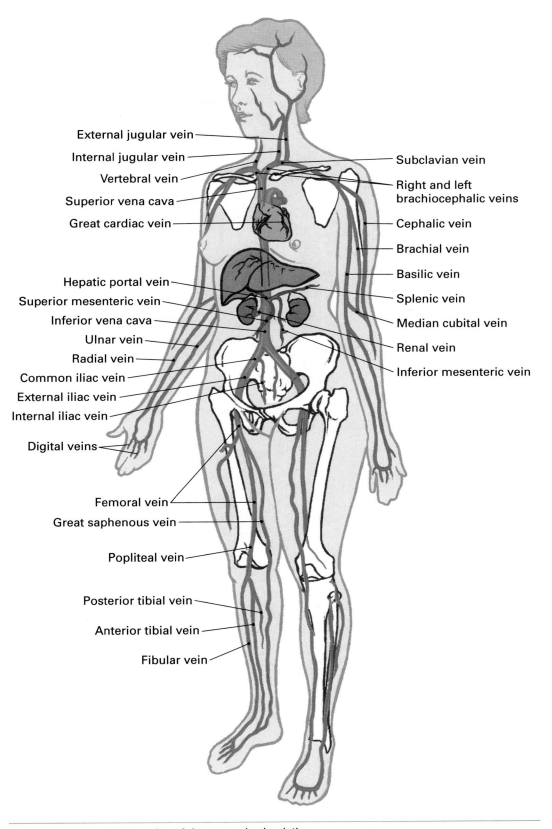

External jugular vein

Internal jugular vein

Vertebral vein

Superior vena cava

Great cardiac vein

Subclavian vein

Right and left brachiocephalic veins

Cephalic vein

Brachial vein

Basilic vein

Hepatic portal vein

Superior mesenteric vein

Inferior vena cava

Ulnar vein

Radial vein

Common iliac vein

External iliac vein

Internal iliac vein

Digital veins

Splenic vein

Median cubital vein

Renal vein

Inferior mesenteric vein

Femoral vein

Great saphenous vein

Popliteal vein

Posterior tibial vein

Anterior tibial vein

Fibular vein

**FIGURE 5.11**   Major veins of the systemic circulation.

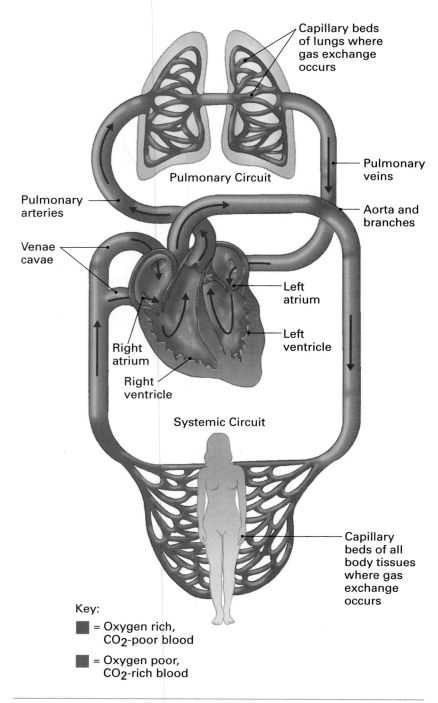

Key:

■ = Oxygen rich, CO$_2$-poor blood

■ = Oxygen poor, CO$_2$-rich blood

■ **FIGURE 5.12** Systemic and pulmonary circulation.

**MED TERM TIP** The instrument used to measure blood pressure is called a **sphygmomanometer** (sfig moh mah **NOM** eh ter). The combining form *sphygm/o* means pulse and the suffix *-manometer* means instrument to measure pressure. A blood pressure reading is reported as two numbers, for example, 120/80. The 120 is the systolic pressure and the 80 is the diastolic pressure (see ■ Figure 5.13). There is not one "normal" blood pressure number. The normal range for blood pressure in an adult is 90/60 to 140/90.

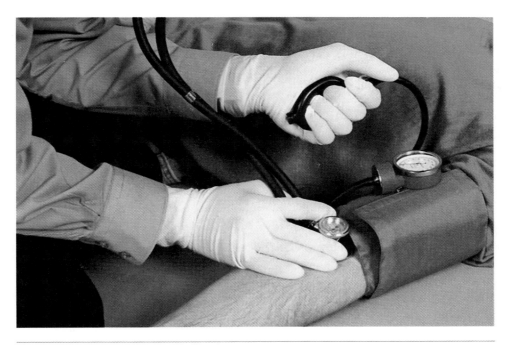

■ **FIGURE 5.13**   Using a sphygmomanometer to measure blood pressure.

## Word Building Relating to the Cardiovascular System

The following list contains examples of medical terms built directly from word parts. The definition for these terms can be determined by a straightforward translation of the word parts.

| Combining Form | Combined With | Medical Term | Definition |
|---|---|---|---|
| angi/o | -graphy | angiography (an jee **OG** rah fee) | making a record of a vessel |
| | -rrhaphy | angiorrhaphy (an jee **OR** rah fee) | suturing a vessel |
| | -spasm | angiospasm (**AN** jee oh spazm) | involuntary muscle contraction of a vessel |
| | -stenosis | angiostenosis (an jee oh sten **OH** sis) | narrowing of a vessel |
| aort/o | -gram | aortogram (ay **OR** toh gram) | record of the aorta |
| | -ic | aortic (ay **OR** tik) | pertaining to the aorta |
| arteri/o | -al | arterial (ar **TEE** ree al) | pertaining to the artery |
| | -ole | arteriole (ar **TEE** ree ohl) | small artery |
| | -rrhexis | arteriorrhexis (ar tee ree oh **REK** sis) | ruptured artery |
| | -sclerosis | arteriosclerosis (ar tee ree oh skleh **ROH** sis) | hardening of an artery |
| ather/o | -ectomy | atherectomy (ath er **EK** toh mee) | excision of fatty substance |
| | -sclerosis | atherosclerosis (ath er oh skleh **ROH** sis) | hardening with fatty substance |
| atri/o | -al | atrial (**AY** tree al) | pertaining to the atrium |
| | inter- -al | interatrial (in ter **AY** tree al) | pertaining to between the atria |

*continued...*

| Combining Form | Combined With | Medical Term | Definition |
|---|---|---|---|
| cardi/o | -ac | cardiac (**CAR** dee ak) | pertaining to the heart |
| | brady- -ia | bradycardia (brad ee **CAR** dee ah) | state of slow heart |
| | -dynia | cardiodynia (car dee oh **DIN** ee ah) | heart pain |
| | electr/o -gram | electrocardiogram (ee lek tro **CAR** dee oh gram) | record of heart electricity |
| | -megaly | cardiomegaly (car dee oh **MEG** ah lee) | enlarged heart |
| | my/o -al | myocardial (my oh **CAR** dee al) | pertaining to heart muscle |
| | my/o -pathy | cardiomyopathy (car dee oh my **OP** ah thee) | heart muscle disease |
| | -ologist | cardiologist (car dee **ALL** oh jist) | specialist in the cardiovascular system |
| | -rrhaphy | cardiorrhaphy (car dee **OR** ah fee) | suture the heart |
| | tachy- -ia | tachycardia (tak ee **CAR** dee ah) | state of fast heart |
| coron/o | -ary | coronary (**KOR** ah nair ee) | pertaining to the heart |
| phleb/o | -itis | phlebitis (fleh **BYE** tis) | inflammation of a vein |
| | -otomy | phlebotomy (fleh **BOT** oh me) | incision in a vein |
| | -rrhaphy | phleborrhaphy (fleh **BOR** ah fee) | suture a vein |
| valvul/o | -itis | valvulitis (val view **LYE** tis) | inflammation of a valve |
| | -ar | valvular (**VAL** view lar) | pertaining to a valve |
| ven/o | -ous | venous (**VEE** nus) | pertaining to a vein |
| | -ule | venule (**VEN** yool) | small vein |
| | -otomy | venotomy (vee **NOT** oh mee) | incision into a vein |
| ventricul/o | -ar | ventricular (ven **TRIK** yoo lar) | pertaining to a ventricle |
| | inter- -ar | interventricular (in ter ven **TRIK** yoo lar) | pertaining to between the ventricles |

# Vocabulary Relating to the Cardiovascular System

| | |
|---|---|
| **auscultation (oss kul TAY shun)** | Process of listening to the sounds within the body by using a stethoscope (see ▦ Figure 5.14). |
| **bruit (brew EE)** | Term used interchangeably with the word *murmur*. A gentle, blowing sound that is heard during auscultation. |
| **cardiology (car dee ALL oh jee)** | The branch of medicine relating to the cardiovascular system. |
| **cyanosis (sigh ah NOH sis)** | Slightly bluish color of the skin due to a deficiency of oxygen and an excess of carbon dioxide in the blood. It is caused by a variety of disorders, ranging from chronic lung disease to congenital and chronic heart problems. |
| **infarct (IN farkt)** | Area of tissue within an organ or part that undergoes necrosis (death) following the loss of its blood supply. |

| | |
|---|---|
| **ischemia (is KEYH mee ah)** | Localized and temporary deficiency of blood supply due to an obstruction to the circulation. |
| **lumen (LOO men)** | The space, cavity, or channel within a tube or tubular organ or structure in the body. |
| **murmur (MUR mur)** | An abnormal heart sound such as a soft blowing sound or harsh click. It may be soft and heard only with a stethoscope, or so loud it can be heard several feet away. Also referred to as a *bruit*. |
| **palpitations (pal pih TAY shunz)** | Pounding, racing heartbeat. |
| **pulse** | Expansion and contraction of a blood vessel wall produced by blood as it moves through an artery. The pulse can be taken at several pulse points throughout the body where an artery is close to the surface. |
| **sphygmomanometer (sfig moh mah NOM eh ter)** | Instrument for measuring blood pressure. Also referred to as a *blood pressure cuff*. |
| **stent** | A stainless steel tube placed within a blood vessel or a duct to widen the lumen (see ▧ Figure 5.15). |
| **stethoscope (STETH oh scope)** | Instrument for listening to body sounds (auscultation), such as the chest, heart, or intestines (see also Figure 5.14). |

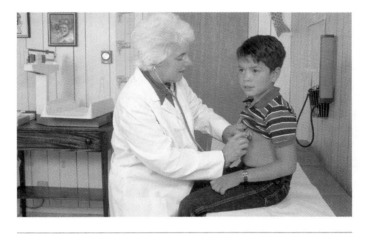

▧ **FIGURE 5.14** Auscultation.

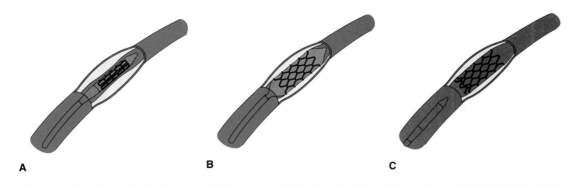

**A**        **B**        **C**

▧ **FIGURE 5.15** Placement of a stent. (A) The stainless steel stent is fitted over a balloon-tipped catheter. (B) The stent is positioned along the blockage and expanded. (C) The balloon is deflated and removed, leaving the stent in place.

# Pathology of the Cardiovascular System

| | |
|---|---|
| **aneurysm (AN yoo rizm)** | Weakness in the wall of an artery that results in localized widening of the artery. Although an aneurysm may develop in any artery, common sites include the aorta in the abdomen and the cerebral arteries in the brain (see ▇ Figure 5.16). |
| **angina pectoris (an JYE nah PECK tor is)** | Condition in which there is severe pain with a sensation of constriction around the heart. Caused by a deficiency of oxygen to the heart muscle. |
| **angiocarditis (an je oh kar DYE tis)** | Inflammation of blood vessels and the heart. |
| **angioma (an jee OH ma)** | Tumor, usually benign, consisting of a network of blood vessels. |
| **angiospasm (AN jee oh spazm)** | Spasm or contraction of smooth muscle in the walls of a blood vessel. |
| **aortic stenosis (ay OR tik steh NOH sis)** | Narrowing of the aorta. |
| **arrhythmia (ah RITH mee ah)** | Irregularity in the heartbeat or action. Comes in many different forms; some are not serious, while others are life threatening. |
| **arteriosclerosis (ar tee ree oh skleh ROH sis)** | Thickening, hardening, and loss of elasticity of the walls of the arteries. Most often due to atherosclerosis. |
| **arteriosclerotic (ar tee ree oh skleh ROT ik) heart disease (ASHD)** | Chronic heart disorder caused by a hardening of the walls of the coronary arteries. May lead to coronary artery disease, angina pectoris, and myocardial infarction. |
| **atherosclerosis (ath er oh skleh ROH sis)** | The most common form of arteriosclerosis. Caused by the formation of yellowish plaques of cholesterol on the inner walls of arteries. |
| **cardiac arrest** | Complete stopping of heart activity. |
| **cardiomyopathy (car dee oh my OP ah thee)** | General term for a disease of the myocardium. Can be caused by alcohol abuse, parasites, viral infection, and congestive heart failure. One of the most common reasons a patient may require a heart transplant. |
| **coarctation (koh ark TAY shun) of the aorta** | Severe congenital narrowing of the aorta. |
| **congenital septal defect (CSD)** | A hole, present at birth, in the septum between two heart chambers; results in a mixture of oxygenated and deoxygenated blood. There can be an atrial septal defect (ASD) and a ventricular septal defect (VSD). |
| **congestive (kon JESS tiv) heart failure (CHF)** | Pathological condition of the heart in which there is a reduced outflow of blood from the left side of the heart because the left ventricle myocardium has become too weak to efficiently pump blood. Results in weakness, breathlessness, and edema. |
| **coronary artery disease (KOR ah nair ee AR ter ee dis EEZ) (CAD)** | Insufficient blood supply to the heart muscle due to an obstruction of one or more coronary arteries. May be caused by atherosclerosis and may cause angina pectoris and myocardial infarction (see ▇ Figure 5.17). |
| **embolus (EM boh lus)** | The obstruction of a blood vessel by a blood clot that has broken off from a thrombus somewhere else in the body and traveled to the point of obstruction. If it occurs in a coronary artery, it may result in a myocardial infarction (see ▇ Figure 5.18). |
| **endocarditis (en doh car DYE tis)** | Inflammation of the lining membranes of the heart. May be due to bacteria or to an abnormal immunological response. In bacterial endocarditis, the mass of bacteria that forms is referred to as *vegetation*. |
| **fibrillation (fih brill AY shun)** | An extremely serious arrhythmia characterized by an abnormal quivering or contractions of heart fibers. When this occurs in the ventricles, cardiac arrest and death can occur. Emergency equipment to defibrillate, or convert the heart to a normal beat, is necessary. |
| **flutter** | An arrhythmia in which the atria beat too rapidly, but in a regular pattern. |

| | |
|---|---|
| **heart block** | Occurs when the electrical impulse is blocked from traveling down the bundle of His or bundle branches. Results in the ventricles beating at a different rate than the atria. Also called a *bundle branch block (BBB)*. |
| **heart valve prolapse (PROH laps)** | The cusps or flaps of the heart valve are too loose and fail to shut tightly, allowing blood to flow backward through the valve when the heart chamber contracts. Most commonly occurs in the mitral valve, but may affect any of the heart valves. |
| **heart valve stenosis (steh NOH sis)** | The cusps or flaps of the heart valve are too stiff. Therefore, they are unable to open fully, making it difficult for blood to flow through, or shut tightly, allowing blood to flow backward. This condition may affect any of the heart valves. |
| **hemangioma (he man gee OH ma)** | A benign mass of blood vessels. Often causing a visible dark red lesion present from birth. Also called a *birthmark*. |
| **hemorrhoid (HIM oh royd)** | Varicose veins in the anal region. |
| **hypertension (high per TEN shun) (HTN)** | Blood pressure above the normal range. |
| **hypertensive (high per TEN siv) heart disease** | Heart disease as a result of persistently high blood pressure, which damages the blood vessels and ultimately the heart. |
| **hypotension (high poh TEN shun)** | Decrease in blood pressure. Can occur in shock, infection, cancer, anemia, or as death approaches. |
| **myocardial infarction (my oh CAR dee al in FARC shun) (MI)** | Condition caused by the partial or complete occlusion or closing of one or more of the coronary arteries (see ■ Figure 5.19). Symptoms include a squeezing pain or heavy pressure in the middle of the chest (angina pectoris). A delay in treatment could result in death. Also referred to as a *heart attack*. |
| **myocarditis (my oh car DYE tis)** | Inflammation of the muscle layer of the heart wall. |
| **patent ductus arteriosus (PAY tent DUCK tus ar tee ree OH sis) (PDA)** | Congenital heart anomaly in which the fetal connection between the pulmonary artery and the aorta fails to close at birth. This condition requires surgery. |
| **pericarditis (pair ih car DYE tis)** | Inflammation of the pericardial sac around the heart. |
| **peripheral vascular disease (PVD)** | Any abnormal condition affecting blood vessels outside the heart. Symptoms may include pain, pallor, numbness, and loss of circulation and pulses. |
| **polyarteritis (pol ee ar ter EYE tis)** | Inflammation of several arteries. |
| **Raynaud's (ray NOZ) phenomenon** | Periodic ischemic attacks affecting the extremities of the body, especially the fingers, toes, ears, and nose. The affected extremities become cyanotic and very painful. These attacks are brought on by arterial constriction due to extreme cold or emotional stress. Named after a French physician, Maurice Raynaud. |
| **rheumatic (roo MAT ik) heart disease** | Valvular heart disease as a result of having had rheumatic fever. |
| **tetralogy of Fallot (teh TRALL oh jee of fal LOH)** | Combination of four congenital anomalies: pulmonary stenosis, an interventricular septal defect, improper placement of the aorta, and hypertrophy of the right ventricle. Needs immediate surgery to correct. Named for Etienne-Louis Fallot, a French physician. |
| **thrombophlebitis (throm boh fleh BYE tis)** | Inflammation of a vein that results in the formation of blood clots within the vein. |
| **thrombus (THROM bus)** | A blood clot forming within a blood vessel (see ■ Figure 5.20). May partially or completely occlude the blood vessel. |
| **varicose (VAIR ih kohs) veins** | Swollen and distended veins, usually in the legs. |

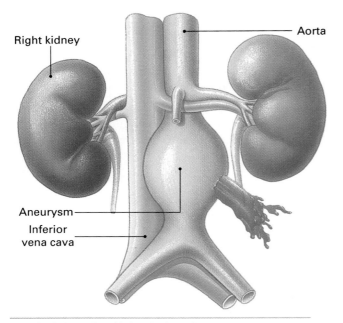

**FIGURE 5.16** Abdominal aortic aneurysm.

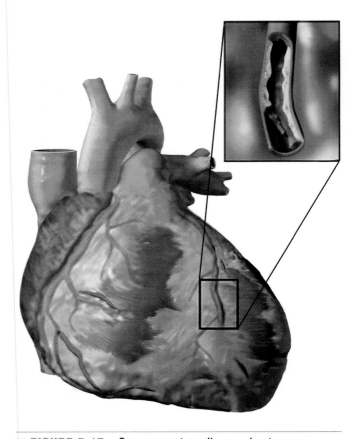

**FIGURE 5.17** Coronary artery disease due to atherosclerosis.

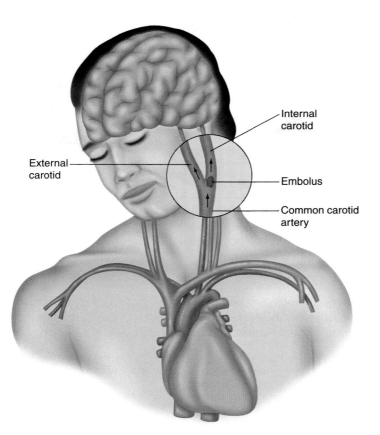

**FIGURE 5.18** Embolus.

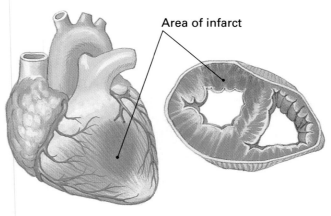

**FIGURE 5.19** Cross section of myocardial infarction.

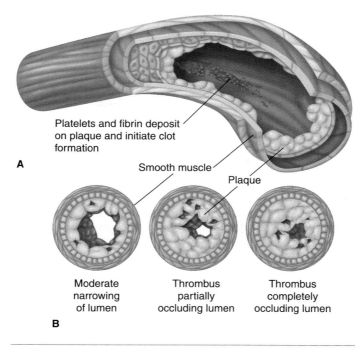

Platelets and fibrin deposit on plaque and initiate clot formation

**A**

Smooth muscle

Plaque

Moderate narrowing of lumen

Thrombus partially occluding lumen

Thrombus completely occluding lumen

**B**

■ **FIGURE 5.20** Thrombus formation in an atherosclerotic vessel. Depicted are (A) the initial clot formation and (B) the varying degrees of occlusion.

# Diagnostic Procedures Relating to the Cardiovascular System

| | |
|---|---|
| **angiography**<br>**(an jee OG rah fee)** | X-rays taken after the injection of an opaque material into a blood vessel. Can be performed on the aorta as an aortic angiogram, on the heart as an angiocardiogram, and on the brain as a cerebral angiogram. |
| **cardiac catheterization**<br>**(CAR dee ak**<br>**cath eh ter ih ZAY shun)** | Passage of a thin tube (catheter) through a blood vessel leading to the heart. Done to detect abnormalities, to collect cardiac blood samples, and to determine the blood pressure within the heart. |
| **cardiac enzymes**<br>**(CAR dee ak EN zyms)** | Blood test to determine the level of enzymes specific to heart muscles in the blood. An increase in the enzymes may indicate heart muscle damage such as a myocardial infarction. These enzymes include creatine phosphokinase (CPK), lactate dehydrogenase (LDH), and glutamic oxaloacetic transaminase (GOT). |
| **cardiac scan** | Patient is given radioactive thallium intravenously and then scanning equipment is used to visualize the heart. It is especially useful in determining myocardial damage. |
| **coronary angiography**<br>**(an jee OG rah fee)** | Radiographic X-ray of the heart and large vessels after the injection of a radiopaque solution. X-rays are taken in rapid sequence as the material moves through the heart. |
| **Doppler ultrasonography**<br>**(DOP ler ul trah son OG rah fee)** | Measurement of sound-wave echoes as they bounce off tissues and organs to produce an image. Can assist in determining heart and blood vessel damage. Named for Christian Doppler, an Austrian physicist. |
| **echocardiography**<br>**(ek oh car dee OG rah fee)** | Noninvasive diagnostic method using ultrasound to visualize internal cardiac structures. Cardiac valve activity can be evaluated using this method. |
| **electrocardiography**<br>**(ee lek troh car dee OG rah fee)**<br>**(ECG, EKG)** | Record of the electrical activity of the heart. Useful in the diagnosis of abnormal cardiac rhythm and heart muscle (myocardium) damage. |

*continued...*

| | |
|---|---|
| **Holter monitor** | Portable ECG monitor worn by a patient for a period of a few hours to a few days to assess the heart and pulse activity as the person goes through the activities of daily living. Used to assess a patient who experiences chest pain and unusual heart activity during exercise and normal activities. Named for Norman Holter, an American biophysicist. |
| **serum lipoprotein (SEE rum lip oh PROH teen) level** | Blood test to measure the amount of cholesterol and triglycerides in the blood. An indicator of atherosclerosis risk. |
| **stress testing** | Method for evaluating cardiovascular fitness. The patient is placed on a treadmill or a bicycle and then subjected to steadily increasing levels of work. An EKG and oxygen levels are taken while the patient exercises. The test is stopped if abnormalities occur on the EKG. Also called an *exercise test* or a *treadmill* test. |
| **venography (vee NOG rah fee)** | X-ray of the veins by tracing the venous pulse. Also called *phlebography*. |

# Therapeutic Procedures Relating to the Cardiovascular System

| | |
|---|---|
| **aneurysmectomy (an yoo riz MEK toh mee)** | Surgical removal of the sac of an aneurysm. |
| **angioplasty (AN jee oh plas tee)** | Surgical procedure of altering the structure of a vessel by dilating it using a balloon inside the vessel (see ▪ Figure 5.21). |
| **arterial anastomosis (ar tee REE all ah nas toe MOE sis)** | Surgical joining together of two arteries. Performed if an artery is severed or if a damaged section of an artery is removed. |
| **cardiopulmonary resuscitation (car dee oh PULL mon air ee ree suss ih TAY shun) (CPR)** | Procedure to restore cardiac output and oxygenated air to the lungs for a person in cardiac arrest. A combination of chest compressions (to push blood out of the heart) and artificial respiration (to blow air into the lungs) performed by one or two CPR-trained rescuers. |
| **commissurotomy (com ih shur OT oh mee)** | Surgical incision to change the size of an opening. For example, in mitral commissurotomy, a stenosis or narrowing is treated by cutting away at the adhesions around the mitral opening (orifice). |
| **coronary (KOR ah nair ee) artery bypass graft (CABG)** | Open-heart surgery in which a blood vessel from another location in the body (often a leg vein) is grafted to route blood around a blocked coronary artery. |
| **defibrillation (dee fib rih LAY shun)** | A procedure that converts serious irregular heartbeats, such as fibrillation, by giving electric shocks to the heart using an instrument called a defibrillator. Also called *cardioversion* (see ▪ Figure 5.22). |
| **embolectomy (em boh LEK toh mee)** | Removal of an embolus or clot from a blood vessel. |
| **endarterectomy (end ar teh REK toh mee)** | Excision of the diseased or damaged inner lining of an artery. Usually performed to remove atherosclerotic plaques. |
| **extracorporeal (EX tra core poor EE al) circulation (ECC)** | During open-heart surgery, the routing of blood to a heart-lung machine so it can be oxygenated and pumped to the rest of the body. |
| **heart transplantation** | Replacement of a diseased or malfunctioning heart with a donor's heart. |

| | |
|---|---|
| **intracoronary artery (in trah KOR ah nair ee AR ter ee) stent** | Placing a stent within a coronary artery to treat coronary ischemia due to atherosclerosis. |
| **ligation (lye GAY shun) and stripping** | Surgical treatment for varicose veins. The damaged vein is tied off (ligation) and removed (stripping). |
| **open-heart surgery** | Surgery that involves incision of the heart, coronary arteries, or heart valves. |
| **pacemaker implantation** | Electrical device that substitutes for the natural pacemaker of the heart (see ■ Figure 5.23A). It controls the beating of the heart by a series of rhythmic electrical impulses. An external pacemaker has the electrodes on the outside of the body. An internal pacemaker has the electrodes surgically implanted within the chest wall (see ■ Figure 5.23B). |
| **percutaneous transluminal coronary angioplasty (per kyoo TAY nee us trans LOO mih nal KOR ah nair ee AN jee oh plas tee) (PTCA)** | Method for treating localized coronary artery narrowing. A balloon catheter is in serted through the skin into the coronary artery and inflated to dilate the narrow blood vessel. |
| **pericardiocentesis (pair ih CAR dee oh sin tee sis)** | Insertion of a needle into the pericardial sac for the purpose of aspirating excess fluid around the heart. |
| **phlebotomy (fleh BOT oh mee)** | Creating an opening into a vein (inserting a needle) to withdraw blood. |
| **thrombectomy (throm BEK toh mee)** | Surgical removal of a thrombus or blood clot from a blood vessel. |
| **thrombolytic therapy (throm boh LIT ik THAIR ah pee)** | Drugs, such as streptokinase (SK) or tissue-type plasminogen activator (tPA), are injected into a blood vessel to dissolve clots and restore blood flow. |
| **valve replacement** | Excision of a diseased heart valve and replacement with an artificial valve. |
| **venipuncture (VEEN ih punk cher)** | Puncture into a vein to withdraw fluids or insert medication and fluids. |

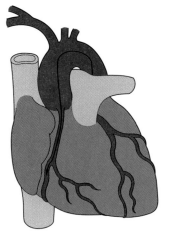 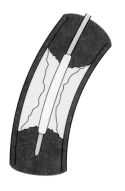 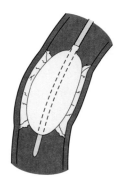 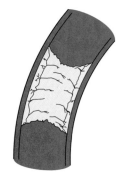

**A**  1.  2.  3.  4.

■ **FIGURE 5.21** (A) Balloon angioplasty: 1. The balloon catheter is threaded into the affected coronary artery. 2. The balloon is positioned across the area of obstruction. 3. The balloon is then inflated, flattening the plaque against the arterial wall. 4. Plaque remains flattened after balloon catheter is removed.

*(continued)*

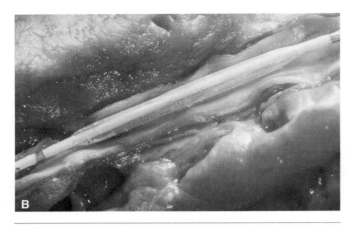

**■ FIGURE 5.21 (continued)** (B) Balloon catheter.
(Southern Illinois University/Photo Researchers, Inc.)

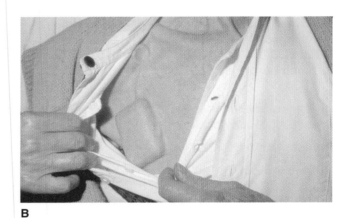

**■ FIGURE 5.22** Defibrillator (cardioverter).

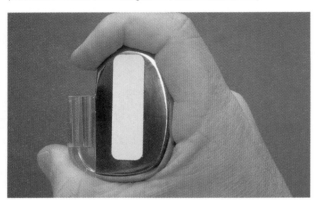

A

B

**■ FIGURE 5.23** (A) Heart pacemaker. (Science Photo Library/Photo Researchers, Inc.) (B) Pacemaker implanted into a patient's chest.
(Yoav Levy/Phototake NYC)

# Pharmacology Relating to the Cardiovascular System

| | |
|---|---|
| **antiarrhythmic** (an tye a RHYTH mik) | Reduces or prevents cardiac arrhythmias. |
| **anticoagulant** (an tye koh AG you lant) | Prevent blood clot formation. |
| **antihypertensive** (an tye hye per TEN sive) | Lowers blood pressure. |
| **antilipidemic** (an tye lip ih DEM ik) | Reduces amount of cholesterol and lipids in the bloodstream. Treats hyperlipidemia. |
| **cardiotonic (card ee oh TAHN ik)** | Increases the force of cardiac muscle contraction. Treats congestive heart failure. |
| **diuretic (dye you RET ik)** | Increases urine production by the kidneys, which works to reduce plasma and therefore blood volume. This results in lower blood pressure. |
| **thrombolytic (throm boh LIT ik)** | Dissolves existing blood clots. |
| **vasoconstrictor** (vaz oh kon STRICK tor) | Contracts smooth muscle in walls of blood vessels. Raises blood pressure. |
| **vasodilator** (vaz oh DYE late or) | Relaxes the smooth muscle in the walls of arteries, thereby increasing diameter of the blood vessel. Used for two main purposes: increasing circulation to an ischemic area and reducing blood pressure. |

# Abbreviations Relating to the Cardiovascular System

| | | | | |
|---|---|---|---|---|
| **AF** | atrial fibrillation | | **ICU** | intensive care unit |
| **AMI** | acute myocardial infarction | | **IV** | intravenous |
| **AS** | aortic stenosis, arteriosclerosis | | **JVP** | jugular venous pulse |
| **ASCVD** | arteriosclerotic cardiovascular disease | | **LDH** | lactate dehydrogenase |
| **ASD** | atrial septal defect | | **LDL** | low-density lipoproteins |
| **ASHD** | arteriosclerotic heart disease | | **LVAD** | left ventricular assist device |
| **AV, A-V** | atrioventricular | | **LVH** | left ventricular hypertrophy |
| **BBB** | bundle branch block (L for left; R for right) | | **MI** | myocardial infarction, mitral insufficiency |
| **BP** | blood pressure | | **mm Hg** | millimeters of mercury |
| **bpm** | beats per minute | | **MR** | mitral regurgitation |
| **CABG** | coronary artery bypass graft | | **MS** | mitral stenosis |
| **CAD** | coronary artery disease | | **MVP** | mitral valve prolapse |
| **cath** | catheterization | | **NSR** | normal sinus rhythm |
| **CC** | cardiac catheterization, chief complaint | | **P** | pulse |
| **CCU** | coronary care unit | | **PAC** | premature atrial contraction |
| **CHF** | congestive heart failure | | **PDA** | patent ductus arteriosus |
| **CoA** | coarctation of the aorta | | **PTCA** | percutaneous transluminal coronary angioplasty |
| **CP** | chest pain | | | |
| **CPK** | creatine phosphokinase | | **PVC** | premature ventricular contraction |
| **CPR** | cardiopulmonary resuscitation | | **S1** | first heart sound |
| **CSD** | congenital septal defect | | **S2** | second heart sound |
| **CV** | cardiovascular | | **SA, S-A** | sinoatrial |
| **DVT** | deep vein thrombosis | | **SGOT** | serum glutamic oxaloacetic transaminase |
| **ECC** | extracorporeal circulation | | **SK** | streptokinase |
| **ECG, EKG** | electrocardiogram | | **tPA** | tissue-type plasminogen activator |
| **ECHO** | echocardiogram | | **Vfib** | ventricular fibrillation |
| **GOT** | glutamic oxaloacetic transaminase | | **VLDL** | very low density lipoproteins |
| **HDL** | high-density lipoproteins | | **VSD** | ventricular septal defect |
| **HTN** | hypertension | | **VT** | ventricular tachycardia |

# Chapter Review

## Pronunciation Practice

*You will find the pronunciation for each term on the enclosed CD-ROM. Check each one off as you master it.*

- ❑ amino acids
- ❑ aneurysm (**AN** yoo rizm)
- ❑ aneurysmectomy (an yoo riz **MEK** toh mee)
- ❑ angina pectoris (an **JYE** nah **PECK** tor is)
- ❑ angiocarditis (an jee oh kar **DYE** tis)
- ❑ angiography (an jee **OG** rah fee)
- ❑ angioma (an jee **OH** mah)
- ❑ angioplasty (**AN** jee oh plas tee)
- ❑ angiorrhaphy (an jee **OR** rah fee)
- ❑ angiospasm (**AN** jee oh spazm)
- ❑ angiostenosis (an jee oh sten **OH** sis)
- ❑ antiarrhythmic (an tye a **RHYTH** mik)
- ❑ anticoagulant (an tye koh **AG** you lant)
- ❑ antihypertensive (an tye hye per **TEN** sive)
- ❑ antilipidemic (an tye lip ih **DEM** ik)
- ❑ aorta (ay **OR** tah)
- ❑ aortic (ay **OR** tik)
- ❑ aortic stenosis (ay **OR** tik steh **NOH** sis)
- ❑ aortic (ay **OR** tik) valve
- ❑ aortogram (ay **OR** toh gram)
- ❑ apex (**AY** peks)
- ❑ arrhythmia (ah **RITH** mee ah)
- ❑ arterial (ar **TEE** ree al)
- ❑ arterial anastomosis (ar **TEE** ree all ah nas toe **MOE** sis)
- ❑ arteries (**AR** teh reez)
- ❑ arteriole (ar **TEE** ree ohl)
- ❑ arteriorrhexis (ar tee ree oh **REK** sis)
- ❑ arteriosclerosis (ar tee ree oh skleh **ROH** sis)
- ❑ arteriosclerotic (ar tee ree oh skleh **ROT** ik) heart disease
- ❑ atherectomy (ath er **EK** toh mee)
- ❑ atherosclerosis (ath er oh skleh **ROH** sis)
- ❑ atria (**AY** tree ah)
- ❑ atrial (**AY** tree al)
- ❑ atrioventricular (ay tree oh ven **TRIK** yoo lar) node

- ❑ atrioventricular (ay tree oh ven **TRIK** yoo lar) valve
- ❑ auscultation (oss kul **TAY** shun)
- ❑ autonomic nervous system (aw toh **NOM** ik **NER** vus **SIS** tem)
- ❑ bicuspid (bye **CUSS** pid) valve
- ❑ blood pressure
- ❑ blood vessels
- ❑ bradycardia (brad ee **CAR** dee ah)
- ❑ bruit (brew **EE**)
- ❑ bundle branches
- ❑ bundle of His (**HISS**)
- ❑ capillaries (**CAP** ih lair eez)
- ❑ capillary bed
- ❑ carbon dioxide
- ❑ cardiac (**CAR** dee ak)
- ❑ cardiac (**CAR** dee ak) arrest
- ❑ cardiac catheterization (**CAR** dee ak cath eh ter ih **ZAY** shun)
- ❑ cardiac enzymes (**CAR** dee ak **EN** zyms)
- ❑ cardiac (**CAR** dee ak) muscle
- ❑ cardiac (**CAR** dee ak) scan
- ❑ cardiodynia (car dee oh **DIN** ee ah)
- ❑ cardiologist (car dee **ALL** oh jist)
- ❑ cardiology (car dee **ALL** oh jee)
- ❑ cardiomegaly (car dee oh **MEG** ah lee)
- ❑ cardiomyopathy (car dee oh my **OP** ah thee)
- ❑ cardiopulmonary resuscitation (car dee oh **PULL** mon air ee ree suss ih **TAY** shun)
- ❑ cardiorrhaphy (car dee **OR** ah fee)
- ❑ cardiotonic (car dee oh **TAHN** ik)
- ❑ circulatory system
- ❑ coarctation (koh ark **TAY** shun) of the aorta
- ❑ commissurotomy (com ih shur **OT** oh me)
- ❑ congenital septal defect
- ❑ congestive (kon **Jess** tiv) heart failure
- ❑ coronary (**KOR** ah nair ee)

- ❏ coronary angiography (**KOR** ah nair ee an jee **OG** rah fee)
- ❏ coronary arteries (**KOR** ah nair ee **AR** te reez)
- ❏ coronary artery (**KOR** ah nair ee **AR** ter ee) bypass graft
- ❏ coronary artery disease (**KOR** ah nair ee **AR** ter ee dis **EEZ**)
- ❏ cusps
- ❏ cyanosis (sigh ah **NOH** sis)
- ❏ defibrillation (dee fib rih **LAY** shun)
- ❏ deoxygenated (dee **OK** sih jen ay ted)
- ❏ diastole (dye **ASS** toe lee)
- ❏ diastolic (dye ah **STOL** ik) pressure
- ❏ diuretic (dye you **RET** ik)
- ❏ Doppler ultrasonography (**DOP** ler ul trah son **OG** rah fee)
- ❏ echocardiography (ek oh car dee **OG** rah fee)
- ❏ electrocardiogram (ee lek troh **CAR** dee oh gram)
- ❏ electrocardiography (ee lek troh car dee **OG** rah fee)
- ❏ embolectomy (em boh **LEK** toh mee)
- ❏ embolus (**EM** boh lus)
- ❏ endarterectomy (end ar teh **REK** toh mee)
- ❏ endocarditis (en doh car **DYE** tis)
- ❏ endocardium (en doh **CAR** dee um)
- ❏ epicardium (ep ih **CAR** dee um)
- ❏ extracorporeal (**EX** tra core poor **EE** al) circulation
- ❏ fibrillation (fih brill **AY** shun)
- ❏ flutter
- ❏ glucose (**GLOO** kohs)
- ❏ heart
- ❏ heart block
- ❏ heart transplantation
- ❏ heart valve prolapse (**PROH** laps)
- ❏ heart valve stenosis (steh **NOH** sis)
- ❏ hemangioma (he man gee **OH** ma)
- ❏ hemorrhoid (**HIM** oh royd)
- ❏ Holter monitor
- ❏ hypertension (high per **TEN** shun)
- ❏ hypertensive (high per **TEN** siv) heart disease
- ❏ hypotension (high poh **TEN** shun)
- ❏ infarct (**IN** farkt)
- ❏ inferior vena cava (in **FEE** ree or **VEE** nah **KAY** vah)
- ❏ interatrial (in ter **AY** tree al)
- ❏ interatrial septum (in ter **AY** tree al **SEP** tum)
- ❏ interventricular (in ter ven **TRIK** yoo lar)
- ❏ interventricular septum (in ter ven **TRIK** yoo lar **SEP** tum)
- ❏ intracoronary artery (in trah **KOR** ah nair ee **AR** ter ee) stent
- ❏ ischemia (is **KEYH** mee ah)
- ❏ ligation (lye **GAY** shun) and stripping
- ❏ lumen (**LOO** men)
- ❏ metabolism (meh **TAB** oh lizm)
- ❏ mitral (**MY** tral) valve
- ❏ murmur (**MUR** mur)
- ❏ myocardial (my oh **CAR** dee al)
- ❏ myocardial infarction (my oh **CAR** dee al in **FARC** shun)
- ❏ myocarditis (my oh car **DYE** tis)
- ❏ myocardium (my oh **CAR** dee um)
- ❏ open-heart surgery
- ❏ oxygen (**OK** sih jen)
- ❏ oxygenated (**OK** sih jen ay ted)
- ❏ pacemaker
- ❏ pacemaker implantation
- ❏ palpitations (pal pih **TAY** shunz)
- ❏ parietal pericardium (pah **RYE** eh tal pair ih **CAR** dee um)
- ❏ patent ductus arteriosus (**PAY** tent **DUCK** tus ar tee ree **OH** sis)
- ❏ percutaneous transluminal coronary angioplasty (per kyoo **TAY** nee us trans **LOO** mih nal **KOR** ah nair ree **AN** jee oh plas tee)
- ❏ pericardiocentesis (pair ih **CAR** dee oh sin tee sis)
- ❏ pericarditis (pair ih car **DYE** tis)
- ❏ pericardium (pair ih **CAR** dee um)
- ❏ peripheral vascular disease
- ❏ phlebitis (fleh **BYE** tis)
- ❏ phleborrhaphy (fleh **BOR** ah fee)
- ❏ phlebotomy (fleh **BOT** oh mee)
- ❏ polyarteritis (pol ee ar ter **EYE** tis)
- ❏ pulmonary (**PULL** mon air ee) artery
- ❏ pulmonary circulation (**PULL** mon air ee ser kew **LAY** shun)
- ❏ pulmonary (**PULL** mon air ee) valve
- ❏ pulmonary (**PULL** mon air ee) veins
- ❏ pulse
- ❏ Purkinje (per **KIN** gee) fibers
- ❏ Raynaud's (ray **NOZ**) phenomenon

- ❑ rheumatic (roo **MAT** ik) heart disease
- ❑ semilunar (sem ih **LOO** nar) valve
- ❑ serum lipoprotein (**SEE** rum lip oh **PROH** teen) level
- ❑ sinoatrial (sigh noh **AY** tree al) node
- ❑ sphygmomanometer (sfig moh mah **NOM** eh ter)
- ❑ stent
- ❑ stethoscope (**STETH** oh scope)
- ❑ stress testing
- ❑ superior vena cava (soo **PEE** ree or **VEE** nah **KAY** vah)
- ❑ systemic circulation (sis **TEM** ik ser kew **LAY** shun)
- ❑ systole (**SIS** toe lee)
- ❑ systolic (sis **TOL** ik) pressure
- ❑ tachycardia (tak ee **CAR** dee ah)
- ❑ tetralogy of Fallot (teh **TRALL** oh jee of fal **LOH**)
- ❑ thrombectomy (throm **BEK** toh mee)
- ❑ thrombolytic (throm boh **LIT** ik)
- ❑ thrombolytic therapy (throm boh **LIT** ik **THAIR** ah pee)
- ❑ thrombophlebitis (throm boh fleh **BYE** tis)
- ❑ thrombus (**THROM** bus)
- ❑ tricuspid (try **CUSS** pid) valve
- ❑ valve replacement
- ❑ valvular (**VAL** view lar)
- ❑ valvulitis (val view **LYE** tis)
- ❑ varicose (**VAIR** ih kohs) veins
- ❑ vasoconstrictor (vaz oh kon **STRICK** tor)
- ❑ vasodilator (vaz oh **DYE** late or)
- ❑ veins (**VAYNS**)
- ❑ venipuncture (**VEEN** ih punk cher)
- ❑ venography (vee **NOG** rah fee)
- ❑ venotomy (vee **NOT** oh mee)
- ❑ venous (**VEE** nus)
- ❑ ventricles (**VEN** trik lz)
- ❑ ventricular (ven **TRIK** yoo lar)
- ❑ venules (**VEN** yools)
- ❑ visceral pericardium (**VISS** er al pair ih **CAR** dee um)

# Case Study

**Admitting Diagnosis:** Difficulty breathing, hypertension, tachycardia

**Final Diagnosis:** CHF secondary to mitral valve prolapse

**History of Present Illness:** Patient was brought to the Emergency Room by her family because of SOB, tachycardia (a racing heart rate), and anxiety. Patient reports that she has experienced these symptoms for the past 6 months, brought on by exertion. The current episode began while she was cleaning house and is more severe than any previous episode. Upon admission in the ER, HR was 120 beats per minute and blood pressure was 180/110. The patient was cyanotic around the lips and nail beds and had severe edema in feet and lower legs. The results of an EKG and cardiac enzyme blood tests were normal. Medication improved the symptoms but she was admitted for observation and a complete cardiac workup for tachycardia, hypertension.

**Summary of Hospital Course:** Patient underwent a full battery of cardiac diagnostic tests. A prolapsed mitral valve was observed on an echocardiogram. A treadmill test had to be stopped early due to onset of severe difficulty in breathing and cyanosis of the lips. Arterial blood gases showed low oxygen, and supplemental oxygen per nasal canula was required to resolve cyanosis. Angiocardiography failed to demonstrate significant coronary artery thrombosis. Blood pressure, tachycardia, anxiety, and pitting edema were controlled with medications. Patient took Lopressor to control blood pressure, Norpace to slow heart rate, Valium for the anxiety, and Lasix to reduce edema. At discharge, HR was 88 beats per minute, blood pressure was 165/98, and there was no evidence of edema unless she was on her feet too long.

**Discharge Plans:** There was no evidence of a myocardial infarction and with lack of significant coronary thrombosis, angioplasty is not indicated for this patient. Patient was placed on a low-salt and low-cholesterol diet. She received instructions on beginning a carefully graded exercise program. She is to continue Lasix, Norpace, Valium, and Lopressor. If symptoms are not controlled by these measures, a mitral valve replacement will be considered.

## Critical Thinking Questions

1. List the four medications this patient was given in the hospital and describe in your own words what condition each medication treats.
   a.
   b.
   c.
   d.

2. Two diagnostic tests conducted in the Emergency Room were normal. List them and describe each test in your own words. Because the results from these two tests were normal, a very serious heart condition could be ruled out. This is noted in the discharge plans. Identify the serious heart condition and describe it in your own words.

3. Explain in your own words why the treadmill test had to be stopped.

4. Which of the following is NOT one of the admitting diagnoses?
   a. high blood pressure
   b. dizziness
   c. difficulty breathing
   d. fast heartbeat

5. The physician has two treatment options for this patient: medication and surgery. If the medication fails to control her condition, then describe what surgery will be considered.

6. Compare and contrast valve stenosis and valve prolapse.

# Chart Note Transcription

## Chart Note

The chart note below contains 11 phrases that can be reworded with a medical term that you learned in this chapter. Each phrase is identified with an underline. Determine the medical term and write your answers in the space provided.

**Current Complaint:** A 56-year-old male was admitted to the Cardiac Care Unit from the Emergency Room with left arm pain, severe pain around the heart,① an abnormally slow heartbeat,② nausea, and vomiting.

**Past History:** Patient reports no heart problems prior to this episode. He has taken medication for high blood pressure③ for the past 5 years. His family history is significant for a father and brother who both died in their 50s from death of heart muscle.④

**Signs and Symptoms:** Patient reports severe pain around the heart that radiates into his left jaw and arm. A record of the heart's electrical activity⑤ and a blood test to determine the amount of heart damage⑥ were abnormal.

**Diagnosis:** An acute death of heart muscle resulting from a blood clot in a coronary vessel.⑦

**Treatment:** First, provide supportive care during the acute phase. Second, evaluate heart damage by passing a thin tube through a blood vessel into the heart to detect abnormalities⑧ and evaluate heart fitness by having patient exercise on a treadmill.⑨ Finally, perform surgical intervention by either inflating a balloon catheter to dilate a narrow vessel⑩ or by open heart surgery to create a shunt around a blocked vessel.⑪

1. _____
2. _____
3. _____
4. _____
5. _____
6. _____
7. _____
8. _____
9. _____
10. _____
11. _____

# Practice Exercises

## A. Complete the following statements.

1. The study of the heart is called _____ .

2. The three layers of the heart are _____ , _____ , and _____ .

3. The impulse for the heartbeat (the pacemaker) originates in the _____ .

4. The artery that does not carry oxygenated blood is the _____ .

5. The four heart valves are _____ , _____ , _____ , and _____ .

6. The _____ are the receiving chambers of the heart and the _____ are the pumping chambers.

## B. State the terms described using the combining forms provided.

The combining form *cardi/o* refers to the heart. Use it to write a term that means

1. pain in the heart _____
2. disease of the heart muscle _____
3. enlargement of the heart _____
4. abnormally fast heart rate _____
5. abnormally slow heart rate _____
6. inflammation of the heart _____

The combining form *phleb/o* refers to the vein. Use it to write a term that means

7. inflammation of a vein _____
8. opening a vein (to withdraw blood) _____
9. suture a vein _____

The combining form *arteri/o* refers to the artery. Use it to write a term that means

10. pertaining to an artery _____
11. hardening of an artery _____

## C. Add a prefix to *-carditis* to form the term for

1. inflammation of the inner lining of the heart _____
2. inflammation of the outer layer of the heart _____
3. inflammation of the muscle of the heart _____

## D. Define each combining form and provide an example of its use.

|  | Definition | Example |
|---|---|---|
| 1. ciardi/o | | |
| 2. valvul/o | | |
| 3. steth/o | | |
| 4. arteri/o | | |
| 5. phleb/o | | |
| 6. angi/o | | |
| 7. ventricul/o | | |

8. thromb/o _____

9. atri/o _____

10. ather/o _____

## E. Write medical terms for the following definitions.

1. pertaining to a vein _____

2. fast heartbeat _____

3. specialist in treating the heart _____

4. recording electrical activity of heart _____

5. high blood pressure _____

6. low blood pressure _____

7. inflammation of inner lining of heart _____

8. bluish coloring to skin _____

9. destruction of a clot _____

10. narrowing of the arteries _____

## F. Write the suffix for each expression and provide an example of its use.

| | Suffix | Example |
|---|---|---|

1. pressure _____

2. abnormal narrowing _____

3. instrument to measure pressure _____

4. small _____

5. hardening _____

## G. Identify the following abbreviations.

1. BP _____

2. CHF _____

3. MI _____

4. CCU _____

5. PVC _____

6. CPR _____

7. CAD _____

8. CP _____

9. EKG _____

10. S1 _____

## H. Write the abbreviations for the following terms.

1. mitral valve prolapse _____

2. ventricular septal defect _____

3. percutaneous transluminal coronary angioplasty _____

4. ventricular fibrillation _____

5. deep vein thrombosis _____

6. lactate dehydrogenase _____

7. coarctation of the aorta _____

8. tissue-type plasminogen activator _____

9. cardiovascular _____

10. extracorporeal circulation _____

## I. Match the terms in column A with the definitions in column B.

|  | A |  | B |
|---|---|---|---|
| 1. | _____ arrhythmia | a. | swollen, distended veins |
| 2. | _____ thrombus | b. | inflammation of vein |
| 3. | _____ bradycardia | c. | serious congenital anomaly |
| 4. | _____ bruit | d. | slow heart rate |
| 5. | _____ phlebitis | e. | insert thin tubing |
| 6. | _____ commissurotomy | f. | irregular heartbeat |
| 7. | _____ varicose vein | g. | murmur |
| 8. | _____ tetralogy of Fallot | h. | clot in blood vessel |
| 9. | _____ catheterization | i. | to change the size of an opening |
| 10. | _____ sphygmomanometer | j. | blood pressure cuff |

## J. Use the following terms in the sentences that follow.

| angioma | angina pectoris | echocardiogram | MI |
|---|---|---|---|
| angiography | varicose veins | hypertension | CHF |
| defibrillation | Holter monitor | pacemaker | CCU |
| murmur | | | |

1. Tiffany was born with a congenital condition that results in an abnormal heart sound. This is called a(n) _____ .

2. Joseph suffered an arrhythmia while hospitalized that resulted in a cardiac arrest. The emergency physician and team used an instrument to give electric shocks to the heart in an attempt to create a normal heart rhythm. This procedure is called _____ .

3. Marguerite has been placed on a low-sodium diet and medication to bring her blood pressure down to a normal range. She suffers from _____ .

4. Tony has had an artificial device called a(n) _____ inserted to control the beating of his heart by producing rhythmic electrical impulses.

5. Derrick's physician determined that he had _____ after examining his legs and finding swollen, tortuous veins.

6. Laura has persistent chest pains that require medication. The term for the pain is _____ .

7. La Tonya is going to have surgery to correct her heart condition. She will be admitted to what hospital unit after her surgery? _____

8. Stephen is going to have a coronary artery bypass graft to correct the blockage in his coronary arteries. He recently suffered a heart attack as a result of this occlusion. His attack is called a(n) _____ .

9. Stephen's physician scheduled an X-ray to determine the extent of his blood vessel damage. This test is called a(n) _____ .

10. A patient who is scheduled to have a diagnostic procedure that uses ultrasound to produce an image of the heart valves is going to have a(n) _____ .

11. Rolando has been diagnosed with a benign tumor of the blood vessels. This is called a(n) _____ .

12. Eric must wear a device for 24 hours that will keep track of his heart activity as he performs his normal daily routine. This device is called a(n) _____ .

13. Lydia is 82 years old and is suffering from a heart condition that causes weakness, edema, and breathlessness. Her heart failure is the cause of her lung congestion. This condition is called _____ .

# Professional Journal

In this exercise you will now have an opportunity to put the words you have learned into practice. Imagine yourself in the role of a cardiology technologist, electrocardiogram technician, or a cardiac sonographer. If you refer back to the Professional Profile at the beginning of this chapter, you will see that these health care professionals are responsible for performing diagnostic tests and treatments such as invasive heart procedures, EKGs, and echocardiograms. Use the 10 words listed below, or any other new terms from this chapter, to write sentences to describe the patients you and the whole cardiology technology team saw today.

An example of a sentence is *Mr. Brown's heart rate was so slow he will require a* **pacemaker implantation**.

1. aneurysm _____

2. angiography _____

3. cardiac catheterization _____

4. electrocardiogram _____

5. arrhythmia _____

6. mitral valve prolapse _____

7. cardiomegaly _____

8. stent _____

9. fibrillation _____

10. coronary artery disease _____

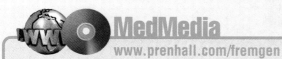

**MedMedia**
www.prenhall.com/fremgen

Use the CD-ROM enclosed with your textbook to gain additional reinforcement through interactive word building exercises, spelling games, labeling activities, and additional quizzes.

Use the above address to access the free, interactive Companion Website created for this textbook. Get hints, instant feedback, and textbook references to chapter-related multiple-choice questions, as well as labeling and matching exercises. In addition, you will find an audio glossary, case studies, and Internet exploration exercises.

***For more information regarding cardiovascular diseases, visit the following websites:***

American College of Cardiology at **www.acc.org**

National Heart, Lung, and Blood Institute at **www.nhlbi.nih.gov**

American Heart Association at **www.americanheart.org**

Centers for Disease Control and Prevention—Cardiovascular Health at
    **www.cdc.gov/cvh/aboutcardio/htm**

Karolinska Institute Library, Stockholm, Sweden—Cardiovascular Disease Resources List at
    **www.mic.ki.se/diseases/index/html**

# Chapter 6

# Blood and the Lymphatic and Immune System

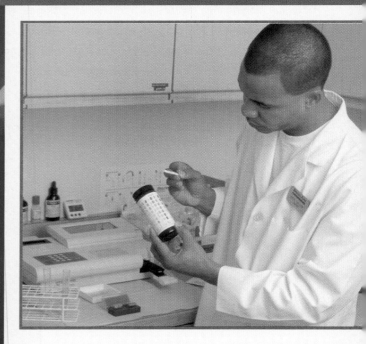

## Learning Objectives

*Upon completion of this chapter, you will be able to:*

- Recognize the combining forms and suffixes introduced in this chapter.

- Gain the ability to pronounce medical terms and major anatomical structures.

- List the major components, structures, and organs of the blood and lymphatic and immune systems and their functions.

- Discuss the immune response.

- Describe the blood typing systems.

- Build blood and lymphatic and immune system medical terms from word parts.

- Define vocabulary, pathology, diagnostic, and therapeutic medical terms relating to the blood and lymphatic and immune systems.

- Recognize types of medication associated with blood and the lymphatic and immune systems.

- Interpret abbreviations associated with blood and the lymphatic and immune systems.

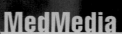

## MedMedia
### www.prenhall.com/fremgen
Additional interactive resources and activities for this chapter can be found on the Companion Website. For animations, audio glossary, and review, access the accompanying CD-ROM in this book.

## Professional Profile

### Clinical Laboratory Science

Clinical laboratory scientists perform a variety of tests using laboratory equipment, microscopes, and computers. These laboratory tests include chemical analyses on body tissues, blood, and other body fluids; growing bacterial cultures; and typing and cross-matching blood for transfusions. Medical laboratory technologists play a key role in patient care because physicians study and use the results of these tests to make their diagnoses. Medical laboratories are found in acute-care facilities, physicians' offices, clinics, private laboratories, public health facilities, and research facilities.

### Medical Technologist (MT) or Clinical Laboratory Scientist (CLS)

- Performs laboratory tests as ordered by a physician
- Graduates from an accredited 4-year college or university program
- Passes a national certification exam

### Medical Laboratory Technician (MLT) or Clinical Laboratory Technician (CLT)

- Works under the supervision of a medical technologist
- Graduates from an accredited 2-year laboratory technician program at a community college or vocational education program
- Passes a national certification exam

### Phlebotomist

- A specialist in drawing venous blood
- Does not conduct laboratory tests
- Completes a vocational education program or on-the-job training program
- Certification exam is available

***For more information regarding these health careers, visit the following websites:***
American Medical Technologists at **www.amt1.com**
American Society for Clinical Laboratory Science at **www.ascls.org**
American Society for Clinical Pathology at **www.ascp.org**

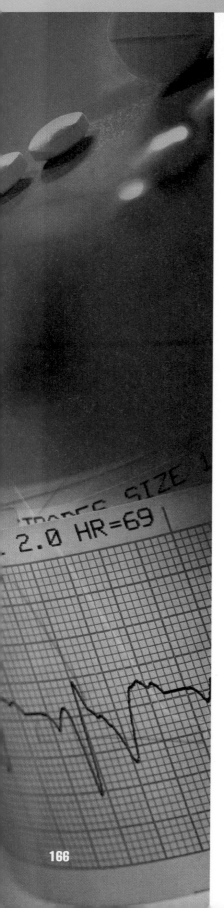

## Overview

## Part I: Blood

### Components of Blood

blood cells (formed elements)
    erythrocytes
    platelets
    leukocytes
plasma

### Combining Forms Relating to Blood

| | | | |
|---|---|---|---|
| agglutin/o | clumping | hemat/o | blood |
| chrom/o | color | leuk/o | white |
| coagul/o | clotting | morph/o | shape |
| erythr/o | red | myel/o | bone marrow |
| fibrin/o | fibers, fibrous | phag/o | eat, swallow |
| granul/o | granules | sanguin/o | blood |
| hem/o | blood | thromb/o | clot |

### Suffixes Relating to Blood

| Suffix | Meaning | Example |
|---|---|---|
| -apheresis | removal, carry away | plasmapheresis |
| -cyte | cell | erythrocyte |
| -cytosis | more than the normal number of cells | erythrocytosis |
| -emia | blood condition | leukemia |
| -globin | protein | hemoglobin |
| -penia | abnormal decrease, too few | hematocytopenia |
| -poiesis | formation | hematopoiesis |
| -stasis | standing still | hemostasis |

## Anatomy and Physiology of Blood

| | | |
|---|---|---|
| **erythrocytes** | **leukocytes** | **red blood cells** |
| **formed elements** | **plasma** | **white blood cells** |
| **hematopoiesis** | **platelets** | |

The average adult has about 5 liters of blood. It circulates throughout the body within the blood vessels of the cardiovascular system. Blood is a mixture of cells floating in watery **plasma** (**PLAZ** mah). As a group these cells are referred to as **formed elements,** but there are three different kinds: **erythrocytes** (eh **RITH** roh sights) or **red blood cells, leukocytes** (**LOO** koh sights) or **white blood cells,** and **platelets** (**PLAYT** lets). Blood cells are produced in the red bone marrow by a process called **hematopoiesis** (hee mah toh poy **EE** sis). Plasma and erythrocytes are responsible for transporting substances, leukocytes protect the body from invading microrganisms and platelets play a role in controlling bleeding.

## Plasma

| | | |
|---|---|---|
| albumin | fibrinogen | potassium |
| amino acids | gamma globulin | serum |
| calcium | globulins | sodium |
| creatinine | glucose | urea |
| fats | plasma proteins | |

Liquid plasma composes about 55 percent of whole blood in the average adult and is 90 to 92 percent water. The remaining 8 to 10 percent portion of plasma is dissolved substances, especially **plasma proteins** such as **albumin** (al **BEW** min), **globulins** (**GLOB** yew lenz), and **fibrinogen** (fye **BRIN** oh jen). Albumin helps transport fatty substances that cannot dissolve in the watery plasma. There are three main types of globulins. One of these, **gamma globulins** (**GAM** ah **GLOB** yoo linz), acts as antibodies. Fibrinogen is a blood-clotting protein. In addition to the plasma proteins, smaller amounts of other important substances are also dissolved in the plasma for transport: **calcium** (**KAL** see um), **potassium** (poh **TASS** ee um), **sodium, glucose** (**GLOO** kohs), **amino** (ah **MEE** noh) **acids, fats,** and waste products such as **urea** (yoo **REE** ah) and **creatinine** (kree AT in in).

> **MED TERM TIP**
> Plasma and **serum** (**SEE** rum) are not interchangeable words. Serum is plasma, but with fibrinogen removed or inactivated. This way it can be handled and tested without it clotting. The term *serum* is also sometimes used to mean antiserum or antitoxin.

## Erythrocytes

| | | |
|---|---|---|
| bilirubin | enucleated | hemoglobin |

Erythrocytes are also called red blood cells (RBCs) (see ▦ Figure 6.1). They are biconcave disks and are **enucleated** (ee **NEW** klee ate ed), which means they no longer contain a nucleus. Red blood cells appear red in color because they contain **hemoglobin** (hee moh **GLOH** bin), which is an iron-containing pigment. Hemoglobin is the part of the red blood cell that picks up oxygen from the lungs and delivers it to the tissues of the body.

There are about 5 million erythrocytes per cubic millimeter of blood. The total number in an average-sized adult is 35 trillion, with males having more red blood cells than females. Erythrocytes have an average life span of 120 days and then the spleen removes the worn-out and damaged ones from circulation. Much of the red blood cell, such as the iron, can be reused, but one portion, **bilirubin** (bil ly **ROO** bin), is disposed of by the liver.

## Leukocytes

| | | |
|---|---|---|
| agranulocytes | lymphocytes | pathogens |
| basophils | monocytes | phagocyte |
| eosinophils | neutrophils | phagocytosis |
| granulocytes | | |

Leukocytes, also referred to as white blood cells (WBCs), provide protection against the invasion of **pathogens** (**PATH** oh ginz) such as bacteria, viruses, and other foreign material. In general, WBCs have a spherical shape with a large nucleus and there are about 8,000 per cubic millimeter of blood (refer to Figure 6.1). There are five different types of WBCs, each with its own strategy for protecting the body. The five can be subdivided into two categories: **granulocytes** (**GRAN** yew loh sights) (with granules in the cytoplasm) and **agranulocytes** (ah **GRAN** yew loh sights) (without granules in the cytoplasm). The name and function of each type is presented in Table 6.1.

> **MED TERM TIP**
> A **phagocyte** (**FAG** oh sight) is a cell that has the ability to ingest (eat) and digest bacteria and other foreign particles. This process, **phagocytosis** (fag oh sigh **TOH** sis), is critical for the control of bacteria within the body.

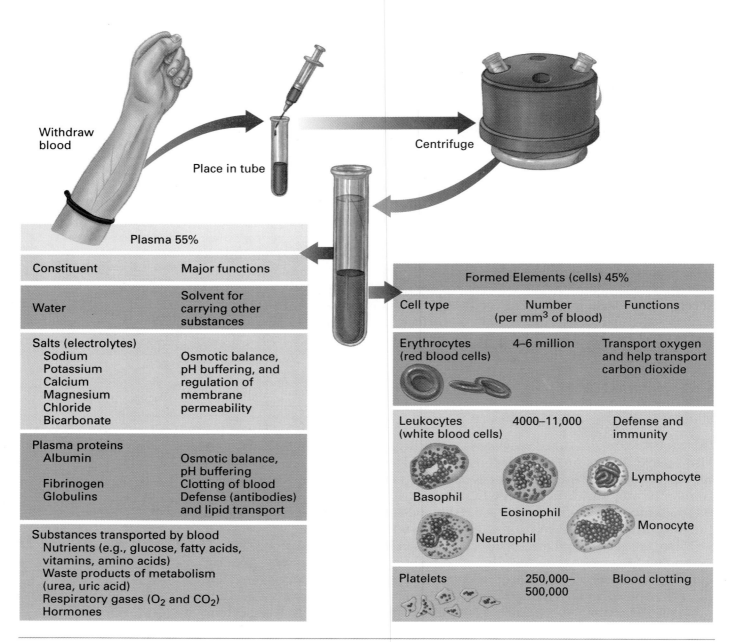

**FIGURE 6.1** Composition of blood.

| Table 6.1 | Leukocyte Classification |
|---|---|
| **Leukocyte** | **Function** |
| Granulocytes | |
| **Basophils** (**BAY** soh fillz) (**basos**) | Release histamine and heparin to damaged tissues |
| **Eosinophils** (ee oh **SIN** oh fillz) (**eosins**) | Destroy parasites and increase during allergic reactions |
| **Neutrophils** (**NOO** troh fillz) | Important for phagocytosis; most numerous of the leukocytes |
| Agranulocytes | |
| **Monocytes** (**MON** oh sights) (**monos**) | Important for phagocytosis |
| **Lymphocytes** (**LIM** foh sights) (**lymphs**) | Provide protection through an immunity activity |

# Platelets

**agglutinate**

**fibrin**

**hemostasis**

**prothrombin**

**thrombin**

**thrombocyte**

**thromboplastin**

*Platelet* is the modern term for **thrombocyte (THROM** boh sight). Platelets are the smallest of all the formed blood elements. They are also not whole cells, but rather are formed when the cytoplasm of a large precursor cell shatters into small plate-like fragments (refer to Figure 6.1). There are between 200,000 and 300,000 per cubic millimeter in the body.

Platelets play a critical part in the blood-clotting process or **hemostasis** (hee moh **STAY** sis). They **agglutinate** (ah **GLOO** tih nayt) or clump together into small clusters when a blood vessel is cut or damaged. Platelets release a substance called **thromboplastin** (throm boh **PLAS** tin), which, in the presence of calcium, reacts with **prothrombin** (proh **THROM** bin) to form **thrombin** (**THROM** bin). Then thrombin, in turn, works to convert fibrinogen to **fibrin** (**FYE** brin), which eventually becomes the mesh-like blood clot.

# Blood Typing

**ABO system**

**blood typing**

**Rh factor**

Each person's blood is different from others' due to the presence of marker proteins on the surface of his or her erythrocytes. Before a person receives a blood transfusion it is important to do a **blood typing.** This is a laboratory test to determine if the donated blood is compatible with the recipient's blood. There are many different subgroups of blood markers, but the two most important ones are the **ABO system** and **Rh factor.**

## ABO System

**type A**

**type AB**

**type B**

**type O**

**universal donor**

**universal recipient**

In the ABO blood system there are two possible RBC markers, A and B. A person with an A marker is said to have **type A** blood. Type A blood produces anti-B antibodies. The presence of a B marker gives **type B** blood and anti-A antibodies. The absence of either an A or a B marker results in **type O** blood, which contains both anti-A and anti-B antibodies. If both markers are present, the blood is **type AB** and does not result in any antibodies.

Because type O blood does not have either marker A or B, it will not react with anti-A or anti-B antibodies. For this reason a person with type O blood is referred to as a **universal donor.** In an emergency, type O blood may be given to a person with any of the other blood types. Similarly, type AB blood is the **universal recipient.** A person with type AB blood has no antibodies against the other blood types and, therefore, in an emergency, can receive any type of blood.

## Rh Factor

**Rh-negative**

**Rh-positive**

**type and crossmatch**

Rh factor is not as difficult to understand as the ABO system. A person with the Rh factor on his or her red blood cells is said to be **Rh-positive (Rh+).** Since this person has the factor, he or she will not make anti-Rh antibodies. A person without the Rh factor is **Rh-negative (Rh-)** and will produce anti-Rh antibodies. Therefore, an Rh+ person may receive both an Rh+ and an Rh- transfusion, but an Rh- person can receive only Rh- blood.

> **MED TERM TIP**
> Before a patient receives a blood transfusion, the laboratory performs a **type and crossmatch.** This test first double checks the blood type of both the donor's and recipient's blood. Then a crossmatch is performed. This process mixes together small samples of both bloods and observes the mixture for adverse reactions.

## Word Building Relating to Blood

The following list contains examples of medical terms built directly from word parts. Their definitions can be determined by a straightforward translation of the word parts.

| Combining Form | Combined With | Medical Term | Definition |
|---|---|---|---|
| fibrin/o | -gen | fibrinogen (fye **BRIN** oh jen) | fiber producing |
|  | -lysis | fibrinolysis (fye brin oh **LYE** sis) | destruction of fibers |
| hem/o | -globin | hemoglobin (hee moh **GLOH** bin) | blood protein |
|  | -lysis | hemolysis (hee **MALL** ih sis) | blood destruction |
|  | -rrhage | hemorrhage (**HEM** er rij) | rapid flow of blood |
|  | -stasis | hemostasis (hee moh **STAY** sis) | stopping blood |
| hemat/o | -ology | hematology (hee mah **TALL** oh jee) | study of blood |
|  | -oma | hematoma (hee mah **TOH** mah) | blood swelling |
|  | -poiesis | hematopoiesis (hee mah toh poy **EE** sis) | blood producing |
| sanguin/o | -ous | sanguinous (**SANG** gwih nus) | pertaining to blood |

| Suffix | Combined With | Medical Term | Definition |
|---|---|---|---|
| -cyte | erythr/o | erythrocyte (eh **RITH** roh sight) | red cell |
|  | leuk/o | leukocyte (**LOO** koh sight) | white cell |
|  | thromb/o | thrombocyte (**THROM** boh sight) | clotting cell |
|  | granul/o | granulocyte (**GRAN** yew loh sight) | granular cell |
|  | a- granul/o | agranulocyte (ah **GRAN** yew loh sight) | nongranular cell |
| -cytosis | erythr/o | erythrocytosis (ee **RITH** row sigh toe sis) | too many red cells |
|  | leuk/o | leukocytosis (**LOO** koh sigh toh sis) | too many white cells |
|  | thromb/o | thrombocytosis (throm boh sigh **TOH** sis) | too many clotting cells |
| -penia | erythr/o | erythropenia (ee **RITH** row pen ee ah) | too few red (cells) |
|  | leuk/o cyt/o | leukocytopenia (**LOO** koh sigh toh pen ee ah) | too few white cells |
|  | thromb/o cyt/o | thrombocytopenia (**THROM** boh sigh toh pen ee ah) | too few clotting cells |
|  | pan- cyt/o | pancytopenia (pan sigh toe **PEN** ee ah) | too few of all cells |
|  | hemat/o cyt/o | hematocytopenia (hee mah toh sigh toh **PEE** nee ah) | too few blood cells |

## Vocabulary Relating to Blood

| | |
|---|---|
| **blood clot** | The hard collection of fibrin, blood cells, and tissue debris that is the end result of hemostasis or the blood-clotting process (see ▇ Figure 6.2). |
| **coagulate (koh ag YOO late)** | When a liquid is converted to a gel or solid, as in blood coagulation. |
| **dyscrasia (dis CRAZ ee ah)** | A general term indicating the presence of a disease affecting blood. |
| **erythropoiesis (eh rith roh poy EE sis)** | The process of forming erythrocytes in the red bone marrow. |
| **hematologist (hee mah TALL oh jist)** | A physician who specializes in treating diseases and conditions of the blood. |
| **hematoma (hee mah TOH mah)** | The collection of blood under the skin as the result of blood escaping into the tissue from damaged blood vessels. Commonly referred to as a *bruise*. |
| **hemostasis (hee moh STAY sis)** | To stop bleeding or the stagnation of blood flow through the tissues. |
| **packed cells** | A transfusion of only the formed elements and without plasma. |
| **whole blood** | Refers to the mixture of both plasma and formed elements. |

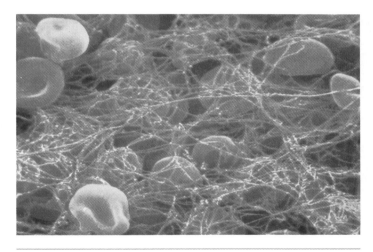

▇ **FIGURE 6.2**  Blood clot.

## Pathology Relating to Blood

| | |
|---|---|
| **anemia (an NEE mee ah)** | A large group of conditions characterized by a reduction in the number of red blood cells or the amount of hemoglobin in the blood; results in less oxygen reaching the tissues. |
| **aplastic anemia (a PLAS tik an NEE mee ah)** | Severe form of anemia that develops as a consequence of loss of functioning red bone marrow. Results in a decrease in the number of all the formed elements. Treatment may eventually require a bone marrow transplant. |
| **erythroblastosis fetalis (eh rith roh blass TOH sis fee TAL is)** | Condition in which antibodies in the mother's blood enter the fetus' blood and cause anemia, jaundice, edema, and enlargement of the liver and spleen. Also called *hemolytic disease of the newborn*. |
| **hemolytic anemia (hee moh LIT ik an NEE mee ah)** | An anemia that develops as the result of the excessive loss of erythrocytes. |

*continued...*

| | |
|---|---|
| **hemolytic (hee moh LIT ik) disease of the newborn** | Condition that may develop during pregnancy if the mother is Rh-negative, in which antibodies in the mother's blood enter the fetus' bloodstream, damaging fetal blood cells. Results in anemia, jaundice, edema, and enlargement of the liver and spleen. Also called *erythroblastosis fetalis*. |
| **hemophilia (hee moh FILL ee ah)** | Hereditary blood disease in which blood-clotting time is prolonged. It is transmitted by a sex-linked trait from females to males. It appears almost exclusively in males. |
| **hyperlipidemia (HYE per lip id ee mee ah)** | Condition of having too high a level of lipids such as cholesterol in the bloodstream. A risk factor for developing atherosclerosis and coronary artery disease. |
| **hypochromic anemia (hi poe CHROME ik an NEE mee ah)** | Anemia resulting from having insufficient hemoglobin in the erythrocytes. Named because the hemoglobin molecule is responsible for the dark red color of the erythrocytes. |
| **iron-deficiency anemia** | Anemia that results from having insufficient iron to manufacture hemoglobin. |
| **leukemia (loo KEE mee ah)** | Cancer of the WBC-forming red bone marrow; results in a large number of abnormal and immature WBCs circulating in the blood. |
| **pernicious anemia (per NISH us an NEE mee ah) (PA)** | Anemia associated with insufficient absorption of vitamin $B_{12}$ by the digestive system. Vitamin $B_{12}$ is necessary for erythrocyte production. |
| **polycythemia vera (pol ee sigh THEE mee ah VAIR rah)** | Production of too many red blood cells by the bone marrow. Blood becomes too thick to easily flow through the blood vessels. |
| **septicemia (sep tih SEE mee ah)** | Having bacteria in the bloodstream. Commonly referred to as *blood poisoning*. |
| **sickle cell anemia** | A genetic disorder in which erythrocytes take on an abnormal curved or "sickle" shape. These cells are fragile and are easily damaged, leading to a hemolytic anemia (see ▧ Figure 6.3). |
| **thalassemia (thal ah SEE mee ah)** | A genetic disorder in which the person is unable to make functioning hemoglobin, resulting in anemia. |

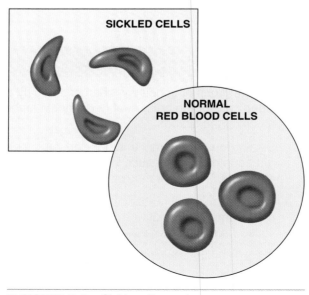

▧ **FIGURE 6.3**   Sickle cell anemia.

# Diagnostic Procedures Relating to Blood

| | |
|---|---|
| **bleeding time** | Test to measure the amount of time it takes for blood to coagulate. |
| **blood culture and sensitivity (C&S)** | Sample of blood is incubated in the laboratory to check for bacterial growth. If bacteria are present, they are identified and tested to determine which antibiotics they are sensitive to. |
| **bone marrow aspiration (as pih RAY shun)** | Sample of bone marrow is removed by aspiration with a needle and examined for diseases such as leukemia or aplastic anemia. |
| **complete blood count (CBC)** | Blood test that consists of five tests: red blood cell count (RBC), white blood cell count (WBC), hemoglobin (Hgb), hematocrit (Hct), and white blood cell differential. |
| **erythrocyte sedimentation (eh RITH roh sight sed ih men TAY shun) rate (ESR)** | Blood test to determine the rate at which mature red blood cells settle out of the blood after the addition of an anticoagulant. This is an indicator of the presence of an inflammatory disease. |
| **hematocrit (hee MAT oh krit) (HCT, Hct, crit)** | Blood test to measure the volume of red blood cells (erythrocytes) within the total volume of blood. |
| **hemoglobin (hee moh GLOH bin) (Hgb, hb)** | A blood test to measure the amount of hemoglobin present in a given volume of blood. |
| **phlebotomy (fleh BOT oh me)** | Incision into a vein in order to remove blood for a diagnostic test. Also called *venipuncture* (see ▇ Figure 6.4). |
| **platelet (PLAYT let) count** | Blood test to determine the number of platelets in a given volume of blood. |
| **prothrombin (proh THROM bin) time (Pro time, PT)** | A measure of the blood's coagulation abilities by measuring how long it takes for a clot to form after prothrombin has been activated. |
| **red blood cell count (RBC)** | Blood test to determine the number of erythrocytes in a volume of blood. A decrease in red blood cells may indicate anemia; an increase may indicate polycythemia. |
| **red blood cell morphology** | Examination of a specimen of blood for abnormalities in the shape (morphology) of the erythrocytes. Used to determine diseases like sickle cell anemia. |
| **sequential multiple analyzer computer (SMAC)** | Machine for doing multiple blood chemistry tests automatically. |
| **white blood cell count (WBC)** | Blood test to measure the number of leukocytes in a volume of blood. An increase may indicate the presence of infection or a disease such as leukemia. A decrease in WBCs may be caused by radiation therapy or chemotherapy. |
| **white blood cell differential (diff er EN shal) (diff)** | Blood test to determine the number of each variety of leukocytes. |

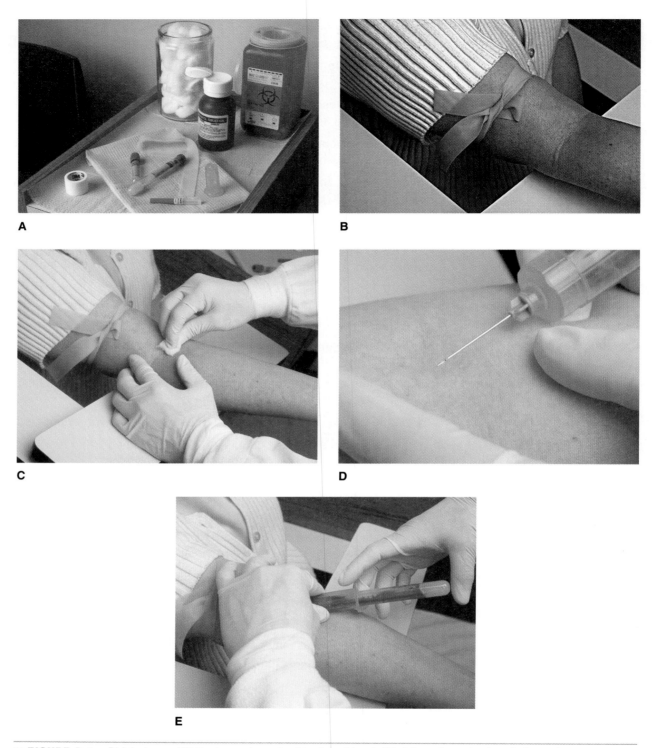

**■ FIGURE 6.4** Phlebotomy. (A) Equipment required to draw blood. (B) A tourniquet is placed above the vein. (C) The area is sterilized with alcohol. (D) The needle is inserted into the vein. (E) Blood fills the vacutube.

## Therapeutic Procedures Relating to Blood

| | |
|---|---|
| **autologous transfusion** (aw TALL oh gus trans FYOO zhun) | Procedure for collecting and storing a patient's own blood several weeks prior to the actual need. It can then be used to replace blood lost during a surgical procedure. |
| **blood transfusion** (trans FYOO zhun) | Artificial transfer of blood into the bloodstream (see ▦ Figure 6.5). |
| **bone marrow transplant (BMT)** | Patient receives red bone marrow from a donor after the patient's own bone marrow has been destroyed by radiation or chemotherapy. |
| **homologous transfusion** (hoh MALL oh gus trans FYOO zhun) | Replacement of blood by transfusion of blood received from another person. |
| **plasmapheresis** (plaz mah fah REE sis) | Method of removing plasma from the body without depleting the formed elements. Whole blood is removed and the cells and plasma are separated. The cells are returned to the patient along with a donor plasma transfusion. |

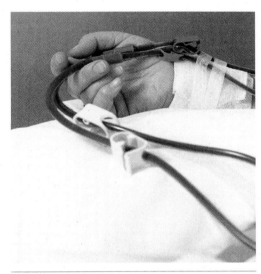

▦ **FIGURE 6.5**   Blood transfusion in process.
(Photo Researchers, Inc. Gaillard/Jerrican)

## Pharmacology Relating to Blood

| | |
|---|---|
| **anticoagulant** (an tih koh AG yoo lant) | Prevents blood clot formation. |
| **antihemorrhagic** (an tih hem er RAJ ik) | Substance that prevents or stops hemorrhaging; a *hemostatic agent*. |
| **antiplatelet** (an tih PLATE let) **agents** | Interferes with the action of platelets. Prolongs bleeding time. Commonly referred to as *blood thinners*. |
| **hematinic (hee mah TIN ik)** | Substance that increases the number of erythrocytes or the amount of hemoglobin in the blood. |
| **hemostatic** (hee moh STAT ik) **agent** | Stops the flow of blood; an *antihemorrhagic*. |
| **thrombolytic** (throm boh LIT ik) | Able to dissolve existing blood clots. |

# Abbreviations Relating to Blood

| | | | |
|---|---|---|---|
| **AHF** | antihemophilic factor | **Hgb, Hb, HGB** | hemoglobin |
| **ALL** | acute lymphocytic leukemia | **lymphs** | lymphocytes |
| **AML** | acute myelogenous leukemia | **MCV** | mean corpuscular volume |
| **basos** | basophils | **monos** | monocytes |
| **BMT** | bone marrow transplant | **PA** | pernicious anemia |
| **CBC** | complete blood count | **PCV** | packed cell volume |
| **CLL** | chronic lymphocytic leukemia | **PMN, polys** | polymorphonuclear neutrophil |
| **CML** | chronic myelogenous leukemia | **PT, pro-time** | prothrombin time |
| **diff** | differential | **RBC** | red blood cell |
| **eosins, eos** | eosinophils | **Rh+** | Rh-positive |
| **ESR, SR, sed rate** | erythrocyte sedimentation rate | **Rh−** | Rh-negative |
| **HCT, Hct, crit** | hematocrit | **SMAC** | sequential multiple analyzer computer |
| **HDN** | hemolytic disease of the newborn | **WBC** | white blood cell |

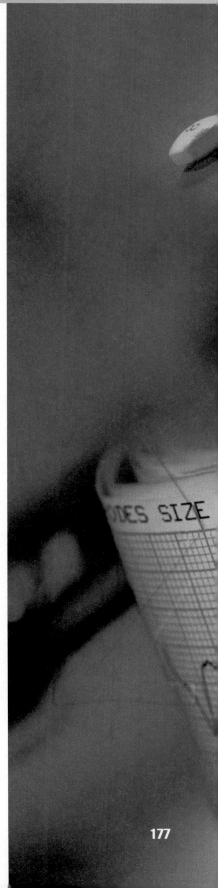

# Overview

## Part II: The Lymphatic and Immune System

**Organs of the Lymphatic and Immune System**

lymph nodes
lymphatic vessels
spleen
thymus gland
tonsils

**Combining Forms Relating to the Lymphatic and Immune System**

| | | | |
|---|---|---|---|
| aden/o | gland | lymphangi/o | lymph vessel |
| adenoid/o | adenoids | splen/o | spleen |
| immun/o | protection | thym/o | thymus |
| lymph/o | lymph | tonsill/o | tonsils |
| lymphaden/o | lymph node | tox/o | poison |

**Suffixes Relating to the Lymphatic and Immune System**

| Suffix | Meaning | Example |
|---|---|---|
| -globulin | protein | immunoglobulin |
| -phage | eat, swallow | macrophage |

## Anatomy and Physiology of the Lymphatic and Immune System

| | | |
|---|---|---|
| **lymph** | **lymphatic vessels** | **thymus gland** |
| **lymph nodes** | **spleen** | **tonsils** |

The lymphatic and immune systems consist of a network of **lymphatic** (lim **FAT** ik) **vessels, lymph nodes, spleen, thymus** (**THIGH** mus) **gland,** and **tonsils** (**TON** sulls) (see ▣ Figure 6.6). This system performs several quite diverse functions for the body. First, it collects excess tissue fluid throughout the body and returns it to the circulatory system, purifying it as it passes through the system. Fluid within lymphatic vessels is referred to as **lymph** (**LIMF**). Lymph is composed of water, white blood cells, nutrients, hormones, salts, carbon dioxide ($CO_2$), oxygen ($O_2$), and urea. Therefore, this system assists the circulatory system in transporting substances throughout the body. Next, it serves as the body's primary defense system against the invasion of pathogens. Finally, lymph vessels around the small intestines are able to pick up absorbed fats for transport.

### Lymphatic Vessels

| | | |
|---|---|---|
| **lymphatic capillaries** | **right lymphatic duct** | **valves** |
| **lymphatic ducts** | **thoracic duct** | |

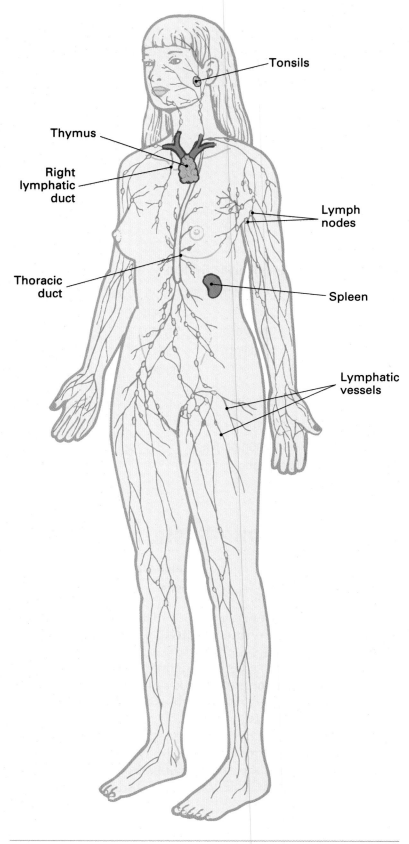

Tonsils

Thymus

Right
lymphatic
duct

Lymph
nodes

Thoracic
duct

Spleen

Lymphatic
vessels

■ **FIGURE 6.6**   Components of the lymphatic system.

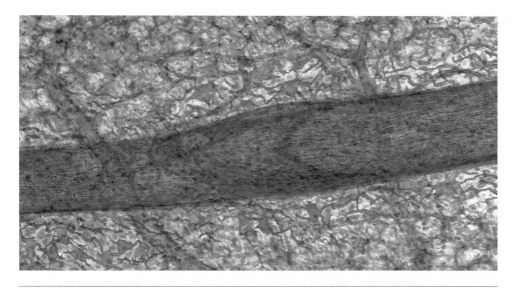

**FIGURE 6.7** Enhanced color microscopic view of lymphatic vessel and valve.
(Michael Abbey/Photo Researchers, Inc.)

The lymphatic vessels form an extensive network of vessels throughout the entire body (refer to Figure 6.6). However, unlike the circulatory system, these vessels are not in a closed loop. Instead, they serve as one-way pipes conducting lymph from the tissues toward the thoracic cavity. These vessels begin as very small **lymphatic capillaries** (**CAP** ih lair eez) in the tissues. Excessive tissue fluid enters these capillaries to begin the trip back to the circulatory system. The capillaries merge into larger lymphatic vessels. These vessels have **valves** along their length to ensure that lymph can only move forward toward the thoracic cavity (see Figure 6.7). These vessels finally drain into one of two large **lymphatic ducts,** the **right lymphatic duct** or the **thoracic duct.** The smaller right lymphatic duct drains the right arm and the right side of the neck and chest. This duct empties lymph into the right subclavian vein. The larger thoracic duct has the responsibility of draining lymph from the rest of the body (see Figure 6.8) and emptying into the left subclavian vein.

> **MED TERM TIP** The term *capillary* is also used to describe the minute blood vessels within the circulatory system. This is one of several general medical terms, such as valves, cilia, and hair, that are used in several systems.

## Lymph Nodes

| | | |
|---|---|---|
| **axillary** | **inguinal** | **mediastinal** |
| **cervical** | **lymph glands** | **metastasized** |

Lymph nodes are small organs composed of lymphatic tissue located along the route of the lymphatic vessels. These nodes, which are also referred to as **lymph glands,** have several functions, including the following:

1. Removing impurities from the lymph as it passes through
2. Manufacturing lymphocytes
3. Producing antibodies to fight disease

Once lymph is drained from the tissue, it is filtered in the node to remove impurities. Lymph nodes also serve to trap and destroy cells from cancerous tumors. Lymph nodes are found throughout the body, but are particularly concentrated in several regions. For example, lymph nodes concentrated in the neck region drain lymph from the head. See Table 6.2 for a list of some of the most important sites for lymph nodes.

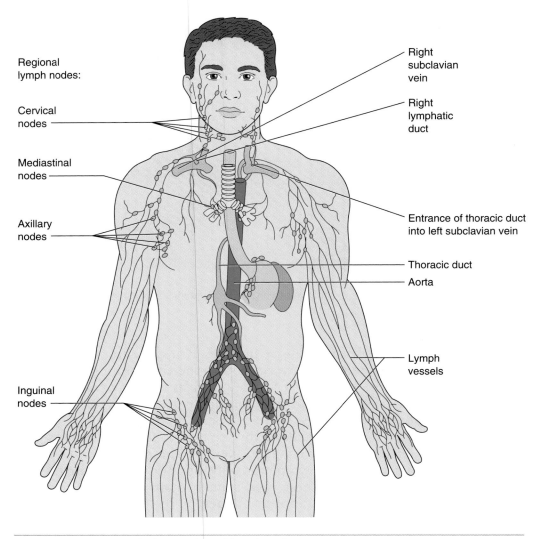

Regional lymph nodes:

Cervical nodes

Mediastinal nodes

Axillary nodes

Inguinal nodes

Right subclavian vein

Right lymphatic duct

Entrance of thoracic duct into left subclavian vein

Thoracic duct

Aorta

Lymph vessels

**■ FIGURE 6.8** Lymphatic vessels and lymph nodes.

**MED TERM TIP** In surgical procedures to remove a malignancy from an organ, such as a breast, the adjacent lymph nodes are also tested for cancer. If cancerous cells are found in the tested lymph nodes, the disease is said to have spread or **metastasized** (meh **TASS** tah sized). Tumor cells may then spread to other parts of the body by means of the lymphatic system.

| Table 6.2 | Sites for Lymph Nodes | |
|---|---|---|
| **Name** | **Location** | **Function** |
| **Axillary (AK** sih lair ee) | Armpits | Become enlarged during infections of arms and breasts; cancer cells from breasts may be present |
| **Cervical (SER** vih kal) | Neck | Drains parts of head and neck; may be enlarged during upper respiratory infections |
| **Inguinal (ING** gwih nal) | Groin | Drains area of the legs and lower pelvis |
| **Mediastinal** (mee dee ass **TYE** nal) | Chest | Assists in draining infection from within the chest cavity |

# Tonsils

**adenoids**        **palatine tonsils**        **pharynx**

**lingual tonsils**        **pharyngeal tonsils**

The tonsils are collections of lymphatic tissue located on each side of the throat or **pharynx** (**FAIR** inks) (refer to Figure 6.6). There are three sets of tonsils: **palatine** (**PAL** ah tyne) **tonsils**; **pharyngeal** (fair **IN** jee al) **tonsils**, commonly referred to as the **adenoids** (**ADD** eh noydz); and **lingual** (**LING** gwal) **tonsils**. All tonsils contain a large number of leukocytes and act as filters to protect the body from the invasion of pathogens through the digestive or respiratory system. Tonsils are not required for life and can safely be removed if they become a continuous site of infection.

# Spleen

**blood sinuses**        **macrophages**

The spleen, located in the upper left quadrant of the abdomen, consists of lymphatic tissue that is highly infiltrated with blood vessels (refer to Figure 6.6). These vessels spread out into slow moving **blood sinuses.** The spleen produces new red blood cells in the unborn baby. In adults it filters out and destroys old red blood cells, recycling the iron, and also stores some of the blood supply for the body. Phagocytic **macrophages** (**MACK** roh fayj ez) line the blood sinuses in the spleen to engulf and remove pathogens. Because the blood is moving through the organ slowly, the macrophages have time to carefully identify pathogens and worn-out RBCs. The spleen is not an essential organ for life and can be removed due to injury or disease. However, without the spleen, a person's susceptibility to a bloodstream infection may be increased.

# Thymus Gland

**T cells**        **T lymphocytes**        **thymosin**

The thymus (**THIGH** mus) gland is located in the upper portion of the mediastinum (refer to Figure 6.6). This gland is essential for the proper development of the immune system. It assists the body with the immune function and the development of antibodies. This organ's hormone, **thymosin** (thigh **MOH** sin), changes lymphocytes to **T lymphocytes** (simply called **T cells**). These cells play an important role in the immune response. The thymus is active in the unborn child and throughout childhood until adolescence, when it begins to shrink in size.

# Immunity

| | | |
|---|---|---|
| **acquired immunity** | **immune response** | **passive acquired immunity** |
| **active acquired immunity** | **immunity** | **protozoans** |
| **bacteria** | **immunizations** | **toxins** |
| **cancerous tumors** | **macrophage** | **vaccinations** |
| **fungi** | **natural immunity** | **viruses** |

**Immunity** (im **YOO** nih tee) is the body's ability to defend itself against pathogens, such as **bacteria** (bak **TEE** ree ah), **viruses, fungi** (**FUN** jee), **protozoans** (proh toh **ZOH** anz), **toxins,** and **cancerous tumors.** Immunity

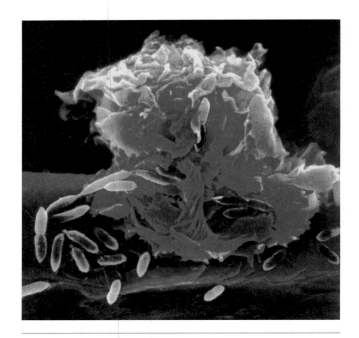

**FIGURE 6.9** Enhanced color photo showing macrophage (purple) on lung blood cell wall attacking bacillus *Escherichia* coli (yellow).

comes in two forms: **natural immunity** and **acquired immunity.** Natural immunity, also called *innate immunity*, is not specific to a particular disease and does not require prior exposure to the pathogenic agent. A good example of natural immunity is the **macrophage.** These leukocytes are present throughout all the tissues of the body, but are concentrated in areas of high exposure to invading bacteria, such as in the lungs and digestive system. They are very active phagocytic cells, ingesting and digesting any pathogen they encounter (see ▦ Figure 6.9).

Acquired immunity is the body's response to a specific pathogen. Acquired immunity may be established either passively or actively. **Passive acquired immunity** results when a person receives protective substances produced by another human or animal. This may take the form of maternal antibodies crossing the placenta to a baby, or an antitoxin or gamma globulin injection. **Active acquired immunity** develops following direct exposure to the pathogenic agent. The agent stimulates the body's **immune response,** a series of different mechanisms all geared to neutralize the agent. **Immunizations** (im yoo nih **ZAY** shuns) or **vaccinations** (vak sih **NAY** shuns) are special types of active acquired immunity. Instead of actually being exposed to the infectious agent and having the disease, a person is exposed to a modified or weakened pathogen that is still capable of stimulating the immune response but not causing the disease.

## Immune Response

| | | |
|---|---|---|
| antibody | B cells | cytotoxic |
| antibody-mediated immunity | B lymphocytes | humoral immunity |
| antigen–antibody complex | cell-mediated immunity | natural killer (NK) cells |
| antigens | cellular immunity | |

Disease-causing agents are recognized as being foreign because they display proteins that are different from a person's own natural proteins. Those foreign proteins, called **antigens** (**AN** tih jens), stimulate the immune response. The immune response consists of two distinct and different processes: **humoral immunity** (**HYOO** mor al im **YOO** nih tee) (also called **antibody-mediated immunity**) and **cellular immunity** (also called **cell-mediated immunity**).

Humoral immunity refers to the production of **B lymphocytes** (**LIM** foh sights), also called **B cells**. B cells respond to antigens by producing a protective protein, an **antibody** (**AN** tih bod ee). Antibodies combine with the antigen to form an **antigen–antibody** (**AN** tih jen **AN** tih bod ee) **complex**. This complex either targets the foreign substance for phagocytosis or prevents the infectious agent from damaging healthy cells.

Cellular immunity involves the production of T cells and **natural killer (NK) cells**. These defense cells are **cytotoxic** (sigh toh **TOK** sik). They physically attack and destroy pathogenic cells.

## Standard Precautions

| | |
|---|---|
| **cross infection** | **reinfection** |
| **nosocomial infection** | **self-inoculation** |
| **Occupational Safety and Health Administration (OSHA)** | |

Hospital and other health care settings contain a large number of infective pathogens. Patients and health care workers are exposed to each other's pathogens and sometimes become infected. An infection acquired in this manner, as a result of hospital exposure, is referred to as a **nosocomial** (no so **KOH** mee all) **infection**. Nosocomial infections can spread in several ways. **Cross infection** occurs when a person, either a patient or health care worker, acquires a pathogen from another patient or health care worker. **Reinfection** takes place when a person becomes infected again with the same pathogen that originally brought him or her to the hospital. **Self-inoculation** occurs when a person becomes infected in a different part of the body by a pathogen from another part of his or her own body—such as intestinal bacteria spreading to the urethra.

With the appearance of the human immunodeficiency virus (HIV) and the hepatitis B virus (HBV) in the mid-1980s, the fight against spreading infections took on even greater significance. In 1987 the **Occupational Safety and Health Administration (OSHA)** issued mandatory guidelines to ensure that all employees at risk of exposure to body fluids are provided with personal protective equipment. These guidelines state that all human blood, tissue, and body fluids must be treated as if they were infected with HIV, HBV, or other blood-borne pathogens. These guidelines were expanded in 1992 and 1996 to encourage the fight against not just blood-borne pathogens, but all nosocomial infections spread by contact with blood, mucous membranes, nonintact skin, and all body fluids (including amniotic fluid, vaginal secretions, pleural fluid, cerebrospinal fluid, peritoneal fluid, pericardial fluid, and semen). These guidelines are commonly referred to as the Standard Precautions. ▧ Figure 6.10 presents a summary of Standard Precaution guidelines.

1. Wash hands before putting on and after removing gloves and before and after working with each patient or patient equipment.
2. Wear gloves when in contact with any body fluid, mucous membrane, or nonintact skin or if you have chapped hands, a rash, or open sores.
3. Wear a nonpermeable gown or apron during procedures that are likely to expose you to any body fluid, mucous membrane, or nonintact skin.
4. Wear a mask and protective eyewear or a face shield when patients are coughing often or if body fluid droplets or splashes are likely.
5. Wear a face mask and eyewear that seal close to the face during procedures that cause body tissues to be vaporized.
6. Remove for proper cleaning any shared equipment—such as a thermometer, stethoscope, or blood pressure cuff—that has come into contact with body fluids, mucous membrane, or nonintact skin.

**FIGURE 6.10**   Summary of Standard Precaution Guidelines.

# Word Building Relating to the Lymphatic and Immune System

The following list contains examples of medical terms built directly from word parts. The definition for these terms can be determined by a straightforward translation of the word parts.

| Combining Form | Combined With | Medical Term | Definition |
|---|---|---|---|
| adenoid/o | -itis | adenoiditis (add eh noyd **EYE** tis) | inflammation of the adenoids |
| | -ectomy | adenoidectomy (add eh noyd **EK** toh mee) | excision of the adenoids |
| immun/o | -globulin | immunoglobulin (im yoo noh **GLOB** yoo lin) | immunity protein |
| | -logy | immunology (im yoo **NALL** oh jee) | study of immunity |
| lymph/o | aden/o –ectomy | lymphadenectomy (lim fad eh **NEK** toh mee) | excision of lymph gland |
| | aden/o -itis | lymphadenitis (lim fad en **EYE** tis) | inflammation of lymph glands |
| | aden/o -pathy | lymphadenopathy (lim fad eh **NOP** ah thee) | lymph gland disease |
| | angi/o -gram | lymphangiogram (lim **FAN** jee oh gram) | record of lymph vessels |
| | -oma | lymphoma (lim **FOH** mah) | lymph tumor |
| | -tic | lymphatic (lim **FAT** ik) | pertaining to lymph |
| path/o | -genic | pathogenic (path oh **JEN** ik) | disease producing |
| | -logy | pathology (path **OL** oh gee) | study of disease |
| splen/o | -ectomy | splenectomy (splee **NEK** toh mee) | excision of spleen |
| | -megaly | splenomegaly (splee noh **MEG** ah lee) | enlarged spleen |
| | -pexy | splenopexy (**SPLEE** noh pek see) | surgical fixation of the spleen |
| thym/o | -ectomy | thymectomy (thigh **MEK** toh mee) | excision of the thymus |
| | -oma | thymoma (thigh **MOH** mah) | thymus tumor |
| tonsill/o | -ectomy | tonsillectomy (ton sih **LEK** toh mee) | excision of the tonsils |
| | -itis | tonsillitis (ton sil **EYE** tis) | inflammation of the tonsils |

# Vocabulary Relating to the Lymphatic and Immune System

| | |
|---|---|
| **allergen (AL er jin)** | An antigen that causes an allergic reaction. |
| **allergist (AL er jist)** | A physician who specializes in testing for and treating allergies. |
| **allergy (AL er jee)** | Hypersensitivity to a common substance in the environment or to a medication. |
| **anaphylaxis (an ah fih LAK sis)** | Severe, potentially life-threatening, allergic reaction to an antigen. |
| **atypical (ay TIP ih kal)** | Abnormal. |
| **autoimmune disease** | A disease that results from the body's immune system attacking its own cells as if they were pathogens. Examples include systemic lupus erythematosus, rheumatoid arthritis, and multiple sclerosis. |
| **Epstein-Barr (EP steen BAR) virus** | Virus that is believed to be the cause of infectious mononucleosis. It was discovered by Anthony Epstein, a British virologist, and Yvonne Barr, a French physician. |
| **hives** | Appearance of wheals as part of an allergic reaction. |
| **human immunodeficiency (im yoo noh dee FIH shen see) virus (HIV)** | Virus that causes AIDS; also known as a retrovirus (see ▓ Figure 6.11). |
| **immunocompromised (im you noh KOM pro mized)** | Having an immune system that is unable to respond properly to pathogens. |
| **immunoglobulins (im yoo noh GLOB yoo linz)** | Antibodies secreted by the B cells. All antibodies are immunoglobulins. They assist in protecting the body and its surfaces from the invasion of bacteria. For example, the immunoglobulin IgA in colostrum, the first milk from the mother, helps to protect the newborn from infection. |
| **immunologist (im yoo NALL oh jist)** | A physician who specializes in treating infectious diseases and other disorders of the immune system. |
| **inflammation (in flah MA shun)** | The tissues' response to injury from pathogens or physical agents. Characterized by redness, pain, swelling, and feeling hot to touch (see ▓ Figure 6.12). |
| **lymphedema (limf eh DEE mah)** | Edema appearing in the extremities due to an obstruction of the lymph flow through the lymphatic vessels. |
| **opportunistic infections** | Infectious diseases that are associated with patients who have compromised immune systems and therefore a lowered resistance to infections and parasites. May be the results of HIV infection. |
| **retrovirus (REH troh vi rus)** | Virus, such as HIV, in which the virus copies itself using the host's DNA. |
| **urticaria (er tih KAY ree ah)** | The severe itching associated with hives, usually associated with food allergy, stress, or drug reactions. |

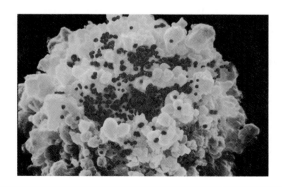

▓ **FIGURE 6.11** Enhanced color scanning electron micrograph of HIV virus (red) infecting T-helper cells (green). (NIBSC/Science Photo Library/Photo Researchers, Inc.)

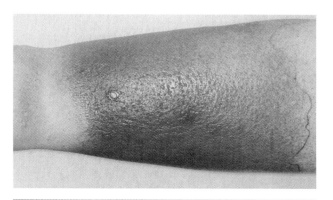

▓ **FIGURE 6.12** Inflammation as illustrated by cellulitis of the arm.

# Pathology Relating to the Lymphatic and Immune System

| | |
|---|---|
| **acquired immunodeficiency syndrome (ac quired im you noh dee FIH shen see SIN drohm) (AIDS)** | Disease that involves a defect in the cell-mediated immunity system. A syndrome of opportunistic infections that occur in the final stages of infection with the human immunodeficiency virus (HIV). This virus attacks $T_4$ lymphocytes and destroys them, which reduces the person's ability to fight infection. |
| **AIDS-related complex (ARC)** | Early stage of AIDS. There is a positive test for the virus but only mild symptoms of weight loss, fatigue, skin rash, and anorexia. |
| **anaphylactic (an ah fih LAK tik) shock** | Life-threatening condition resulting from a severe allergic reaction. Examples of instances that may trigger this reaction include bee stings, medications, or the ingestion of foods. Circulatory and respiratory problems occur, including respiratory distress, hypotension, edema, tachycardia, and convulsions. |
| **elephantiasis (el eh fan TYE ah sis)** | Inflammation, obstruction, and destruction of the lymph vessels that result in enlarged tissues due to edema. |
| **graft vs. host disease (GVHD)** | Serious complication of bone marrow transplant (graft). Immune cells from the donor bone marrow attack the recipient's (host's) tissues. |
| **Hodgkin's disease (HOJ kins dih ZEEZ)** | Also called Hodgkin's lymphoma. Cancer of the lymphatic cells found in concentration in the lymph nodes (see ■ Figure 6.13). Named after Thomas Hodgkin, a British physician, who first described it. |
| **Kaposi's sarcoma (KAP oh seez sar KOH mah)** | Form of skin cancer frequently seen in patients with AIDS. It consists of brownish-purple papules that spread from the skin and metastasize to internal organs. Named for Moritz Kaposi, an Austrian dermatologist. |
| **lymphadenitis (lim fad en EYE tis)** | Inflammation of the lymph nodes. Referred to as *swollen glands*. |
| **malignant lymphoma (lim FOH mah)** | Cancerous tumor of lymphatic tissue; most commonly occurs in lymph nodes, the spleen, or other body sites containing large amounts of lymphatic cells. |
| **mononucleosis (mon oh nook lee OH sis)** | Acute infectious disease with a large number of atypical lymphocytes. Caused by the Epstein–Barr virus. Abnormal liver function may occur. |
| **non-Hodgkin's lymphoma (NHL)** | Cancer of the lymphatic tissues other than Hodgkin's lymphoma. |
| **peritonsillar abscess (pair ih TON sih lar AB sess)** | Infection of the tissues between the tonsils and the pharynx. Also called a *quinsy sore throat*. |
| ***Pneumocystis carinii* pneumonia (noo moh SIS tis kah RYE nee eye new MOH nee ah)** | Pneumonia common in AIDS patients that is caused by infection with an opportunistic parasite. |
| **sarcoidosis (sar koyd OH sis)** | Disease of unknown cause that forms fibrous lesions. Lesions commonly appear in the lymph nodes, liver, skin, lungs, spleen, eyes, and small bones of the hands and feet. |
| **severe combined immunodeficiency syndrome (SCIDS)** | Disease seen in children born with a nonfunctioning immune system. Often forced to live in sealed sterile rooms. |

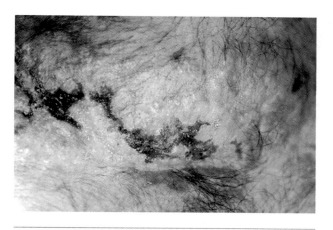

**■ FIGURE 6.13** Late-stage Hodgkin's disease with tumor eroding skin above cancerous lymph node.

## Diagnostic Procedures Relating to the Lymphatic and Immune System

| | |
|---|---|
| **ELISA (enzyme-linked immunosorbent assay) (EN zym LINK'T im yoo noh sor bent ASS say)** | A blood test for an antibody to the AIDS virus. A positive test means that the person has been exposed to the virus. There may be a false-positive reading and then the Western blot test would be used to verify the results. |
| **lymphangiography (lim FAN jee oh graf ee)** | X-ray taken of the lymph vessels after the injection of dye into the foot. The lymph flow through the chest is traced. |
| **Monospot** | Test for infectious mononucleosis. |
| **scratch test** | Form of allergy testing in which the body is exposed to an allergen through a light scratch in the skin (see ■ Figure 6.14). |
| **Western blot** | Test used as a backup to the ELISA blood test to detect the presence of the antibody to HIV (AIDS virus) in the blood. |

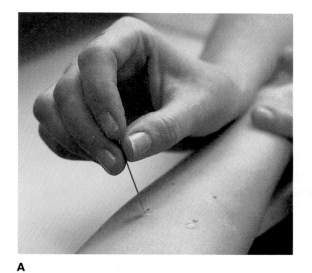

**A**

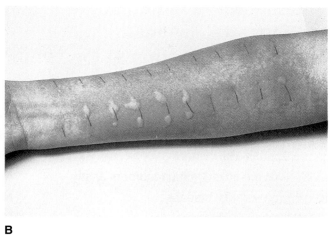

**B**

**■ FIGURE 6.14** (A) Scratch test. (B) Positive scratch test results.
(James King-Holmes/Science Photo Library/Photo Researchers, Inc.; Southern Illinois University/Photo Researchers, Inc.)

## Therapeutic Procedures Relating to the Lymphatic and Immune System

| | |
|---|---|
| **immunization**<br>(im yoo nih ZAY shun) | Exposure to a weakened pathogen that stimulates the immune response and antibody production in order to confer protection against the full-blown disease. Also called *vaccination*. |
| **immunotherapy**<br>(IM yoo noh thair ah pee) | Giving a patient an injection of immunoglobulins or antibodies in order to treat a disease. The antibodies may be produced by another person or animal, for example, antivenom for snake bites. More recent developments include treatments to boost the activity of the immune system, especially to treat cancer and AIDS. |
| **lymphadenectomy**<br>(lim fad eh NEK toh mee) | Excision of a lymph node. This is usually done to test for malignancy. |
| **vaccination**<br>(vak sih NAY shun) | Exposure to a weakened pathogen that stimulates the immune response and antibody production in order to confer protection against the full-blown disease. Also called *immunization*. |

## Pharmacology Relating to the Lymphatic and Immune System

| | |
|---|---|
| **antihistamine**<br>(an tih HIST ah meen) | Blocks the effects of histamine that has been released by the body during an allergic reaction. |
| **anti-inflammatory**<br>(an tih in FLAM ah tore e) | Reduces the body's inflammatory reaction. |
| **antiviral** (an tih VIE ral) | Weakens a viral infection in the body, often by interfering with the virus' ability to replicate. |
| **corticosteroids**<br>(core tih koh STARE royds) | A hormone produced by the adrenal cortex that has very strong anti-inflammatory properties. It is particularly useful in treating autoimmune diseases. |
| **immunosuppressants**<br>(im yoo noh sue PRESS antz) | Blocks certain actions of the immune system. Required to prevent rejection of a transplanted organ. |
| **vasoconstrictors**<br>(vasz oh con STRICT orz) | Produces contraction of the smooth muscles in the walls of arteries. Will raise blood pressure of a patient in anaphylactic shock. |

## Abbreviations Relating to the Lymphatic and Immune System

| | | | |
|---|---|---|---|
| **AIDS** | acquired immunodeficiency syndrome | **Ig** | immunoglobulins (IgA, IgD, IgE, IgG, IgM) |
| **ARC** | AIDS-related complex | **KS** | Kaposi's sarcoma |
| **CD4** | type of T cell affected by HIV infection | **lymphs** | lymphocyte |
| **EBV** | Epstein–Barr virus | **mono** | mononucleosis |
| **ELISA** | enzyme-linked immunosorbent assay | **NHL** | non-Hodgkin's lymphoma |
| **GVHD** | graft vs. host disease | **NK** | natural killer cells |
| **HD** | Hodgkin's disease | **PCP** | *Pneumocystis carinii* pneumonia |
| **HIV** | human immunodeficiency virus (causes AIDS) | **SCIDS** | severe combined immunodeficiency syndrome |

# Chapter Review

## Pronunciation Practice

You will find the pronunciation for each term on the enclosed CD-ROM. Check each one off as you master it.

- ☐ ABO system
- ☐ acquired immunity
- ☐ acquired immunodeficiency syndrome (ac quired im yoo noh dee **FIH** shen see **SIN** drohm)
- ☐ active acquired immunity
- ☐ adenoidectomy (add eh noyd **EK** toh mee)
- ☐ adenoiditis (add eh noyd **EYE** tis)
- ☐ adenoids (**ADD** eh noydz)
- ☐ agglutinate (ah **GLOO** tih nayt)
- ☐ agranulocytes (ah **GRAN** yew loh sights)
- ☐ AIDS-related complex
- ☐ albumin (al **BEW** min)
- ☐ allergen (**AL** er jin)
- ☐ allergist (**AL** er jist)
- ☐ allergy (**AL** er jee)
- ☐ amino (ah **MEE** noh) acids
- ☐ anaphylactic (an ah fih **LAK** tik) shock
- ☐ anaphylaxis (an ah fih **LAK** sis)
- ☐ anemia (an **NEE** mee ah)
- ☐ antibody (**AN** tih bod ee)
- ☐ antibody-mediated immunity (**AN** tih bod ee **MEE** dee ay ted im **YOO** nih tee)
- ☐ anticoagulant (an tih koh **AG** yoo lant)
- ☐ antigen (**AN** tih jen)
- ☐ antigen–antibody (**AN** tih jen **AN** tih bod ee) complex
- ☐ antihemorrhagic (an tih hem er **RAJ** ik)
- ☐ antihistamine (an tih **HIST** ah meen)
- ☐ anti-inflammatory (an tih in **FLAM** ah tore e)
- ☐ antiplatelet (an tih **PLATE** let) agents
- ☐ antiviral (an tih **VIE** ral)
- ☐ aplastic anemia (a **PLAS** tik an **NEE** mee ah)
- ☐ atypical (ay **TIP** ih kal)
- ☐ autoimmune disease
- ☐ autologous transfusion (aw **TALL** oh gus trans **FYOO** zhun)
- ☐ axillary (**AK** sih lair ee)

- ☐ bacteria (bak **TEE** ree ah)
- ☐ basophils (**BAY** soh fillz)
- ☐ B cells
- ☐ B lymphocytes (**LIM** fo sights)
- ☐ bilirubin (billy **ROO** bin)
- ☐ bleeding time
- ☐ blood clot
- ☐ blood culture and sensitivity
- ☐ blood sinuses
- ☐ blood transfusion (trans **FYOO** zhun)
- ☐ blood typing
- ☐ bone marrow aspiration (as pih **RAY** shun)
- ☐ bone marrow transplant
- ☐ calcium (**KAL** see um)
- ☐ cancerous tumor
- ☐ cell-mediated immunity
- ☐ cellular immunity
- ☐ cervical (**SER** vih kal)
- ☐ coagulate (koh ag **YOO** late)
- ☐ complete blood count
- ☐ corticosteroids (core tih koh **STARE** royds)
- ☐ creatinine (kree **AT** in in)
- ☐ cross infection
- ☐ cytotoxic (sigh toh **TOK** sik)
- ☐ dyscrasia (dis **CRAZ** ee ah)
- ☐ elephantiasis (el eh fan **TYE** ah sis)
- ☐ ELISA (enzyme-linked immunosorbent assay) (**EN** zym **LINK'T** im yoo noh sor bent **ASS** say)
- ☐ enucleated (ee **NEW** klee ate ed)
- ☐ eosinophils (ee oh **SIN** oh fillz)
- ☐ Epstein–Barr (**EP** steen **BAR**) virus
- ☐ erythroblastosis fetalis (eh rith roh blass **TOH** sis fee **TAL** iss)
- ☐ erythrocyte (eh **RITH** roh sight)
- ☐ erythrocyte sedimentation (eh **RITH** roh sight sed ih men **TAY** shun) rate

- erythrocytosis (ee **RITH** row sigh toe sis)
- erythropenia (ee **RITH** row pen ee ah)
- erythropoiesis (eh rith roh poy **EE** sis)
- fats
- fibrin (**FYE** brin)
- fibrinogen (fye **BRIN** oh jen)
- fibrinolysis (fye brin oh **LYE** sis)
- formed elements
- fungi (**FUN** jee)
- gamma globulin (**GAM** ah **GLOB** yoo lin)
- globulins (**GLOB** yew lenz)
- glucose (**GLOO** kohs)
- graft vs. host disease
- granulocyte (**GRAN** yew loh sight)
- hematinic (hee mah **TIN** ik)
- hematocrit (hee **MAT** oh krit)
- hematocytopenia (hee mah toh sigh toh **PEE** nee ah)
- hematologist (hee mah **TALL** oh jist)
- hematology (hee mah **TALL** oh jee)
- hematoma (hee mah **TOH** mah)
- hematopoiesis (hee mah toh poy **EE** sis)
- hemoglobin (hee moh **GLOH** bin)
- hemolysis (hee **MALL** ih sis)
- hemolytic anemia (hee moh **LIT** ik an **NEE** mee ah)
- hemolytic (hee moh **LIT** ik) disease of the newborn
- hemophilia (hee moh **FILL** ee ah)
- hemorrhage (**HEM** eh rij)
- hemostasis (hee moh **STAY** sis)
- hemostatic (hee moh **STAT** ik) agent
- hives
- Hodgkin's disease (**HOJ** kins dih **ZEEZ**)
- homologous transfusion (hoh **MALL** oh gus trans **FYOO** zhun)
- human immunodeficiency virus (im yoo noh dee **FIH** shen see)
- humoral immunity (**HYOO** mor al im **YOO** nih tee)
- hyperlipidemia (**HYE** per lip id ee mee ah)
- hypochromic anemia (hi poe **CHROME** ik an **NEE** mee ah)
- immune (im **YOON**) response
- immunity (im **YOO** nih tee)
- immunizations (im yoo nih **ZAY** shuns)
- immunocompromised (im you noh **KOM** pro mized)
- immunoglobulin (im yoo noh **GLOB** yoo lin)

- immunologist (im yoo **NALL** oh jist)
- immunology (im yoo **NALL** oh jee)
- immunosuppressants (im yoo noh sue **PRESS** antz)
- immunotherapy (**IM** yoo noh thair ah pee)
- inflammation (in flah **MA** shun)
- inguinal (**ING** gwih nal)
- innate immunity
- iron-deficiency anemia
- Kaposi's sarcoma (**KAP** oh seez sar **KOH** mah)
- leukemia (loo **KEE** mee ah)
- leukocyte (**LOO** koh sight)
- leukocytopenia (**LOO** koh sight toh pen ee ah)
- leukocytosis (**LOO** koh sigh toh sis)
- lingual tonsils (**LING** gwal **TON** sulls)
- lymph (**LIMF**)
- lymphatic capillaries (**CAP** ih lair eez)
- lymphatic (**LIMF**) ducts
- lymph (**LIMF**) glands
- lymph (**LIMF**) nodes
- lymphadenectomy (lim fad eh **NEK** toh mee)
- lymphadenitis (lim fad en **EYE** tis)
- lymphadenopathy (lim fad eh **NOP** ah thee)
- lymphangiogram (lim **FAN** jee oh gram)
- lymphangiography (lim fan jee **OG** rah fee)
- lymphatic (lim **FAT** ik)
- lymphatic (lim **FAT** ik) vessels
- lymphedema (limf eh **DEE** mah)
- lymphocyte (**LIM** foh sight)
- lymphoma (lim **FOH** mah)
- macrophage (**MACK** roh fayj)
- malignant lymphoma (lim **FOH** mah)
- mediastinal (mee dee ass **TYE** nal)
- metastasized (meh **TASS** tah sized)
- monocytes (**MON** oh sights)
- mononucleosis (mon oh noo klee **OH** sis)
- monospot
- natural immunity (im **YOO** nih tee)
- natural killer cells
- neutrophils (**NOO** troh fills)
- non-Hodgkin's lymphoma (lim **FOH** mah)
- nosocomial (no so **KOH** mee all) infection
- Occupational Safety and Health Administration

- opportunistic infections
  (op or **TOON** is tik in **FEK** shuns)
- packed cells
- palatine tonsils (**PAL** ah tyne **TON** sulls)
- pancytopenia (pan sigh toe **PEN** ee ah)
- passive acquired immunity
- pathogenic (path oh **JEN** ik)
- pathogens (**PATH** oh ginz)
- pathology (path **OL** oh gee)
- peritonsillar abscess (pair ih **TON** sih lar **AB** sess)
- pernicious anemia (per **NISH** us an **NEE** mee ah)
- phagocyte (**FAG** oh sight)
- phagocytosis (fag oh sigh **TOH** sis)
- pharyngeal tonsils (fair **IN** jee al **TON** sulls)
- pharynx (**FAIR** inks)
- phlebotomy (fleh **BOT** oh me)
- plasma (**PLAZ** mah)
- plasma (**PLAZ** mah) proteins
- plasmapheresis (plaz mah fah **REE** sis)
- platelet (**PLAYT** let) count
- platelets (**PLAYT** lets)
- *Pneumocystis carinii* pneumonia (noo moh **SIS** tis kah **RYE** nee eye new **MOH** nee ah)
- polycythemia vera (pol ee sigh **THEE** mee ah **VAIR** ah)
- potassium (poh **TASS** ee um)
- prothrombin (proh **THROM** bin)
- prothrombin (proh **THROM** bin) time
- protozoans (proh toh **ZOH** anz)
- red blood cell count
- red blood cell morphology
- red blood cells
- reinfection
- retrovirus (**REH** troh vi rus)
- Rh factor
- Rh-negative
- Rh-positive
- right lymphatic (lim **FAT** ik) duct
- sanguinous (**SANG** gwih nus)
- sarcoidosis (sar koyd **OH** sis)
- scratch test
- self-innoculation
- septicemia (sep tih **SEE** mee ah)
- sequential multiple analyzer computer
- serum (**SEE** rum)

- severe combined immunodeficiency syndrome
  (im yoo noh dee **FIH** shen see **SIN** drohm)
- sickle cell anemia
- sodium
- spleen
- splenectomy (splee **NEK** toh mee)
- splenomegaly (splee noh **MEG** ah lee)
- splenopexy (**SPLEE** noh pek see)
- T cells
- T lymphocytes (**LIM** foh sights)
- thalassemia (thal ah **SEE** mee ah)
- thoracic (tho **RASS** ik) duct
- thrombin (**THROM** bin)
- thrombocytes (**THROM** boh sights)
- thrombocytopenia (**THROM** boh sigh toh pen ee ah)
- thrombocytosis (throm boh sigh **TOH** sis)
- thrombolytic (throm boh **LIT** ik)
- thromboplastin (throm boh **PLAS** tin)
- thymectomy (thigh **MEK** toh mee)
- thymoma (thigh **MOH** mah)
- thymosin (thigh **MOH** sin)
- thymus (**THIGH** mus) gland
- tonsillectomy (ton sih **LEK** toh mee)
- tonsillitis (ton sil **EYE** tis)
- tonsils (**TON** sulls)
- toxins
- type A
- type AB
- type and crossmatch
- type B
- type O
- universal donor
- universal recipient
- urea (yoo **REE** ah)
- urticaria (er tih **KAY** ree ah)
- vaccinations (vak sih **NAY** shuns)
- valves
- vasoconstrictors (vasz oh con **STRICT** orz)
- viruses
- Western blot
- white blood cell count
- white blood cell differential (diff er **EN** shal)
- white blood cells
- whole blood

# Case Study

## Discharge Summary

**Admitting Diagnosis:** Splenomegaly, weight loss, diarrhea, fatigue, chronic cough

**Final Diagnosis:** Non-Hodgkin's lymphoma, primary site spleen; splenectomy

**History of Present Illness:** Patient is a 36-year-old businessman who was first seen in the office with complaints of feeling generally "run down," intermittent diarrhea, weight loss, and, more recently, a dry cough. He states he has been aware of these symptoms for approximately 6 months, but admits it may have been "coming on" for closer to 1 year. A screening test for mononucleosis was negative. A chest X-ray was negative for pneumonia or bronchitis, but did reveal suspicious nodules in the left thoracic cavity. In spite of a 35-pound weight loss, he has abdominal swelling and splenomegaly detected with abdominal palpation. He was admitted to the hospital for further evaluation and treatment.

**Summary of Hospital Course:** Blood tests were negative for the Epstein–Barr virus and hepatitis B. Abdominal ultrasound confirmed generalized splenomegaly and located a 3-cm encapsulated tumor. A lymphangiogram identified the thoracic nodules to be enlarged lymph glands. Biopsies taken from the spleen tumor and thoracic lymph glands confirmed the diagnosis of non-Hodgkin's lymphoma. A full body MRI failed to demonstrate any additional metastases in the liver or brain. The patient underwent splenectomy for removal of the primary tumor.

**Discharge Plans:** Patient was discharged home following recovery from the splenectomy. The abdominal swelling and diarrhea were resolved, but the dry cough persisted. He was referred to an oncologist for evaluation and establishment of a chemotherapy and radiation therapy protocol to treat the metastatic thoracic lympadenomas and ongoing surveillance for additional metastases.

## Critical Thinking Questions

1. What complaints caused the patient to go to the doctor?
2. Explain in your own words what negative, as in "chest X-ray was negative for pneumonia," means.
3. This discharge summary contains four medical terms that have not been introduced yet. Describe each of these terms in your own words. Use your text as a dictionary.
   a. primary site
   b. encapsulated
   c. ascites
   d. metastases
4. What is the name of a diagnostic procedure that produces an image from high-frequency sound waves? The procedure is _____ .
5. Which of the following pathological conditions was discovered using this procedure?
   a. inflammatory liver disease
   b. an acute infection with a large number of lymphocytes
   c. a malignant tumor of the thymus gland
   d. an enlarged spleen
6. What diagnostic test failed to find any cancer in other organs of the body? Which organs are free of cancer?
7. When the patient was discharged from the hospital, which symptoms were resolved and which persisted?

   Resolved:

   Persisted:

# Chart Note Transcription

## Chart Note

The chart note below contains 10 phrases that can be reworded with a medical term that you learned in this chapter. Each phrase is identified with an underline. Determine the medical term and write your answers in the space provided.

**Current Complaint:** Patient is a 22-year-old female referred to the specialist in treating blood disorders① by her internist. Her complaints include fatigue, weight loss, and easy bruising.

**Past History:** Patient had normal childhood diseases. She is a college student and was feeling well until symptoms gradually appeared starting approximately 3 months ago.

**Signs and Symptoms:** An immunoassay test for AIDS② was normal. The measure of the blood's coagulation abilities③ indicated that the blood took too long to form a clot. A blood test to count all the blood cells④ reported too few red blood cells⑤ and too few clotting cells.⑥ There were too many white blood cells,⑦ but they were immature and atypical. A sample of bone marrow obtained for microscopic examination⑧ found an excessive number of immature white blood cells.

**Diagnosis:** Cancer of the white blood cell forming bone marrow.⑨

**Treatment:** Aggressive chemotherapy for the cancer of the white blood cell forming bone marrow⑩ and replacement blood from another person to replace the erythrocytes and platelets.

1. _____

2. _____

3. _____

4. _____

5. _____

6. _____

7. _____

8. _____

9. _____

10. _____

# Practice Exercises

## A. Complete the following statements.

1. The study of the blood is called _____ .

2. The organs of the lymphatic system other than lymphatic vessels and lymph nodes are the
   _____ , _____ , and _____ .

3. The two lymph ducts are the _____ and _____ .

4. The primary concentrations of lymph nodes are the _____ , _____ ,
   _____ , and _____ regions.

5. The process whereby cells ingest and destroy bacteria within the body is _____ .

6. The formed elements of blood are the _____ , _____ , and _____ .

7. The fluid portion of blood is called _____ .

## B. State the terms described using the combining forms provided.

The combining form *splen/o* refers to the spleen. Use it to write a term that means

1. enlargement of the spleen _____

2. surgical removal of the spleen _____

3. suture of the spleen _____

4. incision into the spleen _____

5. tumor of the spleen _____

6. softening of the spleen _____

The combining form *lymph/o* refers to the lymph. Use it to write a term that means

7. lymph cells _____

8. tumor of the lymph system _____

The combining form *lymphaden/o* refers to the lymph glands. Use it to write a term that means

9. disease of a lymph gland _____

10. tumor of a lymph gland _____

11. inflammation of a lymph gland _____

The combining form *immun/o* refers to the immune system. Use it to write a term that means

12. specialist in the study of the immune system _____

13. immune protein _____

14. study of the immune system _____

The combining form *hemat/o* refers to blood. Use it to write a term that means

15. too few blood cells _____

16. relating to the blood _____

17. blood tumor or mass _____

18. blood formation _____

The combining form *hem/o* refers to blood. Use it to write a term that means

19. blood standing still _____

20. blood destruction _____

**C. Use the following suffixes to create a medical term for the following definitions.**

-penia   -globin   -cytosis   -cyte   -globulin

1. too few white cells _____
2. too few red (cells) _____
3. too few clotting cells _____
4. too few lymph cells _____
5. increase in white cells _____
6. increase in red cells _____
7. increase in clotting cells _____
8. blood protein _____
9. immunity protein _____
10. red cell _____
11. white cell _____
12. lymph cell _____

**D. Write the combining form for each term and use it to form a medical term.**

| | | Combining Form | Medical Term |
|---|---|---|---|
| 1. | bone marrow | _____ | _____ |
| 2. | clot | _____ | _____ |
| 3. | blood | _____ | _____ |
| 4. | gland | _____ | _____ |
| 5. | poison | _____ | _____ |
| 6. | eat/swallow | _____ | _____ |
| 7. | lymph vessel | _____ | _____ |
| 8. | tonsils | _____ | _____ |
| 9. | spleen | _____ | _____ |
| 10. | lymph | _____ | _____ |

**E. Identify the following abbreviations.**

1. basos _____
2. CBC _____
3. Hgb _____
4. PT _____
5. GVHD _____
6. RBC _____
7. PCV _____
8. ESR _____
9. diff _____
10. lymphs _____
11. AIDS _____
12. ARC _____
13. HIV _____

14. ALL _____

15. BMT _____

16. mono _____

17. KS _____

## F. Match the terms in column A with the definitions in column B.

| A | | B | |
|---|---|---|---|
| 1. _____ allergy | | a. | abnormal |
| 2. _____ Rh-positive | | b. | stimulates antibody formation |
| 3. _____ phagocytosis | | c. | decreased RBCs |
| 4. _____ atypical | | d. | mass of blood |
| 5. _____ corticosteroid | | e. | hypersensitivity |
| 6. _____ hematoma | | f. | engulfing |
| 7. _____ anemia | | g. | protective blood protein |
| 8. _____ antibody | | h. | strong anti-inflammatory properties |
| 9. _____ antigen | | i. | presence of blood factor |

## G. Match the terms in column A with the definitions in column B.

| A | | B | |
|---|---|---|---|
| 1. _____ thalassemia | | a. | fluid portion of blood |
| 2. _____ nosocomial | | b. | neutrophil |
| 3. _____ A, B, AB, O | | c. | clotting time test |
| 4. _____ plasma | | d. | blood type |
| 5. _____ serum | | e. | necessary for forming a blood clot |
| 6. _____ phagocyte | | f. | type of anemia |
| 7. _____ hematocrit | | g. | RBCs in total volume |
| 8. _____ prothrombin time | | h. | infection acquired in the hospital |
| 9. _____ vaccination | | i. | has no clotting factors |
| 10. _____ fibrinogen | | j. | immunization |

## H. Use the following terms in the sentences below.

| | | |
|---|---|---|
| Kaposi's sarcoma | mononucleosis | Hodgkin's disease |
| polycythemia vera | anaphylactic shock | AIDS |
| *Pneumocystis carinii* | HIV | peritonsillar abscess |

1. The condition characterized by the production of too many red blood cells is called _____ .

2. The Epstein–Barr virus is thought to be responsible for what infectious disease? _____

3. A life-threatening allergic reaction is _____ .

4. The virus responsible for causing AIDS is _____ .

5. A cancer that is seen frequently in AIDS patients is _____ .

6. An ELISA is used to test for _____ .

7. Malignant tumors concentrate in lymph nodes with this disease: _____ .

8. A type of pneumonia seen in AIDS patients is _____ pneumonia.

9. _____ is also known as quinsy sore throat.

# Professional Journal

In this exercise you will now have an opportunity to put the words you have learned into practice. Imagine yourself in the role of a Clinical Laboratory Scientist. If you refer back to the Professional Profile at the beginning of this chapter, you will see that this health care professional is responsible for performing a variety of tests using laboratory equipment, microscopes, and computers. Use the 10 words listed below, or any other new terms from this chapter, to write sentences to describe the patients you saw today.

An example of a sentence is *The results from the* **CBC** *confirmed that the patient has* **pancytopenia**.

1. aplastic anemia _____

2. blood culture and sensitivity _____

3. bone marrow aspiration _____

4. phlebotomy _____

5. ELISA _____

6. erythropenia _____

7. leukocytosis _____

8. leukemia _____

9. thrombolytic _____

10. hyperlipidemia _____

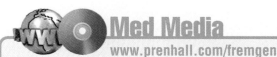

## Med Media
www.prenhall.com/fremgen

Use the CD-ROM enclosed with your textbook to gain additional reinforcement through interactive word building exercises, spelling games, labeling activities, and additional quizzes.

Use the above address to access the free, interactive Companion Website created for this textbook. Get hints, instant feedback, and textbook references to chapter-related multiple-choice questions, as well as labeling and matching exercises. In addition, you will find an audio glossary, case studies, and Internet exploration exercises.

*For more information regarding blood, lymphatic, and immune diseases, visit the following websites:*

American Academy of Allergy, Asthma and Immunology at **www.aaaai.org**

American Society of Hematology at **www.hematology.org**

National Heart, Lung, and Blood Institute at **www.nhlbi.nih.gov**

Centers for Disease Control and Prevention—Health Topics A–Z at **www.cdc.gov**

Stanford Health Library: Diseases and Disorders of the Immune System at **www.healthlibrary.stanford.edu/resources/internet/bodysystems/immune.html**

# Chapter 7
# Respiratory System

## Learning Objectives

*Upon completion of this chapter, you will be able to:*

- Recognize the combining forms and suffixes introduced in this chapter.

- Gain the ability to pronounce medical terms and major anatomical structures.

- List the major organs of the respiratory system and their functions.

- Discuss the process of respiration.

- Build respiratory system medical terms from word parts.

- Define vocabulary, pathology, diagnostic, and therapeutic medical terms relating to the respiratory system.

- Recognize types of medications associated with the respiratory system.

- Interpret abbreviations associated with the respiratory system.

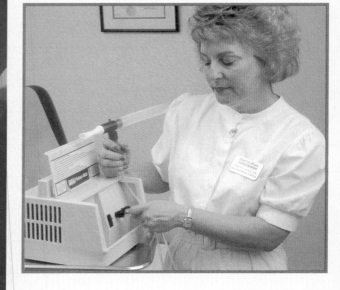

## MedMedia
www.prenhall.com/fremgen
Additional interactive resources and activities for this chapter can be found on the Companion Website. For animations, audio glossary, and review, access the accompanying CD-ROM in this book.

## Professional Profile

### Respiratory Therapy

Respiratory therapists assist patients with respiratory illness and cardiopulmonary disorders. They carry out a wide variety of duties that include performing tests to assess pulmonary function, monitoring oxygen and carbon dioxide levels in the blood, administering breathing treatments, and educating the public on respiratory issues. Often, respiratory therapists are called in to handle emergency situations. They may be responsible for treating victims in distress such as premature babies and drowning victims. Respiratory therapy services are found in acute and long-term care facilities, health maintenance organizations, and home health agencies.

### Registered Respiratory Therapist (RRT)

- Develops and implements respiratory care plans, performs diagnostic tests, provides respiratory treatments, and participates in patient education
- Provides respiratory therapy as ordered by a physician
- Graduates from an accredited 2-year associate or 4-year bachelor's degree respiratory therapy program
- Completes clinical training
- Passes the national registry examination

### Certified Respiratory Therapist (CRT)

- Performs general respiratory care procedures
- Works under the supervision of a physician or registered respiratory therapist
- Completes an accredited 2-year associate degree respiratory therapy program
- Completes clinical training
- Passes the national technician certification examination

***For more information regarding these health careers, visit the following websites:***
American Association for Respiratory Care at **www.aarc.org**
National Board for Respiratory Care at **www.nbrc.org**

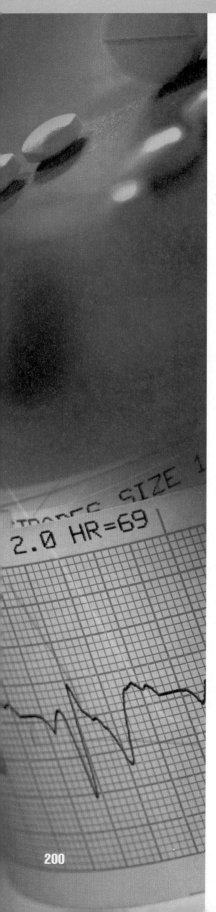

# Overview

## Organs of the Respiratory System

bronchial tubes
larynx
lungs
nose
pharynx
trachea

## Combining Forms Relating to the Respiratory System

| | | | |
|---|---|---|---|
| adenoid/o | adenoids | ox/o | oxygen |
| alveol/o | alveolus; air sac | pharyng/o | pharynx |
| anthrac/o | coal | pleur/o | pleura |
| atel/o | incomplete | pneum/o | lung, air |
| bronch/o | bronchus | pneumon/o | lung, air |
| bronchi/o | bronchus | pulmon/o | lung |
| bronchiol/o | bronchiole | rhin/o | nose |
| coni/o | dust | sinus/o | sinus, cavity |
| diaphragmat/o | diaphragm | spir/o | breathing |
| epiglott/o | epiglottis | steth/o | chest |
| laryng/o | larynx | tonsill/o | tonsils |
| lob/o | lobe | trache/o | trachea, windpipe |
| nas/o | nose | thorac/o | chest |
| orth/o | straight, upright | | |

## Suffixes Relating to the Respiratory System

| Suffix | Meaning | Example |
|---|---|---|
| -capnia | carbon dioxide | hypercapnia |
| -ectasis | dilated, expansion | bronchiectasis |
| -osmia | smell | anosmia |
| -phonia | voice | dysphonia |
| -pnea | breathing | apnea |
| -ptysis | spitting | hemoptysis |
| -thorax | chest | hemothorax |

# Anatomy and Physiology of the Respiratory System

| | | |
|---|---|---|
| bronchial tubes | inspiration | oxygen |
| carbon dioxide | larynx | pharynx |
| exhalation | lungs | trachea |
| expiration | metabolism | |
| inhalation | nose | |

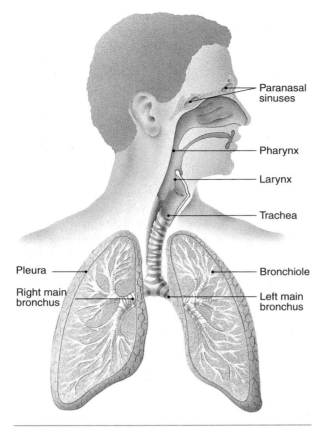

**■ FIGURE 7.1** The respiratory system.

Paranasal sinuses

Pharynx

Larynx

Trachea

Pleura

Right main bronchus

Bronchiole

Left main bronchus

The respiratory system consists of six major organs—the **nose, pharynx (FAIR** inks), **larynx (LAIR** inks), **trachea (TRAY** kee ah), **bronchial (BRONG** key all) **tubes**, and **lungs**—that function together to perform the mechanical and, for the most part, unconscious mechanism of respiration (see ■ Figure 7.1). The body cells require a constant exchange of fresh oxygen and the removal of carbon dioxide. The respiratory system works in conjunction with the cardiovascular system to deliver oxygen to all the cells of the body. The process of respiration must be continuous; interruption for even a few minutes can result in brain damage and/or death.

## Respiration

The process of respiration can be subdivided into three distinct parts: ventilation, external respiration, and internal respiration. Ventilation is the flow of air between the outside environment and the lungs. **Inhalation** (in hah **LAY** shun) is the flow of air into the lungs and **exhalation** (eks hah **LAY** shun) is the flow of air out of the lungs. Inhalation brings fresh **oxygen (OK** sih jen) ($O_2$) into the air sacs, while exhalation removes **carbon dioxide** ($CO_2$) from the body.

External respiration refers to the exchange of oxygen and carbon dioxide that takes place in the lungs. These gases diffuse in opposite directions between the air sacs of the lungs and the bloodstream. Oxygen enters the bloodstream from the air sacs to be delivered throughout the body. Carbon dioxide leaves the bloodstream and enters the air sacs to be expelled from the body during exhalation.

Internal respiration is the process of oxygen and carbon dioxide exchange at the cellular level. At this time oxygen leaves the bloodstream and is delivered

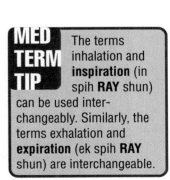

**MED TERM TIP** The terms inhalation and **inspiration** (in spih **RAY** shun) can be used interchangeably. Similarly, the terms exhalation and **expiration** (ek spih **RAY** shun) are interchangeable.

to the tissues. Oxygen is necessary for the body cells' **metabolism** (meh **TAB** oh lizm), all the physical and chemical changes within the body that are necessary for life. The by-product of metabolism is the formation of a waste product, carbon dioxide. The carbon dioxide enters the bloodstream from the tissues and is transported back to the lungs for disposal. Internal respiration is sometimes referred to as *tissue breathing* since the cells within the body also must breathe fresh oxygen or, in other words, have a fresh supply of oxygen to maintain life.

## Nose

| | | |
|---|---|---|
| cilia | nares | palate |
| mucous membrane | nasal cavity | paranasal sinuses |
| mucus | nasal septum | |

> **MED TERM TIP**
> The term *cilia* means hair, and there are other body systems that have cilia or cilia-like processes. For example, when discussing the eye, *cilia* means eyelashes.

The process of ventilation begins with the nose. Air enters the **nasal** (**NAY** zl) **cavity** through two external openings called the two **nares** (**NAIR** eez). The nasal cavity is divided down the middle by the **nasal** (**NAY** zl) **septum**, a cartilaginous plate. The **palate** (**PAL** at) in the roof of the mouth separates the nasal cavity above from the mouth below. The walls of the nasal cavity and the nasal septum are made up of flexible cartilage covered with **mucous** (**MYOO** kus) **membrane**. In fact, much of the respiratory tract is covered with mucous membrane, which secretes a sticky fluid, **mucus** (**MYOO** kus), which cleanses air by trapping dust and bacteria. Since this membrane is also wet, it moisturizes inhaled air as it passes by the surface of the cavity. Very small hairs or **cilia** (**SIL** ee ah) line the opening to the nose (as well as much of the airways), and these filter out large dirt particles before they can enter the nostrils.

> **MED TERM TIP**
> Anyone who has experienced a nosebleed, or *epistaxis*, is aware of the plentiful supply of blood vessels in the nose.

Capillaries in the mucous membranes warm inhaled air as it passes through the nasal cavities. The capillaries or small blood vessels cause the temperature to rise and bring the inhaled air to body temperature. In addition, several **paranasal sinuses** (pair ah **NAY** zl **SIGH** nus es) or air-filled cavities are located within the facial bones. The sinuses act as an echo chamber during sound production and give resonance to the voice.

## Pharynx

| | | |
|---|---|---|
| adenoidectomy | laryngopharynx | palatine tonsils |
| adenoids | lingual tonsils | pharyngeal tonsils |
| auditory tube | nasopharynx | tonsillectomy |
| eustachian tube | oropharynx | tonsils |

Air next enters the pharynx, also called the *throat*, which is used by both the respiratory system and the digestive system. At the end of the pharynx, air enters the trachea while food and liquids are shunted into the esophagus.

The pharynx is about a 5-inch-long tube consisting of three parts: the upper **nasopharynx** (nay zoh **FAIR** inks), middle **oropharynx** (or oh **FAIR** inks), and lower **laryngopharynx** (lair ring goh **FAIR** inks) (see ▪ Figure 7.2). Three pairs of **tonsils** (TON sulls), which are collections of lymphatic tissue, are located in the pharynx. Tonsils are strategically placed to help keep pathogens from entering the body in either the air we breathe or food and liquid we swallow. The nasopharynx, behind the nose, contains the **adenoids** (**ADD** eh noydz) or **pharyngeal tonsils** (fair **IN** jee al **TON** sulls). The oropharynx, behind the mouth, contains the **palatine tonsils** (**PAL** ah tine **TON** sulls) and the **lingual tonsils** (**LING** gwal **TON** sulls). Tonsils are considered a part of the lymphatic system and are discussed in Chapter 6.

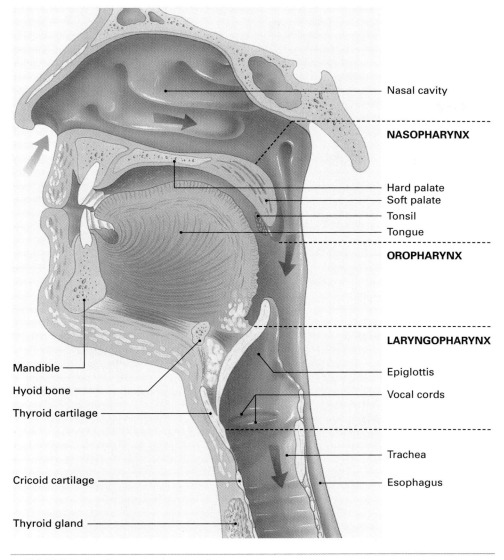

Nasal cavity

**NASOPHARYNX**

Hard palate
Soft palate
Tonsil
Tongue

**OROPHARYNX**

**LARYNGOPHARYNX**

Epiglottis

Vocal cords

Mandible

Hyoid bone

Thyroid cartilage

Trachea

Esophagus

Cricoid cartilage

Thyroid gland

**■ FIGURE 7.2**  Anatomy of upper airway.

> **MED TERM TIP**  *T&A* refers to a **tonsillectomy** (ton sih **LEK** toh mee) and **adenoidectomy** (add eh noyd **EK** toh mee). This procedure of removing the tonsils and the adenoids was once a fairly common childhood surgical procedure. It was thought that if the tonsils were removed, the child would not suffer as many throat and ear infections (see ■ Figure 7.3). However, with the advent of antibiotic treatment for these infections, the T&A procedure is less common. T&As are occasionally performed to correct snoring and breathing problems in adults.

The opening of the **eustachian** (yoo **STAY** she en) or **auditory tube** is also found in the nasopharynx. The other end of this tube is in the middle ear. Each time you swallow, this tube opens to equalize air pressure between the middle ear and the outside atmosphere.

## Larynx

**epiglottis**              **thyroid cartilage**
**glottis**                 **vocal cords**

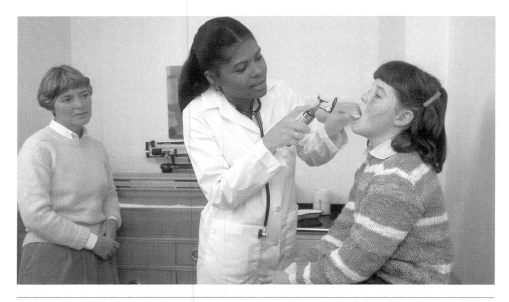

■ **FIGURE 7.3**   Examination of child's tonsils.

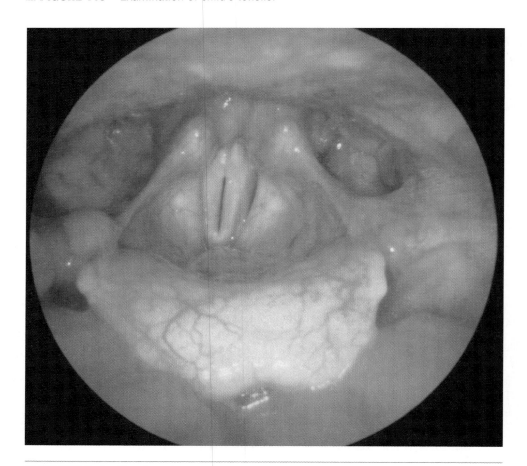

■ **FIGURE 7.4**   Vocal cords.
(CNRI/Phototake NYC)

The larynx or *voice box* is a muscular structure located between the pharynx and the trachea (refer to Figure 7.1). It contains the **vocal cords** (see ■ Figure 7.4). The vocal cords are not actually cord-like in structure. They are folds of membranous tissue that produce sound by vibrating as air passes through the **glottis** (**GLOT** iss), the opening between the two vocal cords.

A flap of cartilaginous tissue, the **epiglottis** (ep ih **GLOT** iss), sits above the glottis. The epiglottis provides protection against food and liquid being inhaled into the lungs since it covers the larynx and trachea during swallowing. This shunts food and liquid from the pharynx into the esophagus. The walls of the larynx are composed of several cartilage plates held together with ligaments and muscles. One of these cartilages, the **thyroid cartilage** (**THIGH** royd **CAR** tih lij), forms what is known as the *Adam's apple*. The thyroid cartilage is generally larger in the male than in the female and helps to produce the deeper voice of the male.

## Trachea

The trachea, also called the *windpipe*, is the passageway for air that extends from the pharynx and larynx down to the main bronchi. It measures approximately 4 inches in length and is composed of smooth muscle and cartilage rings. It is lined by mucous membrane and cilia. Therefore, it also assists in cleansing, warming, and moisturizing air as it travels to the lungs.

## Bronchial Tubes

**alveoli**            **bronchus**                    **respiratory membrane**

**bronchioles**        **pulmonary capillaries**

The distal end of the trachea divides to form the left and right main bronchi. Each **bronchus** (**BRONG** kus) enters one of the lungs and branches repeatedly to form secondary bronchi. Each branch becomes more narrow until the most narrow branches, the **bronchioles** (**BRONG** key ohlz), are formed. Each bronchiole terminates in a small group of air sacs, called **alveoli** (al **VEE** oh lye). Each lung has approximately 150 million alveoli (see ■ Figure 7.5). A network of **pulmonary capillaries** (**CAP** ih lair eez) from the pulmonary blood vessels

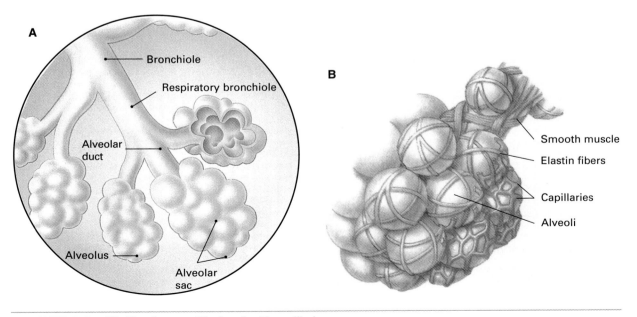

■ **FIGURE 7.5** (A) Alveolar sac; (B) alveoli with capillaries.

tightly encases each alveolus. In fact, the walls of the alveoli and capillaries are so tightly associated with each other they are referred to as a single unit, the **respiratory membrane.** External respiration, the exchange of oxygen ($O_2$) and carbon dioxide ($CO_2$) between the air within the alveolus and the blood inside the capillaries, takes place across the respiratory membrane.

>  **MED TERM TIP** The respiratory system can be thought of as an upside-down tree and its branches. The trunk of the tree consists of the pharynx, larynx, and trachea. The trachea then divides into two branches, the bronchi. Each bronchus divides into smaller and smaller branches. In fact, this branching system of tubes is referred to as the *bronchial tree.*

## Lungs

| | | |
|---|---|---|
| apex | mediastinum | pleural cavity |
| base | parietal pleura | serous fluid |
| hilum | pleura | visceral pleura |

**MED TERM TIP** Some of the abnormal lung sounds heard with a stethoscope, such as crackling and rubbing, are made when the parietal and/or visceral pleura become inflamed and rub against one another.

Each lung is the total collection of the bronchi, bronchioles, and alveoli. They are spongy to the touch because they contain air, like a balloon. The lungs are protected by a double membrane called the **pleura** (**PLOO** rah). The pleura's outer membrane is the **parietal** (pah **RYE** eh tal) **pleura**, which also lines the wall of the chest cavity. The inner membrane or **visceral** (**VISS** er al) **pleura** adheres to the surface of the lungs. The pleura is folded in such a way that it forms a sac around each lung referred to as the **pleural cavity.** There is normally slippery, watery **serous** (**SEER** us) **fluid** between the two layers of the pleura that reduces friction when the two layers rub together during ventilation.

The lungs contain divisions or lobes. There are three lobes in the larger right lung and two in the left lung. The pointed superior portion of each lung is the **apex,** while the broader lower area is the **base.** Entry of structures like the bronchi, pulmonary blood vessels, and nerves into each lung occurs along its medial border in an area called the **hilum** (**HYE** lum). The lungs within the thoracic cavity are protected from puncture and damage by the ribs. The area between the right and left lung is called the **mediastinum** (mee dee ass **TYE** num). The mediastinum contains the heart, aorta, esophagus, thymus gland, and main bronchi. See ■ Figure 7.6 for an illustration of the chest cavity.

## Respiratory Muscles

| | | |
|---|---|---|
| diaphragm | diaphragmatic breathing | intercostal muscles |

The lungs are able to move air in and out due to the difference between the atmospheric pressure and the pressure within the chest cavity. Actually, the **diaphragm** (**DYE** ah fram), which is the muscle separating the abdomen from the thoracic cavity, is able to produce the necessary difference in pressure. To do this the diaphragm contracts and moves down into the abdominal cavity, which causes a decrease of pressure, or negative thoracic pressure, within the chest cavity. Air can then enter the lungs to equalize the pressure during inhalation. The **intercostal** (in ter **COS** tal) **muscles** between the ribs assist in inhalation by raising the rib cage to enlarge the thoracic cavity. The diaphragm and intercostal muscles relax and the thoracic cavity becomes smaller. When this happens, pressure within the cavity increases and air is pushed out of the lungs, resulting in exhalation. Therefore, a quiet, unforced exhalation is a passive process since it does not require any muscle contraction. See ■ Figure 7.7

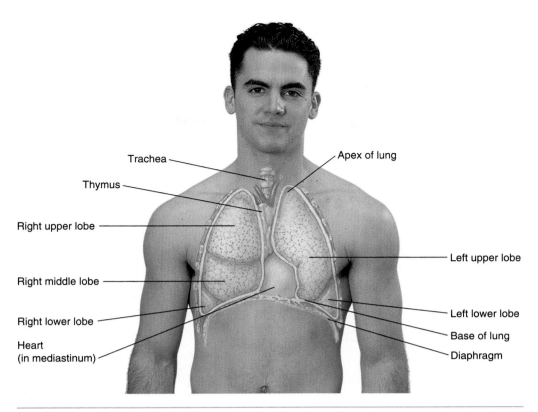

Trachea

Thymus

Right upper lobe

Right middle lobe

Right lower lobe

Heart
(in mediastinum)

Apex of lung

Left upper lobe

Left lower lobe

Base of lung

Diaphragm

**FIGURE 7.6**   The location of the lungs in the thoracic cavity.

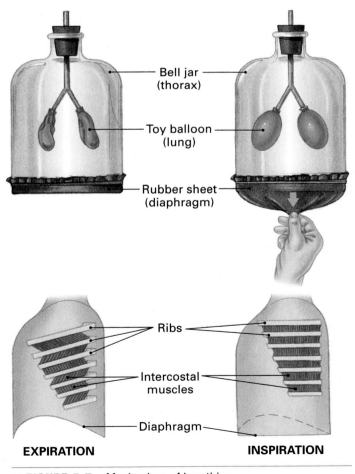

Bell jar
(thorax)

Toy balloon
(lung)

Rubber sheet
(diaphragm)

Ribs

Intercostal
muscles

Diaphragm

**EXPIRATION**

**INSPIRATION**

**FIGURE 7.7**   Mechanism of breathing.

for an illustration of the mechanism of breathing. When a forceful inhalation or exhalation is required, additional chest and neck muscles become active.

 **Diaphragmatic** (dye ah frag **MAT** ik) **breathing** is taught to singers and public speakers. You can practice this type of breathing by allowing your abdomen to expand during inspiration and contract during expiration while your shoulders remain motionless.

## Lung Volumes and Capacities

For some types of medical conditions, such as emphysema, it is important to know the lung capacity and the volume of air that is actually flowing in and out of the lungs. The actual volume of air exchanged in breathing is measured by respiratory therapists to aid in determining the functioning level of the respiratory system. Terminology relating to this measurement is listed in Table 7.1. This volume is measured with pulmonary function equipment.

## Respiratory Rate

### vital signs

**MED TERM TIP** When divers wish to hold their breath longer, they first hyperventilate (breath faster and deeper) in order to get rid of as much $CO_2$ as possible. This will hold off the urge to breath longer, allowing a diver to stay submerged longer.

The respiratory rate is one of our **vital signs** (VS), along with heart rate, temperature, and blood pressure. Respiratory rate is dependent on the level of $CO_2$ in the blood. When the $CO_2$ level is high, we breathe more rapidly to expel the excess. However, if $CO_2$ levels drop, our respiratory rate will also drop.

When a respiratory rate falls outside the range of normal, it could indicate an illness or medical condition. For example, when a patient is running an elevated temperature and has shortness of breath (SOB) due to pneumonia, the respiratory rate may increase dramatically. However, some medications, pain medications in particular, can cause a decrease in the respiratory rate. See Table 7.2 for respiratory rate ranges for different age groups.

| Table 7.1 | Lung Volumes and Capacities |
| --- | --- |
| **Term** | **Definition** |
| Tidal volume (TV) | The amount of air that enters the lungs in a single inhalation or leaves the lungs in a single exhalation of quiet breathing. In an adult this is normally 500 cc.* |
| Inspiratory reserve volume (IRV) | The air that can be forcibly inhaled after a normal respiration has taken place. Also called *complemental air*; generally measures around 3,000 cc.* |
| Expiratory reserve volume (ERV) | The amount of air that can be forcibly exhaled after a normal quiet respiration. This is also called *supplemental air*; approximately 1,000 cc.* |
| Residual volume (RV) | The air remaining in the lungs after a forced exhalation; about 1,500 cc* in the adult. |
| Inspiratory capacity (IC) | The volume of air inhaled after a normal exhale. |
| Functional residual capacity (FRC) | The air that remains in the lungs after a normal exhalation has taken place. |
| Vital capacity (VC) | The total volume of air that can be exhaled after a maximum inhalation. This amount will be equal to the sum of TV, IRV, and ERV. |
| Total lung capacity (TLC) | The volume of air in the lungs after a maximal inhalation. |

*There is a normal range for measurements of the volume of air exchanged. The numbers given are for the average measurement.

## Table 7.2 Respiratory Rates for Different Age Groups

| Age | Respirations per Minute |
| --- | --- |
| Newborn | 30–60 |
| 1-year-old | 18–30 |
| 16-year-old | 16–20 |
| Adult | 12–20 |

# Word Building Relating to the Respiratory System

The following list contains examples of medical terms built directly from word parts. The definition for these terms can be determined by a straightforward translation of the word parts.

| Combining Form | Combined With | Medical Term | Definition |
| --- | --- | --- | --- |
| bronch/o | -gram | bronchogram (**BRONG** koh gram) | record of the bronchus |
| | -itis | bronchitis (brong **KIGH** tis) | inflammation of a bronchus |
| | -plasty | bronchoplasty (**BRONG** koh plas tee) | surgical repair of a bronchus |
| | -scope | bronchoscope (**BRONG** koh scope) | instrument to view inside of bronchus |
| | -spasm | bronchospasm (BRONG koh spazm) | involuntary muscle spasm of bronchi |
| bronchi/o | -ectasis | bronchiectasis (brong key **EK** tah sis) | dilated bronchi |
| laryng/o | -ectomy | laryngectomy (lair in **JEK** toh mee) | excision of the voice box |
| | -itis | laryngitis (lair in **JYE** tis) | inflammation of the voice box |
| | -plasty | laryngoplasty (lair **RING** goh plas tee) | surgical repair of the voice box |
| | -plegia | laryngoplegia (lair **RING** goh plee gee ah) | paralysis of the voice box |
| | -spasm | laryngospasm (lair **RING** goh spazm) | muscle spasms in the voice box |
| lob/o | -ectomy | lobectomy (loh **BEK** toh mee) | excision of a (lung) lobe |
| ox/o | an- -ia | anoxia (ah **NOK** see ah) | condition of no oxygen |
| | hypo- -emia | hypoxemia (high pox **EE** mee ah) | insufficient oxygen in the blood |
| | hypo- -ia | hypoxia (high **POX** ee ah) | insufficient oxygen |
| pleur/o | -centesis | pleurocentesis (ploor oh sen **TEE** sis) | puncture of the pleura |
| | -pexy | pleuropexy (**PLOOR** oh pek see) | surgical fixation of the pleura |
| pulmon/o | -logy | pulmonology (pul mon **ALL** oh jee) | study of the lung |
| | -ary | pulmonary (**PULL** mon air ee) | pertaining to the lung |
| rhin/o | -itis | rhinitis (rye **NYE** tis) | inflammation of the nose |
| | myc/o -osis | rhinomycosis (rye noh my **KOH** sis) | abnormal condition of nose fungus |
| | -plasty | rhinoplasty (**RYE** noh plas tee) | surgical repair of the nose |
| | -rrhagia | rhinorrhagia (rye noh **RAH** jee ah) | rapid flow (of blood) from the nose |
| | -rrhea | rhinorrhea (rye noh **REE** ah) | nose discharge |
| sinus/o | pan- -itis | pansinusitis (pan sigh nus **EYE** tis) | inflammation of all the sinuses |

*continued...*

| Combining Form | Combined With | Medical Term | Definition |
|---|---|---|---|
| thorac/o | -algia | thoracalgia (thor ah **KAL** jee ah) | chest pain |
| | -ic | thoracic (tho **RASS** ik) | pertaining to the chest |
| | -otomy | thoracotomy (thor ah **KOT** oh mee) | incision into the chest |
| trache/o | endo- -al | endotracheal (en doh **TRAY** kee al) | pertaining to inside the trachea |
| | -ostomy | tracheostomy (tray kee **OSS** toh mee) | create an opening in the trachea |
| | -otomy | tracheotomy (tray kee **OTT** oh mee) | incision into the trachea |
| | -stenosis | tracheostenosis (tray kee oh steh **NOH** sis) | narrowing of the trachea |

| Suffix | Combined With | Medical Term | Definition |
|---|---|---|---|
| -phonia | a- | aphonia (a **FOH** nee ah) | no voice |
| | dys- | dysphonia (dis **FOH** nee ah) | abnormal voice |
| -capnia | a- | acapnia (a **CAP** nee ah) | lack of carbon dioxide |
| | hyper- | hypercapnia (high per **CAP** nee ah) | excessive carbon dioxide |
| -pnea | a- | apnea (**AP** nee ah) | not breathing |
| | brady- | bradypnea (bray **DIP** nee ah) | slow breathing |
| | dys- | dyspnea (**DISP** nee ah) | difficult, labored breathing |
| | eu- | eupnea (yoop **NEE** ah) | normal breathing |
| | hyper- | hyperpnea (high per **NEE** ah) | excessive (deep) breathing |
| | hypo- | hypopnea (high **POP** nee ah) | insufficient (shallow) breathing |
| | ortho- | orthopnea (or **THOP** nee ah) | (sitting) straight breathing |
| | tachy- | tachypnea (tak ip **NEE** ah) | rapid breathing |
| -thorax | hem/o | hemothorax (hee moh **THOH** raks) | blood in the chest |
| | py/o | pyothorax (pye oh **THOH** raks) | pus in the chest |
| | pneum/o | pneumothorax (new moh **THOH** raks) | air in the chest |

# Vocabulary Relating to the Respiratory System

| | |
|---|---|
| **anosmia (ah NOZ mee ah)** | Loss of the sense of smell. |
| **asphyxia (as FIK see ah)** | Lack of oxygen that can lead to unconsciousness and death if not corrected immediately. Some of the common causes are drowning, foreign body in the respiratory tract, poisoning, and electric shock. |
| **auscultation (oss kull TAY shun)** | Process of listening for sounds within the body. Generally performed with an instrument to amplify sounds, such as a stethoscope. |
| **Cheyne–Stokes respiration (CHAIN STOHKS res pir AY shun)** | Abnormal breathing pattern in which there are long periods (10 to 60 seconds) of apnea followed by deeper, more rapid breathing. Named for John Cheyne, a Scottish physician, and Sir William Stokes, an Irish surgeon. |

| | |
|---|---|
| **endotracheal intubation (en doh TRAY kee al in too BAY shun)** | Placing a tube through the mouth, through the glottis, and into the trachea to create a patent airway (see ■ Figure 7.8). |
| **epistaxis (ep ih STAKS is)** | Nosebleed. |
| **hemoptysis (hee MOP tih sis)** | Coughing up blood or blood-stained sputum. |
| **hyperventilation (HYE per vent ill a shun)** | To breathe both fast (tachypnea) and deep (hyperpnea). |
| **hypoventilation (HYE poh vent ill a shun)** | To breathe both slow (bradypnea) and shallow (hypopnea). |
| **internist (in TUR nist)** | A physician who specializes in treating diseases and conditions of internal organs such as the respiratory system. |
| **nasal canula (CAN you lah)** | Two-pronged plastic device for delivering oxygen into the nose; one prong is inserted into each nares (see ■ Figure 7.9). |
| **otorhinolaryngology (oh toh rye noh lair in GOL oh jee) (ENT)** | Branch of medicine that treats conditions and diseases of the ear, nose, and throat region. |
| **patent (PAY tent)** | Open or unblocked, such as a patent airway. |
| **percussion (per KUH shun)** | Using the fingertips to tap on a surface to determine the condition beneath the surface. Determined in part by the feel of the surface as it is tapped and the sound generated. |
| **phlegm (FLEM)** | Thick mucus secreted by the membranes that line the respiratory tract. When phlegm is coughed through the mouth, it is called *sputum*. Phlegm is examined for color, odor, and consistency. |
| **pleural (PLOO ral) rub** | Grating sound made when the two layers of the pleura rub together during respiration. It is caused when one of the surfaces becomes thicker as a result of inflammation or other disease conditions. This rub can be felt through the fingertips when they are placed on the chest wall or heard through the stethoscope. |
| **pulmonologist (pull mon ALL oh jist)** | A physician who specializes in treating diseases and disorders of the respiratory system. |
| **purulent (PEWR yoo lent)** | Containing pus or an infection that is producing pus. Pus consists of dead bacteria, white blood cells, and tissue debris. |
| **rales (RALZ)** | Abnormal crackling sound made during inspiration. Usually indicates the presence of fluid or mucus in the airways. |
| **rhonchi (RONG kigh)** | Somewhat musical sound during expiration, often found in asthma or infection. Caused by spasms of the bronchial tubes. Also called *wheezing*. |
| **shortness of breath (SOB)** | Term used to indicate that a patient is having some difficulty breathing. The causes can range from mild SOB after exercise to SOB associated with heart disease. Refer to Figure 7.9 for illustration of patient receiving oxygen for SOB. |
| **sputum (SPEW tum)** | Mucus or phlegm that is coughed up from the lining of the respiratory tract. It is tested to determine what type of bacteria or virus is present as an aid in selecting the proper antibiotic treatment. |
| **stethoscope (STETH oh scope)** | An instrument used to listen to body sounds such as breath sounds or bowel sounds. |
| **stridor (STRIGH dor)** | Harsh, high-pitched, noisy breathing sound that is made when there is an obstruction of the bronchus or larynx. Found in conditions such as croup in children. |
| **thoracic (tho RASS ik) surgeon** | A physician who specializes in treating conditions and diseases of the respiratory system by surgical means. |

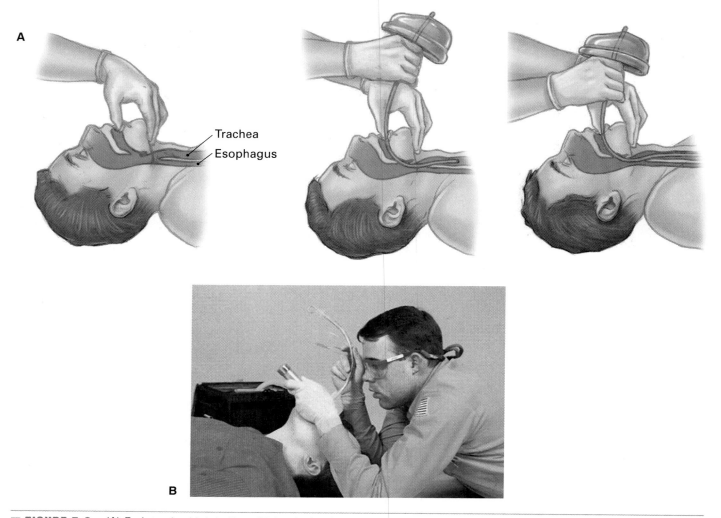

**A**

Trachea

Esophagus

**B**

**FIGURE 7.8**  (A) Endotracheal intubation; (B) intubation into the trachea to ensure an airway.

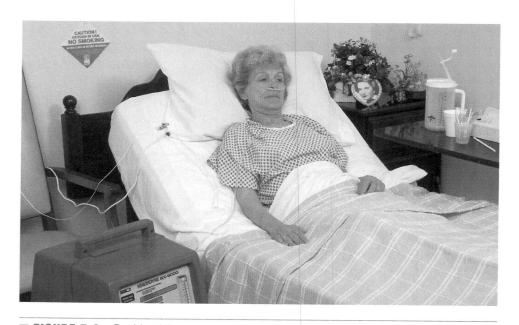

**FIGURE 7.9**  Residential oxygen container with nasal cannula.

# Pathology Relating to the Respiratory System

| | |
|---|---|
| **adult respiratory (RES pih rah tor ee) distress syndrome (ARDS)** | Acute respiratory failure in adults characterized by tachypnea, dyspnea, cyanosis, tachycardia, and hypoxemia. |
| **anthracosis (an thra KOH sis)** | A type of pneumoconiosis that develops from the collection of coal dust in the lung. Also called *black lung* or *miner's lung*. |
| **asbestosis (az bes TOH sis)** | A type of pneumoconiosis that develops from collection of asbestos fibers in the lungs. May lead to the development of lung cancer. |
| **asthma (AZ mah)** | Disease caused by various conditions, such as allergens, and resulting in constriction of the bronchial airways and labored respirations. Can cause violent spasms of the bronchi (bronchospasms) but is generally not a life-threatening condition. Medication can be very effective. |
| **atelectasis (at eh LEK tah sis)** | Condition in which the alveoli in a portion of the lung collapse, which prevents the respiratory exchange of oxygen and carbon dioxide. Can be caused by a variety of conditions, including pressure on the lung from a tumor or other object. |
| **bronchiectasis (brong key EK tah sis)** | Results from a dilation of a bronchus or the bronchi, and can be the result of infection. This abnormal stretching can be irreversible and result in destruction of the bronchial walls. The major symptom is a large amount of purulent (pus-filled) sputum. Rales (bubbling chest sound) and hemoptysis may be present. |
| **bronchogenic carcinoma (brong koh JEN ik car sin OH mah)** | Malignant lung tumor that originates in the bronchi. Usually associated with a history of cigarette smoking (see ▓ Figure 7.10). |
| **chronic obstructive pulmonary (PULL mon air ee) disease (COPD)** | Progressive, chronic, and usually irreversible condition in which the lungs have a diminished capacity for inspiration (inhalation) and expiration (exhalation). The person may have difficulty breathing upon exertion (dyspnea) and a cough. Also called *chronic obstructive lung disease (COLD)*. |
| **cor pulmonale (KOR pull moh NAY lee)** | Hypertrophy of the right ventricle of the heart as a result of chronic lung disease. |
| **croup (KROOP)** | Acute respiratory condition found in infants and children that is characterized by a barking type of cough or stridor. |
| **cystic fibrosis (SIS tik fye BROH sis)** | Hereditary condition that causes the exocrine glands to malfunction. The patient produces very thick mucus that causes severe congestion within the lungs and digestive system. Through more advanced treatment, many children are now living into adulthood with this disease. |
| **diaphragmatocele (dye ah frag MAT oh seel)** | Hernia in which the stomach protrudes through a hole in the diaphragm and puts pressure on the organs within the thoracic cavity. Also known as a *hiatal hernia*. |
| **diphtheria (dif THEAR ee ah)** | Bacterial upper respiratory infection characterized by the formation of a thick membranous film across the throat and a high mortality rate. Rare now due to the DPT (diphtheria, pertussis, tetanus) vaccine. |
| **emphysema (em fih SEE mah)** | Pulmonary condition characterized by the destruction of the walls of the alveoli resulting in a large, overexpanded air sac. Can occur as a result of long-term heavy smoking. Air pollution also worsens this disease. The patient may not be able to breathe except in a sitting or standing position. |
| **empyema (em pye EE mah)** | Pus within the pleural space, usually associated with an infection. |
| **histoplasmosis (his toh plaz MOH sis)** | Pulmonary infection caused by a fungus in dust in the droppings of pigeons and chickens. |

*continued...*

| | |
|---|---|
| **influenza (in floo EN za)** | Viral infection of the respiratory system characterized by chills, fever, body aches, and fatigue. Commonly called the *flu*. |
| **Legionnaire's (lee jen AYRZ) disease** | Severe, often fatal disease characterized by pneumonia and gastrointestinal symptoms. Caused by a bacteria and named after people who came down with it at an American Legion convention in 1976. |
| **paroxysmal nocturnal dyspnea (pah rok SIZ mal nok TUR nal disp NEE ah) (PND)** | Attacks of shortness of breath (SOB) that only occur at night and awaken the patient. |
| **pertussis (per TUH is)** | Commonly called *whooping cough*, due to the whoop sound made when coughing. An infectious disease that children receive immunization against as part of their DPT shots. |
| **pharyngitis (fair in JYE tis)** | Inflammation of the mucous membrane of the pharynx; usually caused by a viral or bacterial infection; commonly called a *sore throat*. |
| **pleural effusion (PLOO ral eh FYOO zhun)** | Abnormal presence of fluid in the pleural cavity. Physicians can detect the presence of fluid by tapping the chest (percussion) or listening with a stethoscope (auscultation). |
| **pleurisy (PLOOR ih see)** | Inflammation of the pleura. |
| **pneumoconiosis (noo moh koh nee OH sis)** | Condition that is the result of inhaling environmental particles that become toxic. Can be the result of inhaling coal dust (anthracosis) or asbestos (asbestosis). |
| ***Pneumocystis carinii* pneumonia (noo moh SIS tis kah RYE nee eye new MOH nee ah) (PCP)** | Pneumonia with a nonproductive cough, very little fever, and dyspnea. Seen in persons with weakened immune systems, such as AIDS patients. |
| **pneumonia (new MOH nee ah)** | Inflammatory condition of the lung that can be caused by bacterial and viral infections, diseases, and chemicals. Results in the filling of the alveoli and air spaces with fluid. |
| **pneumothorax (new moh THOH raks)** | Collection of air or gas in the pleural cavity, which may result in collapse of the lung (see ▓ Figure 7.11). |
| **pulmonary edema (PULL mon air ee eh DEE mah)** | Condition in which lung tissue retains an excessive amount of fluid. Results in labored breathing. |
| **pulmonary embolism (PULL mon air ee EM boh lizm)** | Blood clot or air bubble in the pulmonary artery or one of its branches. May cause an infarct in the lung tissue. |
| **rhinorrhea (rye noh REE ah)** | Watery discharge from the nose, especially with allergies or a cold. Commonly called a *runny nose*. |
| **silicosis (sil ih KOH sis)** | A type of pneumoconiosis that develops from the inhalation of silica (quartz) dust. |
| **sudden infant death syndrome (SIDS)** | Unexpected and unexplained death of an apparently well infant. |
| **tuberculosis (too ber kyoo LOH sis) (TB)** | Infectious disease caused by the tubercle bacillus, *Mycobacterium tuberculosis*. Most commonly affects the respiratory system and causes inflammation and calcification of the system. Tuberculosis is on the increase and is seen in many patients who have AIDS. |

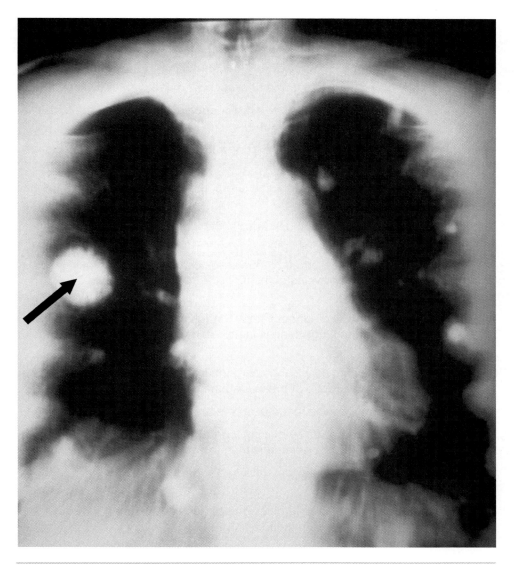

**FIGURE 7.10** X-ray of chest with lung cancer.
(CNR/Phototake NYC)

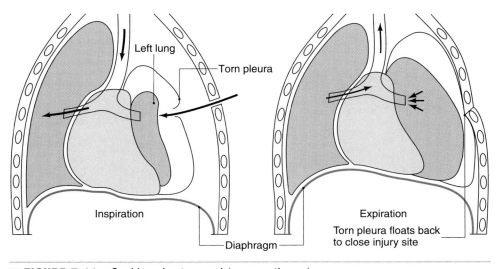

**FIGURE 7.11** Sucking chest wound (pneumothorax).

# Diagnostic Procedures Relating to the Respiratory System

| | |
|---|---|
| **arterial (ar TEE ree al) blood gases (ABGs)** | Testing for the gases present in the blood. Generally used to assist in determining the levels of oxygen ($O_2$) and carbon dioxide ($CO_2$) in the blood. |
| **bronchography (brong KOG rah fee)** | X-ray of the lung after a radiopaque substance has been inserted into the trachea or bronchial tube. |
| **bronchoscopy (brong KOSS koh pee) (Bronch)** | Using a bronchoscope to view inside the bronchi (see ■ Figure 7.12). |
| **chest X-ray (CXR)** | Taking a radiographic picture of the lungs and heart from the back and sides (see ■ Figure 7.13). |
| **laryngoscopy (lair in GOSS koh pee)** | Examination of the interior of the larynx with a lighted instrument. |
| **pulmonary angiography (PULL mon air ee an jee OG rah fee)** | Injecting dye into a blood vessel for the purpose of taking an X-ray of the arteries and veins of the lungs. |
| **pulmonary (PULL mon air ee) function test (PFT)** | A group of diagnostic tests that give information regarding air flow in and out of the lungs, lung volumes, and gas exchange between the lungs and bloodstream. |
| **spirometer (spy ROM eh ter)** | Instrument consisting of a container into which a patient can inhale or exhale for the purpose of measuring the air capacity of the lungs. |
| **spirometry (spy ROM eh tree)** | Using a device to measure the breathing capacity of the lungs. |
| **sputum (SPEW tum) culture and sensitivity (C&S)** | Testing sputum by placing it on a culture medium and observing any bacterial growth. The specimen is then tested to determine antibiotic effectiveness. |
| **sputum cytology (SPEW tum sigh TALL oh jee)** | Testing for malignant cells in sputum. |
| **sweat test** | A test for cystic fibrosis. Patients with this disease have an abnormally large amount of salt in their sweat. |
| **tuberculin (too BER kyoo lin) skin tests (TB test)** | Applying a chemical agent (Tine or Mantoux tests) under the surface of the skin to determine if the patient has been exposed to tuberculosis. |
| **ventilation-perfusion (per FUSE shun) scan** | A nuclear medicine diagnostic test that is especially useful in identifying pulmonary emboli. Radioactive air is inhaled for the ventilation portion to determine if air is filling the entire lung. Radioactive intravenous injection shows whether or not blood is flowing to all parts of the lung. |

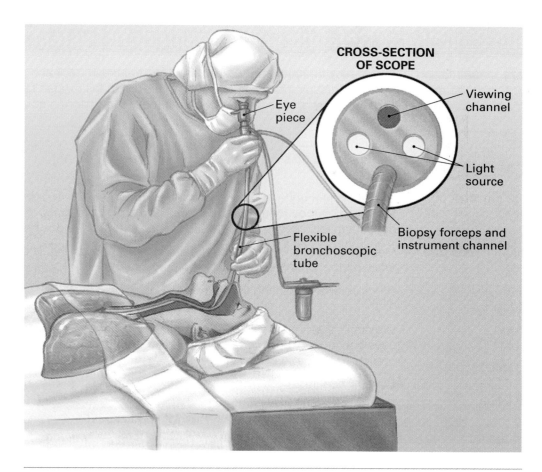

CROSS-SECTION OF SCOPE

Eye piece

Viewing channel

Light source

Biopsy forceps and instrument channel

Flexible bronchoscopic tube

■ **FIGURE 7.12** Bronchoscopy.

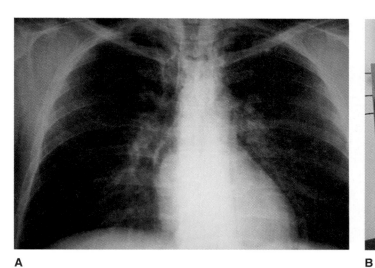

A

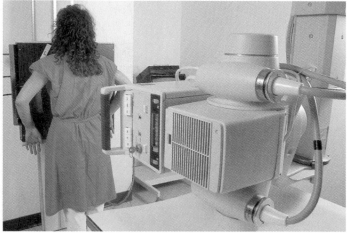

B

■ **FIGURE 7.13** (A) Normal chest X-ray.
(Charles Stewart and Associates)

(B) Patient receiving chest X-ray.
(Bachmann/Photo Researchers, Inc.)

# Therapeutic Procedures Relating to the Respiratory System

| | |
|---|---|
| **cardiopulmonary resuscitation (car dee oh PULL mon air ee ree suss ih TAY shun) (CPR)** | Emergency treatment provided by persons trained in CPR and given to patients when their respirations and heart stop. CPR provides oxygen to the brain, heart, and other vital organs until medical treatment can restore a normal heart and pulmonary function. |
| **Heimlich (HYME lik) maneuver** | Technique for removing a foreign body from the trachea or pharynx by exerting diaphragmatic pressure. Named for Harry Heimlich, an American thoracic surgeon. |
| **hyperbaric (high per BAR ik) oxygen therapy** | Use of oxygen under greater than normal pressure to treat cases of smoke inhalation, carbon monoxide poisoning, and other conditions. In some cases the patient is placed in a hyperbaric oxygen chamber for this treatment. |
| **intermittent positive pressure breathing (IPPB)** | Method for assisting patients in breathing using a mask that is connected to a machine that produces an increased pressure. |
| **pneumonectomy (noo moh NEK toh mee)** | Surgical removal of lung tissue (see ■ Figure 7.14). |
| **postural drainage** | Drainage of secretions from the bronchi by placing the patient in a position that uses gravity to promote drainage. Used for the treatment of cystic fibrosis, bronchiectasis, and before a lobectomy. |
| **thoracentesis (thor ah sen TEE sis)** | Surgical puncture of the chest wall for the removal of fluids (see ■ Figure 7.15). Also called *thoracocentesis*. |
| **thoracostomy (thor ah KOS toh mee)** | Insertion of a tube into the chest for the purpose of draining off fluid or air. Also called *chest tube*. |
| **tracheostomy (tray kee OSS toh mee)** | A surgical procedure, often performed in an emergency, that creates an opening directly into the trachea to allow the patient to breathe easier (see ■ Figure 7.16). |

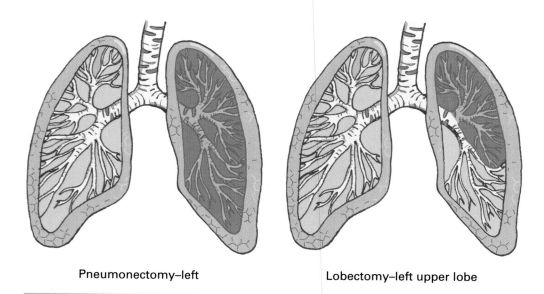

Pneumonectomy–left                    Lobectomy–left upper lobe

■ **FIGURE 7.14**  Lung resection: pneumonectomy and lobectomy.

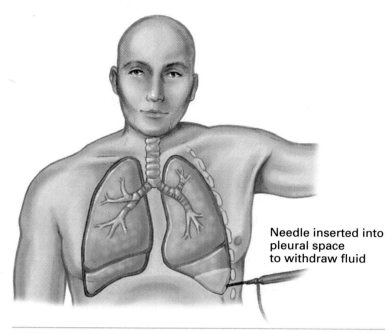

Needle inserted into
pleural space
to withdraw fluid

■ FIGURE 7.15　Thoracentesis.

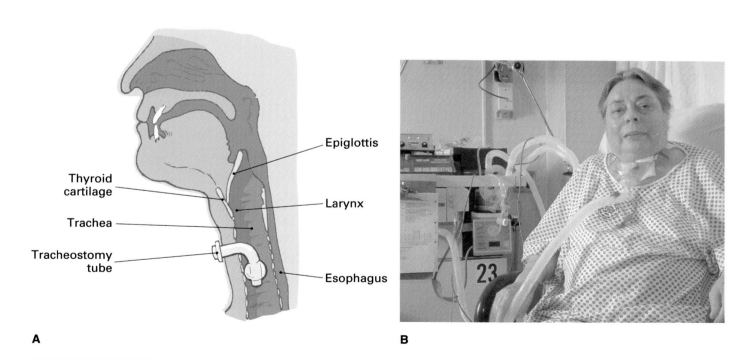

Epiglottis

Thyroid
cartilage

Larynx

Trachea

Tracheostomy
tube

Esophagus

**A**

**B**

■ FIGURE 7.16　(A) Tracheostomy tube in place; (B) patient with tracheostomy tube in place receiving oxygen through mask
placed over ostomy opening.
(Ansell Horn/Phototake NYC)

## Pharmacology Relating to the Respiratory System

| antibiotic (an tih bye AW tic) | Kills bacteria causing respiratory infections. |
|---|---|
| antihistamine (an tih HIST ah meen) | Blocks the effects of histamine that has been released by the body during an allergy attack. |
| antitussive (an tih TUSS ive) | Relieves urge to cough. |
| bronchodilator (BRONG koh dye late or) | Relaxes muscle spasms in bronchial tubes. Used to treat asthma. |
| decongestant (dee kon JES tant) | Reduces stuffiness and congestion throughout the respiratory system. |
| expectorant (ek SPEK toh rant) | Improves the ability to cough up mucus from the respiratory tract. |
| mucolytic (myoo koh LIT ik) | Liquefies mucus so it is easier to cough and clear it from the respiratory tract. |

## Abbreviations Relating to the Respiratory System

| | | | | |
|---|---|---|---|---|
| ABGs | arterial blood gases | IRV | inspiratory reserve volume |
| ARD | acute respiratory disease | LLL | left lower lobe |
| ARDS | adult respiratory distress syndrome | LUL | left upper lobe |
| ARF | acute respiratory failure | MV | minute volume |
| Bronch | bronchoscopy | O$_2$ | oxygen |
| CO$_2$ | carbon dioxide | PCP | *Pneumocystis carinii* pneumonia |
| COLD | chronic obstructive lung disease | PFT | pulmonary function test |
| COPD | chronic obstructive pulmonary disease | PND | paroxysmal nocturnal dyspnea (also postnasal drip) |
| CPR | cardiopulmonary resuscitation | | |
| C&S | culture and sensitivity | PPD | purified protein derivative (tuberculin test) |
| CTA | clear to auscultation | R | respiration |
| CXR | chest X-ray | RD | respiratory disease |
| DOE | dyspnea on exertion | RDS | respiratory distress syndrome |
| DPT | diphtheria, pertussis, tetanus injection | RLL | right lower lobe |
| ENT | ear, nose, and throat | RML | right middle lobe |
| ERV | expiratory reserve volume | RV | reserve volume |
| ET | endotracheal | RUL | right upper lobe |
| FEF | forced expiratory flow | SIDS | sudden infant death syndrome |
| FEV | forced expiratory volume | SOB | shortness of breath |
| FRC | functional residual capacity | T&A | tonsillectomy and adenoidectomy |
| FVC | forced vital capacity | TB | tuberculosis |
| HBOT | hyperbaric oxygen therapy | TLC | total lung capacity |
| HMD | hyaline membrane disease | TPR | temperature, pulse, and respiration |
| IC | inspiratory capacity | TV | tidal volume |
| IPPB | intermittent positive pressure breathing | URI | upper respiratory infection |
| IRDS | infant respiratory distress syndrome | VC | vital capacity |

# Chapter Review

## Pronunciation Practice

 You will find the pronunciation for each term on the enclosed CD-ROM. Check each one off as you master it.

- ❏ acapnia (a **CAP** nee ah)
- ❏ adenoidectomy (add eh noyd **EK** toh mee)
- ❏ adenoids (**ADD** eh noydz)
- ❏ adult respiratory (**RES** pih rah tor ee) distress syndrome
- ❏ alveoli (al **VEE** oh lye)
- ❏ anosmia (ah **NOZ** mee ah)
- ❏ anoxia (ah **NOK** see ah)
- ❏ anthracosis (an thra **KOH** sis)
- ❏ antibiotic (an tih bye **AW** tic)
- ❏ antihistamine (an tih **HIST** ah meen)
- ❏ antitussive (an tih **TUSS** ive)
- ❏ apex
- ❏ aphonia (a **FOH** nee ah)
- ❏ apnea (**AP** nee ah)
- ❏ arterial (ar **TEE** ree al) blood gases
- ❏ asbestosis (az bes **TOH** sis)
- ❏ asphyxia (as **FIK** see ah)
- ❏ asthma (**AZ** mah)
- ❏ atelectasis (at eh **LEK** tah sis)
- ❏ auditory tube
- ❏ auscultation (oss kull **TAY** shun)
- ❏ base
- ❏ bradypnea (bray **DIP** nee ah)
- ❏ bronchial (**BRONG** kee al) tubes
- ❏ bronchiectasis (brong key **EK** tah sis)
- ❏ bronchioles (**BRONG** key ohlz)
- ❏ bronchitis (brong **KIGH** tis)
- ❏ bronchodilator (**BRONG** koh dye late or)
- ❏ bronchogenic carcinoma (brong koh **JEN** ik car sin **OH** mah)
- ❏ bronchogram (**BRONG** koh gram)
- ❏ bronchography (brong **KOG** rah fee)
- ❏ bronchoplasty (**BRONG** koh plas tee)
- ❏ bronchoscope (**BRONG** koh scope)
- ❏ bronchoscopy (brong **KOSS** koh pee)
- ❏ bronchospasm (**BRONG** koh spazm)
- ❏ bronchus (**BRONG** kus)
- ❏ carbon dioxide
- ❏ cardiopulmonary resuscitation (car dee oh **PULL** mon air ee ree suss ih **TAY** shun)
- ❏ chest X-ray
- ❏ Cheyne–Stokes respiration (**CHAIN STOHKS** res pir **AY** shun)
- ❏ chronic obstructive pulmonary (**PULL** mon air ee) disease
- ❏ cilia (**SIL** ee ah)
- ❏ cor pulmonale (**KOR** pull moh **NAY** lee)
- ❏ croup (**KROOP**)
- ❏ cystic fibrosis (**SIS** tik fye **BROH** sis)
- ❏ decongestant (dee kon **JES** tant)
- ❏ diaphragm (**DYE** ah fram)
- ❏ diaphragmatic (dye ah frag **MAT** ik) breathing
- ❏ diaphragmatocele (dye ah frag **MAT** oh seel)
- ❏ diphtheria (dif **THEAR** ee ah)
- ❏ dysphonia (dis **FOH** nee ah)
- ❏ dyspnea (**DISP** nee ah)
- ❏ emphysema (em fih **SEE** mah)
- ❏ empyema (em pye **EE** mah)
- ❏ endotracheal (en doh **TRAY** kee al)
- ❏ endotracheal intubation (en doh **TRAY** kee al in too **BAY** shun)
- ❏ epiglottis (ep ih **GLOT** iss)
- ❏ epistaxis (ep ih **STAKS** is)
- ❏ eupnea (yoop **NEE** ah)
- ❏ eustachian (yoo **STAY** she en) tube
- ❏ exhalation (eks hah **LAY** shun)
- ❏ expectorant (ek **SPEK** toh rant)
- ❏ expiration (ek spih **RAY** shun)
- ❏ glottis (**GLOT** iss)
- ❏ Heimlich (**HYME** lik) maneuver

- hemoptysis (hee **MOP** tih sis)
- hemothorax (hee moh **THOH** raks)
- hilum (**HYE** lum)
- histoplasmosis (his toh plaz **MOH** sis)
- hyperbaric (high per **BAR** ik) oxygen therapy
- hypercapnia (high per **CAP** nee ah)
- hyperpnea (high per **NEE** ah)
- hyperventilation (**HYE** per vent ill a shun)
- hypopnea (high **POP** nee ah)
- hypoventilation (**HYE** poh vent ill a shun)
- hypoxemia (high pox **EE** mee ah)
- hypoxia (high **POX** ee ah)
- influenza (in floo **EN** za)
- inhalation (in hah **LAY** shun)
- inspiration (in spih **RAY** shun)
- intercostal (in ter **COS** tal) muscles
- intermittent positive pressure breathing
- internist (in **TUR** nist)
- laryngectomy (lair in **JEK** toh mee)
- laryngitis (lair in **JYE** tis)
- laryngopharynx (lair ring goh **FAIR** inks)
- laryngoplasty (lair **RING** goh plas tee)
- laryngoplegia (lair **RING** goh plee gee ah)
- laryngoscopy (lair in **GOSS** koh pee)
- laryngospasm (lair **RING** goh spazm)
- larynx (**LAIR** inks)
- Legionnaire's (lee jen **AYRZ**) disease
- lingual tonsils (**LING** gwal **TON** sulls)
- lobectomy (loh **BEK** toh mee)
- lungs
- mediastinum (mee dee ass **TYE** num)
- metabolism (meh **TAB** oh lizm)
- mucolytic (myoo koh **LIT** ik)
- mucous (**MYOO** kus) membrane
- mucus (**MYOO** kus)
- nares (**NAIR** eez)
- nasal canula (**NAY** zl **CAN** you lah)
- nasal (**NAY** zl) cavity
- nasal (**NAY** zl) septum
- nasopharynx (nay zoh **FAIR** inks)
- nose
- oropharynx (or oh **FAIR** inks)

- orthopnea (or **THOP** nee ah)
- otorhinolaryngology (oh toh rye noh lair in **GOL** oh jee)
- oxygen (**OK** sih jen)
- palate (**PAL** at)
- palatine tonsils (**PAL** ah tine **TON** sulls)
- pansinusitis (pan sigh nus **EYE** tis)
- paranasal sinuses (pair ah **NAY** zl **SIGH** nus es)
- parietal pleura (pah **RYE** eh tal **PLOO** rah)
- paroxysmal nocturnal dyspnea (pah rok **SIZ** mal nok **TUR** nal disp **NEE** ah)
- patent (**PAY** tent)
- percussion (per **KUH** shun)
- pertussis (per **TUH** sis)
- pharyngeal tonsils (fair **IN** jee al **TON** sulls)
- pharyngitis (fair in **JYE** tis)
- pharynx (**FAIR** inks)
- phlegm (**FLEM**)
- pleura (**PLOO** rah)
- pleural (**PLOO** ral) cavity
- pleural effusion (**PLOO** ral eh **FYOO** zhun)
- pleural (**PLOO** ral) rub
- pleurisy (**PLOOR** ih see)
- pleurocentesis (ploor oh sen **TEE** sis)
- pleuropexy (**PLOOR** oh pek see)
- pneumoconiosis (noo moh koh nee **OH** sis)
- *Pneumocystis carinii* pneumonia (noo moh **SIS** tis kah **RYE** nee eye new **MOH** nee ah)
- pneumonectomy (noo moh **NEK** toh mee)
- pneumonia (new **MOH** nee ah)
- pneumonomycosis (noo moh noh my **KOH** sis)
- pneumothorax (new moh **THOH** raks)
- postural drainage
- pulmonary (**PULL** mon air ee)
- pulmonary angiography (**PULL** mon air ee an jee **OG** rah fee)
- pulmonary capillaries (**PULL** mon air ee **CAP** ih lair eez)
- pulmonary edema (**PULL** mon air ee eh **DEE** mah)
- pulmonary embolism (**PULL** mon air ee **EM** boh lizm)
- pulmonary (**PULL** mon air ee) function test
- pulmonologist (pull mon **ALL** oh jist)
- pulmonology (pul mon **ALL** oh jee)
- purulent (**PEWR** yoo lent)

- pyothorax (pye oh **THOH** raks)
- rales (**RALZ**)
- respiratory membrane
- rhinitis (rye **NYE** tis)
- rhinomycosis (rye noh my **KOH** sis)
- rhinoplasty (**RYE** noh plas tee)
- rhinorrhagia (rye noh **RAH** jee ah)
- rhinorrhea (rye noh **REE** ah)
- rhonchi (**RONG** kigh)
- serous (**SEER** us) fluid
- shortness of breath
- silicosis (sill ih **KOH** sis)
- spirometer (spy **ROM** eh ter)
- spirometry (spy **ROM** eh tree)
- sputum (**SPEW** tum)
- sputum (**SPEW** tum) culture and sensitivity
- sputum cytology (**SPEW** tum sigh **TALL** oh jee)
- stethoscope (**STETH** oh scope)
- stridor (**STRIGH** dor)
- sudden infant death syndrome
- sweat test
- tachypnea (tak ip **NEE** ah)
- thoracalgia (thor ah **KAL** jee ah)
- thoracentesis (thor ah sen **TEE** sis)
- thoracic (tho **RASS** ik)
- thoracic surgeon (tho **RASS** ik)
- thoracostomy (thor ah **KOS** toh mee)
- thoracotomy (thor ah **KOT** oh mee)
- thyroid cartilage (**THIGH** royd **CAR** tin lij)
- tonsillectomy (ton sih **LEK** toh mee)
- tonsils (**TON** sulls)
- trachea (**TRAY** kee ah)
- tracheostenosis (tray kee oh steh **NOH** sis)
- tracheostomy (tray kee **OSS** toh mee)
- tracheotomy (tray kee **OTT** oh mee)
- tuberculin (too **BER** kyoo lin) skin tests
- tuberculosis (too ber kyoo **LOH** sis)
- ventilation-perfusion (per **FUSE** shun) scan
- visceral pleura (**VISS** er al **PLOO** rah)
- vital signs
- vocal cords

# Case Study

## Pulmonology Consultation Report

**Reason for Consultation:** Evaluation of increasingly severe asthma.

**History of Present Illness:** Patient is currently a 10-year-old male who first presented to the Emergency Room with dyspnea, coughing, and wheezing at 7 years of age. Paroxysmal attacks are increasing in frequency and there do not appear to be any precipitating factors such as exercise. No other family members are asthmatics.

**Results of Physical Examination:** Patient is currently in the ER with a paroxysmal attack with marked dyspnea, cyanosis around the lips, prolonged expiration, and a hacking cough producing thick, nonpurulent phlegm. Thoracic auscultation with stethoscope revealed rhonchi throughout bilateral lung fields. Chest X-ray shows poor pulmonary expansion, with hypoxemia indicated by ABG. A STAT pulmonary function test reveals moderately severe airway obstruction during expiration. This patient responded to oxygen therapy and IV Alupent and steroids, and he is beginning to cough less and breathe with less effort.

**Assessment:** Acute asthma attack with severe airway obstruction. There is no evidence of pulmonary infection. In view of increasing severity and frequency of attacks, all his medications should be reevaluated for effectiveness and all attempts to identify precipitating factors should be made.

**Recommendations:** Patient is to continue to use Alupent for relief of bronchospasms and steroids to reduce general inflammation. Instructions for taking medications and controlling severity of asthma attacks were carefully reviewed with the patient and his family. A referral to an allergist was made to evaluate this young man for presence of environmental allergies.

## Critical Thinking Questions

1. What does the medical term *paroxysmal* mean?
2. What do the following abbreviations stand for?
   a. IV
   b. STAT
   c. ABG
3. The patient was discharged and sent home with two medications. Explain in your own words the purpose of each of these medications.
4. What important information regarding this young man's asthma is unknown to the physician? What does this consulting physician recommend to address this problem?
5. Describe the characteristics related to this patient's cough in your own words.
6. Which of the following is not one of the symptoms seen in the emergency room?
   a. crackling lung sounds
   b. bluish skin
   c. difficulty breathing
   d. extended breathing out time

# Chart Note Transcription

## Chart Note

The chart note below contains 11 phrases that can be reworded with a medical term that you learned in this chapter. Each phrase is identified with an underline. Determine the medical term and write your answers in the space provided.

**Current Complaint:** A 43-year-old female was brought to the Emergency Room by her family. She complained of painful and labored breathing,① rapid breathing,② and fever. Symptoms began 3 days ago, but have become much worse during the past 12 hours.

**Past History:** Patient is a mother of three and a business executive. She has had no surgeries or previous serious illnesses.

**Signs and Symptoms:** Temperature is 103°F, respiratory rate is 20 breaths/minute, blood pressure is 165/98, and heart rate is 90 bpm. A blood test to measure the levels of oxygen in the blood③ indicates a marked low level of oxygen in the blood.④ The process of listening to body sounds⑤ of the lungs revealed abnormal crackling sounds⑥ over the left lower chest. She is producing large amounts of pus-filled⑦ mucus coughed up from the respiratory tract⑧ and a chest X-ray⑨ shows a large cloudy patch in the lower lobe of the left lung.

**Diagnosis:** Left lower lobe inflammatory condition of the lungs caused by bacterial infection.⑩

**Treatment:** Patient was started on intravenous antibiotics. She also required a tube placed through the mouth to create an airway ⑪ for 3 days.

1. _____

2. _____

3. _____

4. _____

5. _____

6. _____

7. _____

8. _____

9. _____

10. _____

11. _____

# Practice Exercises

## A. Complete the following statements.

1. The primary function of the respiratory system is _____ .

2. The movement of air in and out of the lungs is called _____ .

3. Define external respiration: _____ .

4. Define internal respiration: _____ .

5. The organs of the respiratory system are _____ , _____ , _____ , _____ , _____ , and _____ .

6. The passageway for food, liquids, and air is the _____ .

7. The _____ helps to keep food out of the respiratory tract.

8. The function of the cilia in the nose is to _____ .

9. The muscle that divides the thoracic cavity from the abdominal cavity is the _____ .

10. The respiratory rate for an adult is _____ to _____ respirations per minute.

11. The respiratory rate for a newborn is _____ to _____ respirations per minute.

12. The right lung has _____ lobes; the left lung has _____ lobes.

13. The air sacs at the ends of the bronchial tree are called _____ .

14. The term for the double membrane around the lungs is _____ .

15. The nasal cavity is separated from the mouth by the _____ .

16. The small branches of the bronchi are the _____ .

## B. State the terms described using the combining forms provided.

The combining form *rhin/o* refers to the nose. Use it to write a term that means

1. inflammation of the nose _____

2. rapid flow from the nose _____

3. discharge from the nose _____

4. surgical repair of the nose _____

The combining form *laryng/o* refers to the larynx or voice box. Use it to write a term that means

5. inflammation of the larynx _____

6. spasm of the larynx _____

7. visual examination of the larynx _____

8. pertaining to the larynx _____

9. incision of the larynx _____

10. excision of the larynx _____

11. surgical repair of the larynx _____

12. paralysis of the larynx _____

The combining form *bronch/o* refers to the bronchus. Use it to write a term that means

13. bronchial rapid flow _____

14. inflammation of the bronchus _____

15. visually examine the interior of the bronchus _____

16. bronchus disease _____

17. spasm of the bronchus _____

The combining form *thorac/o* refers to the chest. Use it to write a term that means

18. surgical repair of the chest _____

19. incision into the chest _____

20. chest pain _____

21. visual exam inside the chest _____

The combining form *trache/o* refers to the trachea. Use it to write a term that means

22. cutting into the trachea _____

23. surgical repair of the trachea _____

24. narrowing of the trachea _____

25. trachea disease _____

26. suture the trachea _____

27. inflammation of the trachea _____

28. forming an artificial opening into the trachea _____

## C. Define the following combining forms.

1. trache/o _____

2. laryng/o _____

3. bronch/o _____

4. spir/o _____

5. pneumon/o _____

6. rhin/o _____

7. py/o _____

8. pleur/o _____

9. epiglott/o _____

10. alveol/o _____

11. pulmon/o _____

12. tonsill/o _____

13. sinus/o _____

14. lob/o _____

15. nas/o _____

## D. Define each suffix and use it to form a term from the respiratory system.

| | Meaning | Respiratory Term |
|---|---|---|
| 1. -ectasis | _____ | _____ |
| 2. -capnia | _____ | _____ |
| 3. -phonia | _____ | _____ |
| 4. -thorax | _____ | _____ |

5. -pnea     _____     _____

6. -ptysis     _____     _____

7. -osmia     _____     _____

**E. The suffix -pnea means breathing. Use this suffix to write a medical term that means the following:**

1. normal breathing _____

2. difficult or labored breathing _____

3. rapid breathing _____

4. can breathe only in an upright position _____

5. lack of breathing _____

**F. Define the following terms.**

1. total lung capacity _____

2. tidal volume _____

3. residual volume _____

**G. Write the medical term for each definition.**

1. the process of breathing in _____

2. spitting up of blood _____

3. blood clot in the pulmonary artery _____

4. inflammation of a sinus _____

5. sore throat _____

6. air in the pleural cavity _____

7. paralysis of the bronchi _____

8. incision into the pleura _____

9. pain in the pleural region _____

10. hiatal hernia _____

**H. Write the abbreviations for the following terms.**

1. upper respiratory infection _____

2. pulmonary function test _____

3. left lower lobe _____

4. oxygen _____

5. carbon dioxide _____

6. intermittent positive pressure breathing _____

7. chronic obstructive lung disease _____

8. bronchoscopy _____

9. total lung capacity _____

10. tuberculosis _____

11. paroxysmal nocturnal dyspnea _____

## I. Identify the following abbreviations.

1. CXR _____

2. TV _____

3. TPR _____

4. ABGs _____

5. RD _____

6. RUL _____

7. SIDS _____

8. TLC _____

9. ARDS _____

10. HBOT _____

11. CTA _____

12. T & A _____

# Professional Journal

In this exercise you will now have an opportunity to put the words you have learned into practice. Imagine yourself in the role of a registered respiratory therapist. If you refer back to the Professional Profile at the beginning of this chapter, you will see that this health care professional is responsible for performing diagnostic tests, providing respiratory treatments, and participating in patient education. Use the 10 words listed below, or any other new terms from this chapter, to write sentences to describe the patients you saw today.

An example of a sentence is *Following the* **percussion** *treatment, the patient coughed up* **purulent sputum**.

1. oxygen _____

2. adult respiratory distress syndrome _____

3. asthma _____

4. pulmonary function test _____

5. CPR _____

6. cystic fibrosis _____

7. pneumothorax _____

8. dyspnea _____

9. auscultation _____

10. rhonchi _____

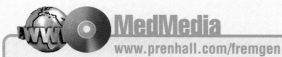

**MedMedia**
www.prenhall.com/fremgen

Use the CD-ROM enclosed with your textbook to gain additional reinforcement through interactive word building exercises, spelling games, labeling activities, and additional quizzes.

Use the above address to access the free, interactive Companion Website created for this textbook. Get hints, instant feedback, and textbook references to chapter-related multiple-choice questions, as well as labeling and matching exercises. In addition, you will find an audio glossary, case studies, and Internet exploration exercises.

***For more information regarding respiratory system diseases, visit the following websites:***

American College of Chest Physicians at **www.chestnet.org**

National Heart, Lung, and Blood Institute at **www.nhlbi.nih.gov**

Pulmonary Channel, an online Health Community at **www.pulmonologychannel.com**

American Lung Association at **www.lungusa.org**

# Chapter 8
# Digestive System

## Learning Objectives

*Upon completion of this chapter, you will be able to:*

- Recognize the combining forms and suffixes introduced in this chapter.
- Gain the ability to pronounce medical terms and major anatomical structures.
- List the major organs of the alimentary canal and their functions.
- Describe the function of the accessory organs of the digestive system.
- Identify the shape and function of each type of tooth.
- Build digestive system medical terms from word parts.
- Define vocabulary, pathology, diagnostic, and therapeutic medical terms relating to the digestive system.
- Recognize types of medications associated with the digestive system.
- Interpret abbreviations associated with the digestive system.

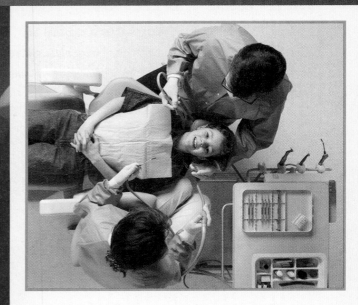

## MedMedia
www.prenhall.com/fremgen

Additional interactive resources and activities for this chapter can be found on the Companion Website. For animations, audio glossary, and review, access the accompanying CD-ROM in this book.

## Professional Profile

### Dental Care

Dental care workers provide care for patients' teeth, gums, tongue, lips, and jaw. Services include treating tooth and gum disease; filling cavities; fabricating and fitting crowns, bridges, and dentures; performing corrective surgery; correcting malocclusions (bad bite) with braces or other appliances; providing preventive care such as teeth cleaning and polishing; and educating the public in good oral hygiene practices.

### Dentist (DDS or DMD)

- Completes prerequisites for dental school at a 4-year college or university
- Graduates from an accredited 4-year dental college
- Receives either a doctor of dental surgery (DDS) or doctor of dental medicine (DMD) degree

### Orthodontist (DDS or DMD)

- Diagnosis, prevention, and treatment of dental and facial irregularities
- Receives a DDS or DMD degree on graduation from dental school
- Completes a minimum of 2 to 3 years of advanced training

### Registered Dental Hygienist (RDH)

- Works under the supervision of a dentist
- Specializes in cleaning teeth and taking X-rays
- Graduates from an accredited dental hygiene program

### Dental Assistant

- Assists with patient care or office management
- Completes on-the-job training, a community college or vocational training program

### Dental Laboratory Technician

- Specialist in fabricating dental prosthetics such as crowns and dentures
- Completes a 2-year vocational program or receives 3 to 4 years of on-the-job training

*For more information regarding these health careers, visit the following websites:*
American Association of Orthodontists at **www.braces.org**
American Dental Assistants Association at **www.dentalassistant.org**
American Dental Association at **www.ada.org**
American Dental Hygienists Association at **www.adha.org**
National Association of Dental Laboratories at **www.nadl.org**

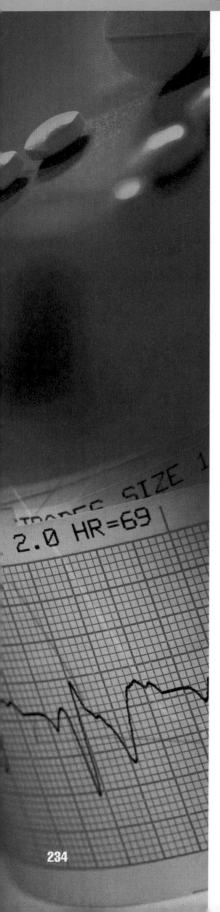

## Organs of the Digestive System

| | |
|---|---|
| anus | pancreas |
| colon | pharynx |
| esophagus | rectum |
| gallbladder (GB) | salivary glands |
| liver | small intestine |
| mouth | stomach |

## Combining Forms Relating to the Digestive System

| | | | |
|---|---|---|---|
| an/o | anus | hepat/o | liver |
| append/o | appendix | ile/o | ileum |
| appendic/o | appendix | jejun/o | jejunum |
| bucc/o | cheek | labi/o | lip |
| cec/o | cecum | lapar/o | abdomen |
| cheil/o | lip | lingu/o | tongue |
| chol/e | bile, gall | lith/o | stone |
| cholangi/o | bile duct | odont/o | tooth |
| cholecyst/o | gallbladder | or/o | mouth |
| choledoch/o | common bile duct | palat/o | palate |
| col/o | colon | pancreat/o | pancreas |
| colon/o | colon | pharyng/o | throat, pharynx |
| dent/o | tooth | proct/o | anus and rectum |
| duoden/o | duodenum | pylor/o | pylorus |
| enter/o | small intestine | rect/o | rectum |
| esophag/o | esophagus | sial/o | saliva, salivary gland |
| gastr/o | stomach | sialaden/o | salivary gland |
| gingiv/o | gums | sigmoid/o | sigmoid colon |
| gloss/o | tongue | stomat/o | mouth |

## Suffixes Relating to the Digestive System

| Suffix | Meaning | Example |
|---|---|---|
| -emesis | vomit | hematemesis |
| -lithiasis | stone | cholelithiasis |
| -orexia | appetite | anorexia |
| -ostomy | surgically create an opening | colostomy |
| -pepsia | digestion | dyspepsia |
| -phagia | eat, swallow | polyphagia |
| -prandial | pertaining to a meal | postprandial |
| -tripsy | surgical crushing | lithotripsy |

# Anatomy and Physiology of the Digestive System

| | | |
|---|---|---|
| accessory organs | gastrointestinal system | pharynx |
| alimentary canal | glucose | rectum |
| amino acids | gut | salivary glands |
| anus | liver | small intestines |
| colon | mouth | stomach |
| esophagus | oral cavity | triglycerides |
| gallbladder | pancreas | |

The digestive system, also known as the **gastrointestinal** (gas troh in **TESS** tih nal) (GI) **system,** includes approximately 30 feet of a continuous muscular tube, called the **gut** or **alimentary canal** (al ih **MEN** tar ree can **NAL**), that stretches between the mouth and the anus. Most of the organs in this system are actually different sections of the gut tubing. In order, starting from the mouth, they are the **mouth** or **oral cavity, pharynx** (**FAIR** inks), **esophagus** (eh **SOFF** ah gus), **stomach** (**STUM** ak), **small intestines, colon** (**COH** lon), **rectum** (**REK** tum), and **anus** (**AY** nus). The **accessory organs** of digestion are those organs in the system that are not part of the continuous gut tube, but rather each organ is connected to the gut by a duct. The accessory organs are the **liver** (**LIV** er), **pancreas** (**PAN** kree ass), **gallbladder,** and **salivary** (**SAL** ih vair ee) **glands.**

This system has three main functions: digesting food, absorbing nutrients, and eliminating waste (see ▓ Figure 8.1). Digestion includes the physical and chemical breakdown of large food particles into simple nutrient molecules like

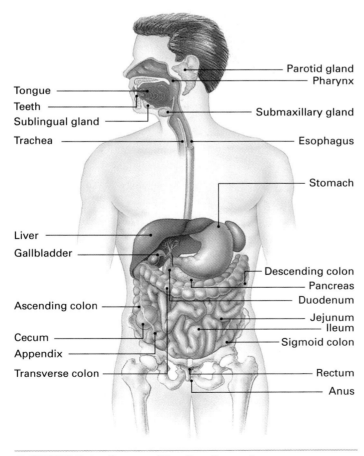

▓ **FIGURE 8.1** Organs of the digestive system.

**glucose, triglycerides,** and **amino acids.** These simple nutrient molecules are absorbed from the intestines and circulated throughout the body by the cardiovascular system. They are used for growth and repair of organs and tissues. Any food that cannot be digested or absorbed becomes a waste product and is expelled.

## Oral Cavity

| | | |
|---|---|---|
| **cheeks** | **saliva** | **tongue** |
| **lips** | **taste buds** | **uvula** |
| **palate** | **teeth** | |

The digestive process begins when food enters the mouth and is mechanically broken up by the chewing movements of the **teeth.** The **tongue,** with its muscular action, moves the food within the mouth and mixes it with **saliva** (suh **LYE** vah) (see ▓ Figure 8.2). Saliva contains digestive enzymes that break down carbohydrates and lubricants that make it easier to swallow the food. **Taste buds** are found on the surface of the tongue and can distinguish the bitter, sweet, sour, and salty flavors in our food. The roof of the oral cavity is known as the **palate** (**PAL** at). The roof of the mouth consists of the hard palate, the bony anterior portion, and the soft palate, the flexible posterior portion. Hanging down from the posterior edge of the soft palate is the **uvula** (**YU** vyu lah). The uvula serves two important functions. It helps in the production of speech and is the location of the gag reflex. The gag reflex helps prevent us from accidentally inhaling food or liquids without first swallowing. The **cheeks** form the lateral walls of this cavity and the **lips** are the anterior opening. The entire oral cavity is lined with mucous membrane (see ▓ Figure 8.3).

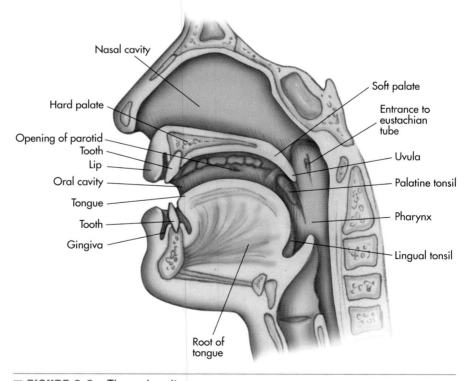

▓ **FIGURE 8.2** The oral cavity.

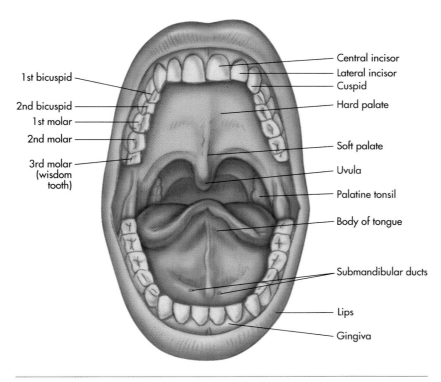

Central incisor
Lateral incisor
Cuspid
Hard palate
Soft palate
Uvula
Palatine tonsil
Body of tongue
Submandibular ducts
Lips
Gingiva

1st bicuspid
2nd bicuspid
1st molar
2nd molar
3rd molar
(wisdom
tooth)

**FIGURE 8.3**   Mouth.

## Teeth

| | | |
|---|---|---|
| **bicuspids** | **dentin** | **permanent teeth** |
| **canines** | **enamel** | **premolars** |
| **crown** | **incisors** | **pulp cavity** |
| **cuspids** | **molars** | **root** |
| **deciduous teeth** | **orthodontics** | **root canal** |

Teeth are important for the first stage of digestion. The teeth in the front of the mouth bite, tear, or cut food into small pieces. These cutting teeth include the **incisors** (in **SIGH** zors) and the **cuspids** (**CUSS** pids) or **canines** (**KAY** nines) (see ▓ Figure 8.4). The remaining teeth grind and crush food into even finer pieces. These grinding teeth include the **bicuspids** (bye **CUSS** pids) or **premolars** (pree **MOH** lars) and the **molars** (**MOH** lars). A tooth can be subdivided into the **crown** and the **root**. The crown is that part of the tooth above the gum line. The root is below the gum line and anchors the tooth in the jaw bone. The crown of the tooth is covered by a layer of **enamel** (en **AM** el), the hardest substance in the body. Under the enamel is **dentin** (**DEN** tin), which makes up the main bulk of the tooth. The hollow interior of a tooth is the **pulp cavity** in the crown and the **root canal** in the root. These cavities contain soft tissue made up of blood vessels, nerves, and lymph vessels (see ▓ Figure 8.5).

> **MED TERM TIP**
> There are three different molars, simply referred to as the first, second, or third molar. However, the third molar has a more common name, the wisdom tooth. Not every person ever forms all four wisdom teeth. Unfortunately, most people do not have enough room in their jaws for the third molars to properly erupt through the gum, a condition referred to as an *impacted wisdom tooth*. This condition requires surgical removal of the third molar.

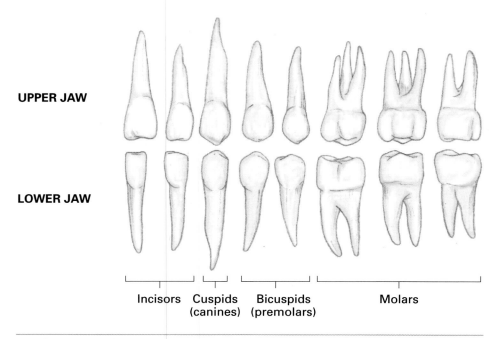

UPPER JAW

LOWER JAW

Incisors  Cuspids  Bicuspids  Molars
(canines)  (premolars)

**FIGURE 8.4**  Adult teeth.

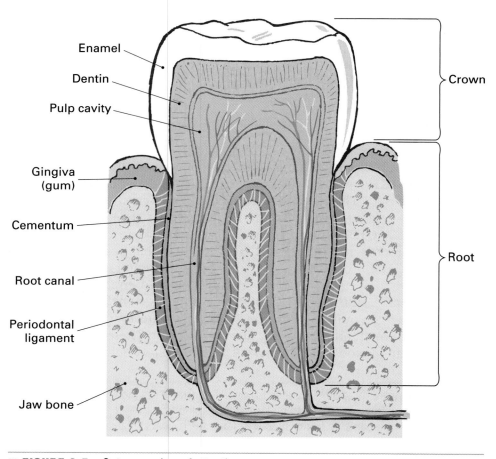

Enamel

Dentin

Pulp cavity

Crown

Gingiva
(gum)

Cementum

Root

Root canal

Periodontal
ligament

Jaw bone

**FIGURE 8.5**  Cut-away view of a tooth.

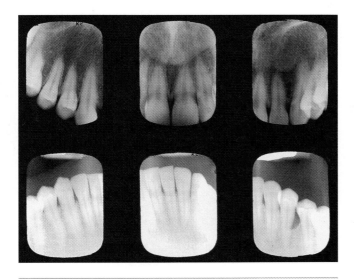

**FIGURE 8.6** Full mouth X-rays.
(Vanessa Vick/Photo Researchers, Inc.)

Humans have two sets of teeth. The first set, often called baby teeth, are the **deciduous (dee SID yoo us) teeth.** There are 20 teeth in this set that erupt through the gums between the ages of 6 to 28 months. At approximately 6 years of age, these teeth begin to fall out and are replaced by the 32 **permanent teeth.** This replacement process will continue until about 18 to 20 years of age. See ▓ Figure 8.6 for a photo of dental X-rays.

## Pharynx

**epiglottis**            **laryngopharynx**            **oropharynx**

After food has left the mouth, it enters the **oropharynx** and then the **laryngopharynx.** Remember from your study of the respiratory system in Chapter 7 that air is also traveling through these portions of the pharynx. The **epiglottis (ep ih GLOT iss)** covers the larynx and trachea so that food is shunted away from the lungs and into the esophagus.

## Esophagus

**peristalsis**

The esophagus is a muscular tube that is about 10 inches long in adults. Food entering the esophagus from the pharynx is delivered to the stomach. The food is propelled along the esophagus by wave-like muscular movements called **peristalsis (pair ih STALL sis).** In fact, peristalsis will work to push food through the entire gut tube.

## Stomach

| | | |
|---|---|---|
| **antrum** | **fundus** | **pyloric sphincter** |
| **body** | **hydrochloric acid** | **rugae** |
| **cardiac sphincter** | **lower esophageal sphincter** | **sphincters** |
| **chyme** | | |

> **MED TERM TIP** The combining term *dent/o* means teeth. Hence we have terms such as dentist and dental care. When the combining form *orth/o*, which means straight, is combined with *dent/o*, we have the specialty of **orthodontics** (or thoh **DON** tiks), or straightening teeth.

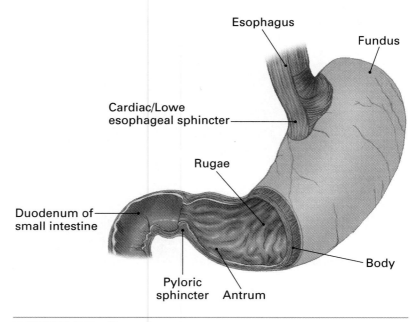

Esophagus

Fundus

Cardiac/Lowe esophageal sphincter

Rugae

Duodenum of small intestine

Body

Pyloric sphincter

Antrum

**FIGURE 8.7** Stomach.

The stomach is a J-shaped muscular organ that acts as a bag or sac to collect, churn, digest, and store food. It is composed of three parts: the **fundus** (**FUN** dus) or upper region, the **body** or main portion, and the **antrum** (**AN** trum) or lower region (see ■ Figure 8.7). The folds in the lining of the stomach are called **rugae** (**ROO** gay). When the stomach is filled with food, the rugae are stretched out and disappear. **Hydrochloric** (high droh **KLOH** rik) **acid (HCl)** is secreted by glands in the mucous membrane lining of the stomach. Food mixes with HCl and other gastric juices to form a liquid mixture called **chyme** (**KIGHM**), which then passes through the remaining portion of the digestive system.

The stomach contains muscular valves called **sphincters** (**SFINGK** ters) that control the flow of food in one direction only. The **cardiac sphincter** (**CAR** dee ak **SFINGK** ter), named after its location near the heart, is located between the esophagus and the fundus. It is also called the **lower esophageal sphincter** (eh soff ah **JEE** al **SFINGK** ter) (LES). It keeps food from backing up into the esophagus.

The antrum tapers off into the **pyloric sphincter** (pigh **LOR** ik **SFINGK** ter). This sphincter opens and closes to control the passage of food into the small intestine. Only a small amount of the chyme is allowed to enter the small intestines with each opening of the sphincter for two important reasons: First, the small intestines are much narrower than the stomach and cannot hold as much as the stomach can. Second, the chyme is highly acidic and must be thoroughly neutralized as it leaves the stomach.

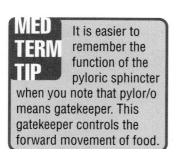

It is easier to remember the function of the pyloric sphincter when you note that pylor/o means gatekeeper. This gatekeeper controls the forward movement of food.

## Small Intestine

| | |
|---|---|
| **duodenum** | **ileum** |
| **ileocecal valve** | **jejunum** |

The small intestine, or small bowel, is the major site of digestion and absorption of nutrients from food (see ■ Figure 8.8). It is located between the pyloric sphincter and the colon. Because the small intestine is concerned with absorption of food products, an abnormality in this organ can cause malnutrition. The

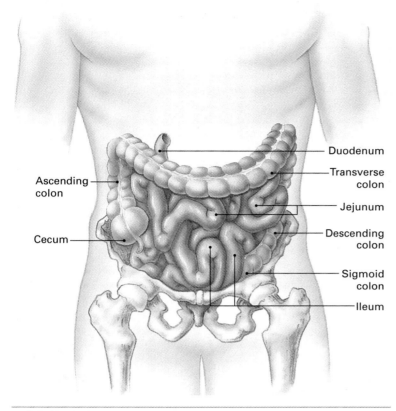

Ascending
colon

Cecum

Duodenum

Transverse
colon

Jejunum

Descending
colon

Sigmoid
colon

Ileum

**FIGURE 8.8** Small intestine.

small intestine contains an average of 20 feet of intestine, making it the longest portion of the alimentary canal. The small intestine has three sections: the **duodenum** (doo oh **DEE** num / doo **OD** eh num), the **jejunum** (jee **JOO** num), and the **ileum** (**ILL** ee um).

- The duodenum, which extends from the pyloric sphincter to the jejunum, is about 10 to 12 inches long. Digestion is completed in the duodenum after the partly digested chyme from the stomach is mixed with digestive juices from the pancreas and gallbladder.

- The jejunum, or middle portion, extends from the middle of the small intestine to the ileum and is about 8 feet long.

- The ileum is the last portion of the small intestine and extends from the jejunum to the colon. At 12 feet in length, it is the longest portion of the small intestine. The ileum connects to the colon through a sphincter called the **ileocecal** (ill ee oh **SEE** kal) **valve**.

**MED TERM TIP** We can live without a portion of the small intestine. For example, in cases of cancer, much of the small intestine and/or colon may have to be removed. The surgeon then creates an opening between the remaining intestine and the abdominal wall. The combining form for the section of intestines connected to the abdominal wall and the suffix *–ostomy* are used to describe this procedure. Therefore, if you know the order of the intestinal parts you can tell what portion has been removed by analyzing the term. For example, if a person has a *jejunostomy,* the jejunum is connected to the abdominal wall, meaning that the ileum (and remainder of the gut tube) have been removed. A person having a *colostomy* means the entire small intestine is present and a portion of the colon has been removed (see Figure 8.9).

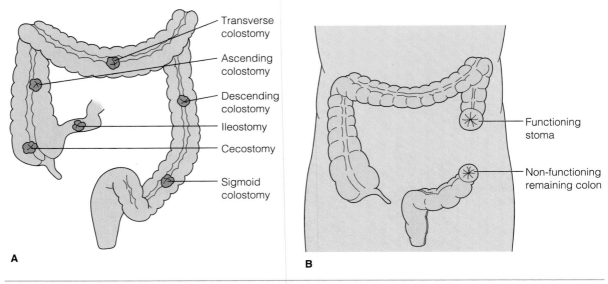

A

B

**FIGURE 8.9** (A) Various -ostomy sites. (B) Descending colostomy with functioning stoma. Also illustrates nonfunctioning sigmoid colon, rectum, and anus.

## Colon

| | | |
|---|---|---|
| anal sphincter | cecum | feces |
| appendix | defecation | sigmoid colon |
| ascending colon | descending colon | transverse colon |

Fluid that remains after the complete digestion and absorption of nutrients in the small intestine enters the colon or large intestine (see ▒ Figure 8.10). Most of this fluid is water and it is reabsorbed into the body. The material that remains after absorption is solid waste called **feces** (**FEE** seez). This is the product evacuated in bowel movements (BM).

The colon is approximately 5 feet long and extends from the ileocecal valve of the small intestine to the anus. The **cecum** (**SEE** kum) is a pouch or sac-like area in the first 2 to 3 inches at the beginning of the colon. The **appendix** (ah **PEN** diks) is a small worm-shaped outgrowth at the end of the cecum. The remaining colon consists of the **ascending colon, transverse colon** (trans **VERS COH** lon), **descending colon,** and **sigmoid colon** (**SIG** moyd **COH** lon). The ascending colon on the right side extends from the cecum to the lower border of the liver. The transverse colon begins where the ascending colon leaves off and moves horizontally across the upper abdomen toward the spleen. The descending colon then travels down the left side of the body to where the sigmoid colon begins. The sigmoid colon leads into the rectum. The rectum is the area for storage of feces. The rectum leads into the anus, which contains the **anal sphincter** (**AY** nal **SFINGK** ter). This sphincter is controlled by muscles that assist in the evacuation of feces or **defecation**.

MED TERM TIP

The term *colon* refers to the large intestine. However, you should be aware that many people use it as a general term referring to the entire intestinal system, both small and large intestines. This is incorrect.

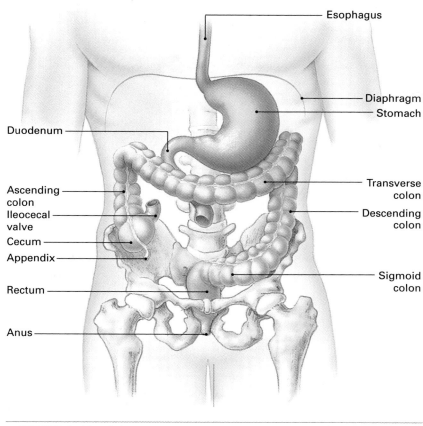

Esophagus

Diaphragm
Stomach

Duodenum

Transverse colon

Ascending colon

Descending colon

Ileocecal valve

Cecum

Appendix

Sigmoid colon

Rectum

Anus

**FIGURE 8.10** Colon.

## Accessory Organs of the Digestive System

gallblader                    pancreas
liver                         salivary glands

The accessory organs of the digestive system, the **salivary** (**SAL** ih vair ee) **glands**, the **liver,** the **pancreas,** and the **gallbladder,** generally function by producing much of the digestive fluids and enzymes necessary for the chemical breakdown of food. Each is attached to the gut tube by a duct.

### Salivary Glands

amylase                  parotid glands               submandibular glands
bolus                    sublingual glands

Salivary glands in the oral cavity produce saliva. This very watery and slick fluid allows food to be swallowed with less danger of choking. Saliva mixed with food in the mouth forms a **bolus** (**BOH** lus), which is then ready to be swallowed. Saliva also contains the digestive enzyme **amylase** (**AM** ill ace) that begins the digestion of carbohydrates. There are three pairs of salivary glands. The **parotid** (pah **ROT** id) **glands** are in front of the ears. The **submandibular** (sub man **DIB** yoo lar) **glands** and **sublingual** (sub **LING** gwal) **glands** are in the floor of the mouth (see Figure 8.11).

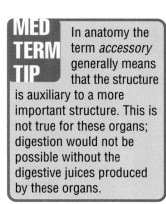

**MED TERM TIP** In anatomy the term *accessory* generally means that the structure is auxiliary to a more important structure. This is not true for these organs; digestion would not be possible without the digestive juices produced by these organs.

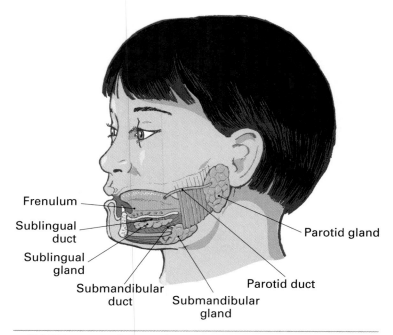

**FIGURE 8.11** Salivary glands.

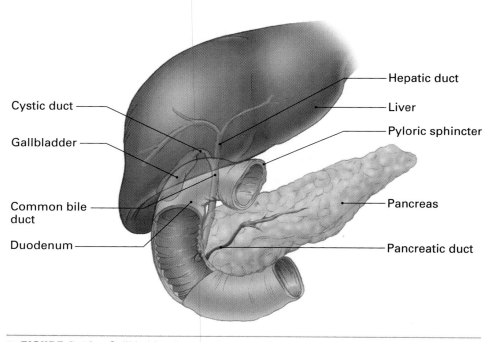

**FIGURE 8.12** Gallbladder, liver, and pancreas.

## Liver

**bile**　　　　　　　　　　　　　　**emulsification**

The liver is a large organ located in the right upper quadrant of the abdomen that has several functions, including processing the nutrients absorbed by the intestines, detoxifying harmful substances in the body, and producing **bile** (**BYE** al) (see ■ Figure 8.12). Bile is important for the digestion of fats and lipids because is makes them more soluble in the watery environment inside the intestines. The process is called **emulsification** (ee mull sih fih **KAY** shun).

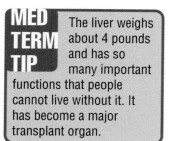

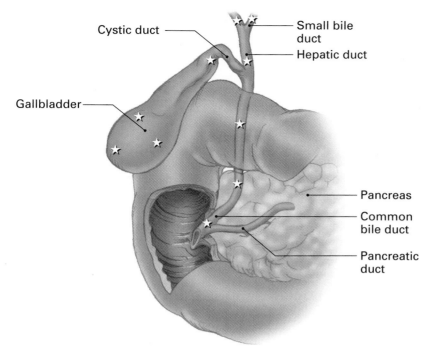

Cystic duct

Small bile duct

Hepatic duct

Gallbladder

Pancreas

Common bile duct

Pancreatic duct

**A**

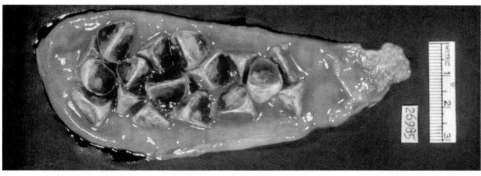

**B**

■ **FIGURE 8.13** (A) Common sites for cholelithiasis. (B) Gallbladder with gallstones.
(Martin Rotker/Phototake NYC)

## Gallbladder

**cholesterol**  **common bile duct**  **gallstones**

The bile produced by the liver is stored in the gallbladder (GB). Bile is released into the duodenum through the **common bile duct (CBD)** (refer to Figure 8.12). If bile contains an excessive amount of **cholesterol** (koh **LES** ter all) **(chol)** and other secretions, it compacts into **gallstones** (see ■ Figure 8.13). There is a higher incidence of stone formation in women than in men, with obesity increasing the risk.

## Pancreas

**pancreatic enzymes**

The pancreas produces **pancreatic enzymes** (pan kree **AT** ik **EN** zimes) that chemically digest carbohydrates, fats, and proteins (refer to Figure 8.12). These enzymes are carried to the duodenum in the pancreatic duct. The pancreas is also an endocrine gland. It produces the hormones insulin and glucagon, which play a role in regulating the level of glucose in the blood.

# Word Building Relating to the Digestive System

The following list contains examples of medical terms built directly from word parts. The definitions for these terms can be determined by a straightforward translation of the word parts.

| Combining Form | Combined With | Medical Term | Definition |
|---|---|---|---|
| append/o | -ectomy | appendectomy (ap en **DEK** toh mee) | excision of the appendix |
| appendic/o | -itis | appendicitis (ah pen dih **SIGH** tis) | inflammation of the appendix |
| bucc/o | -al | buccal (**BYOO** kal) | pertaining to cheeks |
| | labi/o –al | buccolabial (**BYOO** koh labe ee all) | pertaining to cheeks and lips |
| cheil/o | -rrhaphy | cheilorrhaphy (kigh **LOR** ah fee) | suture the lip |
| | -itis | cheilitis (kigh **LYE** tis) | lip inflammation |
| chol/e | -lithiasis | cholelithiasis (koh lee lih **THIGH** ah sis) | condition of gallstones |
| cholecyst/o | -ectomy | cholecystectomy (koh lee sis **TEK** toh mee) | excision of the gallbladder |
| | -gram | cholecystogram (koh lee **SIS** toh gram) | record of the gallbladder |
| | -itis | cholecystitis (koh lee sis **TYE** tis) | inflammation of the gallbladder |
| col/o | -ectomy | colectomy (koh **LEK** toh mee) | excision of the colon |
| | rect/o -al | colorectal (kohl oh **REK** tall) | pertaining to the colon and rectum |
| colon/o | -scope | colonoscope (koh **LON** oh scope) | instrument to view colon |
| | -scopy | colonoscopy (koh lon **OSS** koh pee) | procedure to view colon |
| dent/o | -al | dental (**DENT** al) | pertaining to teeth |
| | -algia | dentalgia (dent **AL** gee ah) | tooth pain |
| enter/o | -rrhaphy | enterorrhaphy (en ter **OR** ah fee) | suture small intestines |
| | -ectomy | enterectomy (en ter **EK** toh mee) | excision of the small intestines |
| | -algia | enteralgia (en ter **AL** jee ah) | small intestine pain |
| | -itis | enteritis (en ter **EYE** tis) | small intestine inflammation |
| gastr/o | -dynia | gastrodynia (gas troh **DIN** ee ah) | stomach pain |
| | enter/o -itis | gastroenteritis (gas troh en ter **EYE** tis) | inflammation of stomach and small intestines |
| | enter/o -ologist | gastroenterologist (gas troh en ter **ALL** oh jist) | specialist in the stomach and small intestines |
| | enter/o -ology | gastroenterology (gas troh en ter **ALL** oh jee) | study of the stomach and small intestines |
| | -malacia | gastromalacia (gas troh mah **LAY** she ah) | softening of the stomach |
| | nas/o -ic | nasogastric (nay zoh **GAS** trik) | pertaining to the nose and stomach |
| | -scope | gastroscope (**GAS** troh scope) | instrument to view inside the stomach |
| | -itis | gastritis (gas **TRY** tis) | stomach inflammation |
| | -ectomy | gastrectomy (gas **TREK** toh mee) | excision of the stomach |

| Combining Form | Combined With | Medical Term | Definition |
|---|---|---|---|
| gingiv/o | -ectomy | gingivectomy (jin gih **VEK** toh mee) | excision of the gums |
| | -itis | gingivitis (jin jih **VIGH** tis) | inflammation of the gums |
| gloss/o | -ectomy | glossectomy (gloss **EK** toh mee) | excision of the tongue |
| | hypo- -al | hypoglossal (high poe **GLOSS** all) | pertaining to under the tongue |
| hepat/o | -itis | hepatitis (hep ah **TYE** tis) | inflammation of the liver |
| | -oma | hepatoma (hep ah **TOH** mah) | liver tumor |
| lapar/o | -otomy | laparotomy (lap ah **ROT** oh mee) | incision into the abdomen |
| | -scope | laparoscope (**LAP** ah roh scope) | instrument to view inside the abdomen |
| lingu/o | sub- -al | sublingual (sub **LING** gwal) | pertaining to under the tongue |
| odont/o | orth/o tic | orthodontic (or thoh **DON** tik) | pertaining to straight teeth |
| or/o | -al | oral (**OR** ral) | pertaining to the mouth |
| pancreat/o | -itis | pancreatitis (pan kree ah **TYE** tis) | inflammation of the pancreas |
| proct/o | -ptosis | proctoptosis (prok top **TOH** sis) | drooping rectum |
| | -scopy | proctoscopy (prok **TOSS** koh pee) | procedure to view the rectum |
| | -plasty | proctoplasty (**PROK** toh plas tee) | surgical repair of the rectum |
| sial/o | -lith | sialolith (sigh **AL** oh lith) | salivary (gland) stone |
| sialaden/o | -itis | sialadenitis (sigh al add eh **NIGH** tis) | inflammation of a salivary gland |
| sigmoid/o | -scope | sigmoidoscope (sig **MOYD** oh scope) | instrument to view inside the sigmoid colon |

| Suffix | Combined With | Medical Term | Definition |
|---|---|---|---|
| -orexia | an- | anorexia (an oh **REK** see ah) | absence of an appetite |
| | dys- | dysorexia (dis oh **REKS** ee ah) | abnormal appetite |
| -ostomy | gastr/o | gastrostomy (gas **TROSS** toh mee) | create an opening in the stomach |
| | duoden/o | duodenostomy (do oh den **OSS** toh mee) | create an opening in the duodenum |
| | jejun/o | jejunostomy (jeh june **OSS** toh mee) | create an opening in the jejunum |
| | ile/o | ileostomy (ill ee **OSS** toh mee) | create an opening in the ileum |
| | col/o | colostomy (koh **LOSS** toh mee) | create an opening in the colon |
| -pepsia | brady- | bradypepsia (brad ee **PEP** see ah) | slow digestion |
| | dys- | dyspepsia (dis **PEP** see ah) | difficult digestion |
| -phagia | a- | aphagia (ah **FAY** jee ah) | unable to swallow/eat |
| | dys- | dysphagia (dis **FAY** jee ah) | difficulty swallowing/eating |
| | poly- | polyphagia (pall ee **FAY** jee ah) | many (excessive) eating |

# Vocabulary Relating to the Digestive System

| | |
|---|---|
| **anorexia (an oh REK see ah)** | A general term meaning loss of appetite that may accompany other conditions. Sometimes also used to refer to *anorexia nervosa* which is a personality disorder involving refusal to eat. |
| **ascites (ah SIGH teez)** | Collection or accumulation of fluid in the peritoneal cavity. |
| **borborygmus (bore bow RIG mus)** | Rumbling and gurgling bowel sounds. |
| **bridge** | Dental appliance that is attached to adjacent teeth for support to replace missing teeth. |
| **bruxism (brux ISM)** | Clenching and grinding of teeth, often during sleep. |
| **caries (KAIR eez)** | Gradual decay and disintegration of teeth that can result in inflamed tissue and abscessed teeth. Commonly called a *tooth cavity*. |
| **constipation (kon stih PAY shun)** | Experiencing difficulty in defecation or infrequent defecation. |
| **crown** | An artificial covering for the tooth created to replace the original enamel. |
| **deglutination (de gloo tin AY shun)** | Swallowing. |
| **denture (DEN chur)** | Partial or complete set of artificial teeth that are set in plastic materials. Acts as a substitute for the natural teeth and related structures. |
| **diarrhea (dye ah REE ah)** | Passing of frequent, watery bowel movements. Usually accompanies gastrointestinal (GI) disorders. |
| **diverticulum (dye ver TIK yoo lum)** | An outpouching off the gut. May become inflamed if food becomes trapped within the pouch. |
| **emesis (EM eh sis)** | Vomiting. |
| **eructation (ee rook TAY shun)** | Belching. |
| ***Escherichia coli* (esh eh REE she ah KOH lye) (*E. coli*)** | A bacteria normally found in the intestines, but may cause damage and disease if it is carried to other areas of the body such as the urinary tract. |
| **flatus (FLAY tus)** | Passing gas. |
| **halitosis (hal ih TOH sis)** | Bad or offensive breath, which can often be a sign of disease. |
| ***Helicobacter pylori* (he li koh BACK ter pie LOR eye) (*H. pylori*)** | A bacteria that may cause inflammation of the stomach lining and peptic ulcers in some people. |
| **hematemesis (hee mah TEM eh sis)** | To vomit blood from the gastrointestinal tract, often looks like coffee grounds. |
| **hematochezia (he mat oh KEY zee ah)** | Passing bright red blood in the stools. |
| **ileus (ILL ee us)** | Severe abdominal pain, inability to pass stools, vomiting, and abdominal distension as a result of an intestinal blockage. May require surgery to reverse the blockage. |
| **implant (IM plant)** | Prosthetic device placed in the jaw to which a tooth or denture may be anchored. |

| | |
|---|---|
| **jaundice (JAWN diss)** | Yellow cast to the skin, mucous membranes, and the whites of the eyes caused by the deposit of bile pigment from too much bilirubin in the blood. Bilirubin is a waste product produced when worn-out red blood cells are broken down. May be a symptom of a disorder such as gallstones blocking the common bile duct or carcinoma of the liver. |
| **mastication (mast ih KAY shun)** | Chewing |
| **melena (me LEE nah)** | Passage of dark tarry stools. Color is the result of digestive enzymes working on blood in the gut. |
| **nausea (NAW see ah)** | A feeling of needing to vomit. |
| **plaque (PLAK)** | Gummy mass of microorganisms that grows on the crowns of teeth and spreads along the roots. It is colorless and transparent. |
| **postprandial (post PRAN dee al) (pp)** | Pertaining to after a meal. |
| **regurgitation (ree gur jih TAY shun)** | Return of fluids and solids from the stomach into the mouth. |
| **steatorrhea (stee at oh REE ah)** | Passage of a large amount of fat in the stool. Caused by an inability to digest fats, usually due to a problem with the pancreatic enzymes. |

# Pathology Relating to the Digestive System

| | |
|---|---|
| **anal fissure (FISH er)** | Crack-like split in the rectum or anal canal. |
| **anal fistula (FIH styoo lah)** | Abnormal tube-like passage from the surface around the anal opening directly into the rectum. |
| **cirrhosis (sih ROH sis)** | Chronic disease of the liver associated with failure of the liver to function properly. |
| **cleft (CLEFT) lip** | Congenital anomaly in which the upper lip fails to come together. Often seen along with a cleft palate. Corrected with surgery. |
| **cleft palate (CLEFT PAL at)** | Congenital anomaly in which the roof of the mouth has a split or fissure. Corrected with surgery. |
| **colorectal carcinoma (kohl oh REK tall car ci NOH mah)** | Cancerous tumor along the length of the colon and rectum. |
| **Crohn's disease (KROHNZ dih ZEEZ)** | Form of chronic inflammatory bowel disease affecting the ileum and/or colon. Also called *regional ileitis*. Named for Burrill Crohn, an American gastroenterologist. |
| **diverticulitis (dye ver tik yoo LYE tis)** | Inflammation of a diverticulum or sac in the intestinal tract, especially in the colon (see ▓ Figure 8.14). |
| **dysentery (dis in TARE ee)** | Disease characterized by diarrhea, often with mucus and blood, severe abdominal pain, fever, and dehydration. |
| **esophageal stricture (eh soff ah JEE al STRIK chur)** | Narrowing of the esophagus that makes the flow of fluids and food into the stomach difficult. |
| **esophageal varices (eh soff ah JEE al VAIR ih seez)** | Enlarged and swollen varicose veins in the lower end of the esophagus; they can rupture and result in serious hemorrhage. |

*continued...*

| | |
|---|---|
| **gastric carcinoma** (GAS trik car si NOH mah) | Cancerous tumor in the stomach. |
| **gastroesophageal reflux** (gas troh ee sof ah GEE all REE fluks) **disease (GERD)** | Acid from the stomach backs up into the esophagus causing inflammation and pain. |
| **hemorrhoids (HEM oh roydz)** | Varicose veins in the rectum. |
| **hepatitis (hep ah TYE tis)** | Inflammation of the liver, usually due to a viral infection. Different viruses are transmitted by different routes, such as sexual contact or from exposure to blood or fecally contaminated water or food. |
| **hiatal hernia** (high AY tal HER nee ah) | Protrusion of the stomach through the diaphragm and extending into the thoracic cavity; gastroesophageal reflux disease is a common symptom (see ▨ Figure 8.15). |
| **impacted wisdom tooth** | Wisdom tooth that is tightly wedged into the jaw bone so that it is unable to erupt (see ▨ Figure 8.16). |
| **inflammatory bowel disease** (in FLAM ah tor ee BOW el dih ZEEZ) **(IBD)** | Ulceration of the mucous membranes of the colon of unknown origin. Also known as *ulcerative colitis*. |
| **inguinal hernia** (ING gwih nal HER nee ah) | Hernia or outpouching of intestines into the inguinal (groin) region of the body (see ▨ Figure 8.17). |
| **intussusception** (in tuh suh SEP shun) | Result of the intestine slipping or telescoping into another section of intestine just below it. More common in children (see ▨ Figure 8.18). |
| **irritable bowel syndrome (IBS)** | Disturbance in the functions of the intestine from unknown causes. Symptoms generally include abdominal discomfort and an alteration in bowel activity. Also called *spastic colon* or *functional bowel syndrome*. |
| **malabsorption syndrome** (mal ab SORP shun SIN drohm) | Inadequate absorption of nutrients from the intestinal tract. May be caused by a variety of diseases and disorders, such as infections and pancreatic deficiency. |
| **oral leukoplakia** (loo koh PLAY key ah) | Development of white patches on the mucous membrane inside the mouth. May develop into cancer. |
| **peptic ulcer (PEP tik ULL sir) disease (PUD)** | Ulcer occurring in the lower portion of the esophagus, stomach, and duodenum; thought to be caused by the acid of gastric juices (see ▨ Figure 8.19). |
| **periodontal disease** (pair ee oh DON tal dih ZEEZ) | Disease of the supporting structures of the teeth, including the gums and bones. |
| **polyposis (pall ee POH sis)** | Small tumors that contain a pedicle or stem-like attachment in the mucous membranes of the large intestine (colon). |
| **pyloric stenosis** (pie LORE ik steh NOH sis) | Narrowing of the pyloric sphincter area of the stomach, may be congenital. Results in projectile (forceful) vomiting. |
| **pyorrhea (pye oh REE ah)** | Discharge of purulent material from dental tissue. |
| **temporomandibular** (tem POR oh man DIB yoo lar) **joint (TMJ) disease** | Inflammation of the jaw joint resulting in pain and poor bite. |
| **ulcerative colitis** (ULL sir ah tiv koh LYE tis) | Ulceration of the mucous membranes of the colon of unknown origin. Also known as *inflammatory bowel disease* (IBD). |
| **volvulus (VOL vyoo lus)** | Condition in which the bowel twists upon itself and causes an obstruction. Painful and requires immediate surgery (see ▨ Figure 8.20). |

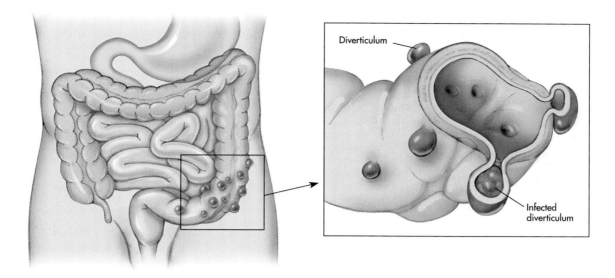

■ **FIGURE 8.14**  Colon with diverticulosis. An infected diverticulum is called diverticulitis.

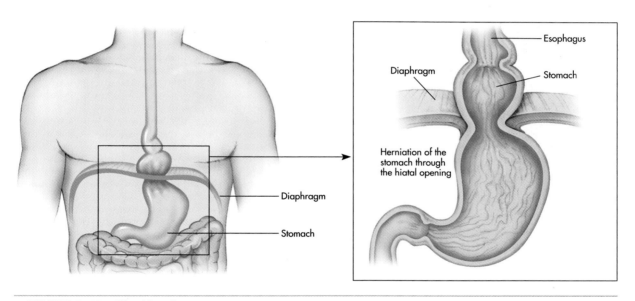

■ **FIGURE 8.15**  Hiatal hernia.

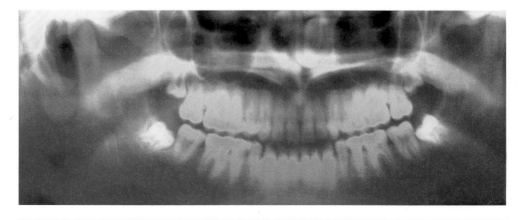

■ **FIGURE 8.16**  Enhanced color X-ray showing impacted wisdom teeth highlighted in yellow.
(Science Photo Library/Photo Researchers, Inc.)

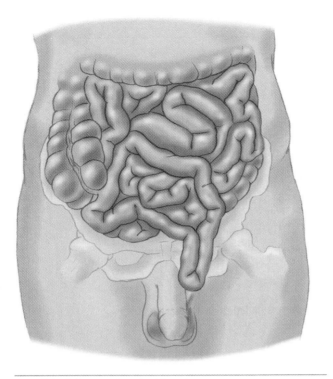

**■ FIGURE 8.17**   Inguinal hernia.

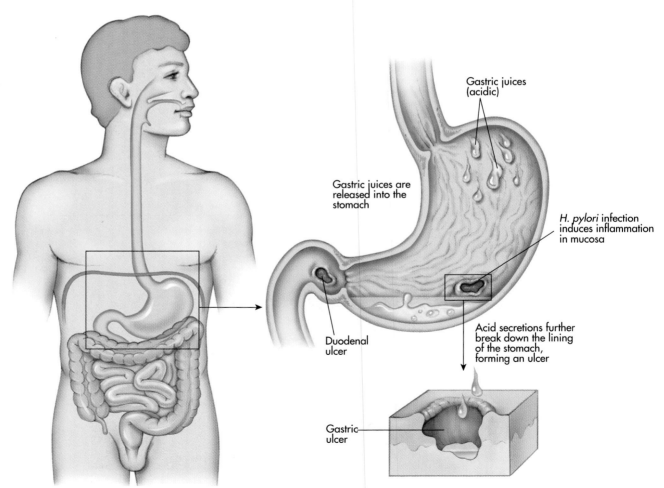

**■ FIGURE 8.18**   Intestinal intussusception.

Gastric juices
(acidic)

Gastric juices are
released into the
stomach

*H. pylori* infection
induces inflammation
in mucosa

Duodenal
ulcer

Acid secretions further
break down the lining
of the stomach,
forming an ulcer

Gastric
ulcer

**■ FIGURE 8.19**   (A) Peptic ulcer disease (PUD).

*(continued)*

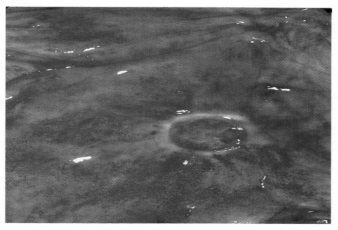

**B**

■ **FIGURE 8.19 (continued)** (B) A superficial gastric ulcer.

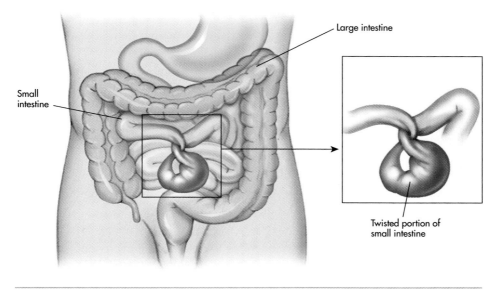

■ **FIGURE 8.20** Volvulus.

## Diagnostic Procedures Relating to the Digestive System

| | |
|---|---|
| **abdominal ultrasonography (ab DOM ih nal ull trah sun OG rah fee)** | Using ultrasound equipment for producing sound waves to create an image of the abdominal organs. |
| **alanine transaminase (AL ah neen trans AM in nase) (ALT)** | An enzyme normally present in the blood. Blood levels are increased in persons with liver disease. |
| **aspartate transaminase (ass PAR tate trans AM in nase) (AST)** | An enzyme normally present in the blood. Blood levels are increased in persons with liver disease. |

*continued...*

| | |
|---|---|
| **barium enema**<br>(BAH ree um EN eh mah) (BE) | Radiographic examination of the small intestine, large intestine, or colon in which an enema containing barium (Ba) is administered to the patient while X-ray pictures are taken (see ■ Figure 8.21). Also called a *lower GI series*. |
| **barium (BAH ree um) swallow** | A barium (Ba) mixture swallowed while X-ray pictures are taken of the esophagus, stomach, and duodenum; used to visualize the upper gastrointestinal tract (upper GI). Also called an *upper GI series*. |
| **bite-wing X-ray** | X-ray taken with a part of the film holder held between the teeth and parallel to the teeth. |
| **cholecystography**<br>(koh lee sis TOG rah fee) | The patient swallows a radiopaque dye so X-ray pictures can be taken that allow visualization of the gallbladder and its components. |
| **colonoscopy**<br>(koh lon OSS koh pee) | A flexible fiberscope passed through the anus, rectum, and colon is used to examine the upper portion of the colon. Polyps and small growths can be removed during this procedure (see ■ Figure 8.22). |
| **endoscopic retrograde cholangiopancreatography**<br>(en doh SKOP ik RET roh grayd koh lan jee oh pan kree ah TOG rah fee) (ERCP) | Using an endoscope to visually examine the hepatic duct, common bile duct, and pancreatic duct. |
| **endoscopy (en DOSS koh pee)** | A general term for a procedure to visually examine the inside of a body cavity or a hollow organ using an instrument called an endoscope. Specific examples of endoscopy relating to the digestive system include colonoscopy, esophagoscopy, gastrointestinal endoscopy, and gastroscopy. |
| **esophagogastroduodenoscopy**<br>(eh soff ah go gas troh duo den OS koh pee) (EGD) | Use of a flexible fiber-optic scope to visually examine the esophagus, stomach, and beginning of the duodenum. |
| **esophagoscopy and biopsy**<br>(eh soff ah GOS koh pee and BYE op see) | The esophagus is visualized by passing an instrument down the esophagus. A tissue sample for biopsy may be taken. |
| **fecal occult (uh CULT) blood test (FOBT)** | Laboratory test on the feces to determine if microscopic amounts of blood are present. Also called *hemoccult* or *stool guaiac* (**GUUY** ak). |
| **gastroscopy**<br>(gas TROS koh pee) | A flexible gastroscope is passed through the mouth and down the esophagus in order to visualize inside the stomach. Used to diagnose peptic ulcers and gastric carcinoma. |
| **intravenous cholangiography**<br>(in trah VEE nus koh LAN jee OG rah fee) (IVC) | A dye is administered intravenously to the patient that allows for X-ray visualization of the bile ducts. |
| **intravenous cholecystography**<br>(in trah VEE nus koh lee sis TOG rah fee) | A dye is administered intravenously to the patient that allows for X-ray visualization of the gallbladder. |
| **laparoscopy**<br>(lap ar OSS koh pee) | A laparoscope is passed into the abdominal wall through a small incision. The abdominal cavity is then visually examined for tumors and other conditions with this lighted instrument. Also called *peritoneoscopy*. |
| **liver biopsy**<br>(LIV er BYE op see) | Excision of a small piece of liver tissue for microscopic examination. Generally used to determine if cancer is present. |

| | |
|---|---|
| **liver (LIV er) scan** | A radioactive substance is administered to the patient by an intravenous (IV) route. This substance enters the liver cells, and this organ can then be visualized. This is used to detect tumors, abscesses, and other pathologies that result in hepatomegaly (an enlarged liver). |
| **lower gastrointestinal series (lower GI series)** | X-ray image of the colon and rectum is taken after the administration of barium (a radiopaque dye) by enema. Also called a *barium enema* (refer to Figure 8.21). |
| **ova and parasites (OH vah and PAR ah sights) (O&P)** | Laboratory examination of feces with a microscope for the presence of parasites or their eggs. |
| **paracentesis (pair ah sin TEE sis)** | Insertion of a needle into the abdominal cavity to withdraw fluid. Test to diagnose disease may be conducted on the fluid. |
| **percutaneous transhepatic cholangiography (per kyoo TAY nee us trans heh PAT ik koh lan jee OG rah fee)(PTC)** | A contrast medium is injected directly into the liver to visualize the bile ducts. Used to detect obstructions. |
| **serum bilirubin (SEE rum BILLY rubin)** | Blood test to determine the amount of the waste product bilirubin in the bloodstream. Elevated levels indicate liver disease. |
| **sigmoidoscopy (sig moid OS koh pee)** | Using a flexible sigmoidoscope to visually examine the sigmoid colon. Commonly done to diagnose cancer and polyps. |
| **stool culture** | A laboratory test of feces to determine if any pathogenic bacteria are present. |
| **upper gastrointestinal (UGI) series** | Administering a barium contrast material orally and then taking an X-ray to visualize the esophagus, stomach, and duodenum. Also called a *barium swallow*. |

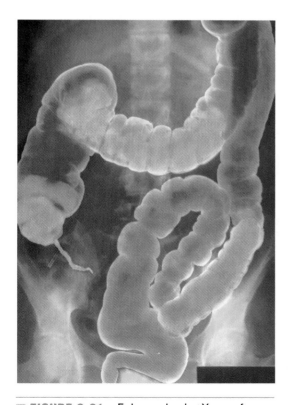

**■ FIGURE 8.21** Enhanced color X-ray of colon during barium enema exam.
(CNRI/Science Photo Library/Photo Researchers, Inc.)

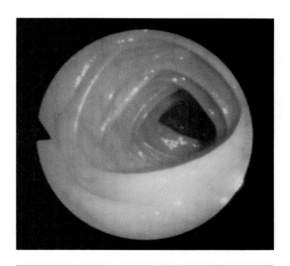

**■ FIGURE 8.22** Colonoscopy examination of the transverse colon.
(CNRI/Science Photo Library/Photo Researchers, Inc.)

# Therapeutic Procedures Relating to the Digestive System

| | |
|---|---|
| **anastomosis** (ah nas toh MOH sis) | Creating a passageway or opening between two organs or vessels. |
| **cholecystectomy** (koh lee sis TEK toh mee) | Surgical excision of the gallbladder. Removal of the gallbladder through the laparoscope is a newer procedure with fewer complications than the more invasive abdominal surgery. The laparoscope requires a small incision into the abdominal cavity (see ■ Figure 8.23). |
| **choledocholithotomy** (koh led oh koh lih THOT oh mee) | Removal of a gallstone through an incision into the common bile duct. |
| **choledocholithotripsy** (koh led oh koh LITH oh trip see) | Crushing of a gallstone in the common bile duct. |
| **colostomy** (koh LOSS toh mee) | Surgical creation of an opening of some portion of the colon through the abdominal wall to the outside surface. The fecal material (stool) drains into a bag worn on the abdomen. |
| **diverticulectomy** (dye ver tik yoo LEK toh mee) | Surgical removal of a diverticulum. |
| **exploratory laparotomy** (ek SPLOR ah tor ee lap ah ROT oh mee) | Abdominal operation for the purpose of examining the abdominal organs and tissues for signs of disease or other abnormalities. |
| **extraction** | Removing or "pulling" of teeth. |
| **fistulectomy** (fis tyoo LEK toh mee) | Excision of a fistula. |
| **gavage** | Using a nasogastric (NG) tube to place liquid nourishment directly into the stomach. |
| **hemorrhoidectomy** (hem oh royd EK toh mee) | Surgical excision of hemorrhoids from the anorectal area. |
| **hepatic lobectomy** (heh PAT ik loh BEK toh mee) | Surgical removal of a lobe of the liver. |
| **hernioplasty** (her nee oh PLAS tee) | Surgical repair of a hernia. Also called *herniorrhaphy*. |
| **lavage** | Using a nasogastric (NG) tube to wash out the stomach. |
| **liver transplant** | Transplant of a liver from a donor. |
| **nasogastric intubation** (NAY zo gas trik in two BAY shun) (NG tube) | A flexible catheter is inserted into the nose and down the esophagus to the stomach. May be used for feeding or to suction out stomach fluids. |
| **root canal** | Dental treatment involving the pulp cavity of the root of a tooth. Procedure is used to save a tooth that is badly infected or abscessed. |
| **vagotomy** (vah GOT oh mee) | Surgical resection of the vagus nerve in an attempt to decrease the amount of acid secretion into the stomach. Used as a method of treatment for ulcer patients. |

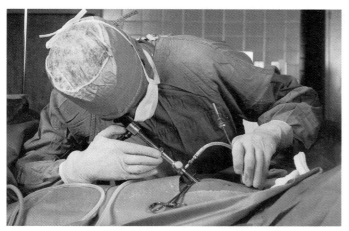

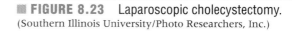

**FIGURE 8.23** Laparoscopic cholecystectomy.
(Southern Illinois University/Photo Researchers, Inc.)

# Pharmacology Relating to the Digestive System

| | |
|---|---|
| **anorexiant (an oh REKS ee ant)** | Treats obesity by suppressing appetite. |
| **antacid** | Used to neutralize stomach acids. |
| **antibiotic** | Used to treat peptic ulcers caused by the *H. pylori* bacteria. |
| **antidiarrheal** | Controls diarrhea. |
| **antiemetic (an tye ee MEH tik)** | Treats nausea, vomiting, and motion sickness. |
| **emetic (ee MEH tik)** | Induces vomiting. |
| **$H_2$-receptor antagonists** | When stimulated, $H_2$-receptors increase the production of stomach acid. Using an antagonist to block these receptors results in a low acid level in the stomach. Used to treat peptic ulcers and gastroesophageal reflux disease. |
| **laxative** | Treats constipation by stimulating a bowel movement. |
| **proton pump inhibitors** | Blocks the stomach's ability to secrete acid. Used to treat peptic ulcers and gastroesophageal reflux disease. |

# Abbreviations Relating to the Digestive System

| | | | | |
|---|---|---|---|---|
| **ac** | before meals | | **HCV** | hepatitis C virus |
| **ALT** | alanine transaminase | | **IBD** | inflammatory bowel disease |
| **AST** | aspartate transaminase | | **IBS** | irritable bowel syndrome |
| **Ba** | barium | | **IVC** | intravenous cholangiography |
| **BE** | barium enema | | **NG** | nasogastric (tube) |
| **BM** | bowel movement | | **NPO** | nothing by mouth |
| **BS** | bowel sounds | | **n&v** | nausea and vomiting |
| **CBD** | common bile duct | | **O&P** | ova and parasites |
| **chol** | cholesterol | | **pc** | after meals |
| **CUC** | chronic ulcerative colitis | | **PEG** | percutaneous endoscopic gastrostomy |
| **E. coli** | *Escherichia coli* | | **PO** | by mouth |
| **EGD** | esophagogastroduodenoscopy | | **pp** | postprandial |
| **ERCP** | endoscopic retrograde cholangiopancreatography | | **PTC** | percutaneous transhepatic cholangiography |
| **FOBT** | fecal occult blood test | | **PUD** | peptic ulcer disease |
| **GB** | gallbladder | | **RDA** | recommended daily allowance |
| **GERD** | gastroesophageal reflux disease | | **SBFT** | small bowel follow-through |
| **GI** | gastrointestinal | | **TPN** | total parenteral nutrition |
| **HAV** | hepatitis A virus | | **UGI** | upper gastrointestinal series |
| **HBV** | hepatitis B virus | | | |

# Chapter Review

## Pronunciation Practice

 *You will find the pronunciation for each term on the enclosed CD-ROM. Check each one off as you master it.*

- ❑ abdominal ultrasonography (ab **DOM** ih nal ull trah sun **OG** rah fee)
- ❑ accessory organs
- ❑ alanine transaminase (AL ah neen trans **AM** in nase)
- ❑ alimentary canal (al ih **MEN** tar ree can **NAL**)
- ❑ amino acids
- ❑ amylase (**AM** ill ace)
- ❑ anal fissure (**FISH** er)
- ❑ anal fistula (**FIH** styoo lah)
- ❑ anal sphincter (**AY** nal **SFINGK** ter)
- ❑ anastomosis (ah nas toh **MOH** sis)
- ❑ anorexia (an oh **REK** see ah)
- ❑ anorexiant (an oh **REKS** ee ant)
- ❑ antacid
- ❑ antibiotic
- ❑ antidiarrheal
- ❑ antiemetic (an tye ee **MEH** tik)
- ❑ antrum (**AN** trum)
- ❑ anus (**AY** nus)
- ❑ aphagia (ah **FAY** jee ah)
- ❑ appendectomy (ap en **DEK** toh mee)
- ❑ appendicitis (ah pen dih **SIGH** tis)
- ❑ appendix (ah **PEN** diks)
- ❑ ascending colon
- ❑ ascites (ah **SIGH** teez)
- ❑ aspartate transaminase (ass **PAR** tate trans **AM** in nase)
- ❑ barium enema (**BAH** ree um **EN** eh mah)
- ❑ barium (**BAH** ree um) swallow
- ❑ bicuspids (bye **CUSS** pids)
- ❑ bile (**BYE** al)
- ❑ bite-wing X-ray
- ❑ body
- ❑ bolus (**BOH** lus)
- ❑ borborygmus (bore bow **RIG** mus)
- ❑ bradypepsia (brad ee **PEP** see ah)
- ❑ bridge
- ❑ bruxism (brux **ISM**)

- ❑ buccal (**BYOO** kal)
- ❑ buccolabial (**BYOO** koh labe ee all)
- ❑ canines (**KAY** nines)
- ❑ cardiac sphincter (**CAR** dee ak **SFINGK** ter)
- ❑ caries (**KAIR** eez)
- ❑ cecum (**SEE** kum)
- ❑ cheeks
- ❑ cheilitis (kigh **LYE** tis)
- ❑ cheilorrhaphy (kigh **LOR** ah fee)
- ❑ cholecystectomy (koh lee sis **TEK** toh mee)
- ❑ cholecystitis (koh lee sis **TYE** tis)
- ❑ cholecystogram (koh lee **SIS** toh gram)
- ❑ cholecystography (koh lee sis **TOG** rah fee)
- ❑ choledocholithotomy (koh led uh koh lih **THOT** oh mee)
- ❑ choledocholithotripsy (koh led oh koh **LITH** oh trip see)
- ❑ cholelithiasis (koh lee lih **THIGH** ah sis)
- ❑ cholesterol (koh **LES** ter all)
- ❑ chyme (**KIGHM**)
- ❑ cirrhosis (sih **ROH** sis)
- ❑ cleft lip (**CLEFT**)
- ❑ cleft palate (**CLEFT PAL** at)
- ❑ colectomy (koh **LEK** toh mee)
- ❑ colon (**COH** lon)
- ❑ colonoscope (koh **LON** oh scope)
- ❑ colonoscopy (koh lon **OSS** koh pee)
- ❑ colorectal (kohl oh **REK** tall)
- ❑ colorectal carcinoma (kohl oh **REK** tall car ci **NOH** mah)
- ❑ colostomy (koh **LOSS** toh mee)
- ❑ common bile duct
- ❑ constipation (kon stih **PAY** shun)
- ❑ Crohn's disease (**KROHNZ** dih **ZEEZ**)
- ❑ crown
- ❑ cuspids (**CUSS** pids)
- ❑ deciduous (dee **SID** yoo us) teeth
- ❑ defecation
- ❑ deglutination (de gloo tin **AY** shun)
- ❑ dental (**DEN** tal)

- dentalgia (dent **AL** gee ah)
- dentin (**DEN** tin)
- denture (**DEN** chur)
- descending colon
- diarrhea (dye ah **REE** ah)
- diverticulectomy (dye ver tik yoo **LEK** toh mee)
- diverticulitis (dye ver tik yoo **LYE** tis)
- diverticulum (dye ver **TIK** yoo lum)
- duodenostomy (do oh den **OSS** toh mee)
- duodenum (doo oh **DEE** num / doo **OD** eh num)
- dysentery (dis in **TARE** ee)
- dysorexia (dis oh **REKS** ee ah)
- dyspepsia (dis **PEP** see ah)
- dysphagia (dis **FAY** jee ah)
- emesis (**EM** eh sis)
- emetic (ee **MEH** tik)
- emulsification (ee mull sih fih **KAY** shun)
- enamel (en **AM** el)
- endoscopic retrograde cholangiopancreatography (en doh **SKOP** ik **RET** roh grayd koh lan jee oh pan kree ah **TOG** rah fee)
- endoscopy (en **DOSS** koh pee)
- enteralgia (en ter **AL** jee ah)
- enterectomy (en ter **EK** toh mee)
- enteritis (en ter **EYE** tis)
- enterorrhaphy (en ter **OR** rah fee)
- epiglottis (ep ih **GLOT** iss)
- eructation (ee rook **TAY** shun)
- *Escherichia coli* (esh eh **REE** she ah **KOH** lye)
- esophageal stricture (eh soff ah **JEE** al **STRIK** chur)
- esophageal varices (eh soff ah **JEE** al **VAIR** ih seez)
- esophagogastroduodenoscopy (eh soff ah go gas troh duo den **OS** koh pee)
- esophagoscopy and biopsy (eh soff ah **GOS** koh pee and **BYE** op see)
- esophagus (eh **SOFF** ah gus)
- exploratory laparotomy (ek **SPLOR** ah tor ee lap ah **ROT** oh mee)
- extraction
- fecal occult (uh **CULT**) blood test
- feces (**FEE** seez)
- fistulectomy (fis tyoo **LEK** toh mee)
- flatus (**FLAY** tus)
- fundus (**FUN** dus)
- gallbladder
- gallstones
- gastrectomy (gas **TREK** toh mee)

- gastric carcinoma (**GAS** trik car si **NOH** mah)
- gastritis (gas **TRY** tis)
- gastrodynia (gas troh **DIN** ee ah)
- gastroenteritis (gas troh en ter **EYE** tis)
- gastroenterologist (gas troh en ter **ALL** oh jist)
- gastroenterology (gas troh en ter **ALL** oh jee)
- gastroesophageal reflux (gas troh ee sof ah **GEE** all **REE** fluks) disease
- gastrointestinal (gas troh in **TESS** tih nal) system
- gastromalacia (gas troh mah **LAY** she ah)
- gastroscope (**GAS** troh scope)
- gastroscopy (gas **TROS** koh pee)
- gastrostomy (gas **TROSS** toh mee)
- gavage
- gingivectomy (jin gih **VEK** toh mee)
- gingivitis (jin jih **VIGH** tis)
- glossectomy (gloss **SEK** toh mee)
- glucose
- gut
- H$_2$-receptor antagonist
- halitosis (hal ih **TOH** sis)
- *Helicobacter pylori* (he li koh **BACK** ter pie **LOR** eye)
- hematemesis (hee mah **TEM** eh sis)
- hematochezia (he mat oh **KEY** zee ah)
- hemorrhoidectomy (hem oh royd **EK** toh mee)
- hemorrhoids (**HEM** oh roydz)
- hepatic lobectomy (heh **PAT** tik loh **BEK** toh mee)
- hepatitis (hep ah **TYE** tis)
- hepatoma (hep ah **TOH** mah)
- hernioplasty (her nee oh **PLAS** tee)
- hiatal hernia (high **AY** tal **HER** nee ah)
- hydrochloric (high droh **KLOH** rik) acid
- hypoglossal (high poe **GLOSS** all)
- ileocecal (ill ee oh **SEE** kal) valve
- ileostomy (ill ee **OSS** toh mee)
- ileum (**ILL** ee um)
- ileus (**ILL** ee us)
- impacted wisdom tooth
- implant (**IM** plant)
- incisors (in **SIGH** zors)
- inflammatory bowel disease (in **FLAM** ah tor ee **BOW** el dih **ZEEZ**)
- inguinal hernia (**ING** gwih nal **HER** nee ah)
- intravenous cholangiography (in trah **VEE** nus koh **LAN** jee **OG** rah fee)
- intravenous cholecystography (in trah **VEE** nus koh lee sis **TOG** rah fee)

- intussusception (in tuh suh **SEP** shun)
- irritable bowel syndrome
- jaundice (**JAWN** diss)
- jejunostomy (jee june **OSS** toh mee)
- jejunum (jee **JOO** num)
- laparoscope (**LAP** ah roh scope)
- laparoscopy (lap ar **OSS** koh pee)
- laparotomy (lap ah **ROT** oh mee)
- laryngopharynx
- lavage
- laxative
- lips
- liver (**LIV** er)
- liver biopsy (**LIV** er **BYE** op see)
- liver (**LIV** er) scan
- liver (**LIV** er) transplant
- lower esophageal sphincter (eh soff ah **JEE** al **SFINGK** ter)
- lower gastrointestinal series
- malabsorption syndrome (mal ab **SORP** shun **SIN** drohm)
- mastication (mast ih **KAY** shun)
- melena (me **LEE** nah)
- molars (**MOH** lars)
- mouth
- nasogastric (nay zoh **GAS** trik)
- nasogastric intubation (**NAY** zo gas trik in two **BAY** shun)
- nausea (**NAW** see ah)
- oral (**OR** al)
- oral (**OR** al) cavity
- oral leukoplakia (**OR** al loo koh **PLAY** key ah)
- oropharynx
- orthodontics (or thoh **DON** tiks)
- ova and parasites (**OH** vah and **PAR** ah sights)
- palate (**PAL** at)
- pancreas (**PAN** kree ass)
- pancreatic enzymes (pan kree **AT** ik **EN** zimes)
- pancreatitis (pan kree ah **TYE** tis)
- paracentesis (pair ah sin **TEE** sis)
- parotid (pah **ROT** id) glands
- peptic ulcers (**PEP** tik **ULL** sirs)
- percutaneous transhepatic cholangiography (per kyoo **TAY** nee us trans heh **PAT** ik koh lan jee **OG** rah fee)
- periodontal disease (pair ee oh **DON** tal dih **ZEEZ**)
- peristalsis (pair ih **STALL** sis)
- permanent teeth

- pharynx (**FAIR** inks)
- plaque (**PLAK**)
- polyphagia (pall ee **FAY** jee ah)
- polyposis (pall ee **POH** sis)
- postprandial (post **PRAN** dee al)
- premolar (pree **MOH** lar)
- proctoplasty (**PROK** toh plas tee)
- proctoptosis (prok top **TOH** sis)
- proctoscopy (prok **TOSS** koh pee)
- proton pump inhibitor
- pulp cavity
- pyloric sphincter (pigh **LOR** ik **SFINGK** ter)
- pyloric stenosis (pigh **LOR** ik steh **NOH** sis)
- pyorrhea (pye oh **REE** ah)
- rectum (**REK** tum)
- regurgitation (ree gur jih **TAY** shun)
- root
- root canal
- rugae (**ROO** gay)
- saliva (suh **LYE** vah)
- salivary (**SAL** ih vair ee) glands
- serum bilirubin (**SEE** rum **BILLY** rubin)
- sialadenitis (sigh al add eh **NIGH** tis)
- sialolith (sigh **AL** oh lith)
- sigmoid colon (**SIG** moyd **COH** lon)
- sigmoidoscope (sig **MOYD** oh scope)
- sigmoidoscopy (sig moid **OS** koh pee)
- small intestine
- sphincters (**SFINGK** ters)
- steatorrhea (stee at oh **REE** ah)
- stomach (**STUM** ak)
- stool culture
- sublingual (sub **LING** gwal)
- sublingual (sub **LING** gwal) glands
- submandibular (sub man **DIB** yoo lar) glands
- taste buds
- teeth
- temporomandibular (tem **POR** oh man **DIB** yoo lar) joint disease
- tongue
- transverse colon (trans **VERS COH** lon)
- triglycerides
- ulcerative colitis (**ULL** sir ah tiv koh **LYE** tis)
- upper gastrointestinal (gas troh in **TESS** tih nal) series
- uvula (**YU** vyu lah)
- vagotomy (vah **GOT** oh mee)
- volvulus (**VOL** vyoo lus)

# Case Study

## Gastroenterology Consultation Report

**Reason for Consultation:** Evaluation of recurrent epigastric and LUQ pain with anemia.

**History of Present Illness:** Patient is a 56-year-old male. He reports a long history of mild dyspepsia characterized by burning epigastric pain, especially when his stomach is empty. This pain has been relieved by over-the-counter antacids. Approximately 2 weeks ago, the pain became significantly worse and he is also nauseated and has vomited several times.

**Past Medical History:** Patient's history is not significant for other digestive system disorders. He had a tonsillectomy at age 8. He sustained a compound fracture of the left ankle in a bicycle accident at age 11 that required surgical fixation. More recently he has been diagnosed with an enlarged prostate gland and surgery has been recommended. However, he would like to resolve this epigastric pain before going forward with the TUR.

**Results of Physical Examination:** CBC indicates anemia and an occult blood test is positive for blood in the feces. A blood test for *Helicobacter pylori* is positive. An erosion in the gastric lining was visualized on an upper GI. Follow-up gastroscopy found evidence of mild reflux esophagitis and an ulcerated lesion in the lining of the pyloric section of the stomach. This ulcer is 1.5 cm in diameter and deep. There is evidence of active bleeding from the ulcer. Multiple biopsies were taken and they were negative for gastric cancer. IV Tagamet relieved the painful symptoms in 2 days.

**Assessment:** Peptic ulcer. Gastric cancer has been ruled out in light of the negative biopsies.

**Recommendations:** A gastrectomy to remove the ulcerated portion of stomach is indicated because ulcer is already bleeding. Patient should continue on Tagamet to reduce stomach acid. Two medications will be added: Keflex to treat the bacterial infection and iron pills to reverse the anemia. Patient was instructed to eat frequent small meals and avoid alcohol and irritating foods.

### Critical Thinking Questions

1. This patient reports LUQ pain. What does LUQ stand for and what organs do you find there?

2. This patient had two diagnostic tests that indicated he was losing blood. Name these two tests and then describe them in your own words.

3. This patient had a procedure to visually examine the ulcer. Name the procedure and then describe in your own words what the physician observed.

4. Name the serious pathological condition that was ruled out.

5. Which of the following is NOT a recommendation of the consulting physician?

   a. medication to reduce stomach acid

   b. surgical removal of a portion of the stomach

   c. an antibiotic

   d. blood transfusion

6. Briefly describe this patient's past medical history in your own words.

# Chart Note Transcription

## Chart Note

The chart note below contains 12 phrases that can be reworded with a medical term that you learned in this chapter. Each phrase is identified with an underline. Determine the medical term and write your answers in the space provided.

**Current Complaint:** Patient is a 74-year-old female seen by a physician who specializes in the treatment of the gastrointestinal tract① with complaints of severe lower abdominal pain and extreme difficulty with having a bowel movement.②

**Past History:** Patient has a history of the presence of gallstones③ requiring a surgical removal of the gallbladder④ 10 years ago and chronic acid backing up from the stomach into the esophagus.⑤

**Signs and Symptoms:** The patient's abdomen is distended with fluid collecting in the abdominal cavity.⑥ X-ray of the colon after inserting barium dye with an enema⑦ revealed the presence of multiple small tumors growing on a stalk⑧ throughout the colon. Visual examination of the colon by a scope inserted through the rectum⑨ was performed, and biopsies taken for microscopic examination located a tumor.

**Diagnosis:** Carcinoma of the section of colon between the descending colon and the rectum.⑩

**Treatment:** Surgical removal of the colon⑪ between the descending colon and the rectum with the surgical creation of an opening of the colon through the abdominal wall.⑫

1. _____
2. _____
3. _____
4. _____
5. _____
6. _____
7. _____
8. _____
9. _____
10. _____
11. _____
12. _____

# Practice Exercises

## A. Define each combining form and provide an example of its use.

| | Definition | Example |
|---|---|---|
| 1. esophag/o | _____ | _____ |
| 2. hepat/o | _____ | _____ |
| 3. ile/o | _____ | _____ |
| 4. proct/o | _____ | _____ |
| 5. gloss/o | _____ | _____ |
| 6. labi/o | _____ | _____ |
| 7. jejun/o | _____ | _____ |
| 8. sigmoid/o | _____ | _____ |
| 9. rect/o | _____ | _____ |
| 10. gingiv/o | _____ | _____ |
| 11. cholecyst/o | _____ | _____ |
| 12. duoden/o | _____ | _____ |
| 13. an/o | _____ | _____ |
| 14. enter/o | _____ | _____ |
| 15. dent/o | _____ | _____ |

## B. State the terms described using the combining forms provided.

The combining form *gastr/o* refers to the stomach. Use it to write a term that means

1. inflammation of the stomach _____
2. study of the stomach and small intestines _____
3. excision of the stomach _____
4. visual exam of the stomach _____
5. suture of the stomach _____
6. enlargement of the stomach _____
7. incision into the stomach _____

The combining form *esophag/o* refers to the esophagus. Use it to write a term that means

8. inflammation of the esophagus _____
9. visual examination of the esophagus _____
10. surgical repair of the esophagus _____
11. pertaining to the esophagus _____
12. excision of the esophagus _____

The combining form *proct/o* refers to the rectum. Use it to write a term that means

13. narrowing of the rectum _____
14. drooping of the rectum _____

15. inflammation of the rectum _____

16. pain in the rectum _____

The combining form *cholecyst/o* refers to the gallbladder. Use it to write a term that means

17. excision of the gallbladder _____

18. condition of having gallbladder stones _____

19. gallbladder stone surgical crushing _____

20. gallbladder inflammation _____

The combining form *lapar/o* refers to the abdomen. Use it to write a term that means

21. instrument to view inside the abdomen _____

22. incision into the abdomen _____

23. visual examination of the abdomen _____

The combining form *hepat/o* refers to the liver. Use it to write a term that means

24. liver tumor _____

25. enlargement of the liver _____

26. pertaining to the liver _____

27. inflammation of the liver _____

The combining form *pancreat/o* refers to the pancreas. Use it to write a term that means

28. inflammation of the pancreas _____

29. pertaining to the pancreas _____

The combining form *col/o* refers to the colon. Use it to write a term that means

30. create an opening in the colon _____

31. inflammation of the colon _____

## C. Use the following suffixes to create a medical term for each definition relating to the digestive system.

-orexia           -phagia           -pepsia

-emesis           -lithiasis           -prandial

1. taken after meals _____

2. gallstones _____

3. no appetite _____

4. difficulty swallowing _____

5. vomiting blood _____

6. slow digestion _____

## D. Identify the following abbreviations

1. BM _____

2. UGI _____

3. BE _____

4. BS _____

5. RDA _____

6. O&P _____

7. PO _____

8. CBD _____

9. NPO _____

10. pp _____

11. NG _____

12. GI _____

13. HBV _____

14. FOBT _____

15. IBD _____

## E. Break apart the medical term *cholangiopancreatography* into its combining forms and suffix. Define the term.

1. Combining forms: (a) _____ (b) _____

2. Suffix: _____

3. Definition:

## F. Match the terms in column A with the definitions in column B.

| A | | B |
|---|---|---|
| 1. _____ eructation | | a. outpouching forming off the colon |
| 2. _____ anorexia | | b. chronic liver disease |
| 3. _____ hematemesis | | c. bad breath |
| 4. _____ halitosis | | d. small colon tumors |
| 5. _____ diverticulum | | e. fluid accumulation in abdominal cavity |
| 6. _____ constipation | | f. vomit blood |
| 7. _____ melena | | g. bowel twists on self |
| 8. _____ ascites | | h. belching |
| 9. _____ cirrhosis | | i. loss of appetite |
| 10. _____ pastic colon | | j. difficulty having BM |
| 11. _____ polyposis | | k. irritable bowel syndrome |
| 12. _____ volvulus | | l. black tarry stool |

## G. Use the following terms in the sentences that follow.

| | | |
|---|---|---|
| colonoscopy | barium swallow | lower GI series |
| gastrectomy | colostomy | colectomy |
| anastomosis | lithotripsy | liver biopsy |
| ileostomy | fecal occult blood test | cholangiography |

1. Excising a small piece of hepatic tissue for microscopic examination is called a(n) _____ .

2. When a surgeon performs a total or partial colectomy for cancer, she may have to create an opening on the surface of the skin for fecal matter to leave the body. This opening is called a(n) _____ .

3. Another name for an upper GI series is a(n) _____ .

4. Mr. White has had a radiopaque material placed into his large bowel by means of an enema for the purpose of viewing his colon. This procedure is called a(n) _____ .

5. A(n) _____ is the surgical removal of the colon.

6. Jessica has been on a red-meat-free diet in preparation for a test of her feces for the presence of hidden blood. This test is called a(n) _____ .

7. Dr. Mendez uses equipment to crush gallstones. This procedure is called _____ .

8. The opening or passageway created surgically between two organs is called a(n) _____ .

9. Removing all or part of the stomach is a(n) _____ .

10. Visualizing the bile ducts by injecting a dye into the patient's arm is called an IV _____ .

11. Passing an instrument into the anus and rectum in order to see the colon is called a(n)
_____ .

12. Ms. Fayne suffers from Crohn's disease, which has necessitated the removal of much of her small intestine. She has had a surgical passage created for the external disposal of waste material from the ileum. This is called a(n) _____ .

## H. Match the terms in column A with the definitions in column B.

| A | B |
|---|---|
| 1. _____ plaque | a. decay |
| 2. _____ pyorrhea | b. prosthetic device used to anchor a tooth |
| 3. _____ root canal | c. inflammation of the gums |
| 4. _____ crown | d. gummy mass of material |
| 5. _____ bridge | e. portion of the tooth covered by enamel |
| 6. _____ implant | f. replacement for missing teeth |
| 7. _____ gingivitis | g. purulent material |
| 8. _____ caries | h. surgery on the tooth pulp |

# Professional Journal

In this exercise you will now have an opportunity to put the words you have learned into practice. Imagine yourself in the role of a dentist. If you refer back to the Professional Profile at the beginning of this chapter, you will see that this health care professional cares for patients' teeth, gums, tongue, lips, and jaw. Use the 10 words listed below, or any other new terms from this chapter, to write sentences to describe the patients you saw today.

An example of a sentence is *Gerald scheduled the surgery to extract his* **impacted wisdom teeth** *over Christmas break.*

1. root canal _____

2. antibiotics _____

3. biscupids _____

4. bite wing x-ray _____

5. bruxism _____

6. caries _____

7. orthodontics _____

8. denture _____

9. oral leukoplakia _____

10. temporomandibular joint _____

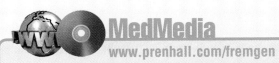

**MedMedia**
www.prenhall.com/fremgen

Use the CD-ROM enclosed with your textbook to gain additional reinforcement through interactive word building exercises, spelling games, labeling activities, and additional quizzes.

Use the above address to access the free, interactive Companion Website created for this textbook. Get hints, instant feedback, and textbook references to chapter-related multiple-choice questions, as well as labeling and matching exercises. In addition, you will find an audio glossary, case studies, and Internet exploration exercises.

***For more information regarding digestive diseases, visit the following websites:***

National Institute of Diabetes and Digestive and Kidney Diseases at **www.niddk.nih.gov**

American Gastroenterological Association's Digestive Health Resource Center at
    **www.gastro/org/public/digestinfo/html**

American College of Gastroenterology at **www.acg.gi.org**

The Medical Consumer Guide for Dental Care at **www.medicalconsumerguide.com/dental/index.html**

# Chapter 9
# Urinary System

## Learning Objectives

*Upon completion of this chapter, you will be able to:*

- Recognize the combining forms and suffixes introduced in this chapter.
- Gain the ability to pronounce medical terms and major anatomical structures.
- List the major organs of the urinary system and their functions.
- Describe the nephron and the mechanisms of urine production.
- Identify the characteristics of urine and a urinalysis.
- Build urinary system medical terms from word parts.
- Define vocabulary, pathology, diagnostic, and therapeutic medical terms relating to the urinary system.
- Recognize types of medications associated with the urinary system.
- Interpret abbreviations associated with the urinary system.

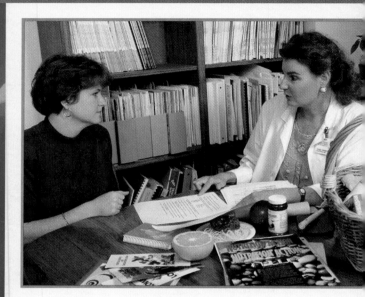

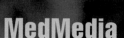

**MedMedia**
www.prenhall.com/fremgen
Additional interactive resources and activities for this chapter can be found on the Companion Website. For animations, audio glossary, and review, access the accompanying CD-ROM in this book.

## Professional Profile

### Dietetics

Registered dietitians are specialists in food and nutrition. Their duties include using diet to prevent and treat diseases, educating the public regarding good nutrition, and advancing the science of how diet and nutrition affect our bodies. Dietitians are found in many settings. Clinical dietitians work in hospitals and nursing homes, evaluating and adjusting patients' diets to treat illness. Consultant dietitians work with individual clients or facilities. Educator dietitians teach the science of nutrition to health care workers and dietitian students. Research dietitians engage in nutritional research for the food industry, government, and pharmaceutical companies. Business and management dietitians work in the food industry ensuring the nutritional quality of food served to the public.

### Registered Dietitian (RD)

- Promotes health and prevents or treats illnesses through diet modification and nutritional education.
- Graduates from a 4-year baccalaureate degree program accredited by the American Dietetic Association
- Completes a 6- to 12-month internship
- Passes a certification exam

### Dietetic Technician, Registered (DTR)

- Assists registered dietitian
- Graduates from an accredited 2-year associate's degree program
- Completes period of supervised practical experience
- Passes registration exam

### Dietetic Assistant

- Assists registered dietitian
- Completes on-the-job training program

*For more information regarding these health careers, visit the following websites:*
American Academy of Nutrition at **www.nutritioneducation.com**
American Dietetic Association at **www.eatright.org**
Society for Nutrition Education at **www.sne.org**

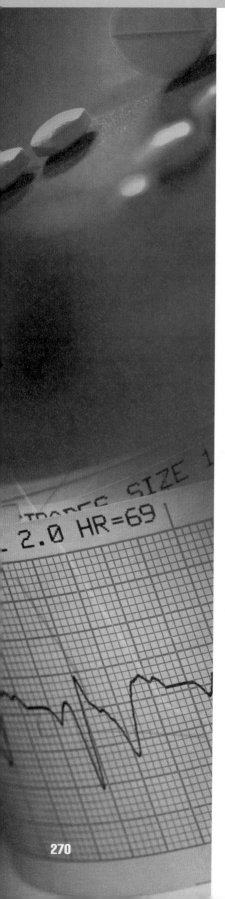

### Organs of the Urinary System

kidneys
ureters
urethra
urinary bladder

### Combining Forms Relating to the Urinary System

| | | | |
|---|---|---|---|
| albumin/o | albumin | noct/i | night |
| azot/o | nitrogenous waste | olig/o | scanty |
| bacteri/o | bacteria | py/o | pus |
| cyst/o | bladder | pyel/o | renal pelvis |
| glomerul/o | glomerulus | ren/o | kidney |
| glycos/o | sugar, glucose | ur/o | urine |
| keton/o | ketones | ureter/o | ureter, urinary tube |
| lith/o | stone | urethr/o | urethra |
| meat/o | meatus | urin/o | urine |
| nephr/o | kidney | vesic/o | bladder |

### Suffixes Relating to the Urinary System

| Suffix | Meaning | Example |
|---|---|---|
| -ectasia | dilation | ureterectasia |
| -lith | stone | nephrolith |
| -lithiasis | condition of stones | nephrolithiasis |
| -ptosis | drooping | nephroptosis |
| -tripsy | surgical crushing | lithotripsy |
| -uria | condition of the urine | hematuria |

## Anatomy and Physiology of the Urinary System

| | | |
|---|---|---|
| bicarbonate | nephrons | urethra |
| chloride | pH | urinary bladder |
| electrolytes | potassium | urinary meatus |
| genitourinary system | sodium | urine |
| homeostasis | uremia | waste products |
| kidneys | ureters | |

You might think of the urinary system, sometimes referred to as the **geni-tourinary** (jen ih toh **YOO** rih nair ee) (GU) **system,** as similar to a water filtration plant. Its main function is to filter and remove **waste products** from the blood. These waste materials result in the production and excretion of **urine** (**YOO** rin) from the body (see ▥ Figure 9.1).

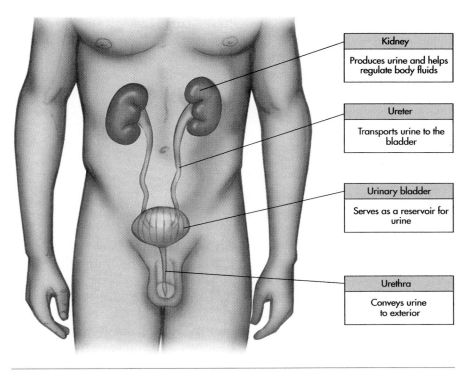

| Kidney |
| Produces urine and helps regulate body fluids |

| Ureter |
| Transports urine to the bladder |

| Urinary bladder |
| Serves as a reservoir for urine |

| Urethra |
| Conveys urine to exterior |

■ **FIGURE 9.1** The organs of the urinary system with major functions.

**MED TERM TIP**  From the time of early man, there has been an interest in urine. Drawings on cave walls and hieroglyphics in Egyptian pyramids reveal interest in urine as a means of determining the physical state of the body. Some of the first doctors, called *pisse prophets*, believed that examining the urine would help treat a patient. We now have physicians in the medical specialty of urology who treat male and female patients with urinary tract problems plus disorders of the male reproductive tract.

The urinary system is one of the hardest working systems of the body. All the body's metabolic processes result in the production of waste products. These waste products are a natural part of all life but quickly become toxic if they stay in the body, resulting in a condition called **uremia** (yoo **REE** mee ah). Waste products in the body are removed through a very complicated system of blood vessels and tubules. The actual filtration or sifting of the waste products takes place in millions of **nephrons** (**NEF** ronz), which make up each of your two **kidneys.** As urine drains from each kidney, the **ureters** (yoo **REE** ters) transport it to the **urinary** (**YOO** rih nair ee) **bladder.** We are constantly producing urine, and our bladders can hold about one quart of this liquid. However, the amount of time before the brain tells us that it is time to empty our bladder varies from one person to another. It then moves from the bladder down the **urethra** (yoo **REE** thrah) to the outside of the body and is excreted through an opening called the **urinary meatus** (**YOO** rih nair ee mee **AY** tus).

Kidneys are responsible for **homeostasis** (hoh mee oh **STAY** sis) or balance in your body. They continually adjust the chemical conditions in the body that allow you to survive. Because of its interaction with the bloodstream and its ability to excrete substances from the body, the urinary system maintains the proper balance of water and chemicals in the body. If the body is low on water, the kidneys conserve it, or in the opposite case, if there is excess water in the body, the kidneys excrete the excess. In addition to water, the kidneys regulate

**MED TERM TIP**

The urinary system and the male reproductive system share some of the same organs, particularly the urethra. Hence the term *genitourinary* (GU) is sometimes used to describe the urinary system. The reproductive system is discussed in Chapter 10.

the level of **electrolytes** (ee **LEK** troh lites)—small biologically important molecules such as **sodium (Na$^+$), potassium (K$^+$), chloride (Cl$^-$),** and **bicarbonate (HCO$_3^-$).** Finally, the kidneys play an important role in maintaining the correct **pH** range within the body, making sure we do not become too acidic or too alkaline.

## Kidneys

| | | |
|---|---|---|
| calyx | peritoneum | renal pyramids |
| cortex | renal artery | renal vein |
| hilum | renal papilla | retroperitoneal |
| medulla | renal pelvis | |

The two kidneys are located in the lumbar region of the back behind the **peritoneum** (pair ih toh **NEE** um), which is the membrane lining the abdominal cavity. The term for this location is **retroperitoneal** (ret roh pair ih toh **NEE** al). Each kidney has a concave or indented area on the edge toward the center that gives the kidney its bean shape (see ▓ Figure 9.2). The center of this concave area is called the **hilum** (**HIGH** lum). The hilum is where the **renal artery** (**REE** nal **AR** teh ree) enters the kidney and the **renal** (**REE** nal) **vein** leaves it. The renal artery delivers the blood that is full of waste products to the kidney (see ▓ Figure 9.3) and the renal vein returns the now cleansed blood to the general circulation. The ureters also leave the kidneys at the hilum. The ureters are narrow tubes that lead from the kidneys to the bladder.

When the surgeon cuts into the kidney, several structures or areas are visible. The outer portion is called the **cortex** (**KOR** teks). The cortex is much like a shell for the kidney. The inner area is called the **medulla** (meh **DULL** ah). Within the medulla are a dozen or so triangular-shaped areas, the **renal pyramids** (**PEER** ah mids), that resemble their namesake, the Egyptian pyramids.

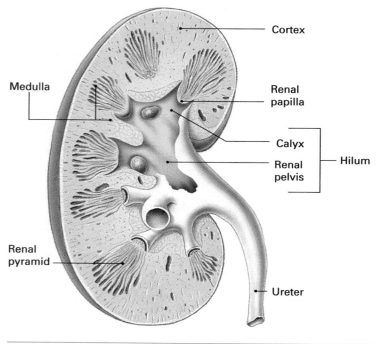

■ **FIGURE 9.2** Sectioned kidney.

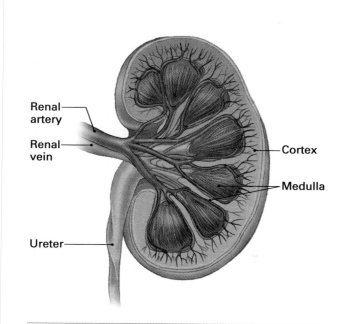

■ **FIGURE 9.3** Renal artery and vein.

The tip of each pyramid points inward toward the hilum. At its tip, called the **renal papilla** (pah **PILL** ah), each pyramid opens into a **calyx** (**KAY** liks) (plural is *calyces*), which is continuous with the **renal pelvis** (**PELL** vis). The calyces and ultimately the renal pelvis collect urine as it is formed. The ureter for each kidney is attached to the renal pelvis.

> **MED TERM TIP**
> The kidney actually resembles a kidney bean in shape. Each weighs 4 to 6 ounces, is 2 to 3 inches wide and approximately 1 inch thick, and is about the size of your fist. In most people the left kidney is slightly higher and larger than the right kidney. Functioning kidneys are necessary for life, but it is possible to live with only one functioning kidney.

## Nephrons

| | | |
|---|---|---|
| afferent arteriole | efferent arteriole | proximal convoluted tubule |
| Bowman's capsule | glomerular capsule | renal corpuscle |
| collecting tubule | glomerulus | renal tubule |
| distal convoluted tubule | loop of Henle | |

The functional or working unit of the kidney is the nephron (see ■ Figure 9.4). You have to examine a small portion of the kidney under a microscope to see these microscopic structures. There are more than one million nephrons in each human kidney.

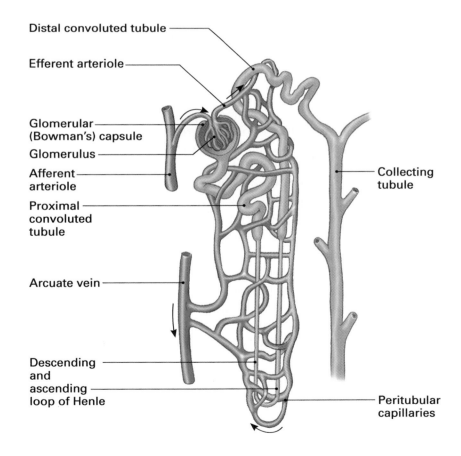

**■ FIGURE 9.4** The structure of a nephron.

Each nephron consists of the **renal corpuscle** (**KOR** pus ehl) and the **renal tubule** (**TOOB** yool) (refer to Figure 9.4). The renal corpuscle is the blood-filtering portion of the nephron. It has a double-walled cuplike structure called the **glomerular** (glom **AIR** yoo lar) or **Bowman's capsule** (**BOW** manz **CAP** sool) that encases a ball of capillaries called the **glomerulus** (glom **AIR** yoo lus). An **afferent arteriole** (**AFF** er ent ar **TEE** ree ol) carries blood to the glomerulus, and an **efferent arteriole** (**EF** er ent ar **TEE** ree ohl) carries blood away from the glomerulus.

Water and substances that were removed from the bloodstream in the renal corpuscle flow into the renal tubules to finish the urine production process. This continuous tubule is divided into four sections: the **proximal convoluted tubule** (**PROK** sim al con voh **LOOT** ed **TOOB** yool), followed by the narrow **loop of Henle,** then the **distal convoluted tubule** (**DISS** tall con voh **LOOT** ed **TOOB** yool), and, finally the **collecting tubule.**

### Stages of Urine Production

| | | |
|---|---|---|
| amino acids | glucose | reabsorption |
| filtration | nutrients | secretion |
| glomerular filtrate | peritubular capillaries | toxins |

Waste products must be eliminated from the body, but some of the glomerular filtrate—water, electrolytes, **nutrients**—must be returned to the bloodstream (see Figure 9.5). Urine, ready for elimination from the body, is the ultimate product of this entire process.

Urine production occurs in three stages: **filtration, reabsorption,** and **secretion.** Each of these steps is performed by a different section of the hard-working nephrons. Following are the three stages of urine production. (See Figure 9.6 for a CAT scan of the working kidneys.)

1. **Filtration.** The first stage is the filtering of particles, which occurs in the renal corpuscle. The pressure of blood flowing through the glomerulus forces material through the glomerular wall of Bowman's capsule and into the renal tubules. This fluid in the tubules is called the **glomerular filtrate** (glom **AIR** yoo lar **FILL** trayt) and consists of water, electrolytes, nutrients such as **glucose** and **amino acids,** wastes, and **toxins.**

2. **Reabsorption.** After filtration, the filtrate passes through the four sections of the tubule. As the filtrate moves along its twisted journey, most of the water and much of the electrolytes and nutrients are reabsorbed into the **peritubular capillaries,** a capillary bed that surrounds the renal tubules. They can then reenter the circulating blood.

3. **Secretion.** The final stage of urine production occurs when the special cells of the renal tubules secrete ammonia, uric acid, and other waste substances directly into the renal tubule. Urine formation is now finished; it passes into the collecting tubules, renal papilla, calyx, and ultimately into the renal pelvis.

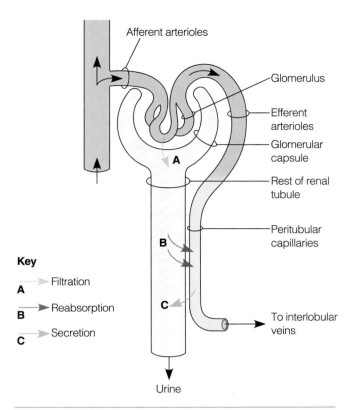

**FIGURE 9.5** Schematic view of the three stages of urine production: (A) filtration; (B) reabsorption; and (C) secretion.

Key

A —→ Filtration

B —→ Reabsorption

C —→ Secretion

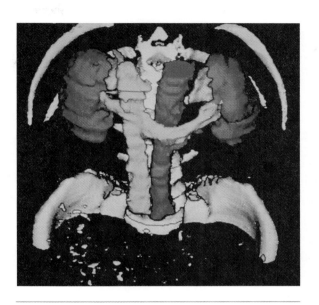

**FIGURE 9.6** Enhanced color CAT scan of kidneys (in red).
(CNRI/GJLP/Phototake NYC)

## Ureters

**cystitis**          **mucous membrane**          **peristaltic waves**

Once urine is formed in the collecting tubules, it drains into the renal pelvis and down the ureter into the urinary bladder. Ureters are very narrow tubes measuring less than 1/4 inch wide and 10 to 12 inches long that extend from the renal pelvis to the urinary bladder. **Mucous membrane** lines the ureters just as it lines most internal passages. ▮ Figure 9.7 shows the kidneys and surrounding structures, including the ureters. Urine goes into the bladder through the ureters every few seconds. It enters as spurts through the ureteral openings into the bladder. This orifice opens and closes through a process of **peristaltic** (pair ih **STALL** tik) **waves.**

**MED TERM TIP**

Mucous membranes will carry infections up the urinary tract from the urinary meatus and urethra into the bladder and eventually up the ureters and into the kidneys if not stopped. It is never wise to ignore a simple bladder infection or what is called **cystitis** (siss **TYE** tis).

## Urinary Bladder

**external sphincter**          **pubic symphysis**          **urination**
**internal sphincter**          **rugae**          **voiding**
**micturition**

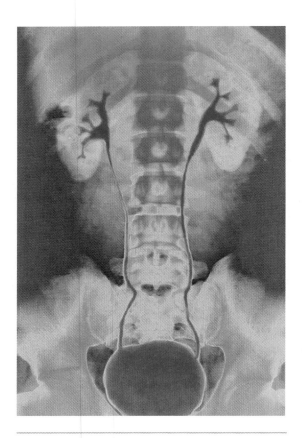

**FIGURE 9.7** Enhanced color three-dimensional model showing kidneys and surrounding structures.
(Clinique Ste. Catherine/ CNRI/Science Photo Library/ Photo Researchers, Inc.)

The bladder is an elastic muscular sac that lies in the base of the pelvis just behind the **pubic symphysis.** It is composed of three layers of smooth muscle tissue lined with mucous membrane containing **rugae** (**ROO** gay) or wrinkles. The bladder receives the urine directly from the ureters, stores urine, and excretes it through the urethra.

Generally, the bladder will hold 250 mL of urine. This amount then creates an urge to void or empty the bladder. Involuntary muscle action causes the bladder to contract and the **internal sphincter** (**SFINGK** ter) to relax. The internal sphincter protects us from having our bladder empty at the wrong time. Voluntary action controls the **external sphincter** (**SFINGK** ter). The act of controlling the emptying of urine is developed sometime after a child is 2 years of age.

## Urethra

semen                    vagina

The urethra is a tubular canal that carries the flow of urine from the bladder to the outside of the body. The external opening is called the urinary meatus. Mucous membrane also lines the urethra as it does the renal pelvis. This is one of the reasons that infection spreads up the urinary tract. The urethra is 1½ inches long in the female and 8 inches long in the male. In a woman it functions only as the outlet for urine and is in front of the **vagina.** In the male, however, it has two functions: an outlet for urine and the passageway for **semen** (**SEE** men) to leave the body.

> The terms *ureter* and *urethra* are frequently confused. Remember that there are two ureters carrying urine from the kidneys into the bladder. There is only one urethra and it carries urine from the bladder to the outside of the body.

## Urine

**albumin**                    **blood**                    **nitrogenous wastes**

Urine is normally straw colored to clear. Although it is 95% water, it also contains many dissolved substances, such as electrolytes, toxins, and **nitrogenous** (nigh **TROJ** eh nus) **wastes.** At times the urine also contains abnormal materials, such as glucose, **blood,** or **albumin** (al **BEW** min). This is the reason that analyzing urine gives medical personnel important information regarding disease processes occurring in a patient. Normally, during a 24-hour period the output of urine will be 1,000 to 2,000 mL, depending on the amount of fluid consumed and the general health of the person. Normal urine is acidic and the specific gravity varies from 1.001 to 1.030.

> The color, odor, volume, and sugar content of urine have been examined for centuries. Color charts for urine were developed by 1140, and "taste testing" was common in the late 17th century. By the 19th century, urinalysis was a routine part of a physical examination.

See Table 9.1 for the normal values for urine testing and Table 9.2 for abnormal findings.

| Table 9.1 | Values for Urinalysis Testing |
|---|---|
| **Element** | **Normal Findings** |
| Color | Straw colored, pale yellow, to deep gold |
| Odor | Aromatic |
| Appearance | Clear |
| Specific gravity | 1.010–1.030 |
| pH | 5.0–8.0 |
| Protein | Negative to trace |
| Glucose | None |
| Ketones | None |
| Blood | Negative |

| Table 9.2 | Abnormal Urinalysis Findings |
| --- | --- |
| Element | Implications |
| Color | Color varies depending on the patient's fluid intake and output or medication. Brown or black urine color indicates a serious disease process. |
| Odor | A fetid or foul odor may indicate infection. For instance, a fruity odor may be found in diabetes mellitus, dehydration, or starvation. Other odors may be due to medication or foods. |
| Appearance | Cloudiness may mean that an infection is present. |
| Specific gravity | Concentrated urine has a higher specific gravity. Dilute urine, such as can be found with diabetes insipidus, acute tubular necrosis, or salt-restricted diets, has a lower specific gravity. |
| pH | A pH value below 7.0 (acidic) is common in urinary tract infections, metabolic or respiratory acidosis, diets high in fruits or vegetables, or administration of some drugs. A pH higher than 7.0 (basic or alkaline) is common in metabolic or respiratory alkalosis, fever, high-protein diets, and taking ascorbic acid. |
| Protein | Protein may indicate glomerulonephritis or preeclampsia in a pregnant woman. |
| Glucose | Small amounts of glucose may be present as the result of eating a high-carbohydrate meal, stress, pregnancy, and taking some medications, such as aspirin or corticosteroids. Higher levels may indicate poorly controlled diabetes, Cushing's syndrome, or infection. |
| Ketones | The presence of ketones may indicate poorly controlled diabetes, dehydration, starvation, or ingestion of large amounts of aspirin. |
| Blood | Blood may indicate some types of anemia, taking of some medications (such as blood thinners), arsenic poisoning, reactions to transfusion, trauma, burns, and convulsions. |

# Word Building Relating to the Urinary System

The following list contains examples of medical terms built directly from word parts. The definition for these terms can be determined by a straightforward translation of the word parts.

| Combining Form | Combined With | Medical Term | Definition |
| --- | --- | --- | --- |
| cyst/o | -algia | cystalgia (sis **TAL** jee ah) | bladder pain |
| | -ectomy | cystectomy (sis **TEK** toh me) | excision of the bladder |
| | -itis | cystitis (siss **TYE** tis) | bladder inflammation |
| | -lith | cystolith (**SIS** toh lith) | bladder stone |
| | -ostomy | cystostomy (sis **TOSS** toh mee) | create a new opening into the bladder |
| | -otomy | cystotomy (sis **TOT** oh mee) | incision into the bladder |
| | -plasty | cystoplasty (**SIS** toh plas tee) | surgical repair of the bladder |
| | -rrhagia | cystorrhagia (sis toh **RAH** jee ah) | rapid bleeding from bladder |
| | -scope | cystoscope (**SIS** toh scope) | instrument used to visually examine the bladder |
| lith/o | -tripsy | lithotripsy (**LITH** oh trip see) | surgical crushing of a stone |
| | -otomy | lithotomy (lith **OT** oh me) | incision to remove a stone |
| nephr/o | -ectomy | nephrectomy (ne **FREK** toh mee) | excision of a kidney |
| | -gram | nephrogram (**NEH** fro gram) | X-ray of the kidney |
| | -itis | nephritis (neh **FRYE** tis) | kidney inflammation |
| | -malacia | nephromalacia (nef roh mah **LAY** she ah) | softening of the kidney |

| | -megaly | nephromegaly (nef roh **MEG** ah lee) | enlarged kidney |
|---|---|---|---|
| | -oma | nephroma (neh **FROH** ma) | kidney tumor |
| | -ptosis | nephroptosis (nef rop **TOH** sis) | drooping kidney |
| | -ostomy | nephrostomy (neh **FROS** toh mee) | create a new opening into the kidney |
| | -otomy | nephrotomy (neh **FROT** oh mee) | incision into a kidney |
| | -pathy | nephropathy (neh **FROP** ah thee) | kidney disease |
| | -pexy | nephropexy (**NEF** roh pek see) | surgical fixation of kidney |
| | -lithiasis | nephrolithiasis (nef roh lith **EE** a sis) | condition of kidney stones |
| | -sclerosis | nephrosclerosis (nef roh skleh **ROH** sis) | hardening of the kidney |
| pyel/o | -gram | pyelogram (**PYE** eh loh gram) | X-ray record of the renal pelvis |
| | -itis | pyelitis (pye eh **LYE** tis) | renal pelvis inflammation |
| | -plasty | pyeloplasty (**PIE** ah loh plas tee) | surgical repair of the renal pelvis |
| ur/o | -logist | urologist (yoo **RALL** oh jist) | specialist in the urinary system |
| | -logy | urology (yoo **RALL** oh jee) | study of the urinary system |
| ureter/o | -ectasis | ureterectasis (yoo ree ter **EK** tah sis) | ureter dilation |
| | -stenosis | ureterostenosis (yoo ree ter oh sten **OH** sis) | narrowing of a ureter |
| urethr/o | -algia | urethralgia (yoo ree **THRAL** jee ah) | urethra pain |
| | -itis | urethritis (yoo ree **THRIGH** tis) | urethra inflammation |
| | -rrhagia | urethrorrhagia (yoo ree throh **RAH** jee ah) | rapid bleeding from the urethra |
| | -scope | urethroscope (yoo **REE** throh scope) | instrument to visually examine the urethra |
| | -stenosis | urethrostenosis (yoo ree throh steh **NOH** sis) | narrowing of the urethra |
| urin/o | -meter | urinometer (yoo rin **OH** meter) | instrument to measure urine |
| | -ary | urinary (yoo rih **NAIR** ee) | pertaining to urine |

| Suffix | Combined With | Medical Term | Definition |
|---|---|---|---|
| -uria | albumin/o | albuminuria (al byoo men **YOO** ree ah) | albumin (protein) in the urine |
| | an- | anuria (an **YOO** ree ah) | condition of no urine |
| | azot/o | azoturia (a zo **TOO** ree ah) | nitrogenous waste in the urine |
| | bacteri/o | bacteriuria (back teer ree **YOO** ree ah) | bacteria in the urine |
| | dys- | dysuria (dis **YOO** ree ah) | condition of difficult or painful urination |
| | glycos/o | glycosuria (glye kohs **YOO** ree ah) | condition of sugar in the urine |
| | hemat/o | hematuria (hee mah **TOO** ree ah) | condition of blood in the urine |
| | keton/o | ketonuria (key tone **YOO** ree ah) | ketones in the urine |
| | noct/i | nocturia (nok **TOO** ree ah) | condition of frequent nighttime urination |
| | olig/o | oliguria (ol ig **YOO** ree ah) | condition of scanty amount of urine |
| | poly- | polyuria (pol ee **YOO** ree ah) | condition of (too) much urine |
| | py/o | pyuria (pye **YOO** ree ah) | condition of pus in the urine |

# Vocabulary Relating to the Urinary System

| | |
|---|---|
| **anuria (an YOO ree ah)** | Complete suppression of urine formed by the kidneys and a complete lack of urine excretion. |
| **calculus (KAL kew lus)** | A stone formed within an organ by an accumulation of mineral salts. Found in the kidney, renal pelvis, ureters, bladder, or urethra. Plural is *calculi* (see ▨ Figure 9.8). |
| **diuresis (dye yoo REE sis)** | Increased formation and secretion of urine. |
| **enuresis (en yoo REE sis)** | Involuntary discharge of urine after the age by which bladder control should have been established. This usually occurs by the age of 5. Also called bed-wetting at night. |
| ***Escherichia coli* (esh eh REE she ah KOH lye) (E. coli)** | Normal bacteria found in the intestinal tract; the most common cause of lower urinary tract infections due to improper hygiene after bowel movements. |
| **frequency** | A greater-than-normal occurrence in the urge to urinate, without an increase in the total daily volume of urine. Frequency is an indication of inflammation of the bladder or urethra. |
| **hesitancy** | A decrease in the force of the urine stream, often with difficulty initiating the flow. It is often a symptom of a blockage along the urethra, such as an enlarged prostate gland. |
| **micturition (mik too RIH shun)** | Another term for urination. |
| **renal colic (REE nal KOL ik)** | Pain caused by a kidney stone. Can be an excruciating pain and generally requires medical treatment. |
| **stricture (STRIK chur)** | Narrowing of a passageway in the urinary system. |
| **uremia (yoo REE me ah)** | Accumulation of waste products (especially nitrogenous wastes) in the bloodstream. Associated with renal failure. |
| **urgency (ER jen see)** | Feeling the need to urinate immediately. |
| **urinary incontinence (YOO rih nair ee in CON tin ens)** | Involuntary release of urine. In some patients an indwelling catheter is inserted into the bladder for continuous urine drainage (see ▨ Figure 9.9). |
| **urinary retention (YOO rih nair ee ree TEN shun)** | An inability to fully empty the bladder, often indicates a blockage in the urethra. |

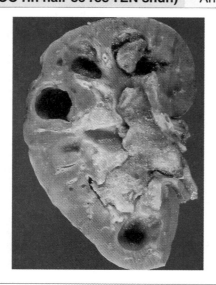

▨ **FIGURE 9.8** Sectioned kidney with calculi.
(Dr. E. Walker/Science Photo Library/Photo Researchers, Inc.)

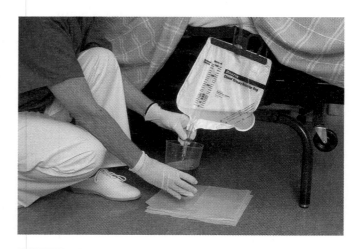

▨ **FIGURE 9.9** Closed urinary drainage system. Urine being measured after it leaves patient's body via catheter.

# Pathology Relating to the Urinary System

| | |
|---|---|
| **acute tubular necrosis (ne KROH sis) (ATN)** | Damage to the renal tubules due to presence of toxins in the urine or to ischemia. Results in oliguria. |
| **bladder neck obstruction (BNO)** | Blockage of the bladder outlet. Often caused by an enlarged prostate gland in males. |
| **cystocele (SIS toh seel)** | Hernia or protrusion of the urinary bladder into the wall of the vagina. |
| **diabetic nephropathy (ne FROH path ee)** | Accumulation of damage to the glomerulus capillaries due to the chronic high blood sugars of diabetes mellitus. |
| **glomerulonephritis (gloh mair yoo loh neh FRYE tis)** | Inflammation of the kidney (primarily of the glomerulus). Since the glomerular membrane is inflamed, it becomes more permeable and will allow protein and blood cells to enter the filtrate. Results in protein in the urine (proteinuria) and hematuria. |
| **hydronephrosis (high droh neh FROH sis)** | Distention of the renal pelvis due to urine collecting in the kidney; often a result of the obstruction of a ureter. |
| **interstitial cystitis (in ter STISH al sis TYE tis)** | Disease of unknown cause in which there is inflammation and irritation of the bladder. Most commonly seen in middle-aged women. |
| **nephrolithiasis (nef roh lith EE a sis)** | The presence of calculi in the kidney. Usually begins with the solidification of salts present in the urine. |
| **polycystic (POL ee sis tik) kidneys** | Formation of multiple cysts within the kidney tissue. Results in the destruction of normal kidney tissue and uremia (see ■ Figure 9.10). |
| **pyelonephritis (pye eh loh neh FRYE tis)** | Inflammation of the renal pelvis and the kidney. One of the most common types of kidney disease. It may be the result of a lower urinary tract infection that moved up to the kidney by way of the ureters. There may be large quantities of white blood cells and bacteria in the urine. Blood (hematuria) may even be present in the urine in this condition. Can occur with any untreated or persistent case of cystitis. |
| **renal failure** | Inability of the kidneys to filter wastes from the blood resulting in uremia. May be acute or chronic. Major reason for a patient being placed on dialysis. |
| **urinary tract infection (UTI)** | Infection, usually from bacteria such as *E. coli*, of any organ of the urinary system. Most often begins with cystitis and may ascend into the ureters and kidneys. Most common in women because of their shorter urethra. |
| **Wilm's tumor (VILMZ TOO mor)** | Malignant kidney tumor found most often in children. |

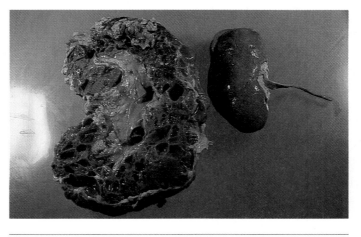

■ **FIGURE 9.10**   A polycystic kidney on the left compared to a normal kidney on the right.

# Diagnostic Procedures Relating to the Urinary System

| | |
|---|---|
| **blood urea nitrogen (BLUD yoo REE ah NIGH troh jen) (BUN)** | Blood test to measure kidney function by the level of nitrogenous waste, urea, that is in the blood. |
| **clean catch specimen** | Urine sample obtained after cleaning off the urinary opening and catching or collecting a sample in midstream (halfway through the urination process) to minimize contamination from the genitalia. |
| **cystography (sis TOG rah fee)** | Process of instilling a contrast material or dye into the bladder by catheter to visualize the urinary bladder on X-ray. |
| **cystoscopy (sis TOSS koh pee)** | Visual examination of the urinary bladder using an instrument called a cystoscope. |
| **excretory urography (EKS kreh tor ee yoo ROG rah fee)** | Injecting dye into the bloodstream and then taking an X-ray to trace the action of the kidney as it excretes the dye. |
| **intravenous pyelogram (in trah VEE nus PYE eh loh gram) (IVP)** | Injecting a contrast medium into a vein and then taking an X-ray to visualize the renal pelvis. |
| **kidneys, ureters, bladder (KUB)** | X-ray taken of the abdomen demonstrating the kidneys, ureters, and bladder without using any contrast dye. Also called a *flat-plate abdomen*. |
| **retrograde pyelogram (RET roh grayd PYE eh loh gram)** | A diagnostic X-ray in which dye is inserted through the urethra to outline the bladder, ureters, and renal pelvis. |
| **urinalysis (yoo rih NAL ih sis) (U/A, UA)** | Laboratory test that consists of the physical, chemical, and microscopic examination of urine. |
| **urine culture and sensitivity (C & S)** | Laboratory test of urine for bacterial infection. Attempt to grow bacteria on a culture medium in order to identify it and determine which antibiotics it is sensitive to. |
| **voiding cystourethrography (sis toh yoo ree THROG rah fee) (VCUG)** | X-ray taken to visualize the urethra while the patient is voiding after a contrast dye has been placed in the bladder. |

# Therapeutic Procedures Relating to the Urinary System

| | |
|---|---|
| **catheterization (kath eh ter ih ZAY shun)** | Insertion of a tube through the urethra and into the urinary bladder for the purpose of withdrawing urine or inserting dye. |
| **extracorporeal shockwave lithotripsy (eks trah cor POR ee al shockwave LITH oh trip see) (ESWL)** | Use of ultrasound waves to break up stones. Process does not require invasive surgery (see ■ Figure 9.11). |
| **hemodialysis (hee moh dye AL ih sis)** | Use of an artificial kidney machine that filters the blood of a person to remove waste products. Use of this technique in patients who have defective kidneys is lifesaving (see ■ Figure 9.12). |
| **lithotomy (lith OT oh mee)** | Surgical incision to remove kidney stones. |
| **lithotripsy (LITH oh trip see)** | Destroying or crushing stones in the bladder or urethra. |
| **meatotomy (mee ah TOT oh me)** | An incision into the meatus in order to enlarge the opening of the urethra. |

| peritoneal dialysis (pair ih TOH nee al dye AL ih sis) | Removal of toxic waste substances from the body by placing warm chemically balanced solutions into the peritoneal cavity. Wastes are filtered out of the blood across the peritoneum. Used in treating renal failure and certain poisonings (see ■ Figure 9.13). |
| --- | --- |
| renal (REE nal) transplant | Surgical placement of a donor kidney (see ■ Figure 9.14). |

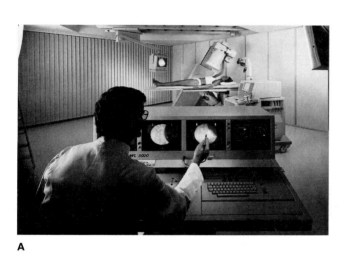

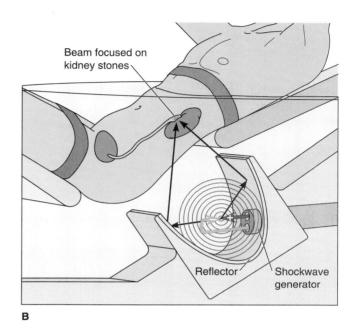

**A**  **B**

■ **FIGURE 9.11**  Extracorporeal shockwave lithotripsy. Acoustic shockwaves created by the shockwave generator travel through soft tissue to shatter the renal stone into fragments, which are then eliminated in the urine. (A) A shockwave generator that does not require water immersion. (B) An illustration of water immersion lithotripsy procedure.

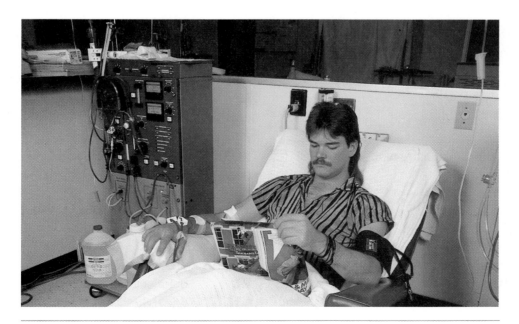

■ **FIGURE 9.12**  Patient undergoing hemodialysis in dialysis unit.
(Southern Illinois University/Photo Researchers, Inc.)

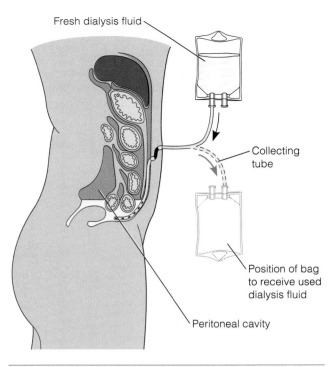

Fresh dialysis fluid

Collecting tube

Position of bag to receive used dialysis fluid

Peritoneal cavity

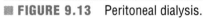

**FIGURE 9.13** Peritoneal dialysis.

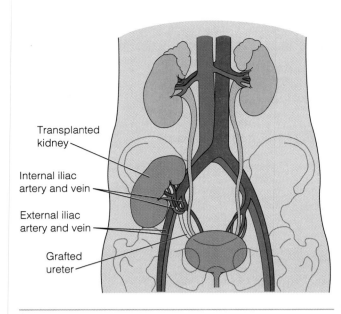

Transplanted kidney

Internal iliac artery and vein

External iliac artery and vein

Grafted ureter

**FIGURE 9.14** Placement of transplanted kidney.

# Pharmacology Relating to the Urinary System

| | |
|---|---|
| **antibiotic** | Used to treat bacterial infections of the urinary tract. |
| **antispasmodic** (an tye spaz MAH dik) | Medication to prevent or reduce bladder muscle spasms. |
| **diuretics (dye yoo REH tiks)** | Medication that increases the volume of urine produced by the kidneys. Useful in the treatment of edema, kidney failure, heart failure, and hypertension. |

# Abbreviations Relating to the Urinary System

| | | | | |
|---|---|---|---|---|
| **AGN** | acute glomerulonephritis | | **H₂O** | water |
| **ARF** | acute renal failure | | **I&O** | intake and output |
| **ATN** | acute tubular necrosis | | **IPD** | intermittent peritoneal dialysis |
| **BNO** | bladder neck obstruction | | **IVP** | intravenous pyelogram |
| **BUN** | blood urea nitrogen | | **K⁺** | potassium |
| **CAPD** | continuous ambulatory peritoneal dialysis | | **KUB** | kidney, ureter, bladder |
| **cath** | catheterization | | **mL** | milliliter |
| **Cl⁻** | chloride | | **Na⁺** | sodium |
| **CRF** | chronic renal failure | | **pH** | acidity or alkalinity of urine |
| **C&S** | culture and sensitivity | | **RP** | retrograde pyelogram |
| **cysto** | cystoscopic exam | | **SG** | specific gravity |
| **E. coli** | *Escherichia coli* | | **U/A, UA** | urinalysis |
| **ESRD** | end-stage renal disease | | **UC** | urine culture |
| **ESWL** | extracorporeal shockwave lithotripsy | | **UTI** | urinary tract infection |
| **GU** | genitourinary | | **VCUG** | voiding cystourethrography |
| **HCO₃⁻** | bicarbonate | | | |

# Chapter Review

## Pronunciation Practice

 *You will find the pronunciation for each term on the enclosed CD-ROM. Check each one off as you master it.*

- ☐ acute tubular necrosis (ne **KROH** sis)
- ☐ afferent arteriole (**AFF** er ent ar **TEE** ree ohl)
- ☐ albumin (al **BEW** min)
- ☐ albuminuria (al byoo men **YOO** ree ah)
- ☐ amino acids
- ☐ antibiotic
- ☐ antispasmodic (an tye spaz **MAH** dik)
- ☐ anuria (an **YOO** ree ah)
- ☐ azoturia (a zo **TOO** ree ah)
- ☐ bacteriuria (back teer ree **YOO** ree ah)
- ☐ bicarbonate
- ☐ bladder neck obstruction
- ☐ blood
- ☐ blood urea nitrogen (**BLUD** yoo **REE** ah **NIGH** troh jen)
- ☐ Bowman's capsule (**BOW** manz **CAP** sool)
- ☐ calculus (**KAL** kew lus)
- ☐ calyx (**KAY** liks)
- ☐ catheterization (kath eh ter ih **ZAY** shun)
- ☐ chloride
- ☐ clean catch specimen
- ☐ collecting tubule (**TOOB** yool)
- ☐ cortex (**KOR** teks)
- ☐ cystalgia (sis **TAL** jee ah)
- ☐ cystectomy (sis **TEK** toh mee)
- ☐ cystitis (sis **TYE** tis)
- ☐ cystocele (**SIS** toh seel)
- ☐ cystography (sis **TOG** rah fee)
- ☐ cystolith (**SIS** toh lith)
- ☐ cystoplasty (**SIS** toh plas tee)
- ☐ cystorrhagia (sis toh **RAH** jee ah)
- ☐ cystoscope (**SIS** toh scope)
- ☐ cystoscopy (sis **TOSS** koh pee)
- ☐ cystostomy (sis **TOSS** toh mee)
- ☐ cystotomy (sis **TOT** oh mee)
- ☐ diabetic nephropathy (ne **FROH** path ee)

- ☐ distal convoluted tubule (**DISS** tall con voh **LOOT** ed **TOOB** yool)
- ☐ diuresis (dye yoo **REE** sis)
- ☐ diuretic (dye yoo **REH** tiks)
- ☐ dysuria (dis **YOO** ree ah)
- ☐ efferent arteriole (**EF** er ent ar **TEE** ree ohl)
- ☐ electrolyte (ee **LEK** troh lite)
- ☐ enuresis (en yoo **REE** sis)
- ☐ *Escherichia coli* (esh eh **REE** she ah **KOH** lye)(*E. coli*)
- ☐ excretory urography (**EKS** kreh tor ee yoo **ROG** rah fee)
- ☐ external sphincter (**SFINGK** ter)
- ☐ extracorporeal shockwave lithotripsy (eks trah cor **POR** ee al shockwave **LITH** oh trip see)
- ☐ filtration
- ☐ frequency
- ☐ genitourinary (jen ih toh **YOO** rih nair ee) system
- ☐ glomerular capsule (glom **AIR** yoo lar **CAP** sool)
- ☐ glomerular filtrate (glom **AIR** yoo lar **FILL** trayt)
- ☐ glomerulonephritis (gloh mair yoo loh neh **FRYE** tis)
- ☐ glomerulus (glom **AIR** yoo lus)
- ☐ glucose
- ☐ glycosuria (glye kohs **YOO** ree ah)
- ☐ hematuria (hee mah **TOO** ree ah)
- ☐ hemodialysis (hee moh dye **AL** ih sis)
- ☐ hesitancy
- ☐ hilum (**HIGH** lum)
- ☐ homeostasis (hoh mee oh **STAY** sis)
- ☐ hydronephrosis (high droh neh **FROH** sis)
- ☐ internal sphincter (**SFINGK** ter)
- ☐ interstitial cystitis (in ter **STISH** al sis **TYE** tis)
- ☐ intravenous pyelogram (in trah **VEE** nus **PYE** eh loh gram)
- ☐ ketonuria (key tone **YOO** ree ah)
- ☐ kidneys
- ☐ kidneys, ureters, bladder
- ☐ lithotomy (lith **OT** oh mee)
- ☐ lithotripsy (**LITH** oh trip see)

- loop of Henle
- meatotomy (mee ah **TOT** oh mee)
- medulla (meh **DULL** ah)
- micturition (mik too **RIH** shun)
- mucous membrane
- nephrectomy (neh **FREK** toh mee)
- nephritis (neh **FRYE** tis)
- nephrogram (**NEH** fro gram)
- nephrolithiasis (nef roh lith **EE** a sis)
- nephroma (neh **FROH** mah)
- nephromalacia (nef roh mah **LAY** she ah)
- nephromegaly (nef roh **MEG** ah lee)
- nephrons (**NEF** ronz)
- nephropathy (neh **FROP** ah thee)
- nephropexy (**NEF** roh pek see)
- nephroptosis (nef rop **TOH** sis)
- nephrosclerosis (nef roh skleh **ROH** sis)
- nephrostomy (neh **FROS** toh mee)
- nephrotomy (neh **FROT** oh mee)
- nitrogenous (nigh **TROJ** eh nus) wastes
- nocturia (nok **TOO** ree ah)
- nutrients
- oliguria (ol ig **YOO** ree ah)
- peristaltic (pair ih **STALL** tik) waves
- peritoneal dialysis (pair ih **TOH** nee al dye **AL** ih sis)
- peritoneum (pair ih toh **NEE** um)
- peritubular capillaries
- pH
- polycystic (**POL** ee sis tik) kidneys
- polyuria (pol ee **YOO** ree ah)
- potassium
- proximal convoluted tubule (**PROK** sim al con voh **LOOT** ed **TOOB** yool)
- pubic symphysis
- pyelitis (pye eh **LYE** tis)
- pyelogram (**PYE** eh loh gram)
- pyelonephritis (pye eh loh neh **FRYE** tis)
- pyeloplasty (**PYE** ah loh plas tee)
- pyuria (pye **YOO** ree ah)
- reabsorption
- renal artery (**REE** nal **AR** teh ree)
- renal colic (**REE** nal **KOL** ik)
- renal corpuscle (**KOR** pus ehl)
- renal (**REE** nal) failure
- renal papilla (pah **PILL** ah)

- renal pelvis (**PELL** vis)
- renal pyramids (**PEER** ah mids)
- renal (**REE** nal) transplant
- renal tubule (**TOOB** yool)
- renal (**REE** nal) vein
- retrograde pyelogram (**RET** roh grayd **PYE** eh loh gram)
- retroperitoneal (ret roh pair ih toh **NEE** al)
- rugae (**ROO** gay)
- secretion
- semen (**SEE** men)
- serum electrolyte (**SEE** rum ee **LEK** troh lite) level
- sodium
- stricture (**STRIK** chur)
- toxins
- uremia (yoo **REE** mee ah)
- ureterectasis (yoo ree ter **EK** tah sis)
- ureterostenosis (yoo ree ter oh sten **OH** sis)
- ureters (yoo **REE** ters)
- urethra (yoo **REE** thrah)
- urethralgia (yoo ree **THRAL** jee ah)
- urethritis (yoo ree **THRIGH** tis)
- urethrorrhagia (yoo ree throh **RAH** jee ah)
- urethroscope (yoo **REE** throh scope)
- urethrostenosis (yoo ree throh steh **NOH** sis)
- urgency (**ER** jen see)
- urinalysis (yoo rih **NAL** ih sis)
- urinary (**YOO** rih nair ee)
- urinary (**YOO** rih nair ee) bladder
- urinary incontinence (**YOO** rih nair ee in **CON** tin ens)
- urinary meatus (**YOO** rih nair ee mee **AY** tus)
- urinary retention (**YOO** rih nair ee ree **TEN** shun)
- urinary tract infection
- urination
- urine (**YOO** rin)
- urine culture and sensitivity
- urinometer (yoo rin **OH** meter)
- urologist (yoo **RALL** oh jist)
- urology (yoo **RALL** oh jee)
- vagina
- voiding
- voiding cystourethrography (sis toh yoo ree **THROG** rah fee)
- waste products
- Wilm's tumor (**VILMZ TOO** mor)

# Case Study

## Discharge Summary

**Admitting Diagnosis:** Severe right side pain, visible blood in his urine.

**Final Diagnosis:** Pyelonephritis right kidney, complicated by chronic cystitis.

**History of Present Illness:** Patient has long history of frequent bladder infections, but denies any recent lower pelvic pain or dysuria. Earlier today he had rapid onset of severe right side pain, and is unable to stand fully erect. His temperature was 101°F and his skin was sweaty and flushed. He was admitted from the ER for further testing and diagnosis.

**Summary of Hospital Course:** Clean catch urinalysis revealed gross hematuria and pyuria, but no albuminuria. A culture and sensitivity was ordered to identify the pathogen and a broad-spectrum IV antibiotic was started. An intravenous pyelogram indicated no calculi or obstructions in the ureters. Cystoscopy discovered evidence of chronic cystitis, bladder irritation, and a bladder neck obstruction. The obstruction appears to be congenital and the probable cause of the chronic cystitis. The patient was catheterized to ensure complete emptying of the bladder, and fluids were encouraged. Patient responded well to the antibiotic therapy and fluids, and his symptoms improved.

**Discharge Plans:** Patient was discharged home after 3 days in the hospital. He was switched to an oral antibiotic for the pyelonephritis and chronic cystitis. A repeat urinalysis is scheduled for next week. After all inflammation is corrected, will repeat cystoscopy to reevaluate bladder neck obstruction. Will discuss if urethroplasty is indicated at that time.

## Critical Thinking Questions

1. This patient has a long history of frequent bladder infections. What did the physician discover that explained this?

2. Describe, in your own words, the patient's condition when he came to the emergency room.

3. This patient has gross hematuria. What do you think the term *gross* means in this context?

4. The following terms are not referred to in this chapter. Define each in your own words, using your text as a dictionary.
   a. congenital
   b. chronic
   c. pathogen
   d. oral

5. Which of the following substances was not found in the patient's urine?
   a. protein
   b. pus
   c. blood

6. How are pyelonephritis and glomerulonephritis alike? How are they different?

# Chart Note Transcription

## Chart Note

The chart note below contains 11 phrases that can be reworded with a medical term that you learned in this chapter. Each phrase is identified with an underline. Determine the medical term and write your answers in the space provided.

**Current Complaint:** A 36-year-old male was seen by the specialist in the treatment of diseases of the urinary system① because of right flank pain and blood in the urine.②

**Past History:** Patient has a history of bladder infection;③ denies experiencing any symptoms for 2 years.

**Signs and Symptoms:** A technique used to obtain an uncontaminated urine sample④ obtained for laboratory analysis of the urine⑤ revealed blood in the urine, but no pus in the urine.⑥ A kidney X-ray made after inserting dye into the bladder⑦ was normal on the left, but dye was seen filling the right tube between the kidney and bladder⑧ only halfway to the kidney.

**Diagnosis:** Stone in the tube between the kidney and the bladder⑨ on the right.

**Treatment:** Patient underwent the use of ultrasound waves to break up stones.⑩ Pieces of dissolved kidney stones⑪ were flushed out, after which symptoms resolved.

1. _____

2. _____

3. _____

4. _____

5. _____

6. _____

7. _____

8. _____

9. _____

10. _____

11. _____

# Practice Exercises

## A. State the terms described using the combining forms indicated.

The combining form *nephr/o* refers to the kidney. Use it to write a term that means

1. surgical fixation of the kidney _____
2. X-ray record of the kidney _____
3. condition of kidney stones _____
4. removal of a kidney _____
5. inflammation of the kidney _____
6. kidney disease _____
7. hardening of the kidney _____

The combining form *cyst/o* refers to the urinary bladder. Use it to write a term that means

8. inflammation of the bladder _____
9. rapid bleeding from the bladder _____
10. surgical repair of the bladder _____
11. instrument to view inside the bladder _____
12. bladder pain _____

The combining form *pyel/o* refers to the renal pelvis. Use it to write a term that means

13. surgical repair of the renal pelvis _____
14. inflammation of the renal pelvis _____
15. X-ray record of the renal pelvis _____

The combining form *ureter/o* refers to one or both of the ureters. Use it to write a term that means

16. a ureteral stone _____
17. surgical repair of a ureter _____
18. surgical removal of a ureter _____

The combining form *urethr/o* refers to the urethra. Use it to write a term that means

19. surgical repair of the urethra _____
20. surgical creation of an opening into the urethra _____

## B. Define the following terms.

1. micturition _____
2. diuretic _____
3. renal colic _____
4. catheterization _____
5. pyelitis _____
6. nephropyelitis _____
7. lithotomy _____
8. enuresis _____
9. meatotomy _____

10. diabetic nephropathy _____

11. urinalysis _____

12. hesitancy _____

## C. Write the medical term that means

1. absence of urine _____

2. blood in the urine _____

3. kidney stone _____

4. crushing a stone _____

5. inflammation of the urethra _____

6. pus in the urine _____

7. bacteria in the urine _____

8. painful urination _____

9. ketones in the urine _____

10. albumin in the urine _____

11. (too) much urine _____

## D. Write the abbreviation for the following terms.

1. potassium _____

2. sodium _____

3. urinalysis _____

4. blood urea nitrogen _____

5. specific gravity _____

6. intravenous pyelogram _____

7. bladder neck obstruction _____

8. intake and output _____

9. acute tubular necrosis _____

10. end stage renal disease _____

## E. Identify the following abbreviations.

1. KUB _____

2. cath _____

3. cysto _____

4. GU _____

5. ESWL _____

6. UTI _____

7. UC _____

8. RP _____

9. ARF _____

10. BUN _____

11. CRF _____

12. $H_2O$ _____

**F. Match the terms in column A with the definitions in column B.**

| | A | | B |
|---|---|---|---|
| 1. | _____ Wilm's tumor | a. | kidney stones |
| 2. | _____ electrolytes | b. | feeling the need to urinate immediately |
| 3. | _____ nephrons | c. | childhood malignant kidney tumor |
| 4. | _____ loop of Henle | d. | swelling of the kidney due to urine collecting in the renal pelvis |
| 5. | _____ calyx | e. | involuntary release of urine |
| 6. | _____ incontinence | f. | collects urine as it is produced |
| 7. | _____ hydronephrosis | g. | sodium and potassium |
| 8. | _____ urgency | h. | functional unit of the kidneys |
| 9. | _____ nephrolithiasis | i. | part of the renal tubule |
| 10. | _____ polycystic kidneys | j. | multiple cysts in the kidneys |

**G. Use the following terms in the sentences that follow.**

| | |
|---|---|
| renal transplant | cystoscopy |
| cystostomy | intravenous pyelogram (IVP) |
| renal biopsy | nephropexy |
| ureterectomy | urinary tract infection |
| pyelolithectomy | |

1. Juan suffered from chronic renal failure. His sister, Maria, donated one of her normal kidneys to him and he had a(n) _____ .

2. Anesha's floating kidney needed surgical fixation. Her physician performed a surgical procedure known as _____ .

3. Kenya's physician stated that she had a general infection that he referred to as a UTI. The full name for this infection is _____ .

4. The surgeons operated on Robert to remove calculus from his renal pelvis. The name of this surgery is _____ .

5. Charles had to have a small piece of his kidney tissue removed so that the physician could perform a microscopic evaluation. This procedure is called a(n) _____ .

6. Naomi had to have one of her ureters removed due to a stricture. This procedure is called _____ .

7. The physician had to create a temporary opening between Eric's bladder and his abdominal wall. This procedure is called _____ .

8. Sally's bladder was visually examined using a special instrument. This procedure is called a(n) _____ .

9. The doctors believe that Jacob has a tumor of the right kidney. They are going to do a test called a(n) _____ that requires them to inject a radiopaque contrast medium intravenously so that they can see the kidney on X-ray.

# Professional Journal

In this exercise you will now have an opportunity to put the words you have learned into practice. Imagine yourself in the role of a dietitian. If you refer back to the Professional Profile at the beginning of this chapter, you will see that this health care professional uses diet to prevent and treat diseases, educates the public regarding good nutrition, and advances the science of how diet and nutrition affect our bodies. Use the 10 words listed below, or any other new terms from this or previous chapters, to write sentences to describe the patients you saw today.

An example of a sentence is *The patient was newly diagnosed with* **hypertension** *and required instruction in a low-salt diet.*

1. renal failure _____

2. glycosuria _____

3. hyperlipidemia _____

4. anaphylactic shock _____

5. pernicious anemia _____

6. alimentary canal _____

7. anorexia _____

8. dyspepsia _____

9. cholecystitis _____

10. constipation _____

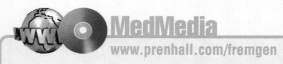
**MedMedia**
www.prenhall.com/fremgen

Use the CD-ROM enclosed with your textbook to gain additional reinforcement through interactive word building exercises, spelling games, labeling activities, and additional quizzes.

Use the above address to access the free, interactive Companion Website created for this textbook. Get hints, instant feedback, and textbook references to chapter-related multiple-choice questions, as well as labeling and matching exercises. In addition, you will find an audio glossary, case studies, and Internet exploration exercises.

***For more information regarding kidney and urinary diseases, visit the following websites:***

National Institutes of Health—select the Kidney and Urinary System link at **www.health.nih.gov**

Stanford Health Library at
   **http://healthlibrary.stanford.edu/resources/internet/bodysystems/urinary.html**

Your Urology Community at **www.urologychannel.com**

# Chapter 10

# Reproductive System

## Learning Objectives

*Upon completion of this chapter, you will be able to:*

- Recognize the combining forms and suffixes introduced in this chapter.

- Gain the ability to pronounce medical terms and major anatomical structures.

- List the major organs of the female and male reproductive systems and their functions.

- Use medical terms to describe circumstances relating to pregnancy.

- Identify the symptoms and origin of sexually transmitted diseases.

- Build female and male reproductive system medical terms from word parts.

- Define vocabulary, pathology, diagnostic, and therapeutic medical terms relating to the female and male reproductive systems.

- Recognize types of medications associated with the female and male reproductive systems.

- Interpret abbreviations associated with the female and male reproductive systems.

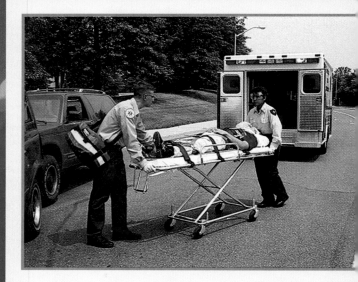

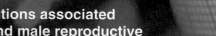

## MedMedia
www.prenhall.com/fremgen
Additional interactive resources and activities for this chapter can be found on the Companion Website. For animations, audio glossary, and review, access the accompanying CD-ROM in this book.

## Professional Profile

### Emergency Medical Service

Emergency medical services provide basic and advanced prehospital emergency care for traumatic or medical emergencies. They evaluate the patient's condition, initiate medical care according to a set of protocols, and stabilize and transport the patient to a hospital. Emergency medical services may work out of rescue, police, and fire departments; hospital emergency rooms; free-standing governmental emergency medical services; and private ambulance services.

### Emergency Medical Technician—Paramedic (EMT-P)

- Performs advanced life support procedures, administers drugs, interprets electrocardiograms, intubates patients, and utilizes the most complex monitoring equipment
- Completes the longest and most rigorous training program, 750 to 2,000 hours of training above the basic emergency medical technician level
- Completes an approved paramedic program in advanced emergency medical techniques
- Completes clinical training period

### Emergency Medical Technician—Intermediate (EMT-I)

- Performs certain advanced life support procedures, completes patient assessments, administers intravenous fluids, and uses a defibrillator
- Completes an approved emergency medical technician intermediate program
- Completes additional hours of training above the basic emergency medical technician level

### Emergency Medical Technician—Basic (EMT-B)

- Performs basic life support procedures such as establishing open airways, treating shock, assisting in childbirth, controlling bleeding, bandaging wounds, immobilizing fractures, and transporting patients
- Completes 140 hours of classroom instruction and a 10-hour internship in a hospital emergency room
- Completes an approved emergency medical technician basic program

*For more information regarding these health careers, visit the following websites:*
National Association of Emergency Medical Technicians at **www.naemt.org**
National Registry of Emergency Medical Technicians at **www.nremt.org**

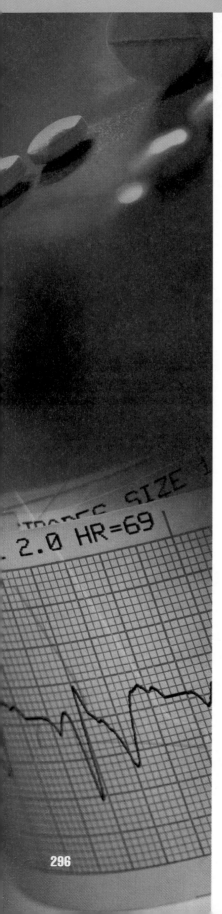

## Introduction

**fertilization**      **ova**
**genitalia**        **sperm**
**impregnation**

The reproductive organs are not necessary to sustain the life of the individual, but they are necessary for a continuation of the human race. The actual reproductive process consists of male cells called **sperm** joining female cells called **ova** (**OH** vah) or eggs. This process is called **fertilization** (fer til ih **ZAY** shun) or **impregnation** (im preg **NAY** shun). The term **genitalia** (jen ih **TAY** lee ah) is a general term used to refer to both male and female reproductive organs.

## Part I: Female Reproductive System

### Organs of the Female Reproductive System

breasts              uterus
fallopian tubes      vagina
ovaries              vulva

### Combining Forms Relating to the Female Reproductive System

| | | | |
|---|---|---|---|
| amni/o | amnion | men/o | menses, menstruation |
| cervic/o | neck, cervix | metr/o | uterus |
| chori/o | chorion | nat/o | birth |
| colp/o | vagina | o/o | egg |
| culd/o | cul-de-sac | omphal/o | navel, umbilicus |
| embry/o | embryo | oophor/o | ovary |
| episi/o | vulva | ov/o | egg |
| fet/o | fetus | ovari/o | ovary |
| gynec/o | woman, female | part/o | childbirth |
| hymen/o | hymen | perine/o | perineum |
| hyster/o | uterus | salping/o | fallopian tubes, uterine tubes |
| lact/o | milk | uter/o | uterus |
| mamm/o | breast | vagin/o | vagina |
| mast/o | breast | vulv/o | vulva |

### Suffixes Relating to the Female Reproductive System

| Suffix | Meaning | Example |
|---|---|---|
| -arche | beginning | menarche |
| -cyesis | state of pregnancy | pseudocyesis |
| -gravida | pregnancy | multigravida |
| -para | to bear (offspring) | nullipara |
| -salpinx | fallopian tube | pyosalpinx |
| -tocia | labor, childbirth | dystocia |

# Anatomy and Physiology of the Female Reproductive System

clitoris

fallopian tubes

labia majora

labia minora

ovaries

perineum

uterus

vagina

vulva

The female reproductive system consists of both internal and external genitalia. The internal genitalia are located in the pelvic cavity and consist of one **uterus** (**YOO** ter us), two **ovaries** (**OH** vah reez), two **fallopian tubes** (fah **LOH** pee an **TOOBS**), and the **vagina** (vah **JIGH** nah), which extends to the external surface of the body (see ■ Figure 10.1).

The external genitalia are also referred to as the **vulva** (**VULL** vah) and contain the **labia majora** (**LAY** bee ah mah **JOR** ah), **labia minora** (**LAY** bee ah mih **NOR** ah), and **clitoris** (**KLIT** oh ris). The region between the vaginal opening and the anus is referred to as the **perineum** (pair ih **NEE** um).

## Internal Genitalia

### Uterus

anteflexion

cervix

corpus

endometrium

fundus

ligaments

menarche

menopause

menstrual period

menstruation

myometrium

ovum

perimetrium

The uterus is a hollow, pear-shaped organ that contains a thick muscular wall, a mucous membrane lining, and a rich supply of blood. It lies in the center of the pelvic cavity between the bladder and the rectum. It is normally bent slightly forward, which is called **anteflexion** (an tee **FLEK** shun), and held in position by strong fibrous **ligaments** (**LIG** ah ments) anchored in the outer layer of the uterus, called the **perimetrium** (pear ee **MEE** tre um). The uterus has three sections: the **fundus** (**FUN** dus) or upper portion, between where the fallopian tubes connect to the uterus; **corpus** (**KOR** pus) or body, which is the central portion; and **cervix** (**SER** viks) (Cx), or lower portion, which is also called the neck of the uterus and opens into the vagina.

> **MED TERM TIP**
> It is important to know the various parts of the uterus since they are used in descriptions of medical examinations and surgical procedures. For instance, during pregnancy, the height of the fundus is an important measurement for estimating the stage of pregnancy and the size of the fetus. Following birth, massaging the fundus with pressure applied in a circular pattern stimulates the uterine muscle to contract to help stop bleeding. Patients may be more familiar with a common term for uterus, *womb*. However, the correct medical term is uterus.

The inner layer, or **endometrium** (en doh **MEE** tre um), of the uterine wall contains a rich blood supply. The endometrium reacts to hormonal changes every month that prepare it to receive a fertilized egg or **ovum** (**OH** vum). The fertilized ovum implants in the endometrium, which can then provide nourishment and protection for the developing baby. Contractions of the thick

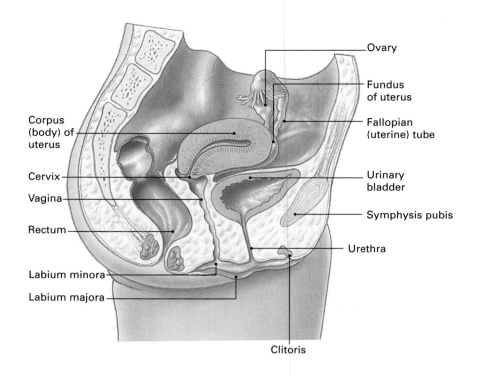

Ovary

Fundus
of uterus

Fallopian
(uterine) tube

Corpus
(body) of
uterus

Cervix

Vagina

Urinary
bladder

Symphysis pubis

Rectum

Urethra

Labium minora

Labium majora

Clitoris

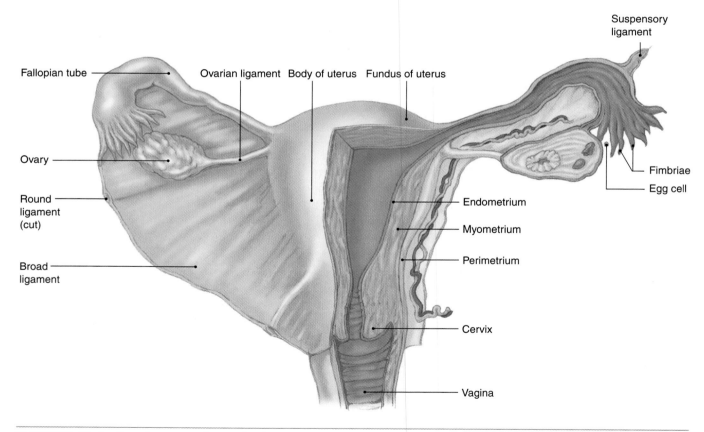

Suspensory
ligament

Fallopian tube

Ovarian ligament

Body of uterus

Fundus of uterus

Ovary

Fimbriae

Egg cell

Round
ligament
(cut)

Endometrium

Myometrium

Broad
ligament

Perimetrium

Cervix

Vagina

**█ FIGURE 10.1**   Female organs of reproduction.

muscular walls of the uterus, called the **myometrium** (my oh **MEE** tre um), assist in propelling the fetus through the birth canal at delivery.

If a pregnancy is not established, the endometrium is sloughed off, resulting in **menstruation** (men stroo **AY** shun) or the **menstrual** (**MEN** stroo all) **period.** During a pregnancy, the lining of the uterus does not leave the body but remains to nourish the unborn child. The girl's first menstrual period (usually during her early teenage years) is called **menarche** (men **AR** kee), while the ending of menstrual activity and childbearing years is called **menopause** (**MEN** oh pawz). This generally occurs between the ages of 40 and 55.

## Ovaries

**estrogen**  
**follicle stimulating hormone**  
**luteinizing hormone**  
**ovulation**  
**progesterone**

There are two ovaries located on each side of the uterus within the pelvic cavity (see ▪ Figure 10.2). These are small almond-shaped glands that produce ova and hormones. In humans, approximately every 28 days, hormones from the anterior pituitary, **follicle** (**FOLL** ih kl) **stimulating hormone** (FSH) and **luteinizing** (loo teh **NIGH** zing) **hormone** (LH), stimulate **ovulation** (ov yoo **LAY** shun), the process by which one ovary releases an ovum (see ▪ Figure 10.3). The principal female hormones produced by the ovaries, **estrogen** (**ESS** troh jen) and **progesterone** (proh **JES** ter ohn), stimulate the endometrium to be prepared to receive a fertilized ovum.

**MED TERM TIP** The singular for egg is *ovum*. The plural term for many eggs is *ova*. The term *ova* is not used exclusively when discussing the human reproductive system. For instance, testing the stool for ova and parasites is used to detect the presence of parasites or their ova in the digestive tract, a common cause for severe diarrhea.

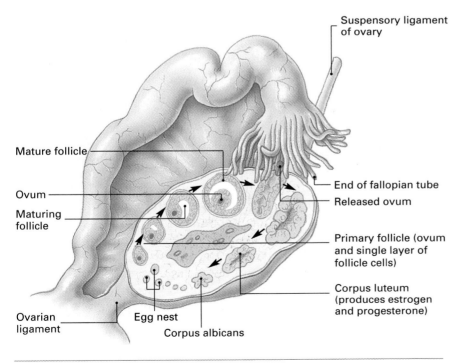

Labels:
- Mature follicle
- Ovum
- Maturing follicle
- Ovarian ligament
- Egg nest
- Corpus albicans
- Suspensory ligament of ovary
- End of fallopian tube
- Released ovum
- Primary follicle (ovum and single layer of follicle cells)
- Corpus luteum (produces estrogen and progesterone)

▪ **FIGURE 10.2**   The ovary.

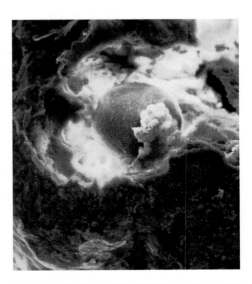

▪ **FIGURE 10.3**   Enhanced color scanning electron micrograph of the ovulation process. The egg (pink in center) has ruptured. The external surface of the ovary is brown in this photo.
(P. M. Motta and J. Van Blekrom/Science Photo Library/Photo Researchers, Inc.)

### Fallopian Tubes

| ectopic pregnancy | oviducts | uterine tubes |
|---|---|---|
| fimbriae | tubal pregnancy | |

The fallopian tubes, also called the **uterine (YOO** ter in) **tubes** or **oviducts (OH** vih ducts), are approximately 5½ inches long and run from the area around each ovary to either side of the upper portion of the uterus. Near the ovaries, the unattached ends of these two tubes expand into finger-like projections, **fimbriae (FIM** bree ay). The fimbriae catch an ovum after ovulation and direct it into the fallopian tube. The fallopian tube can then propel the ovum from the ovary to the uterus so that it can implant. The meeting of the egg and sperm, called *fertilization,* normally takes place within the upper one-half of the fallopian tubes.

> **MED TERM TIP**
> When the fertilized egg adheres or implants to the fallopian tube instead of moving into the uterus, a condition called **tubal pregnancy (TOO** bal **PREG** nan see) exists. There is not enough room in the fallopian tube for the fetus to grow normally. Implantation of the fertilized egg in any location other than the uterus is called an **ectopic pregnancy** (ek **TOP** ik **PREG** nan see). Ectopic is a general term meaning *in the wrong place.*

### Vagina

| hymen | semen |
|---|---|
| penis | vaginal orifice |

The vagina is a muscular tube, lined with mucous membrane, that extends from the cervix of the uterus to the outside of the body. The vagina allows for the passage of the menstrual flow. In addition, during intercourse, it receives the male's **penis (PEE** nis) and **semen (SEE** men), which is the fluid containing sperm. The vagina also serves as the birth canal through which the baby passes during a normal vaginal birth.

The **hymen (HIGH** men) is a thin membranous tissue that covers the external vaginal opening or **vaginal orifice (VAJ** ih nal **OR** ih fis). This membrane is broken during the first sexual encounter of the female and can also be broken prematurely by the use of tampons or during physical activity.

## Vulva

| Bartholin's glands | erectile tissue | urinary meatus |
|---|---|---|

The vulva is a general term meaning the female external genitalia. **Bartholin's (BAR** toh linz) **glands,** which secrete mucus for lubrication, are located on the outer side of the vaginal orifice. The labia majora and labia minora are folds of skin that serve as protection for the genitalia and, in particular, the **urinary meatus (YOO** rih nair ee mee **AY** tus). Since the urinary tract and the reproductive organs are located in proximity to one another and each contains mucous membranes that can transport infection, there is a danger of infection entering the urinary tract. The clitoris is a small organ containing **erectile** (ee **REK** tile) **tissue** that is covered by the labia minora. The clitoris contains sensitive tissue that is aroused during sexual stimulation and corresponds to the penis in the male.

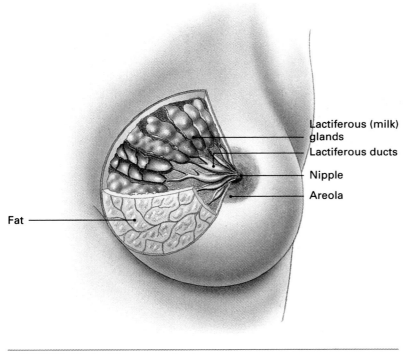

**■ FIGURE 10.4** Mammary gland.

## Breast

| | | |
|---|---|---|
| **areola** | **lactiferous ducts** | **nipple** |
| **breasts** | **lactiferous glands** | **nurse** |
| **lactation** | **mammary glands** | |

The **breasts,** or **mammary** (**MAM** ah ree) **glands** (see ■ Figure 10.4), play a vital role in the reproductive process because they produce milk, a process called **lactation** (lak **TAY** shun), to nourish the newborn. The size of the breasts, which varies greatly from woman to woman, has no bearing on the ability to **nurse** or feed a baby. Milk is produced by the **lactiferous** (lak **TIF** er us) **glands** and is carried to the **nipple** by the **lactiferous** (lak **TIF** er us) **ducts.** The **areola** (ah **REE** oh la) is the pigmented area around the nipple. As long as the breast is stimulated by the nursing infant, the breast will continue to secrete milk.

## Pregnancy

| | | |
|---|---|---|
| **abortion** | **dilation stage** | **placenta** |
| **afterbirth** | **effacement** | **placental stage** |
| **amnion** | **elective abortion** | **pregnancy** |
| **amniotic fluid** | **embryo** | **premature** |
| **breech presentation** | **expulsion stage** | **spontaneous abortion** |
| **chorion** | **fetus** | **therapeutic abortion** |
| **congenital anomalies** | **gestation** | **umbilical cord** |
| **crowning** | **labor** | **viable** |
| **delivery** | **miscarriage** | |

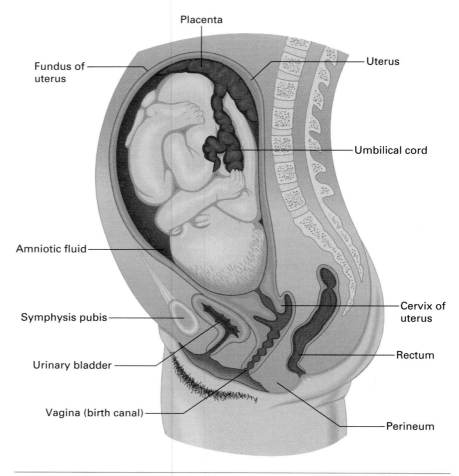

Placenta

Fundus of uterus

Uterus

Umbilical cord

Amniotic fluid

Symphysis pubis

Urinary bladder

Cervix of uterus

Rectum

Vagina (birth canal)

Perineum

**■ FIGURE 10.5** Anatomy of pregnancy.

> **MID TERM TIP**
> The term **abortion** (ah **BOR** shun) (AB) has different meanings for medical professionals and the general population. The general population equates the term *abortion* specifically with the planned termination of a pregnancy. However, to the medical community, abortion is a broader medical term meaning that a pregnancy has ended before a fetus is **viable** (**VYE** ah bull), meaning before it can live on its own. Additional terms must be used in conjunction with abortion to give more information. For instance, a **spontaneous abortion** (ah **BOR** shun) is the unplanned loss of a pregnancy (commonly referred to as a **miscarriage**), a **therapeutic abortion** (thair ah **PEU** tik ah **BOR** shun) is the termination of a pregnancy for the health of the mother, and an **elective abortion** is the legal termination of a pregnancy for nonmedical reasons.

**Pregnancy** (**PREG** nan see) refers to the period of time during which a baby grows and develops in its mother's uterus (see ■ Figure 10.5). The normal length of time for a pregnancy, **gestation** (jess **TAY** shun), is 40 weeks. If a baby is born before completing at least 37 weeks of gestation, it is considered **premature.**

During pregnancy the female body undergoes many changes. In fact, all of the body systems become involved in the development of a healthy infant (see ■ Figures 10.6 to 10.8). From the time the fertilized egg implants in the uterus until approximately the end of the eighth week, the infant is referred to as an **embryo** (**EM** bree oh). This is a period of rapid growth and formation of the major organ systems. Following the embryo stage until birth, the infant is called a **fetus** (**FEE** tus).

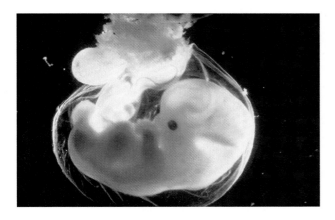

**■ FIGURE 10.6** Embryo at 5 to 6 weeks *in utero.*
(Petit Format/Nestle/Photo Researchers, Inc.)

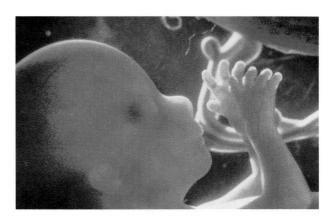

**■ FIGURE 10.7** Fetus at 4 months *in utero.*
(Petit Format/Nestle/Photo Researchers, Inc.)

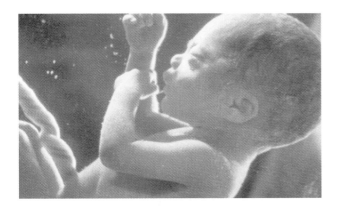

**■ FIGURE 10.8** Fetus 8–9 months (almost full term) *in utero.*
(Petit Format/Nestle/Science Source/Photo Researchers, Inc.)

The fetus receives nourishment from its mother by way of the **placenta** (plah **SEN** tah), which is a spongy structure that forms in the uterus next to the fetus. The placenta is commonly referred to as the **afterbirth**. The fetus is attached to the placenta by way of the **umbilical cord** (um **BILL** ih kal **KORD**). The fetus is surrounded by two membranous sacs, the **amnion** (**AM** nee on) and the **chorion** (**KOR** ree on). The amnion is the innermost sac and it holds the **amniotic** (am nee **OT** ik) **fluid** in which the fetus floats. The chorion is an outer, protective sac and also forms part of the placenta.

**Labor** (**LAY** bor) is the actual process of expelling the fetus from the uterus and through the vagina (see ■ Figure 10.9). The first stage is referred to as the **dilation** (dye **LAY** shun) **stage,** in which the uterine muscles contract strongly to expel the fetus. During this process the fetus presses on the cervix and causes it to dilate or expand. As the cervix dilates, it also becomes thinner, referred to as **effacement** (eh **FACE** ment). When the cervix is completely dilated to 10 centimeters, the second stage of labor begins. This is the **expulsion** (ex **PULL** shun) **stage** and ends with **delivery** of the baby. Generally, the head of the baby appears first, which is referred to as **crowning** (see ■ Figure 10.10). In some cases the baby's buttocks will appear first, and this is referred to as a **breech presentation** (see ■ Figure 10.11). The last stage of labor is the **placental** (plah **SEN** tal) **stage** (see also Figure 10.9). Immediately after childbirth, the uterus continues to contract, causing the placenta to be expelled through the vagina.

> **MED TERM TIP**
> During the embryo stage of gestation, the organs and organ systems of the body are formed. Therefore, this is a very common time for **congenital anomalies** (con **JEN** ih tal ah **NOM** ah lees), or birth defects, to occur. This may happen before the woman is even aware of being pregnant.

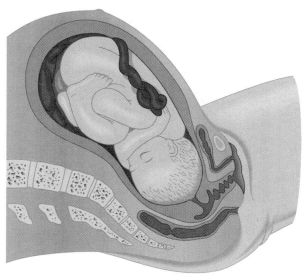

DILATION STAGE:
First uterine contraction to dilation of cervix

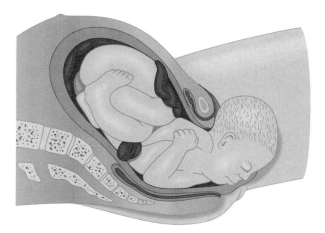

EXPULSION STAGE:
Birth of baby or expulsion

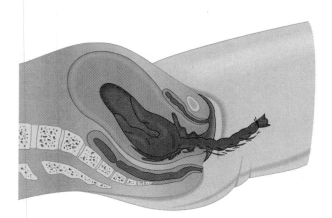

PLACENTAL STAGE:
Delivery of placenta

■ **FIGURE 10.9**   Three stages of labor and delivery.

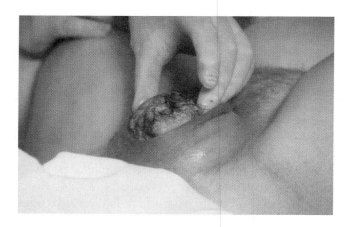

■ **FIGURE 10.10**   Crowning. Baby's head at vaginal opening.
(D. Van Rossum/Petit Format/Photo Researchers, Inc.)

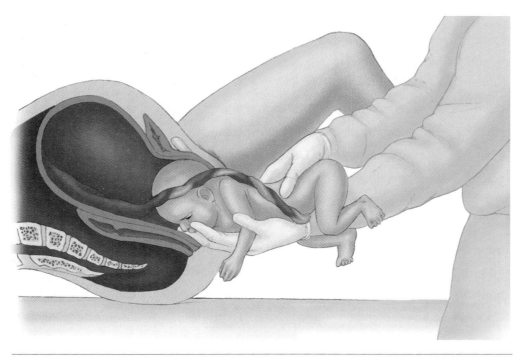

**FIGURE 10.11** Breech presentation.

## Word Building Relating to the Female Reproductive System

The following list contains examples of medical terms built directly from word parts. The definition for these terms can be determined by a straightforward translation of the word parts.

| Combining Form | Combined With | Medical Term | Definition |
|---|---|---|---|
| amni/o | -otomy | amniotomy (am nee **OT** oh mee) | incision into amnion |
| | -rrhea | amniorrhea (am nee oh **REE** ah) | flow of fluid from amnion |
| cervic/o | -ectomy | cervicectomy (ser vih **SEK** toh mee) | excision of cervix |
| | endo- -itis | endocervicitis (en doh ser vih **SIGH** tis) | inflammation within cervix |
| colp/o | -scope | colposcope (**KOL** poh scope) | instrument to view inside vagina |
| | -scopy | colposcopy (kol **POSS** koh pee) | process of viewing vagina |
| episi/o | -otomy | episiotomy (eh peez ee **OT** oh mee) | incision into vulva |
| | -rrhaphy | episiorrhaphy (eh peez ee **OR** ah fee) | suture of vulva |
| gynec/o | -ologist | gynecologist (gigh neh **KOL** oh jist) | specialist in female reproductive system |
| | -ology | gynecology (gigh ne **KOL** oh jee) | study of female reproductive system |
| hyster/o | -ectomy | hysterectomy (hiss ter **EK** toh mee) | excision of the uterus |
| | -pexy | hysteropexy (**HISS** ter oh pek see) | surgical fixation of the uterus |
| | -rrhexis | hysterorrhexis (hiss ter oh **REK** sis) | ruptured uterus |
| lact/o | -ic | lactic (**LAK** tik) | pertaining to milk |
| | -rrhea | lactorrhea (lak toh **REE** ah) | milk discharge |

*continued...*

| Combining Form | Combined With | Medical Term | Definition |
|---|---|---|---|
| mamm/o | -gram | mammogram (**MAM** moh gram) | record of the breast |
| | -plasty | mammoplasty (**MAM** moh plas tee) | surgical repair of breast |
| mast/o | -algia | mastalgia (mas **TAL** jee ah) | breast pain |
| | -ectomy | mastectomy (mass **TEK** toh mee) | excision of the uterus |
| | -itis | mastitis (mas **TYE** tis) | inflammation of the breast |
| men/o | a- -rrhea | amenorrhea (ah men oh **REE** ah) | no menstrual flow |
| | dys- -rrhea | dysmenorrhea (dis men oh **REE** ah) | difficult menstrual flow |
| | oligo- -rrhea | oligomenorrhea (ol lih goh men oh **REE** ah) | scanty menstrual flow |
| | -rrhagia | menorrhagia (men oh **RAY** jee ah) | abnormal, rapid menstrual flow |
| metr/o | endo- -itis | endometritis (en doh meh **TRY** tis) | inflammation within the uterus |
| | peri- -itis | perimetritis (pair ih meh **TRY** tis) | inflammation around the uterus |
| | -rrhea | metrorrhea (meh troh **REE** ah) | flow from uterus |
| | -rrhagia | metrorrhagia (meh troh **RAY** jee ah) | rapid (menstrual) blood flow from uterus |
| nat/o | neo- | neonate (**NEE** oh nayt) | newborn |
| | neo- -ology | neonatology (nee oh nay **TALL** oh jee) | study of the newborn |
| oophor/o | -ectomy | oophorectomy (oh off oh **REK** toh mee) | excision of the ovary |
| | -itis | oophoritis (oh off oh **RIGH** tis) | inflammation of the ovary |
| part/o | ante- -um | antepartum (an tee **PAR** tum) | before birth |
| | post- -um | postpartum (post **PAR** tum) | after birth |
| salping/o | -cyesis | salpingocyesis (sal ping goh sigh **EE** sis) | tubal pregnancy |
| | -ostomy | salpingostomy (sal ping **GOS** toh mee) | create an opening in the fallopian tube |
| | -itis | salpingitis (sal ping **JIGH** tis) | inflammation of the fallopian tubes |

| Prefix | Suffix | Medical Term | Definition |
|---|---|---|---|
| pseudo- | -cyesis | pseudocyesis (soo doh sigh **EE** sis) | false pregnancy |
| nulli- | -gravida | nulligravida (null ih **GRAV** ih dah) | no pregnancies |
| primi- | | primigravida (prem ih **GRAV** ih dah) | first pregnancy |
| multi- | | multigravida (mull tih **GRAV** ih dah) | multiple pregnancies |
| nulli- | -para | nullipara (null **IP** ah rah) | no births |
| primi- | | primipara (prem **IP** ah rah) | first birth |
| multi- | | multipara (mull **TIP** ah rah) | multiple births |
| hemato- | -salpinx | hematosalpinx (hee mah toh **SAL** pinks) | blood in fallopian tube |
| pyo- | | pyosalpinx (pie oh **SAL** pinks) | pus in fallopian tube |
| dys- | -tocia | dystocia (dis **TOH** she ah) | difficult labor and childbirth |

# Vocabulary Relating to the Female Reproductive System

| | |
|---|---|
| **atresia (ah TREE she ah)** | Congenital lack of a normal body opening. |
| **barrier contraception (kon trah SEP shun)** | Prevention of a pregnancy using a device to prevent sperm from meeting an ovum. Examples include condoms, diaphragms, and cervical caps. |
| **breech presentation** | Most correctly refers to the presentation of the buttocks in the birth canal. Commonly used to indicate presentation of any part of the fetus in the birth canal other than crown of the head (refer to Figure 10.11). |
| **colostrum (kuh LOS trum)** | A thin fluid first secreted by the breast after delivery. It does not contain much protein, but is rich in antibodies. |
| **dyspareunia (dis pah ROO nee ah)** | Painful sexual intercourse. |
| **estimated date of confinement (EDC)** | Estimation date when the baby will be born based on a calculation from the last menstrual period of the mother. |
| **fraternal twins** | Twins that develop from two different ova fertilized by two different sperm. Although twins, these siblings do not have identical DNA. |
| **gestation (jess TAY shun)** | Length of time from conception to birth, generally 9 months. Calculated from the first day of the last menstrual period, with a range of from 259 days to 280 days. |
| **identical twins** | Twins that develop from the splitting of one fertilized ovum. These siblings have identical DNA. |
| **infertility** | Inability to produce children. Generally defined as no pregnancy after properly timed intercourse for 1 year. |
| **intrauterine (in trah YOO ter in) device (IUD)** | Device that is inserted into the uterus by a physician for the purpose of contraception (see ▓ Figure 10.12). |
| **last menstrual period (LMP)** | Date when the last menstrual period started. |
| **low birth weight (LBW)** | Abnormally low weight in a newborn. It is usually considered to be less than 5.5 pounds. |
| **meconium (meh KOH nee um)** | The first bowel movement of a newborn. It is greenish in color and consists of mucus and bile. |
| **neonate (NEE oh nayt)** | Term used to describe the newborn infant during the first 4 weeks of life. |
| **obstetrician (ob steh TRISH an)** | A physician specializing in providing care for pregnant women and delivering infants. |
| **obstetrics (ob STET riks) (OB)** | Branch of medicine that treats women during pregnancy and childbirth, and immediately after childbirth. |
| **parturition (par too RISH un)** | Childbirth. |
| **premenstrual syndrome (pre MEN stroo al SIN drohm) (PMS)** | Symptoms that develop just prior to the onset of a menstrual period, which can include irritability, headache, tender breasts, and anxiety. |
| **puberty (PEW ber tee)** | Beginning of menstruation and the ability to reproduce. |
| **puerperium (pew er PEER ee um)** | Term used to refer to the 3 to 6 week period after childbirth. |

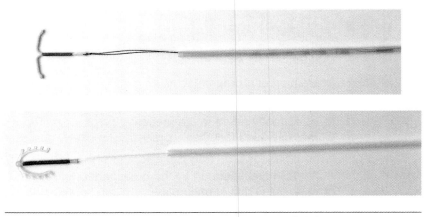

**FIGURE 10.12**   Examples of intrauterine devices (IUDs).

# Pathology Relating to the Female Reproductive System

| | |
|---|---|
| **abruptio placentae**<br>**(ah BRUP tee oh plah SEN tee)** | Emergency condition in which the placenta tears away from the uterine wall before the 20th week of pregnancy. Requires immediate delivery of the baby. |
| **breast cancer** | Malignant tumor of the breast. Usually forms in the milk-producing gland tissue or the lining of the milk ducts (see ■ Figure 10.13A). |
| **candidiasis**<br>**(kan dih DYE ah sis)** | Yeast infection of the skin and mucous membranes that can result in white plaques on the tongue and vagina. |
| **cervical cancer**<br>**(SER vih kal CAN ser)** | Malignant growth in the cervix. An especially difficult type of cancer to treat that causes 5% of the cancer deaths in women. Pap smear tests have helped to detect early cervical cancer. |
| **choriocarcinoma**<br>**(kor ee oh kar sih NOH mah)** | Rare type of cancer of the uterus. May occur following a normal pregnancy or abortion. |
| **condyloma (kon dih LOH ma)** | Wart-like growth on the external genitalia. |
| **cystocele (SIS toh seel)** | Hernia or outpouching of the bladder that protrudes into the vagina. This may cause urinary frequency and urgency. |
| **Down syndrome**<br>**(DOWN SIN drohm)** | Genetic disorder named after J. H. L. Down, a British physician, that produces moderate-to-severe mental retardation and multiple birth defects. The physical characteristics of a child with this disorder are a sloping forehead, flat nose or absent bridge to the nose, low-set eyes, and a generally dwarfed physical growth. The disorder occurs more commonly when the mother is over age 40 (see ■ Figure 10.14). |
| **eclampsia (eh KLAMP see ah)** | Convulsive seizures and coma occurring in the woman between the 20th week of pregnancy and the first week of postpartum. Preceded by preeclampsia. |
| **endometrial cancer**<br>**(en doh MEE tree al CAN ser)** | Cancer of the endometrial lining of the uterus. |
| **endometriosis**<br>**(en doh mee tree OH sis)** | Abnormal condition of endometrium tissue appearing throughout the pelvis or on the abdominal wall. This tissue is normally found within the uterus. |
| **erythroblastosis fetalis**<br>**(eh rithroh blass TOH sis**<br>**fee TAL iss)** | Condition developing in the baby when the mother's blood type is Rh-negative and the baby's blood is Rh-positive. The baby's red blood cells can be destroyed as a result of this condition. Treatment is early diagnosis and blood transfusion. Also called *hemolytic disease of the newborn*. |
| **fibrocystic (figh bro SIS tik)**<br>**breast disease** | Benign cysts forming in the breast (refer to ■ Figure 10.13B). |

| | |
|---|---|
| **fibroid tumor**<br>**(FIGH broyd TOO mor)** | Benign tumor or growth that contains fiber-like tissue. Uterine fibroid tumors are the most common tumors in women (see ■ Figure 10.15). |
| **menorrhagia**<br>**(men oh RAY jee ah)** | Excessive bleeding during the menstrual period. Can be measured either in the total number of days or the amount of blood or both. |
| **ovarian carcinoma**<br>**(oh VAY ree an kar sih NOH mah)** | Cancer of the ovary. |
| **ovarian cyst**<br>**(oh VAY ree an SIST)** | Cyst that develops within the ovary. These may be multiple cysts and may rupture causing pain and bleeding. |
| **pelvic inflammatory disease**<br>**(PELL vik in FLAM mah toh ree dih ZEEZ) (PID)** | Any inflammation of the female reproductive organs, generally bacterial in nature. |
| **placenta previa**<br>**(plah SEN tah PREE vee ah)** | When the placenta has become placed in the lower portion of the uterus and, in turn, blocks the birth canal (see ■ Figure 10.16). |
| **preeclampsia**<br>**(pre eh KLAMP see ah)** | Metabolic disease of pregnancy. If untreated, it may result in true eclampsia. Symptoms include hypertension, headaches, albumin in the urine, and edema. Also called *toxemia*. |
| **prolapsed umbilical**<br>**(pro LAPS'D um BILL ih kal)**<br>**cord** | When the umbilical cord of the baby is expelled first during delivery and is squeezed between the baby's head and the vaginal wall. This presents an emergency situation since the baby's circulation is compromised. |
| **prolapsed uterus**<br>**(pro LAPS'D YOO ter us)** | Fallen uterus that can cause the cervix to protrude through the vaginal opening. Generally caused by weakened muscles from vaginal delivery or as the result of pelvic tumors pressing down. |
| **rectocele (REK toh seel)** | Protrusion or herniation of the rectum into the vagina. |
| **stillbirth** | Birth in which a viable-aged fetus dies before or at the time of delivery. |
| **toxic shock syndrome (TSS)** | Rare and sometimes fatal staphylococcus infection that generally occurs in menstruating women. |

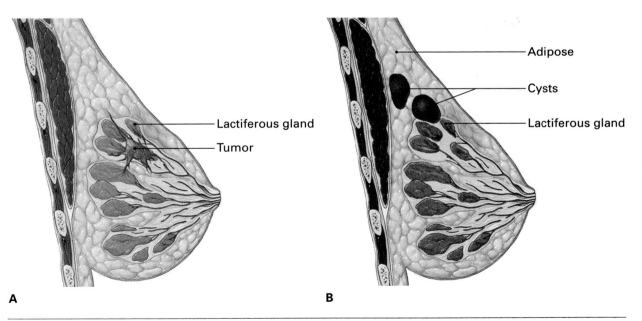

**A**    **B**

■ **FIGURE 10.13** (A) Breast cancer. Tumor is growing within a milk gland. (B) Fibrocystic breast disease. Cysts have formed within the adipose tissue of the breast.

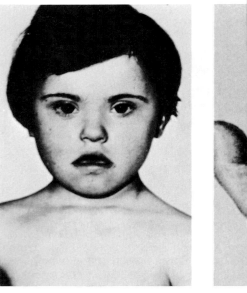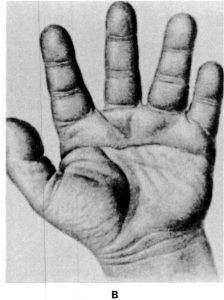

A                                          B

■ **FIGURE 10.14**   (A) Face of a 5-year-old girl with Down syndrome. Note widely set eyes, underdeveloped bridge of the nose, partially open mouth, and protruding tongue. (B) Short, broad hand of a 9-year-old Down syndrome patient, showing shortened fifth finger and transverse crease across palm.

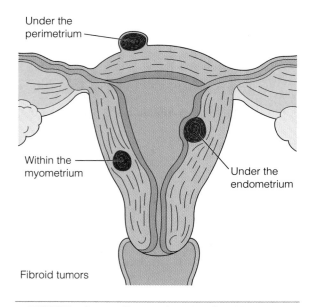

Under the perimetrium

Within the myometrium

Under the endometrium

Fibroid tumors

■ **FIGURE 10.15**   Types of uterine fibroid tumors.

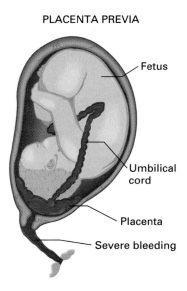

PLACENTA PREVIA

Fetus

Umbilical cord

Placenta

Severe bleeding

■ **FIGURE 10.16**   Placenta previa.

# Diagnostic Procedures Relating to the Female Reproductive System

| | |
|---|---|
| **amniocentesis (am nee oh sen TEE sis)** | Puncturing of the amniotic sac using a needle and syringe for the purpose of withdrawing amniotic fluid for testing. Can assist in determining fetal maturity, development, and genetic disorders. |
| **Apgar (AP gar) score** | Evaluation of a neonate's adjustment to the outside world. Observes color, heart rate, muscle tone, respiratory rate, and response to stimulus. |
| **cervical biopsy (SER vih kal BYE op see)** | Taking a sample of tissue from the cervix to test for the presence of cancer cells. |
| **chorionic villus (kor ree ON ik vill us) sampling (CVS)** | Removal of a small piece of the chorion for genetic analysis. May be done at an earlier stage of pregnancy than amniocentesis. |
| **endometrial biopsy (en doh MEE tre al BYE op see)** | Taking a sample of tissue from the lining of the uterus to test for abnormalities. |
| **fetal (FEE tal) monitoring** | Using electronic equipment placed on the mother's abdomen to check the fetal heart rate (FHR) and fetal heart tone (FHT) during labor. The normal heart rate of the fetus is rapid, ranging from 120 to 160 beats per minute. A drop in the fetal heart rate indicates the fetus is in distress. |
| **hysterosalpingography (hiss ter oh sal pin GOG rah fee) (HSG)** | Taking an X-ray after injecting radiopaque material into the uterus and fallopian tubes. |
| **laparoscopy (lap ar OS koh pee)** | Examination of the peritoneal cavity using an instrument called a laparoscope. The instrument is passed through a small incision made by the surgeon into the abdominopelvic cavity (see ▪ Figure 10.17). |
| **mammography (mam OG rah fee)** | Using X-ray to diagnose breast disease, especially breast cancer. |
| **PAP (Papanicolaou) (pap ah NIK oh low) smear** | Test for the early detection of cancer of the cervix named after the developer of the test, George Papanicolaou, a Greek physician. A scraping of cells is removed from the cervix for examination under a microscope. |
| **pelvic (PELLViK) examination** | Physical examination of the vagina and adjacent organs performed by a physician placing the fingers of one hand into the vagina. A visual examination is performed using a *speculum* (see ▪ Figure 10.18). |
| **pelvic ultrasonography (PELL vik ull trah son OG rah fee)** | Use of ultrasound waves to produce an image or photograph of an organ, such as the uterus, ovaries, or fetus. |
| **pelvimetry (pell VIM eh tree)** | Measurement of the pelvic area that helps in determining if the fetus can be delivered vaginally. |
| **pregnancy (PREG nan see) test** | Chemical test that can determine a pregnancy during the first few weeks. Can be performed in a physician's office or with a home-testing kit. |

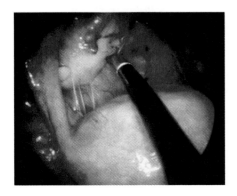

▪ **FIGURE 10.17**   Removal of adhesions between the uterus and ovary during laparoscopic procedure.
(Southern Illinois University/Photo Researchers, Inc.)

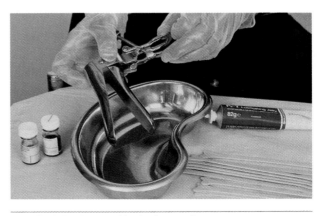

▪ **FIGURE 10.18**   Vaginal speculum.
(Simon Fraser/Science Photo Library/Photo Researchers, Inc.)

# Therapeutic Procedures Relating to the Female Reproductive System

| | |
|---|---|
| **cauterization** (kaw ter ih ZAY shun) | Destruction of tissue using an electric current, a caustic product, a hot iron, or by freezing. |
| **cesarean (see SAYR ee an) section (CS, C-section)** | Surgical delivery of a baby through an incision into the abdominal and uterine walls. Legend has it that the Roman emperor, Julius Caesar, was the first person born by this method. |
| **conization (kon ih ZAY shun)** | Surgical removal of a core of cervical tissue. Also refers to partial removal of the cervix. |
| **cryosurgery** (cry oh SER jer ee) | Exposing tissues to extreme cold to destroy tissues. Used in treating malignant tumors, and to control pain and bleeding. |
| **culdoscopy (kul DOS koh pee)** | Examination of the female pelvic cavity by introducing an endoscope through the wall of the vagina. |
| **dilation and curettage** (dye LAY shun and koo reh TAHZ) (D & C) | Surgical procedure in which the opening of the cervix is dilated and the uterus is scraped or suctioned of its lining or tissue. Often performed after a spontaneous abortion and to stop excessive bleeding from other causes. |
| **episiotomy** (eh peez ee OT oh mee) | Surgical incision of the perineum to facilitate the delivery process. Can prevent an irregular tearing of tissue during birth. |
| **genetic counseling** | Evaluation of parents' potential for producing a child with a genetic disease. Especially important for families with a history of genetic diseases (see ▓ Figure 10.19). |
| **hymenectomy** (high men EK toh mee) | Surgical removal of the hymen. Performed when the hymen tissue is particularly tough. |
| **Kegel (KAY gull) exercises** | Exercises named after A. H. Kegel, an American gynecologist, who developed them to strengthen female pubic muscles. The exercises are useful in treating incontinence and as an aid in the childbirth process. |
| **laparotomy** (lap ah ROT oh mee) | Surgical opening of the abdomen; an abdominal operation. |
| **lumpectomy** (lump EK toh mee) | Excision of only a breast tumor and the tissue immediately surrounding it. |
| **radical mastectomy** (mast EK toh mee) | Surgical removal of the breast tissue plus chest muscles and axillary lymph nodes. |
| **simple mastectomy** (mast EK toh mee) | Surgical removal of the breast tissue. |
| **total abdominal hysterectomy** (hiss ter EK toh me)—**bilateral salpingo-oophorectomy** (sal ping goh ohoh foe REK toh mee) (TAH-BSO) | Removal of the entire uterus, cervix, both ovaries, and both fallopian tubes. |
| **tubal ligation** (TOO bal lye GAY shun) | Surgical tying off of the fallopian tubes to prevent conception from taking place. Results in sterilization of the female. |
| **vaginal hysterectomy** (VAJ ih nal hiss ter EK toh me) | Removal of the uterus through the vagina rather than through an abdominal incision. |

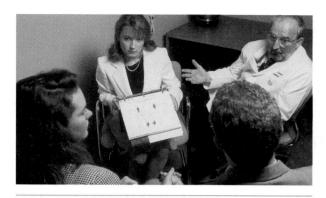

**■ FIGURE 10.19** Genetic counseling with parents.
(Will and Demi McIntyre/Photo Researchers, Inc.)

## Pharmacology Relating to the Female Reproductive System

| | |
|---|---|
| **hormone replacement therapy (HRT)** | Menopause or the surgical loss of the ovaries results in the lack of estrogen production. Replacing this estrogen with an oral medication prevents some of the consequences of menopause, especially in younger woman who have surgically lost their ovaries. |
| **oral contraceptive (kon trah SEP tive) pills (OCPs)** | Birth control medication that uses low doses of female hormones to prevent conception by blocking ovulation. |
| **oxytocin (ox ee TOH sin)** | Oxytocin is a natural hormone that improves uterine contractions during labor and delivery. |

## Abbreviations Relating to the Female Reproductive System

| | | | | |
|---|---|---|---|---|
| **AB** | abortion | | **HSG** | hysterosalpingography |
| **AI** | artificial insemination | | **IUD** | intrauterine device |
| **BSE** | breast self-examination | | **IVF** | *in vitro* fertilization |
| **CPD** | cephalopelvic disproportion | | **LAVH** | laparoscopic assisted vaginal hysterectomy |
| **CS, C-section** | cesarean section | | **LBW** | low birth weight |
| **CVS** | chorionic villus sampling | | **LH** | luteinizing hormone |
| **Cx** | cervix | | **LMP** | last menstrual period |
| **D & C** | dilation and curettage | | **MH** | marital history |
| **DOB** | date of birth | | **NB** | newborn |
| **DUB** | dysfunctional uterine bleeding | | **NGU** | nongonococcal urethritis |
| **ECC** | endocervical curettage | | **OB** | obstetrics |
| **EDC** | estimated date of confinement | | **OCPs** | oral contraceptive pills |
| **EMB** | endometrial biopsy | | **PAP** | Papanicolaou test |
| **ERT** | estrogen replacement therapy | | **PI, para I** | first delivery |
| **FEKG** | fetal electrocardiogram | | **PID** | pelvic inflammatory disease |
| **FHR** | fetal heart rate | | **PKU** | phenylketonuria |
| **FHT** | fetal heart tone | | **PMP** | previous menstrual period |
| **FSH** | follicle-stimulating hormone | | **PMS** | premenstrual syndrome |
| **FTND** | full-term normal delivery | | **TAH-BSO** | total abdominal hysterectomy–bilateral salpingo-oophorectomy |
| **GI, grav I** | first pregnancy | | | |
| **GYN, gyn** | gynecology | | **TSS** | toxic shock syndrome |
| **HCG, hCG** | human chorionic gonadotropin | | **UC** | uterine contractions |
| **HRT** | hormone replacement therapy | | | |

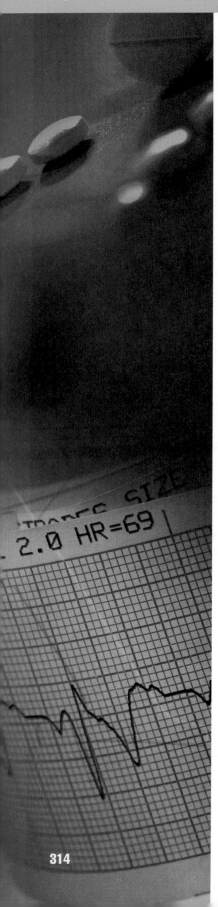

# Part II: Male Reproductive System

## Organs of the Male Reproductive System

bulbourethral gland        scrotum

epididymis                 seminal vesicle

penis                      testes

prostate gland             vas deferens

## Combining Forms Relating to the Male Reproductive System

| | | | |
|---|---|---|---|
| andr/o | male | prostat/o | prostate |
| balan/o | glans penis | spermat/o | sperm |
| crypt/o | hidden | test/o | testes |
| epididym/o | epididymis | testicul/o | testes |
| hydr/o | water, fluid | varic/o | varicose veins |
| orch/o | testes | vas/o | vas deferens |
| orchi/o | testes | vesicul/o | seminal vesicle |
| orchid/o | testes | | |

## Suffixes Relating to the Male Reproductive System

| Suffix | Meaning | Example |
|---|---|---|
| -genesis | produces, generates | spermatogenesis |
| -spermia | condition of sperm | oligospermia |

# Anatomy and Physiology of the Male Reproductive System

**bulbourethral gland**        **scrotum**        **testes**

**epididymis**                 **semen**          **urethra**

**penis**                      **seminal vesicles**   **vas deferens**

**prostate gland**

The male reproductive system is a combination of reproduction and urinary systems. In the male, the major organs of reproduction are located outside the body: the **penis** (**PEE** nis) and the organs located in the **scrotum** (**SKROH** tum). The scrotum contains the two **testes** (**TESS** teez), each with an **epididymis** (ep ih **DID** ih mis). The penis contains the **urethra** (yoo **REE** thrah), which carries both urine and **semen** (**SEE** men) to the outside of the body (see ■ Figure 10.20).

   The internal organs of reproduction include two **seminal vesicles** (**SEM** ih nal **VESS** ih kls), two **vas deferens** (**VAS DEF** er enz), the **prostate** (**PROSS** tayt) **gland,** and two **bulbourethral** (buhl boh yoo **REE** thral) **glands.**

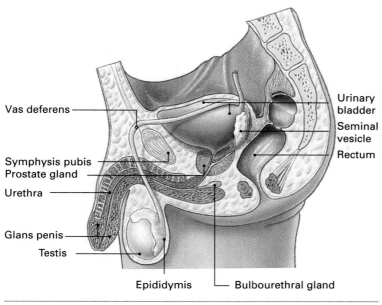

■ **FIGURE 10.20** Male reproductive organs.

# External Organs of Reproduction

## Scrotum

**perineum**                          **testicles**

The scrotum is actually a sac that serves as a container for the testes or **testicles** (**TESS** tih kls). This sac, which is divided by a septum, supports the testicles and lies between the legs and behind the penis. During early childhood, the testes will frequently retract up into the pelvic cavity. However, as the young boy reaches 1 year in age, the testes will remain permanently in the scrotum. The **perineum** (pair ih **NEE** um) of the male is similar to that in the female. It is the area between the anus and the scrotum.

## Testes

**seminiferous tubules**     **spermatogenesis**     **spermatozoon**

**sperm**                          **spermatozoa**          **testosterone**

The testes are oval in shape and are responsible for the development of **sperm** (see ■ Figure 10.21). This process, called **spermatogenesis** (sper mat oh **JEN** eh sis), takes place within the **seminiferous tubules** (sem ih **NIF** er us **TOO** byools). The testes must be maintained at the proper temperature for the sperm to survive. This lower temperature level is achieved by the placement of the testes suspended in the scrotum outside the body. The hormone **testosterone** (tess **TOSS** ter ohn), which is responsible for the growth and development of the male reproductive organs and sperm, is also produced by the testes. The singular for testes is *testis*.

> **MED TERM TIP**
>
> **Spermatozoon** (sper mat oh **ZOH** on) and its plural form, **spermatozoa** (sper mat oh **ZOH** ah), are other terms that mean *sperm*. You have no doubt realized that there can be several terms with the same meaning in medical terminology. You must continue to remain flexible when working with these terms in your career. In some cases, one term will be more commonly used, depending on the type of medical specialty or even what part of the country you are in.

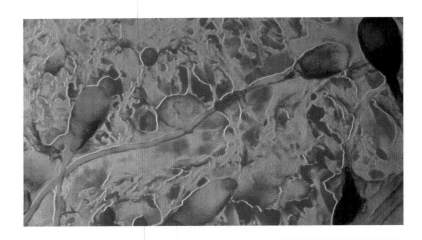

**FIGURE 10.21** Enhanced color photo of sperm through electron microscope.
(Dennis Kunkel/CNRI/Phototake NYC)

### Epididymis

Each epididymis is a coiled tubule that lies on top of the testes within the scrotum. This elongated structure serves to store sperm as they are produced by the testes until they are ready to be released into the vas deferens.

### Penis

| | | |
|---|---|---|
| circumcision | ejaculation | glans penis |
| coitus | erectile tissue | prepuce |
| copulation | foreskin | vagina |

The penis is the male sex organ containing **erectile** (ee **REK** tile) **tissue** that is encased in skin. This organ delivers semen into the female **vagina.** The soft tip of the penis is referred to as the **glans penis** (**GLANS PEE** nis). It is protected by a covering called the **prepuce** (**PREE** pyoos) or **foreskin** (**FOR** skin). It is this covering of skin that is removed during the procedure known as **circumcision** (ser kum **SIH** zhun). The penis becomes erect during sexual stimulation, which allows it to be placed within the female for the **ejaculation** (ee jak yoo **LAY** shun) of semen.

## Internal Organs of Reproduction

### Vas Deferens

| | | |
|---|---|---|
| spermatic cord | vasectomy | vasovasostomy |

Each vas deferens carries sperm from the epididymis up into the pelvic cavity. They travel up in front of the urinary bladder, over the top, and then back down the posterior side of the bladder to empty into the urethra. They, along with nerves, arteries, veins, and lymphatic vessels running between the pelvic cavity and the testes, form the **spermatic cord** (sper **MAT** ik **KORD**).

> **MED TERM TIP**
> During sexual intercourse, which is also referred to as **coitus** (**KOH** ih tus) or **copulation** (kop yoo **LAY** shun), the male can eject up to 100 million sperm cells. The adult male produces nearly 200 million sperm daily.

> **MED TERM TIP**
> The vas deferens is the tubing that is severed during a procedure called a **vasectomy** (vas **EK** toh mee). A vasectomy results in the sterilization of the male since the sperm are no longer able to travel into the urethra and out of the penis during sexual intercourse. The surgical procedure to reverse a vasectomy is a **vasovasostomy** (vas oh vay **ZOS** toh mee). A new opening is created in order to reconnect one section of the vas deferens to another section of the vas deferens, thereby reestablishing an open tube for sperm to travel through.

## Seminal Vesicles

The two seminal vesicles are small glands located at the base of the urinary bladder. These vesicles are connected to the vas deferens just before it empties into the urethra. The seminal vesicles secrete a fluid that nourishes the sperm. This liquid, along with the sperm, constitutes semen, the fluid that is eventually ejaculated during sexual intercourse.

## Prostate Gland

The single prostate gland is located just below the urinary bladder. It surrounds the urethra and when enlarged can cause difficulty in urination. The prostate is important for the reproductive process since it secretes an alkaline fluid that assists in keeping the sperm alive by neutralizing the pH of the urethra and vagina.

## Bulbourethral Glands

**Cowper's glands**

The bulbourethral glands, also known as **Cowper's** (**KOW** perz) **glands,** are two small glands located on either side of the urethra just below the prostate. They produce a mucus-like lubricating fluid that joins with semen to become a part of the ejaculate.

## Urethra

**sphincter**                    **urinary meatus**

The male urethra extends from the urinary bladder to the external opening in the penis, the **urinary meatus** (**YOO** rih nair ee me **AY** tus). It serves a dual function: the elimination of urine and the ejaculation of semen. During the ejaculation process, a **sphincter** (**SFINGK** ter) closes to keep urine from escaping.

## Word Building Relating to the Male Reproductive System

The following list contains examples of medical terms built directly from word parts. The definition for these terms can be determined by a straightforward translation of the word parts.

| Combining Form | Combined With | Medical Term | Definition |
|---|---|---|---|
| andr/o | -gen | androgen (**AN** droh jen) | male producing |
| | -pathy | andropathy (an **DROP** ah thee) | male disease |
| balan/o | -itis | balanitis (bal ah **NYE** tis) | inflammation of glans penis |
| | -plasty | balanoplasty (**BAL** ah noh plas tee) | surgical repair of glans penis |
| | -rrhea | balanorrhea (bah lah noh **REE** ah) | discharge from glans penis |
| epididym/o | -ectomy | epididymectomy (ep ih did ih **MEK** toh mee) | excision of epididymis |
| | -itis | epididymitis (ep ih did ih **MYE** tis) | inflammation of the epididymis |
| orch/o | an- -ism | anorchism (an **OR** kizm) | condition of no testes |
| orchi/o | -ectomy | orchiectomy (or kee **EK** toh mee) | excision of testes |
| | -otomy | orchiotomy (or kee **OT** oh mee) | incision into testes |
| | -plasty | orchioplasty (**OR** kee oh plas tee) | surgical repair of testes |

*continued...*

| Combining Form | Combined With | Medical Term | Definition |
|---|---|---|---|
| orchid/o | crypto- -ism | cryptorchidism (kript **OR** kid izm) | condition of hidden testes |
| | -ectomy | orchidectomy (or kid **EK** toh mee) | excision of the testes |
| | -pexy | orchidopexy (**OR** kid oh peck see) | surgical fixation of testes |
| prostat/o | -itis | prostatitis (pross tah **TYE** tis) | prostate inflammation |
| | -ectomy | prostatectomy (pross tah **TEK** toh mee) | excision of prostate |
| | -lith | prostatolith (pross **TAT** oh lith) | stone in prostate |
| | lith/o -otomy | prostatolithotomy (pross tah toh lih **THOT** oh mee) | prostate stone incision |
| | -rrhea | prostatorrhea (pross tah toh **REE** ah) | discharge from prostate |
| spermat/o | -genesis | spermatogenesis (sper mat oh **JEN** eh sis) | sperm forming |
| | -lysis | spermatolysis (sper mah **TOL** ih sis) | sperm destruction |
| vas/o | -ectomy | vasectomy (vas **EK** toh mee) | excision of vas deferens |
| | vas/o -ostomy | vasovasostomy (vas oh vay **ZOS** toh mee) | create an opening between the one severed end of the vas deferens and the other severed end of the vas deferens (reversal of vasectomy) |

| Prefix | Suffix | Medical Term | Definition |
|---|---|---|---|
| a- | -spermia | aspermia (ah **SPER** mee ah) | condition of no sperm |
| oligo- | | oligospermia (ol ih goh **SPER** mee ah) | condition of scanty (few) sperm |

## Vocabulary Relating to the Male Reproductive System

| | |
|---|---|
| **ejaculation** (ee jak yoo **LAY** shun) | The release of semen through the urethra. |
| **erectile (ee REK tile) dysfunction (ED)** | Inability to engage in sexual intercourse due to inability to maintain an erection. Also called *impotence*. |
| **impotence (IM poh tents)** | Inability to engage in sexual intercourse due to inability to maintain an erection. Also called *erectile dysfunction*. |
| **spermatolytic** (sper mah toh **LIT** ik) | Destruction of sperm. One form of birth control is the use of spermatolytic creams. |
| **sterility** | Inability to father children due to a problem with spermatogenesis. |

# Pathology Relating to the Male Reproductive System

| | |
|---|---|
| **benign prostatic hypertrophy (bee NINE pross TAT ik high PER troh fee) (BPH)** | Noncancerous enlargement of the prostate gland commonly seen in males over age 50. |
| **chancroid (SHANG kroyd)** | Highly infectious nonsyphilitic venereal ulcer (see ▓ Figure 10.22). |
| **chlamydia (klah MID ee ah)** | Parasitic microorganism causing genital infections in males and females. Can lead to pelvic inflammatory disease in females and eventual infertility. |
| **cryptorchidism (kript OR kid izm)** | Failure of the testes to descend into the scrotal sac before birth. Generally, the testes will descend before a boy is 1 year old. A surgical procedure called orchidopexy may be required to bring the testes down into the scrotum permanently. Failure of the testes to descend could result in sterility in the male. |
| **epispadias (ep ih SPAY dee as)** | Congenital opening of the urethra on the dorsal surface of the penis. |
| **genital herpes (JEN ih tal HER peez)** | Creeping skin disease that can appear like a blister or vesicle, caused by a sexually transmitted virus. |
| **genital (JEN ih tal) warts** | Growth of warts on the genitalia of both males and females that can lead to cancer of the cervix in females. Caused by the sexual transmission of the human papilloma virus (HPV). |
| **gonorrhea (gon oh REE ah) (GC)** | Sexually transmitted inflammation of the mucous membranes of either sex. Can be passed on to an infant during the birth process. |
| **hydrocele (HIGH droh seel)** | Accumulation of fluid within the testes. Common in infants. |
| **hypospadias (high poh SPAY dee as)** | Congenital opening of the male urethra on the underside of the penis. |
| **phimosis (fih MOH sis)** | Narrowing of the foreskin over the glans penis that results in difficulty with hygiene. This condition can lead to infection or difficulty with urination. The condition is treated with circumcision, the surgical removal of the foreskin. |
| **prostate cancer (PROSS tayt CAN ser)** | Slow-growing cancer that affects a large number of males after age 50. The PSA (prostate-specific antigen) test is used to assist in early detection of this disease. |
| **sexually transmitted disease (STD)** | Disease usually acquired as the result of sexual intercourse. Formerly more commonly referred to as *venereal disease* (VD). |
| **syphilis (SIF ih lis)** | Infectious, chronic, venereal disease that can involve any organ. May exist for years without symptoms, but is fatal if untreated. Treated with the antibiotic penicillin. |
| **testicular carcinoma (kar sih NOH mah)** | Cancer of one or both testicles. |
| **testicular torsion** | A twisting of the spermatic cord. |
| **trichomoniasis (trik oh moh NYE ah sis)** | Genitourinary infection that is usually without symptoms (asymptomatic) in both males and females. In women the disease can produce itching and/or burning, a foul-smelling discharge, and result in vaginitis. |
| **varicocele (VAIR ih koh seel)** | Enlargement of the veins of the spermatic cord that commonly occurs on the left side of adolescent males. |
| **venereal disease (veh NEER ee al dih ZEEZ) (VD)** | Disease usually acquired as the result of sexual intercourse. More commonly referred to as *sexually transmitted disease* (STD). |

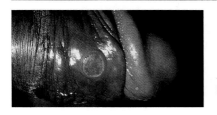

▓ **FIGURE 10.22** Chancroid ulcer on the penis.
(Biophoto Associates/Photo Researchers, Inc.)

## Diagnostic Procedures Relating to the Male Reproductive System

| | |
|---|---|
| **digital rectal (DIJ ih tal REK tal) exam (DRE)** | Manual examination for an enlarged prostate gland performed by palpating (feeling) the prostate gland through the wall of the rectum. |
| **prostate-specific antigen (PROSS tayt-specific AN tih jen) (PSA)** | A blood test to screen for prostate cancer. Elevated blood levels of PSA are associated with prostate cancer. |
| **semen analysis (SEE men ah NAL ih sis)** | This procedure is used when performing a fertility workup to determine if the male is able to produce sperm. Semen is collected by the patient after abstaining from sexual intercourse for a period of 3 to 5 days. The sperm in the semen are analyzed for number, swimming strength, and shape. Also used to determine if a vasectomy has been successful. After a period of 6 weeks, no further sperm should be present in a sample from the patient. |

## Therapeutic Procedures Relating to the Male Reproductive System

| | |
|---|---|
| **castration (kass TRAY shun)** | Excision of the testicles in the male or the ovaries in the female. |
| **circumcision (ser kum SIH zhun)** | Surgical removal of the end of the prepuce or foreskin of the penis. Generally performed on the newborn male at the request of the parents. The primary reason is for ease of hygiene. Circumcision is also a ritual practice in some religions. |
| **orchidopexy (OR kid oh peck see)** | Surgical fixation to move undescended testes into the scrotum, and to attach them to prevent retraction. Used to treat cryptorchidism. |
| **sterilization (ster ih lih ZAY shun)** | Process of rendering a male or female sterile or unable to conceive children. |
| **transurethral resection of the prostate (trans yoo REE thral REE sek shun of the PROSS tayt) (TUR, TURP)** | Surgical removal of the prostate gland by inserting a device through the urethra and removing prostate tissue. |
| **vasectomy (vas EK toh mee)** | Removal of a segment or all of the vas deferens to prevent sperm from leaving the male body. Used for contraception purposes (see ■ Figure 10.23). |

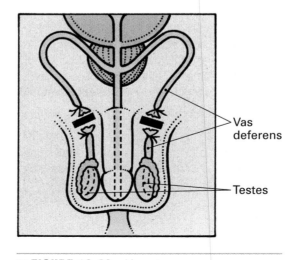

■ **FIGURE 10.23**   Vasectomy.

## Pharmacology Relating to the Male Reproductive System

| | |
|---|---|
| **androgen (AN droh jen) therapy** | Replacement male hormones to treat patients who produce insufficient hormone naturally. |
| **antiprostatic (an tye pross TAT ik) agents** | Medication to treat early cases of benign prostatic hypertrophy. May prevent surgery for mild cases. |
| **erectile (ee REK tile) dysfunction agents** | Medication that temporarily produces an erection in patients with erectile dysfunction. |

## Abbreviations Relating to the Male Reproductive System

| | | | |
|---|---|---|---|
| **BPH** | benign prostatic hypertrophy | **PSA** | prostate-specific antigen |
| **DRE** | digital rectal exam | **RPR** | rapid plasma reagin (test for syphilis) |
| **ED** | erectile dysfunction | **SPP** | suprapubic prostatectomy |
| **GC** | gonorrhea | **STD** | sexually transmitted disease |
| **GU** | genitourinary | **TUR** | transurethral resection |
| **HPV** | human papilloma virus | **TURP** | transurethral resection of the prostate |
| **HSV** | *Herpes simplex* virus | **VD** | venereal disease |
| **NGU** | nongonococcal urethritis | | |

# Chapter Review

## Pronunciation Practice

*You will find the pronunciation for each term on the enclosed CD-ROM. Check each one off as you master it.*

- ❑ abortion (ah **BOR** shun)
- ❑ abruptio placentae (ah **BRUP** tee oh plah **SEN** tee)
- ❑ afterbirth
- ❑ amenorrhea (ah men oh **REE** ah)
- ❑ amniocentesis (am nee oh sen **TEE** sis)
- ❑ amnion (**AM** nee on)
- ❑ amniorrhea (am nee oh **REE** ah)
- ❑ amniotic (am nee **OT** ik) fluid
- ❑ amniotomy (am nee **OT** oh mee)
- ❑ androgen (**AN** droh jen)
- ❑ androgen (**AN** droh jen) therapy
- ❑ andropathy (an **DROP** ah thee)
- ❑ anorchism (an **OR** kizm)
- ❑ anteflexion (an tee **FLEK** shun)
- ❑ antepartum (an tee **PAR** tum)
- ❑ antiprostatic (an tye pross **TAT** ik) agents
- ❑ Apgar (**AP** gar) score
- ❑ areola (ah **REE** oh la)
- ❑ aspermia (ah **SPER** mee ah)
- ❑ atresia (ah **TREE** she ah)
- ❑ balanitis (bal ah **NYE** tis)
- ❑ balanoplasty (**BAL** ah noh plas tee)
- ❑ balanorrhea (bah lah noh **REE** ah)
- ❑ barrier contraception (kon trah **SEP** shun)
- ❑ Bartholin's (**BAR** toh linz) glands
- ❑ benign prostatic hypertrophy (bee **NINE** pross **TAT** ik high **PER** troh fee)
- ❑ breast cancer
- ❑ breasts
- ❑ breech presentation
- ❑ bulbourethral (buhl boh yoo **REE** thral) gland
- ❑ candidiasis (kan dih **DYE** ah sis)
- ❑ castration (kass **TRAY** shun)
- ❑ cauterization (kaw ter in **ZAY** shun)
- ❑ cervical biopsy (**SER** vih kal **BYE** op see)

- ❑ cervical cancer (**SER** vih kal **CAN** ser)
- ❑ cervicectomy (ser vih **SEK** toh mee)
- ❑ cervix (**SER** viks)
- ❑ cesarean (see **SAYR** ee an) section
- ❑ chancroid (**SHANG** kroyd)
- ❑ chlamydia (klah **MID** ee ah)
- ❑ choriocarcinoma (kor ee oh kar sih **NOH** mah)
- ❑ chorion (**KOR** ree on)
- ❑ chorionic villus (kor ree **ON** ik vill us) sampling
- ❑ circumcision (ser kum **SIH** zhun)
- ❑ clitoris (**KLIT** oh ris)
- ❑ coitus (**KOH** ih tus)
- ❑ colostrum (kuh **LOS** trum)
- ❑ colposcope (**KOL** poh scope)
- ❑ colposcopy (kol **POSS** koh pee)
- ❑ condyloma (kon dih **LOH** mah)
- ❑ congenital anomalies (con **JEN** ih tal ah **NOM** ah lees)
- ❑ conization (kon ih **ZAY** shun)
- ❑ copulation (kop yoo **LAY** shun)
- ❑ corpus (**KOR** pus)
- ❑ Cowper's (**KOW** perz) glands
- ❑ crowning
- ❑ cryosurgery (cry oh **SER** jer ee)
- ❑ cryptorchidism (kript **OR** kid izm)
- ❑ culdoscopy (kul **DOS** koh pee)
- ❑ cystocele (**SIS** toh seel)
- ❑ delivery
- ❑ digital rectal (**DIJ** ih tal **REK** tal) exam
- ❑ dilation and curettage (dye **LAY** shun and koo reh **TAHZ**)
- ❑ dilation (dye **LAY** shun) stage
- ❑ Down syndrome (**DOWN SIN** drohm)
- ❑ dysmenorrhea (dis men oh **REE** ah)
- ❑ dyspareunia (dis pah **ROO** nee ah)

- dystocia (dis **TOH** she ah)
- eclampsia (eh **KLAMP** see ah)
- ectopic pregnancy (ek **TOP** ik **PREG** non see)
- effacement (eh **FACE** ment)
- ejaculation (ee jak yoo **LAY** shun)
- elective abortion (ah **BOR** shun)
- embryo (**EM** bree oh)
- endocervicitis (en doh ser vih **SIGH** tis)
- endometrial biopsy (en doh **MEE** tree al **BYE** op see)
- endometrial cancer (en doh **MEE** tree al **CAN** ser)
- endometriosis (en doh mee tree **OH** sis)
- endometritis (en doh meh **TRY** tis)
- endometrium (en doh **MEE** tree um)
- epididymectomy (ep ih did ih **MEK** toh mee)
- epididymis (ep ih **DID** ih mis)
- epididymitis (ep ih did ih **MYE** tis)
- episiorrhaphy (eh peez ee **OR** ah fee)
- episiotomy (eh peez ee **OT** oh mee)
- epispadias (ep ih **SPAY** dee as)
- erectile (ee **REK** tile) dysfunction
- erectile (ee **REK** tile) dysfunction agents
- erectile (ee **REK** tile) tissue
- erythroblastosis fetalis (eh rith roh blass **TOH** sis fee **TAL** iss)
- estimated date of confinement
- estrogen (**ESS** troh jen)
- expulsion (ex **PULL** shun) stage
- fallopian tubes (fah **LOH** pee an **TOOBS**)
- fertilization (fer til ih **ZAY** shun)
- fetal (**FEE** tal) monitoring
- fetus (**FEE** tus)
- fibrocystic (figh bro **SIS** tik) breast disease
- fibroid tumor (**FIGH** broyd **TOO** mor)
- fimbriae (**FIM** bree ay)
- follicle (**FOLL** ih kl) stimulating hormone
- foreskin (**FOR** skin)
- fraternal twins
- fundus (**FUN** dus)
- genetic counseling
- genital herpes (**JEN** ih tal **HER** peez)
- genital (**JEN** ih tal) warts
- genitalia (jen ih **TAY** lee ah)
- gestation (jess **TAY** shun)

- glans penis (**GLANS PEE** nis)
- gonorrhea (gon oh **REE** ah)
- gynecologist (gigh neh **KOL** oh jist)
- gynecology (gigh neh **KOL** oh jee)
- hematosalpinx (hee mah toh **SAL** pinks)
- hormone replacement therapy
- hydrocele (**HIGH** droh seel)
- hymen (**HIGH** men)
- hymenectomy (high men **EK** toh mee)
- hypospadias (high poh **SPAY** dee as)
- hysterectomy (hiss ter **EK** toh mee)
- hysteropexy (**HISS** ter oh pek see)
- hysterorrhexis (hiss ter oh **REK** sis)
- hysterosalpingography (hiss ter oh sal pin **GOG** rah fee)
- identical twins
- impotence (**IM** poh tents)
- impregnation (im preg **NAY** shun)
- infertility
- intrauterine (in trah **YOO** ter in) device
- Kegel (**KAY** gull) exercises
- labia majora (**LAY** bee ah mah **JOR** ah)
- labia minora (**LAY** bee ah mih **NOR** ah)
- labor (**LAY** bor)
- lactation (lak **TAY** shun)
- lactic (**LAK** tik)
- lactiferous (lak **TIF** er us) ducts
- lactiferous (lak **TIF** er us) glands
- lactorrhea (lak toh **REE** ah)
- laparoscopy (lap ar **OS** koh pee)
- laparotomy (lap ah **ROT** oh mee)
- last menstrual period
- ligaments (**LIG** ah ments)
- low birth weight
- lumpectomy (lump **EK** toh mee)
- luteinizing (loo teh **NIGH** zing) hormone
- mammary (**MAM** ah ree) glands
- mammogram (**MAM** moh gram)
- mammography (mam **OG** rah fee)
- mammoplasty (**MAM** moh plas tee)
- mastalgia (mas **TAL** jee ah)
- mastectomy (mass **TEK** toh mee)
- mastitis (mas **TYE** tis)

- meconium (meh **KOH** nee um)
- menarche (men **AR** kee)
- menopause (**MEN** oh pawz)
- menorrhagia (men oh **RAY** jee ah)
- menstrual (**MEN** stroo all) period
- menstruation (men stroo **AY** shun)
- metrorrhagia (meh troh **RAY** jee ah)
- metrorrhea (meh troh **REE** ah)
- miscarriage
- multigravida (mull tih **GRAV** ih dah)
- multipara (mull **TIP** ah rah)
- myometrium (my oh **MEE** tre um)
- neonate (**NEE** oh nayt)
- neonatology (nee oh nay **TALL** oh jee)
- nipple
- nulligravida (null ih **GRAV** ih dah)
- nullipara (null **IP** ah rah)
- nurse
- obstetrician (ob steh **TRISH** an)
- obstetrics (ob **STET** riks)
- oligomenorrhea (ol ih goh men oh **REE** ah)
- oligospermia (ol ih goh **SPER** mee ah)
- oophorectomy (oh oh foe **REK** toh mee)
- oophoritis (oh off oh **RIGH** tis)
- oral contraceptive (kon trah **SEP** tive) pills
- orchidectomy (or kid **EK** toh mee)
- orchidopexy (**OR** kid oh peck see)
- orchiectomy (or kee **EK** toh mee)
- orchioplasty (**OR** kee oh plas tee)
- orchiotomy (or kee **OT** oh mee)
- ova (**OH** vah)
- ovarian carcinoma (oh **VAY** ree an kar sih **NOH** mah)
- ovarian cyst (oh **VAY** ree an **SIST**)
- ovaries (**OH** vah reez)
- oviducts (**OH** vih ducts)
- ovulation (ov yoo **LAY** shun)
- ovum (**OH** vum)
- oxytocin (ox ee **TOH** sin)
- PAP (Papanicolaou) (pap ah **NIK** oh low) smear
- parturition (par too **RISH** un)
- pelvic (**PELL** vik) examination
- pelvic inflammatory disease (**PELL** vik in **FLAM** mah toh ree dih **ZEEZ**)
- pelvic ultrasonography (**PELL** vik ull trah son **OG** rah fee)
- pelvimetry (pell **VIM** eh tree)
- penis (**PEE** nis)
- perimetritis (pair ih meh **TRY** tis)
- perimetrium (pear ee **MEE** tre um)
- perineum (pair ih **NEE** um)
- phimosis (fih **MOH** sis)
- placenta (plah **SEN** tah)
- placenta previa (plah **SEN** tah **PRE** vee ah)
- placental (plah **SEN** tal) stage
- postpartum (post **PAR** tum)
- preeclampsia (pre eh **KLAMP** see ah)
- pregnancy (**PREG** nan see)
- pregnancy (**PREG** nan see) test
- premature
- premenstrual syndrome (pre **MEN** stroo al **SIN** drohm)
- prepuce (**PREE** pyoos)
- primigravida (prem ih **GRAV** ih dah)
- primipara (prem **IP** ah rah)
- progesterone (proh **JES** ter ohn)
- prolapsed umbilical (pro **LAPS'D** um **BILL** ih kal) cord
- prolapsed uterus (pro **LAPS'D YOO** ter us)
- prostate cancer (**PROSS** tayt **CAN** ser)
- prostate (**PROSS** tayt) gland
- prostatectomy (pross tah **TEK** toh mee)
- prostate-specific antigen (**PROSS** tayt-specific **AN** tih jen)
- prostatitis (pross tah **TYE** tis)
- prostatolith (pross **TAT** oh lith)
- prostatolithotomy (pross tah toh lih **THOT** oh mee)
- prostatorrhea (pross tah toh **REE** ah)
- pseudocyesis (soo doh sigh **EE** sis)
- puberty (**PEW** ber tee)
- puerperium (pew er **PEER** ee um)
- pyosalpinx (pie oh **SAL** pinks)
- radical mastectomy (mast **EK** toh mee)
- rectocele (**REK** toh seel)
- salpingitis (sal pin **JIGH** tis)
- salpingocyesis (sal ping goh sigh **EE** sis)
- salpingostomy (sal ping **GOS** toh mee)
- scrotum (**SKROH** tum)
- semen (**SEE** men)

- semen analysis (**SEE** men ah **NAL** ih sis)
- seminal vesicles (**SEM** ih nal **VESS** ih kls)
- seminiferous tubules (sem ih **NIF** er us **TOO** byools)
- sexually transmitted disease
- simple mastectomy (mast **EK** toh mee)
- sperm
- spermatic cord (sper **MAT** ik **KORD**)
- spermatogenesis (sper mat oh **JEN** eh sis)
- spermatolysis (sper mah **TOL** ih sis)
- spermatolytic (sper mah toh **LIT** ik)
- spermatozoa (sper mat oh **ZOH** ah)
- spermatozoon (sper mat oh **ZOH** on)
- sphincter (**SFINGK** ter)
- spontaneous abortion (ah **BOR** shun)
- sterility
- sterilization (ster ih lih **ZAY** shun)
- stillbirth
- syphilis (**SIF** ih lis)
- testes (**TESS** teez)
- testicles (**TESS** tih kls)
- testicular carcinoma (kar sih **NOH** mah)
- testicular torsion
- testosterone (tess **TOSS** ter ohn)
- therapeutic abortion (thair an **PEU** tik ah **BOR** shun)

- total abdominal hysterectomy (hiss ter **EK** toh me)–bilateral salpingo-oophorectomy (sal ping goh oh oh foe **REK** toh mee)
- toxic shock syndrome
- transurethral resection of the prostate (trans yoo **REE** thrall **REE** sek shun of the **PROSS** tayt)
- trichomoniasis (trik oh moh **NYE** ah sis)
- tubal ligation (**TOO** bal lye **GAY** shun)
- tubal pregnancy (**TOO** bal **PREG** nan see)
- umbilical cord (um **BILL** ih kal **KORD**)
- urethra (yoo **REE** thrah)
- urinary meatus (**YOO** rih nair ee mee **AY** tus)
- uterine (**YOO** ter in) tubes
- uterus (**YOO** ter us)
- vagina (vah **JIGH** nah)
- vaginal hysterectomy (**VAJ** ih nal hiss ter **EK** toh me)
- vaginal orifice (**VAJ** ih nal **OR** ih fis)
- varicocele (**VAIR** ih koh seel)
- vas deferens (**VAS DEF** er enz)
- vasectomy (vas **EK** toh mee)
- vasovasostomy (vas oh vay **ZOS** toh mee)
- venereal disease (veh **NEER** ee al dih **ZEEZ**)
- viable (**VYE** ah bull)
- vulva (**VULL** vah)

# Case Study

## High-Risk Obstetrics Consultation Report

**Reason for Consultation:** High-risk pregnancy with late-term bleeding

**History of Present Illness:** Patient is 23 years old. She is currently estimated to be at 240 days of gestation. She has had a 23-lb weight gain with this pregnancy. Amniocentesis at 20 weeks indicated male fetus with no evidence of genetic or developmental disorders. She noticed a moderate degree of vaginal bleeding this morning but denies any cramping or pelvic pain. She immediately saw her obstetrician who referred her for high-risk evaluation.

**Past Medical History:** This patient is multigravida but nullipara with three early miscarriages without obvious cause. She was diagnosed with cancer of the left ovary 4 years ago. It was treated with a left oophorectomy and chemotherapy. She continues to undergo full-body CT scan every 6 months, and there has been no evidence of metastasis since that time. Menarche was at age 13 and her menstrual history is significant for menorrhagia resulting in chronic anemia.

**Results of Physical Examination:** Patient appears well nourished and abdominal girth appears consistent with length of gestation. She is understandably quite anxious regarding the sudden spotting. Pelvic ultrasound indicates placenta previa with placenta almost completely overlying cervix. However, there is no evidence of abruptio placentae at this time. Fetal size estimate is consistent with 25 weeks of gestation. The fetus is turned head down and the umbilical cord is not around the neck. The fetal heart tones are strong with a rate of 90 beats/minute. There is no evidence of cervical effacement or dilation at this time.

**Recommendations:** Fetus appears to be developing well and in no distress at this time. The placenta appears to be well attached on ultrasound, but the bleeding is cause for concern. With the extremely low position of the placenta, this patient is at very high risk for abruptio placentae when cervix begins effacement and dilation. She may require early delivery by cesarean section at that time. She will definitely require C-section at onset of labor. At this time, recommend bed rest with bathroom privileges. She is to return every other day for 2 weeks and every day after that for evaluation of cervix and fetal condition. She is to call immediately if she notes any further bleeding or change in activity level of the fetus.

## Critical Thinking Questions

1. Describe in your own words the treatment this patient received for her ovarian cancer. What procedure does she continue to have every 6 months?

2. Describe in your own words this patient's menstrual history.

3. Which of the following choices describes this patient (choose all that apply)?
   a. She has never been pregnant.
   b. She has several live children.
   c. She has no live children.
   d. She has been pregnant several times.

4. This patient has placenta previa. What procedure discovered this condition? The physician, however, is much more concerned about abruptio placentae. Explain why.

5. Describe the condition of the fetus.

6. The following two phrases are not specifically defined by your text. Explain what you believe them to mean based on the context of this consultation report.
   a. high-risk pregnancy
   b. abdominal girth appears consistent with length of gestation

# Chart Note Transcription

## Chart Note

The chart note below contains 10 phrases that can be reworded with a medical term that you learned in this chapter. Each phrase is identified with an underline. Determine the medical term and write your answers in the space provided.

**Current Complaint:** Patient is a 77-year-old male seen by the urologist with complaints of nocturia and difficulty with the release of semen from the urethra.① 

**Past History:** Medical history revealed that the patient had failure of the testes to descend into the scrotum② at birth, which was repaired by surgical fixation of the testes.③ He had also undergone elective sterilization by removal of a segment of the vas deferens④ at the age of 41.

**Signs and Symptoms:** Patient states he first noted these symptoms about 5 years ago. They have become increasingly severe and now he is not able to sleep without waking up to urinate up to 20 times a night and has difficulty completing the process of sexual relations.⑤ Palpation of the prostate gland through the rectum⑥ revealed multiple round firm nodules in prostate gland. A needle biopsy was negative for slow-growing cancer that frequently affects males over 50⑦ and a blood test for prostate cancer⑧ was normal.

**Diagnosis:** Noncancerous enlargement of the prostate gland.⑨

**Treatment:** Patient was scheduled for a surgical removal of prostate tissue through the urethra.⑩

1. _____

2. _____

3. _____

4. _____

5. _____

6. _____

7. _____

8. _____

9. _____

10. _____

# Practice Exercises

## A. Complete the following statements.

1. The study of the female reproductive system is the medical specialty of _____ .

2. A physician who specializes in the treatment of women is called a(n) _____ .

3. A general term that refers to both the male and female reproductive organs is _____ .

4. The time required for the development of a fetus is called _____ .

5. The cessation of menstruation is called _____ .

6. The female sex cell is a(n) _____ .

7. The inner lining of the uterus is called the _____ .

8. The organ in which the developing fetus resides is called the _____ .

9. The tubes that extend from the outer edges of the uterus and assist in transporting the ova and sperm are called _____ .

10. One of the longest terms used in medical terminology refers to the removal of the uterus, cervix, ovaries, and fallopian tubes. This term is _____ .

## B. State the terms described using the combining forms provided.

The combining form *colp/o* refers to the vagina. Use it to write a term that means

1. visual examination of the vagina _____

2. instrument used to examine the vagina _____

3. suture of the vagina _____

The combining form *cervic/o* refers to the cervix. Use it to write a term that means

4. inflammation of the cervix _____

5. pertaining to the cervix _____

The combining form *hyster/o* also refers to the uterus. Use it to write a term that means

6. uterine disease _____

7. surgical fixation of the uterus _____

8. removal of the uterus _____

9. rupture of the uterus _____

10. suture of the uterus _____

The combining form *oophor/o* refers to the ovaries. Use it to write a term that means

11. inflammation of an ovary _____

12. excision of an ovary _____

The suffix *-gravida* refers to pregnancy. Use it to write a term that means

13. multiple pregnancies _____

14. no pregnancies _____

15. first pregnancy _____

The suffix –*para* refers to bear (offspring). Use it to write a term that means

16. never bearing offspring _____

17. to bear multiple offspring _____

18. to bear first offspring _____

## C. Identify the following abbreviations.

1. Cx _____

2. LMP _____

3. MH _____

4. PID _____

5. DOB _____

6. CS _____

7. NB _____

8. PMS _____

9. TSS _____

10. LBW _____

## D. Write the abbreviations for the following terms.

1. phenylketonuria _____

2. artificial insemination _____

3. uterine contractions _____

4. full-term normal delivery _____

5. intrauterine device _____

6. dilation and curettage _____

7. dysfunctional uterine bleeding _____

8. gynecology _____

9. abortion _____

10. oral contraception pills _____

## E. Define the following combining terms.

1. metr/o _____

2. hyster/o _____

3. gynec/o _____

4. episi/o _____

5. oophor/o _____

6. ovari/o _____

7. salping/o _____

8. men/o _____

9. vagin/o _____

10. mamm/o _____

**F. Match the terms in column A with the definitions in column B.**

|     | A                      |     | B                                    |
|-----|------------------------|-----|--------------------------------------|
| 1.  | _____ erythroblastosis fetalis | a.  | lack of a normal body opening        |
| 2.  | _____ ovary            | b.  | hemolytic disease of the newborn     |
| 3.  | _____ vagina           | c.  | top of uterus                        |
| 4.  | _____ fundus           | d.  | female erectile tissue               |
| 5.  | _____ placenta         | e.  | produces eggs                        |
| 6.  | _____ endometrium      | f.  | normal place for fertilization       |
| 7.  | _____ clitoris         | g.  | beginning of menstruation            |
| 8.  | _____ miscarry         | h.  | birth canal                          |
| 9.  | _____ lactation        | i.  | nourishes fetus                      |
| 10. | _____ fallopian tube   | j.  | uterine lining                       |
| 11. | _____ dysmenorrhea     | k.  | cessation of menstruation            |
| 12. | _____ menarche         | l.  | nursing                              |
| 13. | _____ menopause        | m.  | newborn                              |
| 14. | _____ neonate          | n.  | abort                                |
| 15. | _____ atresia          | o.  | painful menstruation                 |

**G. Use the following terms in the sentences that follow.**

| premenstrual syndrome | puberty          | eclampsia   |
|-----------------------|------------------|-------------|
| D & C                 | cesarean section | laparoscopy |
| fibroid tumor         | conization       |             |
| stillbirth            | endometriosis    |             |

1. Kesha had a core of tissue from her cervix removed for testing. This is called _____ .

2. Joan delivered a baby that had died while still in the uterus. She had a(n) _____ .

3. Ashley has just started her first menstrual cycle. She is said to have entered _____ .

4. Kimberly is experiencing tender breasts, headaches, and some irritability just prior to her monthly menstrual cycle. This may be _____ .

5. Ana has been scheduled for an examination in which her physician will use an instrument to observe her abdominal cavity to rule out the diagnosis of severe endometriosis. The physician will insert the instrument through a small incision. This procedure is called a(n) _____ .

6. Lenora is scheduled to have a hysterectomy as a result of a long history of large benign growths in her uterus that have caused pain and bleeding. Lenora has a(n) _____ .

7. Tiffany's physician has recommended that she have a uterine scraping to stop excessive bleeding after a miscarriage. She will be scheduled for a _____ .

8. Stacey is having frequent prenatal checkups to prevent the serious condition of pregnancy called _____ .

9. Marion has experienced painful menstrual periods as a result of the lining of her uterus being displaced into her pelvic cavity. This is called _____ .

10. The results of Shataundra's pelvimetry indicate that she will probably require a(n) _____ for her baby's delivery.

**H. Match the terms in column A with the definitions in column B.**

|  | A |  | B |
|---|---|---|---|
| 1. | _____ gonorrhea | a. | also called STD |
| 2. | _____ genital herpes | b. | caused by parasitic microorganism |
| 3. | _____ candidiasis | c. | treated with penicillin |
| 4. | _____ syphilis | d. | caused by human papilloma virus |
| 5. | _____ venereal disease | e. | can pass to infant during birth |
| 6. | _____ genital warts | f. | genitourinary infection |
| 7. | _____ chancroid | g. | venereal ulcer |
| 8. | _____ chlamydia | h. | yeast infection |
| 9. | _____ trichomoniasis | i. | skin disease with vesicles |

**I. Complete the following statements.**

1. The male reproductive system is a combination of the _____ and _____ systems.

2. The male's external organs of reproduction consist of the _____ and the _____ .

3. Another term for the prepuce is the _____ .

4. The organs responsible for developing the sperm cells are the _____ .

5. The glands of lubrication and fluid production at each side of the male urethra are the _____ .

6. The male sex hormone is _____ .

7. The area between the scrotum and the anus is called the _____ .

**J. State the terms described using the combining forms provided.**

The combining form *prostat/o* refers to the prostate. Use this to write a term that means

1. removal of prostate _____

2. pertaining to the prostate _____

3. inflammation of the prostate _____

4. flow from the prostate _____

The combining form *orchi/o* refers to the testes. Use this to write a term that means

5. excision of the testes _____

6. surgical repair of the testes _____

7. incision into the testes _____

8. disease of the testes _____

The combining form *vesicul/o* refers to the seminal vesicle. Use this to write a term that means

9. disease of the seminal vesicle _____

10. inflammation of the seminal vesicle _____

**K. Identify the following abbreviations.**

1. SPP _____

2. TUR _____

3. GU _____

4. BPH _____

5. DRE _____

6. PSA _____

**L. Define the following terms.**

1. spermatogenesis _____

2. hydrocele _____

3. transurethral resection of the prostate (TURP) _____

4. aspermia _____

5. orchiectomy _____

6. vasectomy _____

7. cauterization _____

# Professional Journal

In this exercise you will now have an opportunity to put the words you have learned into practice. Imagine yourself in the role of a paramedic. If you refer back to the Professional Profile at the beginning of this chapter, you will see that this health care professional performs advanced life support procedures. Use the 10 words listed below, or any other new terms from this chapter or previous chapters, to write sentences to describe the patients you saw today.

An example of a sentence is *A diagnosis of* **hysterorrhexis** *was suspected because the woman in labor was experiencing severe bleeding.*

1. abruptio placentae _____

2. breech presentation _____

3. C-section _____

4. dilation stage _____

5. pulmonary embolism _____

6. dyspnea _____

7. myocardial infarction _____

8. defibrillation _____

9. greenstick fracture _____

10. hemorrhage _____

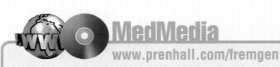
MedMedia
www.prenhall.com/fremgen

Use the CD-ROM enclosed with your textbook to gain additional reinforcement through interactive word building exercises, spelling games, labeling activities, and additional quizzes.

Use the above address to access the free, interactive Companion Website created for this textbook. Get hints, instant feedback, and textbook references to chapter-related multiple-choice questions, as well as labeling and matching exercises. In addition, you will find an audio glossary, case studies, and Internet exploration exercises.

***For more information regarding reproductive system diseases, check the links to men's health topics and women's health topics at the following websites:***

Centers for Disease Control and Prevention Health Topics at **www.cdc.gov/health/default.htm**

Intelihealth featuring Harvard Medical School's Consumer Health Information at
**www.intelihealth.com**

Stanford University's Health Library at
**http://healthlibrary.stanford.edu/resources/internet/bodysys.htm**

# Chapter 11
# Endocrine System

## Learning Objectives

*Upon completion of this chapter, you will be able to:*

- Recognize the combining forms and suffixes introduced in this chapter.
- Gain the ability to pronounce medical terms and major anatomical structures.
- List the major glands of the endocrine system.
- List the major hormones secreted by each endocrine gland and discuss their functions.
- Build endocrine system medical terms from word parts.
- Define vocabulary, pathology, diagnostic, and therapeutic medical terms relating to the endocrine system.
- Recognize types of medications associated with the endocrine system.
- Interpret abbreviations associated with the endocrine system.

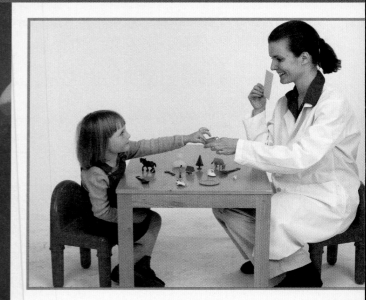

## MedMedia
www.prenhall.com/fremgen

Additional interactive resources and activities for this chapter can be found on the Companion Website. For animations, audio glossary, and review, access the accompanying CD-ROM in this book.

## Professional Profile

### Speech-Language Pathology

Speech-language pathologists evaluate and treat communication disorders. They are found in hospitals, long-term care facilities, home health agencies, schools, and rehabilitation facilities. Professionals in this field work with patients of all ages, some having problems from birth—such as cleft palate or cerebral palsy—while others have problems that occur at any stage of life—such as brain injury or stroke. The range of problems treated by speech-language pathologists includes stuttering, swallowing difficulties, or difficulty comprehending or producing language. Speech-language pathologists are responsible for evaluating patients to identify their specific problems and designing and carrying out a treatment program.

### Speech-Language Pathologist (CCC)

- Evaluates and treats communication disorders
- Graduates from an accredited master's degree program
- Completes a clinical fellowship
- Passes a national examination to receive Certificate of Clinical Competence (CCC)

*For more information regarding this health career, visit the following website:* American Speech-Language Hearing Association at **www.asha.org**

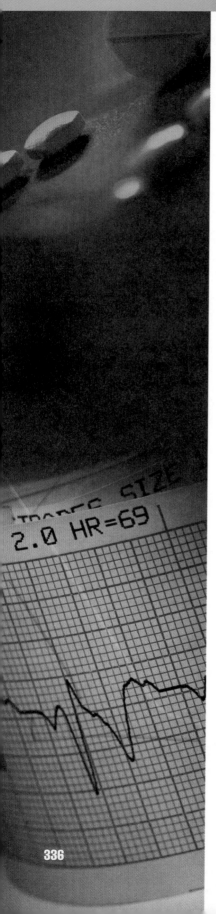

### Organs of the Endocrine System

adrenal glands
ovaries
pancreas (islets of Langerhans)
parathyroid glands
pineal gland
pituitary gland
testes
thymus gland
thyroid gland

### Combining Forms Relating to the Endocrine System

| | | | |
|---|---|---|---|
| acr/o | extremities | kal/i | potassium |
| aden/o | gland | natr/o | sodium |
| adren/o | adrenal glands | ophthalm/o | eye |
| adrenal/o | adrenal glands | pancreat/o | pancreas |
| andr/o | male | parathyroid/o | parathyroid gland |
| calc/o | calcium | pineal/o | pineal gland |
| crin/o | secrete | pituitar/o | pituitary gland |
| estr/o | female | somat/o | body |
| glyc/o | sugar | thym/o | thymus gland |
| glycos/o | sugar | thyr/o | thyroid gland |
| gonad/o | sex glands | thyroid/o | thyroid gland |
| home/o | sameness | tox/o | poison |

### Suffixes Relating to the Endocrine System

| Suffix | Meaning | Example |
|---|---|---|
| -crine | to secrete | endocrine |
| -dipsia | thirst | polydipsia |
| -emia | blood condition | hyperkalemia |
| -tropin | stimulate | adrenocorticotropin |
| -uria | urine condition | polyuria |

## Anatomy and Physiology of the Endocrine System

| | | |
|---|---|---|
| adrenal glands | hormones | pituitary gland |
| endocrine glands | ovaries | target organs |
| endocrine system | pancreas | testes |
| exocrine glands | parathyroid glands | thymus gland |
| glands | pineal gland | thyroid gland |
| homeostasis | | |

The **endocrine** (**EN** doh krin) **system** is a collection of **glands** that secrete **hormones** (**HOR** mohnz) directly into the bloodstream. Hormones are chemicals that act on their **target organs** to either increase or decrease the target's activity level. In this way the endocrine system is instrumental in maintaining **homeostasis** (hoe me oh **STAY** sis), that is, adjusting the activity level of most of the tissues and organs of the body to maintain a stable internal environment.

The body actually has two distinct types of glands: **exocrine** (**EKS** oh krin) **glands** and **endocrine** (**EN** doh krin) **glands.** Exocrine glands release their secretions into a duct that carries them to the outside of the body. For example, sweat glands release sweat into a sweat duct that travels to the surface of the body. Endocrine glands, however, release hormones directly into the bloodstream. The secretion of the thyroid gland directly enters the bloodstream. Because they have no ducts, they are referred to as *ductless glands.*

The endocrine system consists of the following glands: two **adrenal** (ad **REE** nal) **glands,** two **ovaries** (**OH** vah reez) in the female, four **parathyroid** (pair ah **THIGH** royd) **glands,** the **pancreas** (**PAN** kree ass), the **pineal** (pih **NEAL**) **gland,** the **pituitary** (pih **TOO** ih tair ee) **gland,** two **testes** (**TESS** teez) in the male, the **thymus** (**THIGH** mus) **gland,** and the **thyroid** (**THIGH** royd) **gland.** The endocrine glands as a whole affect the functions of the entire body (see ▇ Figure 11.1). Table 11.1 presents a description of the endocrine glands, their hormones, and their functions.

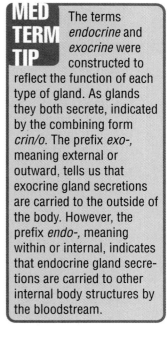

**MED TERM TIP** The terms *endocrine* and *exocrine* were constructed to reflect the function of each type of gland. As glands they both secrete, indicated by the combining form *crin/o.* The prefix *exo-*, meaning external or outward, tells us that exocrine gland secretions are carried to the outside of the body. However, the prefix *endo-*, meaning within or internal, indicates that endocrine gland secretions are carried to other internal body structures by the bloodstream.

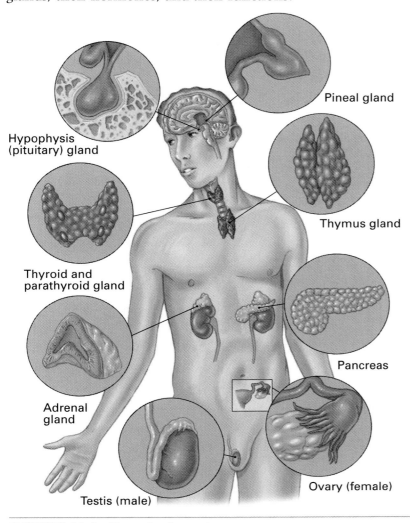

Pineal gland

Hypophysis (pituitary) gland

Thymus gland

Thyroid and parathyroid gland

Adrenal gland

Pancreas

Testis (male)

Ovary (female)

▇ **FIGURE 11.1** The endocrine system.

## Table 11.1    Endocrine Glands and Their Hormones

| Gland and Hormone | Function |
|---|---|
| **Adrenal cortex** | |
| Glucocorticoids | |
| Cortisol | Regulates carbohydrate levels in the body |
| Mineralcorticoids | |
| Aldosterone | Regulates electrolytes and fluid volume in body |
| Steroid sex hormones | |
| Androgen, estrogen, progesterone | Responsible for reproduction and secondary sexual characteristics |
| **Adrenal medulla** | |
| Epinephrine (adrenaline) | Intensifies response during stress; "fight or flight" response |
| Norepinephrine | Chiefly a vasoconstrictor |
| **Ovaries** | |
| Estrogen | Stimulates development of secondary sex characteristics in females; regulates menstrual cycle |
| Progesterone | Prepares for conditions of pregnancy |
| **Pancreas** | |
| Glucagon | Stimulates liver to release glucose into the blood |
| Insulin | Regulates and promotes entry of glucose into cells |
| **Parathyroid glands** | |
| Parathyroid hormone | Stimulates bone breakdown; regulates calcium level in the blood |
| **Pituitary anterior lobe** | |
| Adrenocorticotropic hormone (ACTH) | Regulates function of adrenal cortex |
| Follicle-stimulating hormone (FSH) | Stimulates growth of eggs in female and sperm in males |
| Growth hormone (GH) | Stimulates growth of the body |
| Luteinizing hormone (LH) | Regulates function of male and female gonads and plays a role in releasing ova in females |
| Melanocyte-stimulating hormone (MSH) | Stimulates pigment in skin |
| Prolactin | Stimulates milk production |
| Thyroid-stimulating hormone (TSH) | Regulates function of thyroid gland |
| **Pituitary posterior lobe** | |
| Antidiuretic hormone (ADH) | Stimulates reabsorption of water by the kidneys |
| Oxytocin | Stimulates uterine contractions and releases milk into ducts |
| **Testes** | |
| Testosterone | Promotes sperm production and development of secondary sex characteristics in males |
| **Thymus** | |
| Thymosin | Promotes development of cells in immune system |
| **Thyroid gland** | |
| Calcitonin | Stimulates deposition of calcium into bone |
| Thyroxine ($T_4$) | Stimulates metabolism in cells |
| Triiodothyronine ($T_3$) | Stimulates metabolism in cells |

# Adrenal Glands

| adrenal cortex | corticosteroids | mineralocorticoids |
|---|---|---|
| adrenal medulla | cortisol | norepinephrine |
| adrenaline | epinephrine | progesterone |
| aldosterone | estrogen | steroid sex hormones |
| androgens | glucocorticoids | |

MED TERM TIP The term *cortex* is frequently used in anatomy to indicate the outer portion of an organ such as the adrenal gland or the kidney. The term *cortex* means *bark*, as in the bark of a tree. The term *medulla* means *marrow*. Because marrow is found in the inner cavity of bones, the term came to stand for the middle of an organ.

The two adrenal glands are located above each of the kidneys (see ▪ Figure 11.2). Each gland is composed of two sections: **adrenal cortex** (**KOR** tex) and **adrenal medulla** (meh **DOOL** lah).

The outer adrenal cortex manufactures several different families of hormones: **mineralocorticoids** (min er al oh **KOR** tih koydz), **glucocorticoids** (gloo koh **KOR** tih koydz), and **steroid** (**STAIR** oyd) **sex hormones.** However, because they are all produced by the cortex they are collectively referred to as **corticosteroids** (kor tih koh **STAIR** oydz). The mineralocorticoid hormone, **aldosterone** (al **DOSS** ter ohn), regulates sodium (Na$^+$) and potassium (K$^+$) levels in the body. The glucocorticoid hormone, **cortisol** (**KOR** tih sal), regulates carbohydrates in the body. The adrenal cortex of both men and women secretes steroid sex hormones: **androgens** (**AN** druh jenz), **estrogen**

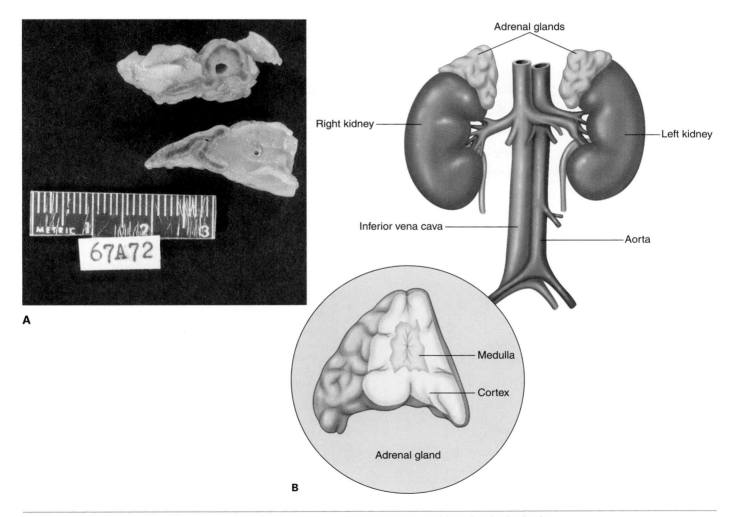

A

67A72

Adrenal glands

Right kidney

Left kidney

Inferior vena cava

Aorta

Medulla

Cortex

Adrenal gland

B

▪ **FIGURE 11.2**  The adrenal glands: (A) actual specimen; (B) appearance and location in the body.
(Martin Rotker/Phototake NYC)

(**ESS** troh jen), and **progesterone** (proh **JESS** ter ohn). These hormones regulate secondary sexual characteristics. All hormones secreted by the adrenal cortex are steroid hormones.

The inner portion of the adrenal medulla is responsible for secreting the hormones **epinephrine** (ep ih **NEF** rin) and **norepinephrine** (nor ep ih **NEF** rin). Epinephrine is also called **adrenaline** (ah **DREN** ah lin). These hormones are critical during emergency situations because they increase blood pressure, heart rate, and respiration levels. This helps the body perform better during emergencies or otherwise stressful times.

## Ovaries

| | | |
|---|---|---|
| estrogen | gonads | ova |
| gametes | menstrual cycle | progesterone |

The two ovaries are located in the lower abdominopelvic cavity of the female. They are the female **gonads** (**GOH** nadz). Gonads are organs that produce **gametes** (gam **EATS**), or the reproductive sex cells. In the case of females, the gametes are the **ova** (**OH** vah). Of importance to the endocrine system, the ovaries produce the female sex hormones, **estrogen** and **progesterone**. Estrogen is responsible for the appearance of the female sexual characteristics and regulation of the **menstrual** (men **STROO** all) **cycle** (see ■ Figure 11.3). Progesterone helps to maintain a suitable uterine environment for pregnancy.

## Pancreas

| | | |
|---|---|---|
| diabetes insipidus | hypoglycemia | non-insulin-dependent diabetes mellitus |
| diabetes mellitus | insulin | |
| digestive enzymes | insulin-dependent diabetes mellitus | type 1 |
| glucagon | | type 2 |
| hyperglycemia | islets of Langerhans | |

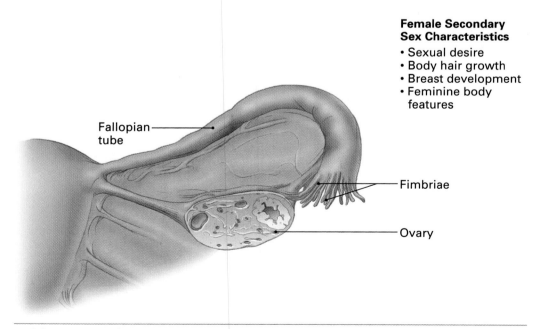

**Female Secondary Sex Characteristics**
- Sexual desire
- Body hair growth
- Breast development
- Feminine body features

Fallopian tube

Fimbriae

Ovary

■ **FIGURE 11.3**  Structure and functions of the ovary.

The pancreas is located along the lower curvature of the stomach (see ▨ Figure 11.4). It is the only organ in the body that has both endocrine and exocrine functions. The exocrine portion of the pancreas releases **digestive enzymes** through a duct into the duodenum of the small intestines. The endocrine sections of the pancreas, **islets of Langerhans** (EYE lets of **LAHNG** er hahnz), are named after Dr. Paul Langerhans, a German anatomist. The islets cells produce two different hormones: **insulin** (**IN** suh lin) and **glucagon** (**GLOO** koh gon). Insulin, produced by β islet cells, stimulates the cells of the body to take in glucose from the bloodstream. Loss or impairment of the function of insulin results in **diabetes mellitus** (dye ah **BEE** teez **MELL** ih tus) (DM) and **hyperglycemia** (high per glye **SEE** mee ah), which is a high blood sugar level. In contrast, overproduction of insulin will result in **hypoglycemia** (high poh glye **SEE** mee ah), or a low blood sugar level.

There are two distinctly different types of diabetes mellitus: **type 1** and **type 2**. In type 1 there is a destruction of the islet cells and the person fails to produce an adequate amount of insulin. Therefore, he or she must take insulin injections to replace the insulin the pancreas is unable to produce. Type 1 is also called **insulin-dependent diabetes mellitus** (IDDM). In type 2 diabetes mellitus the person makes a sufficient amount of insulin, but it has lost its ability to influence the cells of the body. These patients (except in severe cases) do not take insulin. Therefore type 2 is also called **non–insulin-dependent diabetes mellitus** (NIDDM). This type of DM is usually treated by diet, exercise, and oral hypoglycemic agents—medications that result in a more normal blood sugar level.

Another set of islet cells, the α cells, secrete a different hormone, glucagon, in response to hypoglycemia. Glucagon stimulates the liver to release glucose, thereby raising the blood glucose level. Glucagon is released when the body needs more sugar, such as at the beginning of strenuous activity or several hours after the last meal has been digested. Insulin and glucagon have opposite effects on blood sugar level. Insulin will reduce the blood sugar level, while glucagon will increase it.

> **MED TERM TIP** Many people just use the term *diabetes* to refer to diabetes mellitus (DM). But there is another type of diabetes, called **diabetes insipidus** (dye ah **BEE** teez in **SIP** ih dus) (DI), that is a result of the inadequate secretion of the antidiuretic hormone (ADH) from the pituitary gland.

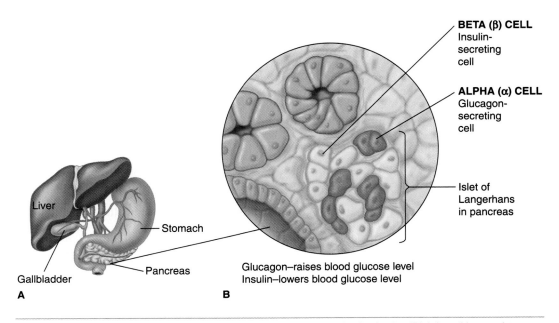

BETA (β) CELL
Insulin-secreting cell

ALPHA (α) CELL
Glucagon-secreting cell

Islet of Langerhans in pancreas

Liver

Stomach

Gallbladder

Pancreas

Glucagon–raises blood glucose level
Insulin–lowers blood glucose level

A

B

▨ **FIGURE 11.4** The pancreas: (A) appearance and location in the body; (B) islet of Langerhans.

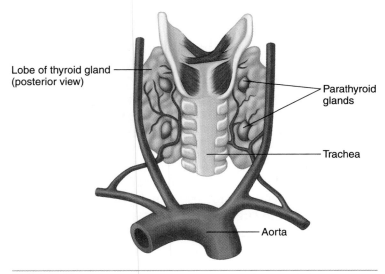

Lobe of thyroid gland
(posterior view)

Parathyroid
glands

Trachea

Aorta

■ **FIGURE 11.5** The parathyroid glands and their relation to the thyroid gland and trachea.

## Parathyroid Glands

**calcium**              **parathyroid hormone**         **tetany**

**MED TERM TIP** A calcium deficiency in the system can result in a condition called **tetany** (**TET** ah nee) or muscle excitability and tremors. If the parathyroid glands are removed during thyroid surgery, calcium replacement in the body is often necessary.

The four tiny parathyroid glands are located on the dorsal surface of the thyroid gland (see ■ Figure 11.5). The **parathyroid hormone** (pair ah **THIGH** royd **HOR** mohn) (**PTH**) secreted by these glands regulates the amount of **calcium** in the blood. If calcium levels in the blood fall too low, parathyroid hormone levels in the blood are increased and will stimulate bone breakdown to release more calcium into the blood.

## Pineal Gland

**circadian rhythm**         **melatonin**            **thalamus**

**MED TERM TIP** The pineal gland is an example of an organ named for its shape. *Pineal* means shaped like a pine cone.

The pineal gland is a small pine cone-shaped gland that is part of the **thalamus** (**THALL** mus) region of the brain. The pineal gland secretes **melatonin** (mel ah **TOH** nin). This hormone is not well understood, but plays a role in regulating the body's **circadian** (seer **KAY** dee an) **rhythm.** This is the 24-hour clock that governs our periods of wakefulness and sleepiness.

## Pituitary Gland

| | | |
|---|---|---|
| **adrenocorticotropin hormone** | **growth hormone** | **posterior lobe** |
| **anterior lobe** | **hypothalamus** | **prolactin** |
| **antidiuretic hormone** | **luteinizing hormone** | **somatotropin** |
| **follicle-stimulating hormone** | **melanocyte-stimulating hormone** | **thyroid-stimulating hormone** |
| | **oxytocin** | **vasopressin** |

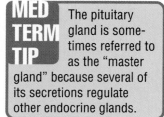

**MED TERM TIP** The pituitary gland is sometimes referred to as the "master gland" because several of its secretions regulate other endocrine glands.

The pituitary gland is located on the underneath side of the brain (see ■ Figure 11.6). The small marble-shaped gland is divided into an **anterior lobe** and a **posterior lobe.** Both lobes are controlled by the **hypothalamus** (high poh **THAL** ah mus) in the brain.

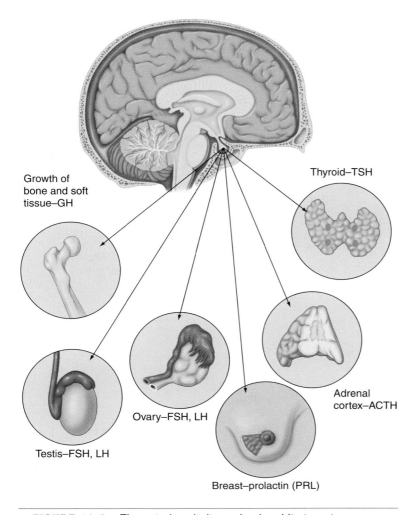

Growth of bone and soft tissue–GH

Thyroid–TSH

Testis–FSH, LH

Ovary–FSH, LH

Breast–prolactin (PRL)

Adrenal cortex–ACTH

**FIGURE 11.6**   The anterior pituitary gland and its target organs.

The anterior pituitary secretes several different hormones (see ▓ Figure 11.7). **Growth hormone** (GH), also called **somatotropin** (so mat oh **TROH** pin), promotes growth of the body by stimulating cells to rapidly increase in size and divide. **Thyroid-stimulating hormone** (TSH) regulates the function of the thyroid gland. **Adrenocorticotropin hormone** (ah dree noh kor tih koh **TROH** pin **HOR** mohn) (ACTH) regulates the function of the adrenal cortex. **Prolactin** (proh **LAK** tin) (PRL) stimulates milk production in the breast following pregnancy and birth. **Follicle-stimulating hormone** (**FOLL** ih kl **STIM** yoo lay ting **HOR** mohn) (FSH) and **luteinizing hormone** (**LOO** tee in eye zing **HOR** mohn) (LH) both exert their influence on the male and female gonads. FSH is responsible for the development of ova in ovaries and sperm in testes. It also stimulates the ovary to secrete estrogen. LH stimulates secretion of sex hormones in both males and females and plays a role in releasing ova in females. **Melanocyte-stimulating hormone** (MSH) stimulates melanocytes to produce more melanin, thereby darkening the skin.

The posterior pituitary secretes two hormones, **antidiuretic** (an tye dye yoo **RET** ik) **hormone** (ADH) and **oxytocin** (ok see **TOH** sin). ADH, also called **vasopressin** (vaz oh **PRESS** in), promotes water reabsorption by the kidney tubules. Oxytocin stimulates uterine contractions during labor and delivery, and after birth the release of milk from the mammary glands.

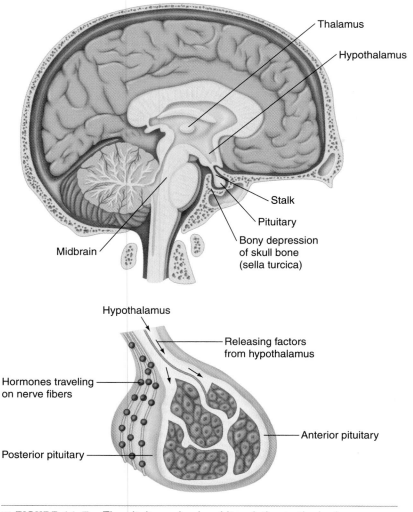

**FIGURE 11.7**  The pituitary gland and its relation to the brain.

## Testes

**sperm**                         **testosterone**

The testes are two oval glands located in the scrotal sac of the male. They are the male gonads, which produce the male gametes, **sperm,** and the male sex hormone, **testosterone** (tess **TOSS** ter own). Testosterone produces the male secondary sexual characteristics and regulates sperm production (see ▥ Figure 11.8)

## Thymus Gland

**T cells**                        **thymosin**

In addition to its role as part of the immune system, the thymus is also one of the endocrine glands because it secretes the hormone **thymosin** (thigh **MOH** sin). Thymosin, like the rest of the thymus gland, is important for proper development of the immune system. The thymus gland is located in the mediastinal cavity anterior and superior to the heart (see ▥ Figure 11.9). The thymus is present at birth and grows to its largest size during puberty. At puberty it begins to shrink and eventually is replaced with connective and adipose tissue.

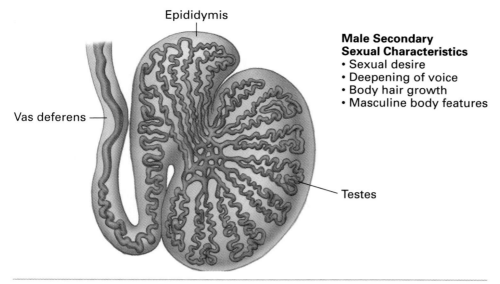

Epididymis

**Male Secondary
Sexual Characteristics**
• Sexual desire
• Deepening of voice
• Body hair growth
• Masculine body features

Vas deferens

Testes

**FIGURE 11.8**   Structure and function of male testes.

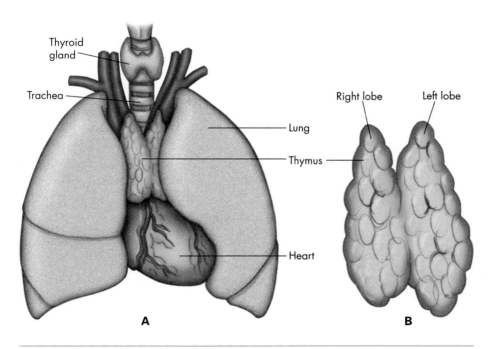

Thyroid
gland

Trachea

Lung

Thymus

Heart

Right lobe       Left lobe

A                                    B

**FIGURE 11.9**   The thymus gland: (A) appearance and position; (B) with anatomical structures.

The most important function of the thymus is the development of the immune system in the newborn. It is essential to the growth and development of thymic lymphocytes or **T cells,** which are critical for the body's immune system. The complete function of the thymus gland is not very well understood.

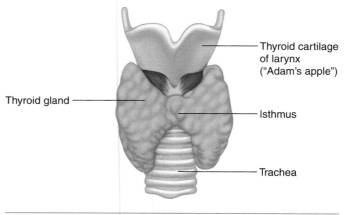

Thyroid cartilage
of larynx
("Adam's apple")

Thyroid gland

Isthmus

Trachea

■ **FIGURE 11.10** The thyroid gland and its relation to the trachea and larynx.

## Thyroid Gland

| | | |
|---|---|---|
| **calcitonin** | **T₃** | **thyroxine** |
| **goiter** | **T₄** | **triiodothyronine** |
| **iodine** | | |

The thyroid gland (see ■ Figure 11.10), which resembles a butterfly in shape, has right and left lobes. It is located on either side of the trachea and larynx. The thyroid cartilage, or Adam's apple, is located just above the thyroid gland. This gland produces the hormones **thyroxine** (thigh **ROKS** in), which is also known as **T₄,** and **triiodothyronine** (try eye oh doh **THIGH** roh neen), which is called **T₃.** These hormones are produced in the thyroid gland from the mineral **iodine** (**EYE** oh dine). T₃ and T₄ help to regulate the production of energy and heat in the body to adjust the metabolic rate of the body.

**MED TERM TIP** Iodine is found in many foods, including vegetables and seafood. It is also present in iodized salt, which is one of the best sources of iodine for people living in the Goiter belt, composed of states located away from saltwater. A lack of iodine in the diet can lead to thyroid disorders, including **goiter** (**GOY** ter).

The thyroid gland also secretes **calcitonin** (kal sih **TOH** nin) in response to hypercalcemia (too high blood calcium level). Its action is the opposite of parathyroid hormone and stimulates the increased deposition of calcium into bone, thereby lowering blood levels of calcium.

# Word Building Relating to the Endocrine System

The following list contains examples of medical terms built directly from word parts. The definitions of these terms can be determined by a straightforward translation of the word parts.

| Combining Form | Combined With | Medical Term | Definition |
|---|---|---|---|
| aden/o | -oma | adenoma (ad eh **NOH** mah) | gland tumor |
| adren/o | -megaly | adrenomegaly (ad ree noh **MEG** ah lee) | enlarged adrenal gland |
| | -pathy | adrenopathy (ad ren **OP** ah thee) | adrenal gland disease |
| adrenal/o | -ectomy | adrenalectomy (ad ree nal **EK** toh mee) | excision of adrenal glands |
| | -itis | adrenalitis (ad ree nal **EYE** tis) | inflammation of an adrenal gland |
| andr/o | -gen | androgen (**AN** druh jen) | male forming |
| calc/o | hyper- -emia | hypercalcemia (high per kal **SEE** mee ah) | excessive calcium in the blood |
| | hypo- -emia | hypocalcemia (high poh kal **SEE** mee ah) | low calcium in the blood |
| crin/o | endo- -ologist | endocrinologist (en doh krin **ALL** oh jist) | specialist in the endocrine system |
| | endo- -ology | endocrinology (en doh krin **ALL** oh jee) | study of the endocrine system |
| | endo- -pathy | endocrinopathy (en doh krin **OP** ah thee) | endocrine system disease |
| estr/o | -gen | estrogen (**ESS** troh jen) | female forming |
| glyc/o | hyper- -emia | hyperglycemia (high per glye **SEE** mee ah) | excessive sugar in the blood |
| | hypo- -emia | hypoglycemia (high poh glye **SEE** mee ah) | low sugar in the blood |
| kal/i | hyper- -emia | hyperkalemia (high per kal **EE** mee ah) | excessive potassium in the blood |
| natr/o | hypo- -emia | hyponatremia (high poh nah **TREE** mee ah) | low sodium in the blood |
| parathyroid/o | -ectomy | parathyroidectomy (pair ah thigh royd **EK** toh mee) | excision of the parathyroid gland |
| | -oma | parathyroidoma (pair ah thigh royd **OH** ma) | parathyroid gland tumor |
| thyr/o | -megaly | thyromegaly (thigh roh **MEG** ah lee) | enlarged thyroid |
| | toxic/o -osis | thyrotoxicosis (thigh roh toks ih **KOH** sis) | abnormal condition of poisoning by the thyroid |
| thyroid/o | -ectomy | thyroidectomy (thigh royd **EK** toh mee) | excision of the thyroid |
| | eu- | euthyroid (yoo **THIGH** royd) | normal thyroid |
| | hyper- -ism | hyperthyroidism (hi per **THIGH** royd izm) | state of excessive thyroid |
| | hypo- -ism | hypothyroidism (high poh **THIGH** royd izm) | state of low thyroid |
| | -otomy | thyroidotomy (thigh royd **OTT** oh mee) | incision into thyroid gland |

| Suffix | Combined With | Medical Term | Definition |
|---|---|---|---|
| -dipsia | poly- | polydipsia (pall ee **DIP** see ah) | many (excessive) thirst |
| -uria | poly- | polyuria (pall ee **YOO** ree ah) | condition of (too) much urine |
| | glycos/o | glycosuria (glye kohs **YOO** ree ah) | sugar in the urine |

## Vocabulary Relating to the Endocrine System

| | |
|---|---|
| **edema (eh DEE mah)** | Condition in which the body tissues contain excessive amounts of fluid. |
| **exophthalmos (eks off THAL mohs)** | Condition in which the eyeballs protrude, such as in Graves' disease. This is generally caused by an overproduction of thyroid hormone (see ▦ Figure 11.11). |
| **gynecomastia (gigh neh koh MAST ee ah)** | The development of breast tissue in males. May be a symptom of adrenal feminization. |
| **hirsutism (HER soot izm)** | Condition of having an excessive amount of hair. Term generally used to describe females who have the adult male pattern of hair growth. Can be the result of a hormonal imbalance. |
| **hypersecretion** | Excessive hormone production by an endocrine gland. |
| **hyposecretion** | Deficient hormone production by an endocrine gland. |
| **metabolism (meh TAB oh lizm)** | Sum of all chemical and physical changes that take place in the body. |
| **obesity (oh BEE sih tee)** | Having an abnormal amount of fat in the body. |
| **syndrome (SIN drohm)** | Group of symptoms and signs that, when combined, present a clinical picture of a disease or condition. |

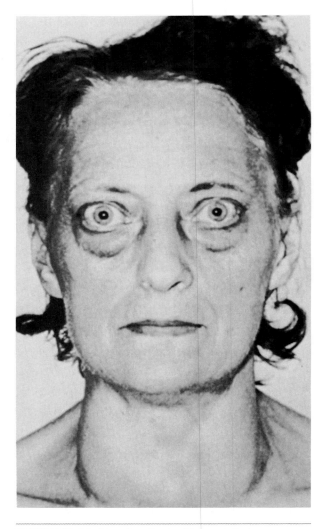

▦ **FIGURE 11.11** A patient with exophthalmos.

# Pathology Relating to the Endocrine System

| | |
|---|---|
| **acidosis (as ih DOH sis)** | Excessive acidity of body fluids due to the accumulation of acids, as in diabetic acidosis. |
| **acromegaly (ak roh MEG ah lee)** | Chronic disease of adults that results in an elongation and enlargement of the bones of the head and extremities. There can also be mood changes. Due to an excessive amount of growth hormone in an adult. |
| **Addison's disease (AD ih sons dih ZEEZ)** | Disease named for Thomas Addison, a British physician, that results from a deficiency in adrenocortical hormones. There may be an increased pigmentation of the skin, generalized weakness, and weight loss. |
| **adenocarcinoma (ad eh no car sih NO mah)** | A cancerous tumor in a gland that is capable of producing the hormones secreted by that gland. One cause of hypersecretion pathologies. |
| **adrenal feminization (ad REE nal fem ih nigh ZAY shun)** | Development of female secondary sexual characteristics (such as breasts) in a male. Often as a result of increased estrogen secretion by the adrenal cortex. |
| **adrenal virilism (ad REE nal VIR ill izm)** | Development of male secondary sexual characteristics (such as deeper voice and facial hair) in a female. Often as a result of increased androgen secretion by the adrenal cortex. |
| **cretinism (KREE tin izm)** | Congenital condition in which a lack of thyroid may result in arrested physical and mental development (see ■ Figure 11.12). |
| **Cushing's syndrome (CUSH ings SIN drohm)** | Set of symptoms named after Harvey Cushing, an American neurosurgeon, that result from hypersecretion of the adrenal cortex. This may be the result of a tumor of the adrenal glands. The syndrome may present symptoms of weakness, edema, excess hair growth, skin discoloration, and osteoporosis (see ■ Figure 11.13). |
| **diabetes insipidus (dye ah BEE teez in SIP ih dus) (DI)** | Disorder caused by the inadequate secretion of a hormone by the posterior lobe of the pituitary gland. There may be polyuria and polydipsia. This is more common in the young. |
| **diabetes mellitus (dye ah BEE teez MELL ih tus) (DM)** | Chronic disorder of carbohydrate metabolism that results in hyperglycemia and glycosuria. There are two distinct forms of diabetes mellitus: insulin-dependent diabetes mellitus (IDDM) or type 1, and non–insulin-dependent diabetes mellitus (NIDDM) or type 2. |
| **diabetic retinopathy (dye ah BET ik ret in OP ah thee)** | Secondary complication of diabetes that affects the blood vessels of the retina, resulting in visual changes and even blindness. |
| **dwarfism (DWARF izm)** | Condition of being abnormally short in height. It may be the result of a hereditary condition or a lack of growth hormone. |
| **gigantism (JYE gan tizm)** | Excessive development of the body due to the overproduction of the growth hormone by the pituitary gland in a child or teenager. The opposite of *dwarfism* (see ■ Figure 11.14). |
| **goiter (GOY ter)** | Enlargement of the thyroid gland (see ■ Figure 11.15). |
| **Graves' disease** | Condition named for Robert Graves, an Irish physician, that results in overactivity of the thyroid gland and can cause a crisis situation. Also called *hyperthyroidism.* |
| **Hashimoto's disease (hash ee MOH tohz dih ZEEZ)** | Chronic form of thyroiditis, named for a Japanese surgeon. |
| **hyperthyroidism (hi per THIGH royd izm)** | Condition that results from overactivity of the thyroid gland and can cause a crisis situation. Also called *Graves' disease.* |

*continued...*

| | |
|---|---|
| **hypothyroidism (high poh THIGH royd izm)** | Result of a deficiency in secretion by the thyroid gland. This results in a lowered basal metabolism rate with obesity, dry skin, slow pulse, low blood pressure, sluggishness, and goiter. Treatment is replacement with synthetic thyroid hormone. |
| **insulin-dependent diabetes mellitus (dye ah BEE teez MELL ih tus)** | Also called *type 1 diabetes mellitus.* It develops early in life when the pancreas stops insulin production. Persons with IDDM must take daily insulin injections. |
| **insulinoma (in sue lin OH mah)** | Tumor of the islets of Langerhans cells of the pancreas that secretes an excessive amount of insulin. |
| **ketoacidosis (kee toh ass ih DOH sis)** | Acidosis due to an excess of acidic ketone bodies (waste products). A serious condition requiring immediate treatment that can result in death for the diabetic patient if not reversed. Also called *diabetic acidosis.* |
| **myxedema (miks eh DEE mah)** | Condition resulting from a hypofunction of the thyroid gland. Symptoms can include anemia, slow speech, enlarged tongue and facial features, edematous skin, drowsiness, and mental apathy (see ▣ Figure 11.16). |
| **non–insulin-dependent diabetes mellitus (dye ah BEE teez MELL ih tus)** | Also called *type 2 diabetes mellitus.* It develops later in life when the pancreas produces insufficient insulin. Persons may take oral hypoglycemics to stimulate insulin secretion, or may eventually have to take insulin. |
| **panhypopituitarinism (pan high poh pih TOO ih tair ee nizm)** | Deficiency in all the hormones secreted by the pituitary gland. Often recognized because of problems with the glands regulated by the pituitary–adrenal cortex, thyroid, ovaries, and testes. |
| **peripheral neuropathy (per IF eh rall new ROP ah thee)** | Damage to the nerves in the lower legs and hands as a result of diabetes mellitus. Symptoms include either extreme sensitivity or numbness and tingling. |
| **pheochromocytoma (fee oh kroh moh sigh TOH ma)** | Usually benign tumor of the adrenal medulla that secretes epinephrine. Symptoms include anxiety, heart palpitations, dyspnea, profuse sweating, headache, and nausea. |
| **tetany (TET ah nee)** | Painful muscle cramps that result from hypocalcemia. |
| **thyrotoxicosis (thigh roh toks ih KOH sis)** | Condition that results from overproduction of the thyroid gland. Symptoms include a rapid heart action, tremors, enlarged thyroid gland, exophthalmos, and weight loss. |
| **von Recklinghausen's (REK ling how zenz) disease** | Excessive production of parathyroid hormone, which results in degeneration of the bones. Named for Friedrich von Recklinghausen, a German histologist. |

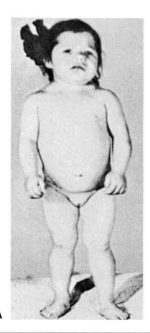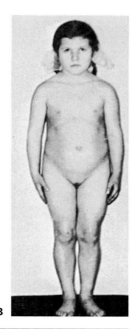

**■ FIGURE 11.12** (A) A 6-year-old child with congenital hypothyroidism, cretinism, exhibiting marked mental and physical retardation. (B) The same patient after 3 years of thyroxine therapy, which resulted in a spurt of growth and regression of pathological manifestations. Mental retardation is delayed.

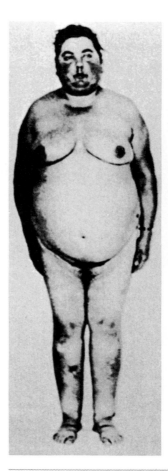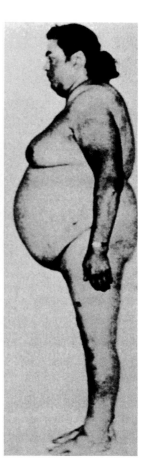

**■ FIGURE 11.13** Cushing's syndrome patient showing round, red face; stocky neck; and marked obesity of the trunk with protruding abdomen. Note bruises on trunk and legs and also stretch marks. Note fat pads above the collar bone and on the back of the neck, which produces the "buffalo hump."

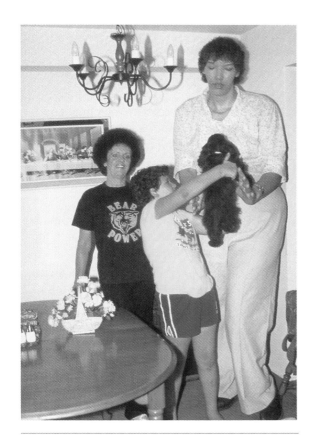

**■ FIGURE 11.14** Gigantism of mother with normal son.

(Bettina Cirrone/Photo Researchers, Inc.)

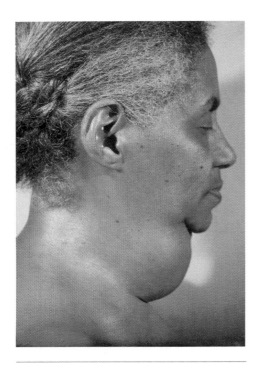

**FIGURE 11.15**   Goiter.
(Martin Rotker/Phototake NYC)

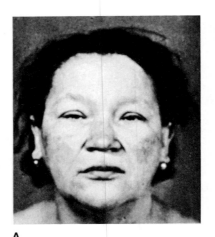

A

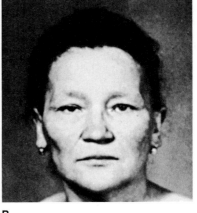

B

**FIGURE 11.16**   (A) A 62-year-old patient with myxedema exhibiting marked edema of the face and a somnolent look. The hair is stiff and without luster. (B) The same patient after 3 months of treatment with thyroxine.

## Diagnostic Procedures Relating to the Endocrine System

| | |
|---|---|
| **basal metabolic (BAY sal met ah BOLL ik) rate (BMR)** | Somewhat outdated test to measure the energy used when the body is in a state of rest. |
| **blood serum test** | Blood test to measure the level of substances such as calcium, electrolytes, testosterone, insulin, and glucose. Used to assist in determining the function of various endocrine glands. |
| **fasting blood sugar (FBS)** | Blood test to measure the amount of sugar circulating throughout the body after a 12-hour fast. |
| **glucose (GLOO kohs) tolerance test (GTT)** | Test to determine the blood sugar level. A measured dose of glucose is given to a patient either orally or intravenously. Blood samples are then drawn at certain intervals to determine the ability of the patient to use glucose. Used for diabetic patients to determine their insulin response to glucose. |
| **protein-bound iodine test (PBI)** | Blood test to measure the concentration of thyroxine ($T_4$) circulating in the bloodstream. The iodine becomes bound to the protein in the blood and can be measured. Useful in establishing thyroid function. |
| **radioactive iodine uptake test (RAIU)** | Test in which radioactive iodine is taken orally (PO) or intravenously (IV). The amount that is eventually taken into the thyroid gland (the uptake) is measured to assist in determining thyroid function. |
| **radioimmunoassay (RIA) (ray dee oh im yoo noh ASS ay)** | Test used to measure the levels of hormones in the plasma of the blood. |

| | |
|---|---|
| serum glucose (SEE rum GLOO kohs) tests | Blood test performed to assist in determining insulin levels and useful for adjusting medication dosage. |
| thyroid echogram (THIGH royd EK oh gram) | Ultrasound examination of the thyroid that can assist in distinguishing a thyroid nodule from a cyst. |
| thyroid (THIGH royd) function test (TFT) | Blood test used to measure the levels of $T_3$, $T_4$, and TSH in the bloodstream to assist in determining thyroid function. |
| thyroid (THIGH royd) scan | Test in which a radioactive iodine is administered that localizes in the thyroid gland. The gland can then be visualized with a scanning device to detect pathology such as tumors. |
| total calcium | Blood test to measure the total amount of calcium to assist in detecting parathyroid and bone disorders. |
| two-hour postprandial (post PRAN dee al) glucose tolerance test | Blood test to assist in evaluating glucose metabolism. The patient eats a high carbohydrate diet and fasts overnight before the test. A blood sample is then taken 2 hours after a meal. |

## Therapeutic Procedures Relating to the Endocrine System

| | |
|---|---|
| chemical thyroidectomy (thigh royd EK toh mee) | Large dose of radioactive iodine is given in order to kill thyroid gland cells without having to actually do surgery. |
| laparoscopic adrenalectomy (lap row SKOP ik ad ree nal EK toh mee) | Excision of the adrenal gland through a small incision in the abdomen and using endoscopic instruments. |
| lobectomy (lobe EK toh mee) | Excision of only one lobe of the thyroid gland. |
| parathyroidectomy (pair ah thigh royd EK toh mee) | Excision of one or more of the parathyroid glands. This is performed to halt the progress of hyperparathyroidism. |
| thymectomy (thigh MEK toh mee) | Removal of the thymus gland. |
| thyroidectomy (thigh royd EK toh mee) | Removal of the entire thyroid or a portion (partial thyroidectomy) to treat a variety of conditions, including nodes, cancer, and hyperthyroidism. |
| thyroparathyroidectomy (thigh roh pair ah thigh royd EK toh mee) | Surgical removal (excision) of the thyroid and parathyroid glands. |

# Pharmacology Relating to the Endocrine System

| | |
|---|---|
| **corticosteroids (kor tih koh STAIR oydz)** | Although the function of these hormones in the body is to regulate carbohydrate metabolism, they also have a strong anti-inflammatory action. Therefore they are used to treat severe chronic inflammatory diseases such as rheumatoid arthritis. Long-term use of corticosteroids has adverse side effects such as osteoporosis and the symptoms of Cushing's disease. |
| **epinephrine (ep ih NEF rin)** | As a medication, epinephrine is used to constrict blood vessels and block severe allergic reactions. |
| **human growth hormone therapy** | Therapy with human growth hormone in order to stimulate skeletal growth. Used to treat children with abnormally short stature. |
| **insulin (IN suh lin)** | Administered to replace insulin for type 1 diabetics or to treat severe type 2 diabetics. |
| **oral hypoglycemic (high poh glye SEE mik) agents** | Medications taken by mouth that cause a decrease in blood sugar. This is not used for insulin-dependent patients. There is no proof that this medication will prevent the agent long-term complications of diabetes mellitus. |
| **thyroid replacement hormone** | Given to replace thyroid in patients with hypothyroidism or who have had a thyroidectomy. |
| **vasopressin (vaz oh PRESS in)** | Given to control diabetes insipidus and promote reabsorption of water in the kidney tubules. |

# Abbreviations Relating to the Endocrine System

| | | | |
|---|---|---|---|
| **ACTH** | adrenocorticotropic hormone | **NIDDM** | non–insulin-dependent diabetes mellitus |
| **ADH** | antidiuretic hormone | **NPH** | neutral protamine Hagedorn (insulin) |
| **BMR** | basal metabolic rate | **PBI** | protein-bound iodine |
| **DI** | diabetes insipidus | **PRL** | prolactin |
| **DM** | diabetes mellitus | **PTH** | parathyroid hormone |
| **FBS** | fasting blood sugar | **RAI** | radioactive iodine |
| **FSH** | follicle-stimulating hormone | **RAIU** | radioactive iodine uptake |
| **GH** | growth hormone | **RIA** | radioimmunoassay |
| **GTT** | glucose tolerance test | **T$_3$** | triiodothyronine |
| **IDDM** | insulin-dependent diabetes mellitus | **T$_4$** | thyroxine |
| **K$^+$** | potassium | **T$_7$** | free thyroxine index |
| **LH** | luteinizing hormone | **TFT** | thyroid function test |
| **MSH** | melanocyte-stimulating hormone | **TSH** | thyroid-stimulating hormone |
| **Na$^+$** | sodium | | |

# Chapter Review

## Pronunciation Practice

 *You will find the pronunciation for each term on the enclosed CD-ROM. Check each one off as you master it.*

- ☐ acidosis (ass ih **DOH** sis)
- ☐ acromegaly (ak roh **MEG** ah lee)
- ☐ Addison's disease (**AD** ih sons dih **ZEEZ**)
- ☐ adenocarcinoma (ad eh no car sih **NO** mah)
- ☐ adenoma (ad eh **NOH** mah)
- ☐ adrenal cortex (**KOR** tex)
- ☐ adrenal feminization (ad **REE** nal fem ih nigh **ZAY** shun)
- ☐ adrenal (ad **REE** nal) glands
- ☐ adrenal medulla (ad **REE** nal meh **DOOL** lah)
- ☐ adrenal virilism (ad **REE** nal **VIR** ill izm)
- ☐ adrenalectomy (ad ree nal **EK** toh mee)
- ☐ adrenaline (ah **DREN** ah lin)
- ☐ adrenalitis (ad ree nal **EYE** tis)
- ☐ adrenocorticotropin hormone (ah dree noh kor tih koh **TROH** pin **HOR** mohn)
- ☐ adrenomegaly (ad ree noh **MEG** ah lee)
- ☐ adrenopathy (ad ren **OP** ah thee)
- ☐ aldosterone (al **DOSS** ter ohn)
- ☐ androgens (**AN** druh jenz)
- ☐ anterior lobe
- ☐ antidiuretic hormone (an tye dye yoo **RET** ik **HOR** mohn)
- ☐ basal metabolic (**BAY** sal met ah **BOLL** ik) rate
- ☐ blood serum test
- ☐ calcitonin (kal sih **TOH** nin)
- ☐ calcium
- ☐ chemical thyroidectomy (thigh royd **EK** toh mee)
- ☐ circadian (seer **KAY** dee an) rhythm
- ☐ corticosteroids (kor tih koh **STAIR** oydz)
- ☐ cortisol (**KOR** tih sal)
- ☐ cretinism (**KREE** tin izm)
- ☐ Cushing's syndrome (**CUSH** ings **SIN** drohm)
- ☐ diabetes insipidus (dye ah **BEE** teez in **SIP** ih dus)
- ☐ diabetes mellitus (dye ah **BEE** teez **MELL** ih tus)
- ☐ diabetic retinopathy (dye ah **BET** ik ret in **OP** ah thee)

- ☐ digestive enzymes
- ☐ dwarfism (**DWARF** izm)
- ☐ edema (eh **DEE** mah)
- ☐ endocrine (**EN** doh krin) glands
- ☐ endocrine (**EN** doh krin) system
- ☐ endocrinologist (en doh krin **ALL** oh jist)
- ☐ endocrinology (en doh krin **ALL** oh jee)
- ☐ endocrinopathy (en doh krin **OP** ah thee)
- ☐ epinephrine (ep ih **NEF** rin)
- ☐ estrogen (**ESS** troh jen)
- ☐ euthyroid (yoo **THIGH** royd)
- ☐ exocrine (**EKS** oh krin) glands
- ☐ exophthalmos (eks off **THAL** mohs)
- ☐ fasting blood sugar
- ☐ follicle-stimulating hormone (**FOLL** ih kl **STIM** yoo lay ting **HOR** mohn)
- ☐ gametes (gam **EATS**)
- ☐ gigantism (**JYE** gan tizm)
- ☐ glands
- ☐ glucagon (**GLOO** koh gon)
- ☐ glucocorticoids (gloo koh **KOR** tih koydz)
- ☐ glucose (**GLOO** kohs) tolerance test
- ☐ glycosuria (glye kohs **YOO** ree ah)
- ☐ goiter (**GOY** ter)
- ☐ gonads (**GOH** nadz)
- ☐ Graves' disease
- ☐ growth hormone
- ☐ gynecomastia (gigh neh koh **MAST** ee ah)
- ☐ Hashimoto's disease (hash ee **MOH** tohz dih **ZEEZ**)
- ☐ hirsutism (**HER** soot izm)
- ☐ homeostasis (hoe me oh **STAY** sis)
- ☐ hormones (**HOR** mohnz)
- ☐ human growth hormone therapy
- ☐ hypercalcemia (high per kal **SEE** mee ah)
- ☐ hyperglycemia (high per glye **SEE** mee ah)

- ❏ hyperkalemia (high per kal **EE** mee ah)
- ❏ hypersecretion
- ❏ hyperthyroidism (high per **THIGH** royd izm)
- ❏ hypocalcemia (high poh kal **SEE** mee ah)
- ❏ hypoglycemia (high poh glye **SEE** mee ah)
- ❏ hyponatremia (high poh nah **TREE** mee ah)
- ❏ hyposecretion
- ❏ hypothalamus (high poh **THAL** ah mus)
- ❏ hypothyroidism (high poh **THIGH** royd izm)
- ❏ insulin (**IN** suh lin)
- ❏ insulin-dependent diabetes mellitus
- ❏ insulinoma (in sue lin **OH** mah)
- ❏ iodine (**EYE** oh dine)
- ❏ islets of Langerhans (**EYE** lets of **LAHNG** er hahnz)
- ❏ ketoacidosis (kee toh ass ih **DOH** sis)
- ❏ laparoscopic adrenalectomy (lap row **SKOP** ik ad ree nal **EK** toh mee)
- ❏ lobectomy (lobe **EK** toh mee)
- ❏ luteinizing hormone (**LOO** tee in eye zing **HOR** mohn)
- ❏ melanocyte-stimulating hormone
- ❏ melatonin (mel ah **TOH** nin)
- ❏ menstrual (men **STROO** all) cycle
- ❏ metabolism (meh **TAB** oh lizm)
- ❏ mineralocorticoids (min er al oh **KOR** tih koydz)
- ❏ myxedema (miks eh **DEE** mah)
- ❏ non–insulin-dependent diabetes mellitus
- ❏ norepinephrine (nor ep ih **NEF** rin)
- ❏ obesity (oh **BEE** sih tee)
- ❏ oral hypoglycemic (high poh glye **SEE** mik) agent
- ❏ ova (**OH** vah)
- ❏ ovaries (**OH** vah reez)
- ❏ oxytocin (ok see **TOH** sin)
- ❏ pancreas (**PAN** kree ass)
- ❏ panhypopituitarinism (pan high poh pih **TOO** ih tair ee nizm)
- ❏ parathyroid (pair ah **THIGH** royd) glands
- ❏ parathyroid hormone (pair ah **THIGH** royd **HOR** mohn)
- ❏ parathyroidectomy (pair ah thigh royd **EK** toh mee)
- ❏ parathyroidoma (pair ah thigh royd **OH** mah)
- ❏ peripheral neuropathy (per **IF** eh rall new **ROP** ah thee)
- ❏ pheochromocytoma (fee oh kroh moh sigh **TOH** ma)
- ❏ pineal (pih **NEAL**) gland
- ❏ pituitary (pih **TOO** ih tair ee) gland
- ❏ polydipsia (pall ee **DIP** see ah)

- ❏ polyuria (pall ee **YOO** ree ah)
- ❏ posterior lobe
- ❏ progesterone (proh **JESS** ter ohn)
- ❏ prolactin (proh **LAK** tin)
- ❏ protein-bound iodine test
- ❏ radioactive iodine uptake test
- ❏ radioimmunoassay (ray dee oh im yoo noh **ASS** ay)
- ❏ serum glucose (**SEE** rum **GLOO** kohs) tests
- ❏ somatotropin (so mat oh **TROH** pin)
- ❏ sperm
- ❏ steroid (**STAIR** oyd) sex hormones
- ❏ syndrome (**SIN** drohm)
- ❏ $T_3$
- ❏ $T_4$
- ❏ T cells
- ❏ target organs
- ❏ testes (**TESS** teez)
- ❏ testosterone (tess **TOSS** ter own)
- ❏ tetany (**TET** ah nee)
- ❏ thalamus (**THALL** mus)
- ❏ thymectomy (thigh **MEK** toh mee)
- ❏ thymosin (thigh **MOH** sin)
- ❏ thymus (**THIGH** mus) gland
- ❏ thyroid echogram (**THIGH** royd **EK** oh gram)
- ❏ thyroid (**THIGH** royd) function tests
- ❏ thyroid (**THIGH** royd) gland
- ❏ thyroid (**THIGH** royd) replacement hormone
- ❏ thyroid (**THIGH** royd) scan
- ❏ thyroid-stimulating hormone
- ❏ thyroidectomy (thigh royd **EK** toh mee)
- ❏ thyroidotomy (thigh royd **OTT** oh mee)
- ❏ thyromegaly (thigh roh **MEG** ah lee)
- ❏ thyroparathyroidectomy (thigh roh pair ah thigh royd **EK** toh mee)
- ❏ thyrotoxicosis (thigh roh toks ih **KOH** sis)
- ❏ thyroxine (thigh **ROKS** in)
- ❏ total calcium
- ❏ triiodothyronine (try eye oh doh **THIGH** roh neen)
- ❏ two-hour postprandial (post **PRAN** dee al) glucose tolerance test
- ❏ type 1
- ❏ type 2
- ❏ vasopressin (vaz oh **PRESS** in)
- ❏ von Recklinghausen's (**REK** ling how zenz) disease

# Case Study

## Discharge Summary

**Admitting Diagnosis:** Hyperglycemia, ketoacidosis, glycosuria

**Final Diagnosis:** New-onset type 1 diabetes mellitus

**History of Present Illness:** Patient presented to pediatrician's office with a 2-month history of weight loss, fatigue, polyuria, and polydipsia. Her family history is significant for a grandfather, mother, and older brother with type 1 diabetes mellitus. The pediatrician found hyperglycemia with a fasting blood sugar and glycosuria with a urine dipstick. Patient was also noted to be dehydrated and extremely lethargic. She is being admitted at this time for management of new-onset diabetes mellitus.

**Summary of Hospital Course:** At the time of admission, the FBS was 300 mg/100 mL and she was in ketoacidosis. She rapidly improved after receiving insulin; her serum glucose level normalized, and her lethargy disappeared. The next day a 2-hour postprandial glucose tolerance test confirmed the diagnosis of diabetes mellitus while an abdominal X-ray and a pancreas CT scan were normal. There was no evidence of diabetic retinopathy. Attempts to control hyperglycemia with oral hypoglycemics were not successful and patient was started on insulin injections. She was discharged 3 days later on a protocol of b.i.d. (twice a day) insulin injections. The patient and her family were instructed in diet, exercise, symptoms of hypoglycemic coma, and long-term complications of diabetes mellitus.

**Discharge Plans:** Patient was discharged to home with her parents. She is on a 2,000-calorie ADA diet with three meals and two snacks. She may engage in any activity and may return to school next Monday. Her parents are to check her serum glucose levels b.i.d. and call the office for insulin dosage. She is to return to the office in 2 weeks.

## Critical Thinking Questions

1. The patient's admitting diagnosis is three symptoms related to her final diagnosis. List the three symptoms and describe each in your own words.

   a.

   b.

   c.

2. This patient has type 1 diabetes mellitus. Use your text to explain the difference between type 1 and type 2.

3. This discharge summary contains four medical terms that have not been introduced yet. Describe each of these terms in your own words. Use your text as a dictionary.

   a. retinopathy

   b. protocol

   c. coma

   d. b.i.d.

4. This patient had three different types of blood tests during her hospital stay. List the three blood tests and describe the differences among them in your own words.

   a.

   b.

   c.

5. This patient had two imaging procedures conducted by the radiology department while she was in the hospital. List them and describe the differences between the two.

   a.

   b.

6. Describe the patient's discharge instructions in your own words.

# Chart Note Transcription

## Chart Note

The chart note below contains 11 phrases that can be reworded with a medical term that you learned in this chapter. Each phrase is identified with an underline. Determine the medical term and write your answers in the space provided.

**Current Complaint:** A 56-year-old female was referred to the <u>specialist in the treatment of diseases of the endocrine glands</u>① for evaluation of weakness, edema, <u>an abnormal amount of fat in the body,</u>② and <u>an excessive amount of hair for a female</u>.③

**Past History:** Patient reports she has been overweight most of her life in spite of a healthy diet and regular exercise. She was diagnosed with osteoporosis after incurring a pathological rib fracture following a coughing attack.

**Signs and Symptoms:** Patient has moderate edema in bilateral feet and lower legs as well as a puffy face and an upper lip moustache. She is 100 lbs. over normal body weight for her age and height. She moves slowly and appears generally lethargic. A test to <u>measure the hormone levels in the blood plasma</u>④ reports increased <u>steroid hormone that regulates carbohydrates in the body</u>⑤ levels in the blood. A CT scan demonstrates a <u>gland tumor</u>⑥ in the right <u>outer layer of the adrenal gland.</u>⑦

**Diagnosis:** <u>A group of symptoms associated with hypersecretion of the adrenal cortex</u>⑧ secondary to a <u>gland tumor</u>⑨ in the right <u>outer layer of the adrenal gland.</u>⑩

**Treatment:** <u>Surgical removal of the right adrenal gland.</u>⑪

1. _____

2. _____

3. _____

4. _____

5. _____

6. _____

7. _____

8. _____

9. _____

10. _____

11. _____

# Practice Exercises

## A. Complete the following statements.

1. The study of the endocrine system is called _____ .

2. The master endocrine gland is the _____ .

3. _____ is a general term for the sexual organs that produce gametes.

4. The term for the hormones produced by the outer portion of the adrenal cortex is _____ .

5. The hormone produced by the testes is _____ .

6. The two hormones produced by the ovaries are _____ and _____ .

7. An inadequate supply of the hormone _____ causes diabetes insipidus.

8. Another term for thyroxine is _____ .

9. The term for a protrusion of the eyeballs in Graves' disease is _____ .

10. A general medical term for a hormone-secreting cancerous tumor is _____ .

## B. State the terms described using the combining forms provided.

The combining form *thyroid/o* refers to the thyroid. Use it to write a term that means

1. excision of the thyroid _____

2. inflammation of the thyroid _____

3. normal thyroid _____

4. incision of the thyroid _____

The combining form *pancreat/o* refers to the pancreas. Use it to write a term that means

5. inflammation of the pancreas _____

6. removal of the pancreas _____

7. incision into the pancreas _____

The combining form *adrenal/o* refers to the adrenal glands. Use it to write a term that means

8. excision of an adrenal gland _____

9. inflammation of the adrenal glands _____

The combining form *thym/o* refers to the thymus glands. Use it to write a term that means

10. tumor of the thymus gland _____

11. removal of the thymus gland _____

## C. Match the terms in column A with the definitions in column B.

| | A | | B |
|---|---|---|---|
| 1. | _____ Cushing's disease | a. | enlarged thyroid |
| 2. | _____ goiter | b. | overactive adrenal cortex |
| 3. | _____ acidosis | c. | hyperthyroidism |
| 4. | _____ gigantism | d. | underactive adrenal cortex |
| 5. | _____ cretinism | e. | associated with diabetes |
| 6. | _____ myxedema | f. | causes polyuria and polydipsia |
| 7. | _____ diabetes mellitus | g. | thyroiditis |
| 8. | _____ diabetes insipidus | h. | arrested growth |
| 9. | _____ Hashimoto's disease | i. | poor carbohydrate metabolism |
| 10. | _____ Graves' disease | j. | enlarged facial features and edematous skin |
| 11. | _____ Addison's disease | k. | excessive growth hormone |

## D. Identify the following abbreviations.

1. PBI _____

2. $K^+$ _____

3. $T_4$ _____

4. GTT _____

5. DM _____

6. BMR _____

7. $Na^+$ _____

8. ADH _____

## E. Write the abbreviations for the following terms.

1. non–insulin-dependent diabetes mellitus _____

2. insulin-dependent diabetes mellitus _____

3. adrenocorticotropin hormone _____

4. parathyroid hormone _____

5. triiodothyronine _____

6. thyroid stimulating hormone _____

7. fasting blood sugar _____

8. prolactin _____

**F. Build an endocrine system term using one of the following suffixes.**

-crine              -uria

-dipsia           -emia

1. the presence of sugar or glucose in the urine _____

2. the glandular system that secretes directly into the bloodstream _____

3. excessive urination _____

4. condition of excessive calcium in the blood _____

5. excessive thirst _____

**G. Define the following terms.**

1. corticosteroid _____

2. hirsutism _____

3. tetany _____

4. diabetic retinopathy _____

5. hyperglycemia _____

6. hypoglycemia _____

7. adrenaline _____

8. insulin _____

9. thyrotoxicosis _____

10. parathyroid glands _____

# Professional Journal

In this exercise you will now have an opportunity to put the words you have learned into practice. Imagine yourself in the role of an endocrinologist. Physicians in this medical specialty are trained to diagnose and treat diseases related to the endocrine glands. Use the 10 words listed below, or any other new terms from this chapter, to write sentences to describe the patients you saw today.

An example of a sentence is *A diagnosis of* **adrenal feminization** *was suspected when the patient developed* **gynecomastia.**

1.  adenocarcinoma _____

2.  chemical thyroidectomy _____

3.  gigantism _____

4.  ketoacidosis _____

5.  radioimmunoassay _____

6.  polydipsia _____

7.  glucose tolerance test _____

8.  panhypopituitarinism _____

9.  hypercalcemia _____

10. dwarfism _____

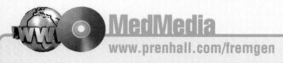

## MedMedia
www.prenhall.com/fremgen

Use the CD-ROM enclosed with your textbook to gain additional reinforcement through interactive word building exercises, spelling games, labeling activities, and additional quizzes.

Use the above address to access the free, interactive Companion Website created for this textbook. Get hints, instant feedback, and textbook references to chapter-related multiple-choice questions, as well as labeling and matching exercises. In addition, you will find an audio glossary, case studies, and Internet exploration exercises.

***For more information regarding endocrine system diseases, visit the following websites:***

Centers for Disease Control and Prevention's Health Topics A to Z at **www.cdc.gov/health/default.htm**

Health Information provided by the National Institutes of Health at **http://health.nih.gov**

Health Information provided by the Stanford Health Library at **http://healthlibrary.stanford.edu**

InteliHealth featuring Harvard Medical School's Consumer Health Information at **www.intelihealth.com**

Medical Encyclopedia provided by University of Maryland Medicine at **www.umm.edu/ency**

University of Iowa Health Care's Virtual Hospital at **www.vh.org**

## Learning Objectives

*Upon completion of this chapter, you will be able to:*

- Recognize the combining forms, prefixes, and suffixes introduced in this chapter.

- Gain the ability to pronounce medical terms and major anatomical structures.

- List the major organs of the nervous system and their functions.

- Describe the components of a nerve.

- Distinguish between the central nervous system, peripheral nervous system, and autonomic nervous system.

- Build nervous system medical terms from word parts.

- Define vocabulary, pathology, diagnostic, and therapeutic medical terms relating to the nervous system.

- Recognize types of medications associated with the nervous system.

- Interpret abbreviations associated with the nervous system.

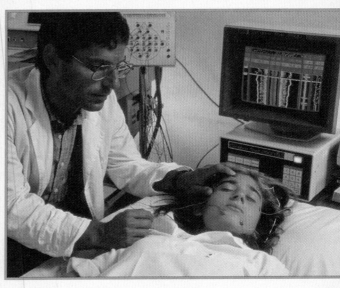

(Larry Mulvehill/Science Source/Photo Researchers, Inc.)

## MedMedia
www.prenhall.com/fremgen

Additional interactive resources and activities for this chapter can be found on the Companion Website. For animations, audio glossary, and review, access the accompanying CD-ROM in this book.

## Professional Profile

### Electroneurodiagnostics

Electroneurodiagnostics (END) is the science that studies and records electrical activity of the brain and nervous system, with tests performed by END technologists who conduct diagnostic tests using electronic equipment and machines. Potential areas of specialization include electroencephalography (recording the electrical activity of the brain), electromyography (recording the electrical activity of muscles), polysomnography (recording brain activity, respiratory rate, and heart rate during stages of sleep), evoked potential tests (recording the brain's response to different types of sensory stimuli), and nerve conduction tests (recording how fast electrical messages travel along a nerve). These tests are useful in diagnosing brain, spinal cord, and nerve diseases and conditions such as strokes, tumors, and pinched nerves. The majority of electroneurodiagnostic technologists work in hospitals, but they are also found in clinics and physicians' offices.

### Electroneurodiagnostic Technologists

- Performs diagnostic tests as ordered by a physician
- Graduates from a 2-year associate's degree or certification program
- May choose to become a Registered Electroencephalography Technologist (R. EEG T.), a Registered Evoked Potential Technologist (R. EP T.), a Registered Polysomnographic Technologist (RPSGT), or a Certification in Neurophysiologic Intraoperative Monitoring (CNIM), if qualification criteria are met
- Some facilities provide on-the-job training sufficient for persons to qualify for some of these positions, especially if the person has training or experience in other health care fields

***For more information regarding this health career, visit the following websites:***
American Society of Electroneurodiagnostic Technologists at **www.aset.org**
Association of Polysomnographic Technologists at **www.aptweb.org**

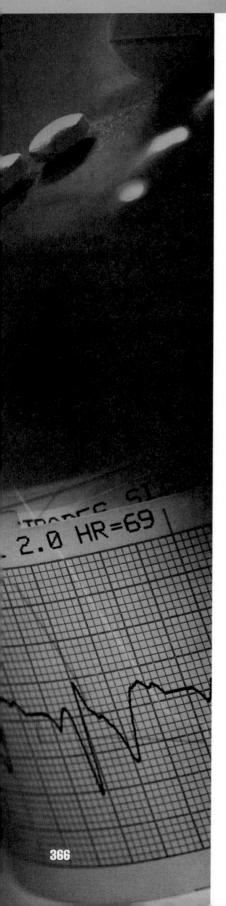

### Organs of the Nervous System

brain
nerves
spinal cord

### Combining Forms Relating to the Nervous System

| | | | |
|---|---|---|---|
| cephal/o | head | narc/o | stupor |
| cerebell/o | cerebellum | neur/o | nerve |
| cerebr/o | cerebrum | phas/o | speech |
| encephal/o | brain | poli/o | gray matter |
| gli/o | glue | pont/o | pons |
| medull/o | medulla | radicul/o | nerve root |
| mening/o | meninges | thalam/o | thalamus |
| meningi/o | meninges | ventricul/o | ventricle |
| myel/o | spinal cord | | |

### Suffixes Relating to the Nervous System

| Suffix | Meaning | Example |
|---|---|---|
| -algesia | pain, sensitivity | analgesia |
| -esthesia | feeling, sensation | anesthesia |
| -kinesia | movement | bradykinesia |
| -lepsy | seizure | narcolepsy |
| -paresis | weakness | hemiparesis |
| -phasia | speech | dysphasia |
| -plegia | paralysis | paraplegia |
| -sthenia | strength | myasthenia |
| -taxia | muscle coordination | ataxia |

## Anatomy and Physiology of the Nervous System

| | | |
|---|---|---|
| brain | glands | sensory receptors |
| central nervous system | muscles | spinal cord |
| cranial nerves | peripheral nervous system | spinal nerves |

The nervous system is responsible for coordinating all the activity of the body. To do this it first receives information from both external and internal **sensory receptors** and then uses that information to adjust the activity of **muscles** and **glands** to match the needs of the body.

The nervous system can be subdivided into the **central nervous system (CNS)** and the **peripheral** (per **IF** er al) **nervous system (PNS)** (see ■ Figure 12.1). The CNS consists of the **brain** and **spinal cord.** Sensory information comes into the CNS, where it is processed. Motor messages then exit the CNS

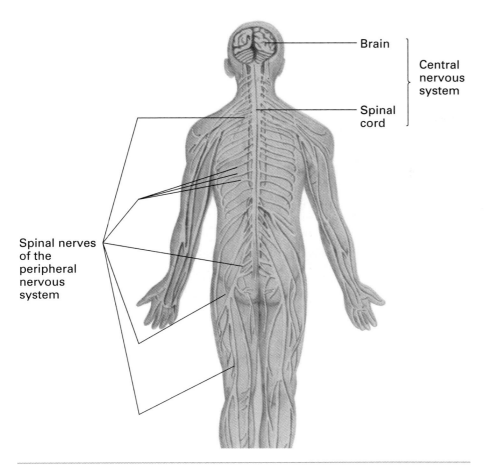

Brain

Central nervous system

Spinal cord

Spinal nerves of the peripheral nervous system

**FIGURE 12.1** The nervous system.

carrying commands to muscles and glands. The PNS contains the **cranial** (**KRAY** nee al) **nerves** and **spinal nerves.** Sensory nerves carry information to the CNS and motor nerves carry commands away from the CNS. All portions of the nervous system are composed of nervous tissue.

## Nervous Tissue

| axon | nerve cell body | neurotransmitter |
|------|-----------------|------------------|
| dendrites | neuroglial cells | synapse |
| myelin | neuron | synaptic cleft |

Nervous tissue consists of two basic types of cells: **neurons** (**NOO** ronz) and **neuroglial** (noo **ROH** glee all) **cells.** Neurons are individual nerve cells (see Figure 12.2). These are the cells that are capable of conducting electrical impulses in response to a stimulus. Neurons have three basic parts: **dendrites** (**DEN** drights), a **nerve cell body,** and an **axon** (**AK** son) (see Figure 12.3). Dendrites are highly branched projections that receive impulses. The nerve cell body contains the nucleus and many of the other organelles of the cell. A neuron has only a single axon, a projection from the nerve cell body that conducts the electrical impulse toward its destination. The point at which the axon of one neuron meets the dendrite of the next neuron is called a **synapse** (sih **NAPSE**). Electrical impulses cannot pass directly across the gap between two neurons, called the **synaptic** (sih **NAP** tik) **cleft.** They instead require the help of a chemical messenger, called a **neurotransmitter** (noo roh **TRANS** mit ter).

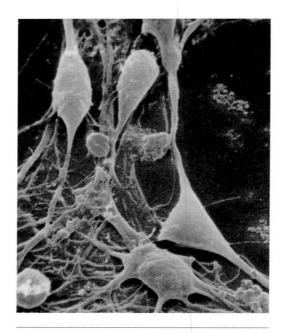

**FIGURE 12.2** Enhanced color scanning electron micrograph of neurons.
(CNRI/Science Photo Library/Photo Researchers, Inc.)

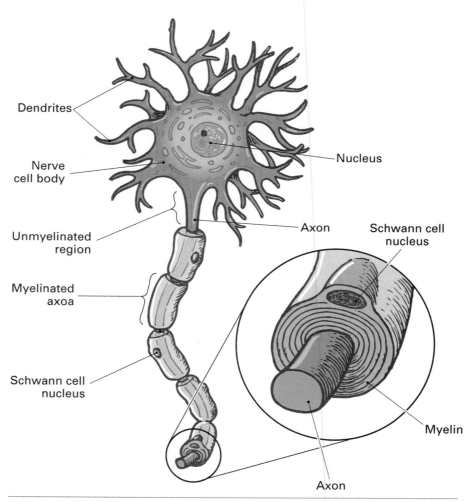

Dendrites

Nerve
cell body

Unmyelinated
region

Myelinated
axoa

Schwann cell
nucleus

Nucleus

Axon

Schwann cell
nucleus

Myelin

Axon

**FIGURE 12.3** Neuron.

A variety of neuroglial cells are found in nervous tissue. Each has a different support function for the neurons. For example, some neuroglial cells produce **myelin** (**MY** eh lin), a fatty substance that acts as insulation for many axons. They do not conduct electrical impulses.

## Central Nervous System

| | | |
|---|---|---|
| gray matter | myelinated | tract |
| meninges | poliomyelitis | white matter |

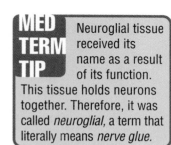
Because the central nervous system (CNS) is a combination of the brain and spinal cord, it is able to receive impulses from all over the body, process this information, and then respond with an action. This system consists of both **gray** and **white matter**. Gray matter is comprised of unsheathed or uncovered cell bodies and dendrites. White matter is **myelinated** (**MY** eh lih nayt ed) nerve fibers (see ▪ Figure 12.4). Bundles of nerve fibers interconnecting different parts of the CNS are called **tracts.** The CNS is encased and protected by three membranes known as the **meninges** (men **IN** jeez).

### The Brain

| | | |
|---|---|---|
| brain stem | frontal lobe | parietal lobe |
| cerebellum | gyri | pons |
| cerebral cortex | hypothalamus | sulci |
| cerebral hemisphere | medulla oblongata | temporal lobe |
| cerebrospinal fluid | midbrain | thalamus |
| cerebrum | occipital lobe | ventricles |
| diencephalon | | |

**MED TERM TIP** Certain disease processes attack the gray matter and the white matter of the central nervous system. For instance, **poliomyelitis** (poh lee oh my ell **EYE** tis) is a viral infection of the gray matter of the spinal cord. The combining term *poli/o* means gray matter. This disease has almost been conquered, due to the polio vaccine.

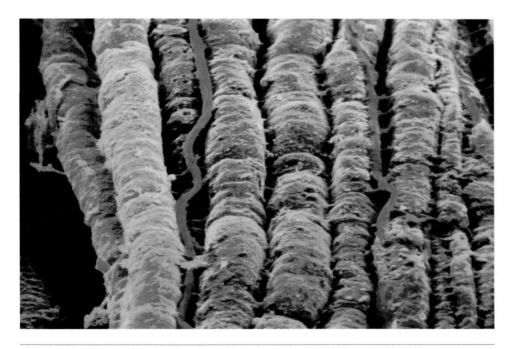

▪ **FIGURE 12.4**  Enhanced color nerve fibers.
(Prof. P. Motto/Photo Researchers, Inc.)

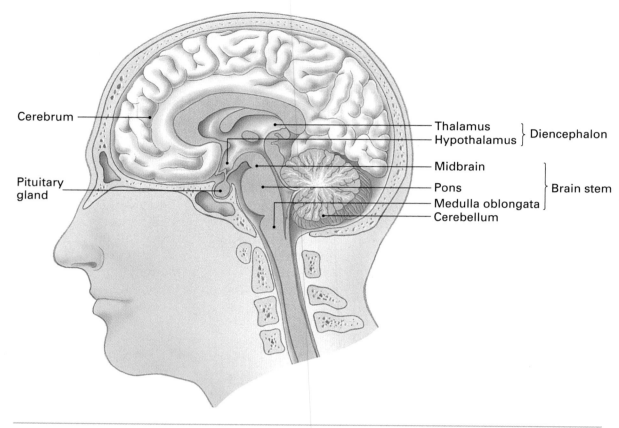

Cerebrum

Pituitary
gland

Thalamus  } Diencephalon
Hypothalamus

Midbrain
Pons            } Brain stem
Medulla oblongata
Cerebellum

**FIGURE 12.5**  Sagittal section of the brain.

The brain is one of the largest organs in the body and coordinates most body activities. It is the center for all thought, memory, judgment, and emotion. Each part of the brain is responsible for controlling different body functions, such as temperature regulation and breathing. There are four sections to the brain: **cerebrum** (**SER** eh brum), **cerebellum** (ser eh **BELL** um), **diencephalon** (dye en **SEFF** ah lon), and **brain stem** (see █ Figure 12.5).

The largest section of the brain is the cerebrum. It is located in the upper portion of the brain and is the area that processes thoughts, judgment, memory, association skills, and the ability to discriminate between items. The outer layer of the cerebrum is the **cerebral cortex** (seh **REE** bral **KOR** teks), which is composed of folds of gray matter. The elevated portions of the cerebrum, or convolutions, are called **gyri** (**JYE** rye) and are separated by fissures, or valleys, called **sulci** (**SULL** kye). The cerebrum is subdivided into left and right halves called **cerebral hemispheres** (**HEM** is feerz). Each hemisphere has four lobes. The lobes and their locations and functions are as follows (see █ Figure 12.6):

1. **Frontal lobe:** Most anterior portion of the cerebrum; controls motor function, personality, and speech.

2. **Parietal** (pah **RYE** eh tal) **lobe:** The most superior portion of the cerebrum; receives and interprets nerve impulses from sensory receptors and interprets language.

3. **Occipital** (ock **SIP** ih tal) **lobe:** The most posterior portion of the cerebrum; controls vision.

4. **Temporal** (**TEM** por al) **lobe:** The left and right lateral portion of the cerebrum; controls hearing and smell.

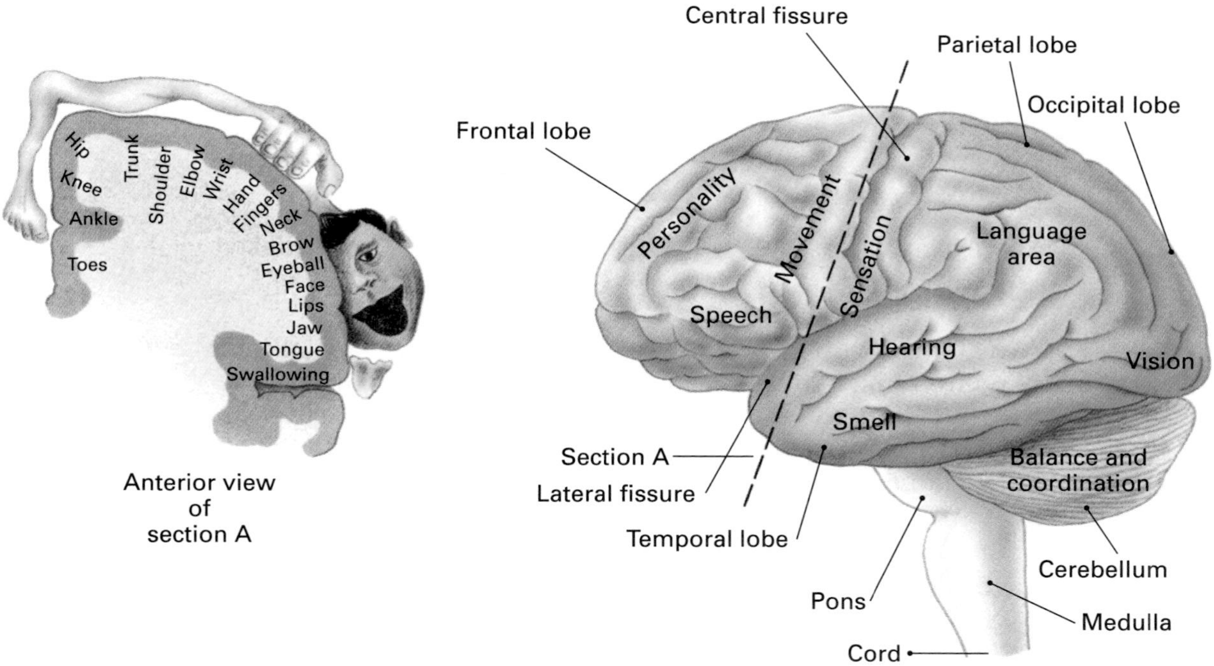
Hip
Knee
Ankle
Toes
Trunk
Shoulder
Elbow
Wrist
Hand
Fingers
Neck
Brow
Eyeball
Face
Lips
Jaw
Tongue
Swallowing
Anterior view of section A
Central fissure
Parietal lobe
Occipital lobe
Frontal lobe
Personality
Movement
Sensation
Language area
Speech
Hearing
Vision
Smell
Section A
Lateral fissure
Temporal lobe
Balance and coordination
Cerebellum
Pons
Medulla
Cord

**FIGURE 12.6** The brain: lateral view.

The diencephalon, located below the cerebrum, contains two of the most critical areas of the brain, the **thalamus** (**THAL** ah mus) and the **hypothalamus** (high poh **THAL** ah mus). The thalamus is composed of gray matter and acts as a center for relaying impulses from the eyes, ears, and skin to the cerebrum. Our pain perception is controlled by the thalamus. The hypothalamus, lying just below the thalamus, controls body temperature, appetite, sleep, sexual desire, and emotions, such as fear. The hypothalamus is actually responsible for controlling the autonomic nervous system, cardiovascular system, the gastrointestinal system, and the release of hormones from the pituitary gland.

The cerebellum, the second largest portion of the brain, is located beneath the posterior part of the cerebrum. This part of the brain aids in coordinating voluntary body movements and maintaining balance and equilibrium. The cerebellum refines the muscular movement that is initiated in the cerebrum.

The final portion of the brain is the brain stem. This area has three components: **midbrain, pons** (**PONZ**), and **medulla oblongata** (meh **DULL** ah ob long **GAH** tah). The midbrain acts as a pathway for impulses to be conducted between the brain and the spinal cord. The pons—a term that means bridge—connects the cerebellum to the rest of the brain. The medulla oblongata is the most inferior positioned portion of the brain; it connects the brain to the spinal cord. However, this vital area contains the centers that control respiration, heart rate, temperature, and blood pressure. Additionally this is the site where nerve tracts cross from one side of the brain to control functions and movement on the other side of the body.

**MED TERM TIP**

Because nerve tracts cross from one side of the body to the other side of the brain, damage to one side of the brain results in symptoms appearing on the opposite side of the body. Since nerve cells that control the movement of the right side of the body are located in the left side of the medulla oblongata, a stroke that paralyzed the right side of the body would actually have occurred in the left side of the brain.

The brain has four interconnected cavities called **ventricles** (**VEN** trik lz): one in each cerebral hemisphere, one in the thalamus, and one in front of the cerebellum. These contain **cerebrospinal fluid** (ser eh broh **SPY** nal **FLOO** id) (CSF), which is the watery, clear fluid that provides protection from shock or sudden motion to the brain.

### Spinal Cord

| | | |
|---|---|---|
| **ascending tracts** | **spinal cavity** | **vertebral column** |
| **descending tracts** | **vertebral canal** | |

The function of the spinal cord is to provide a pathway for impulses traveling to and from the brain. The spinal cord is actually a column of nervous tissue that extends from the medulla oblongata of the brain down to the level of the second lumbar vertebra within the **vertebral** (**VER** teh bral) **column.** The vertebral column consists of the 33 vertebrae of the backbone. They line up to form a continuous canal for the spinal cord called the **spinal cavity** or **vertebral** (**VER** teh bral) **canal** (see ■ Figures 12.7 and 12.8).

> **MED TERM TIP**
>
> The combining form *myel/o* means marrow and is used for both the spinal cord and bone marrow. To the ancient Greek philosophers and physicians, the spinal cord appeared to be much like the marrow found in the medullary cavity of a long bone.

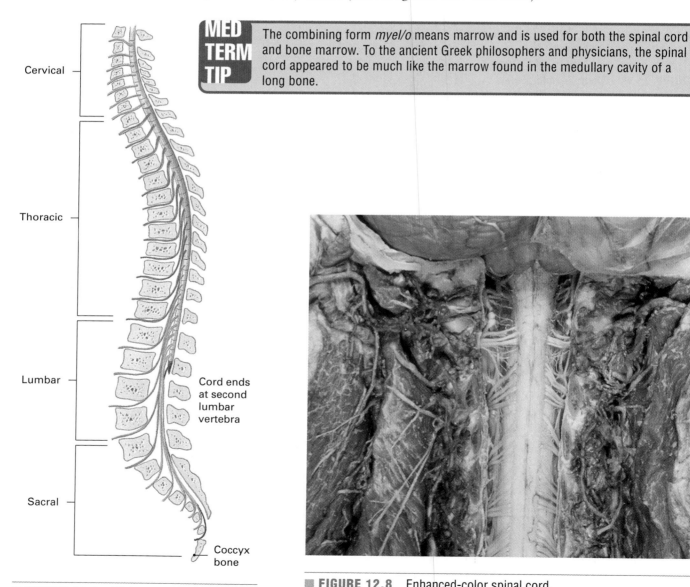

Cervical

Thoracic

Lumbar

Cord ends at second lumbar vertebra

Sacral

Coccyx bone

■ **FIGURE 12.7**  Divisions of the spinal cord.

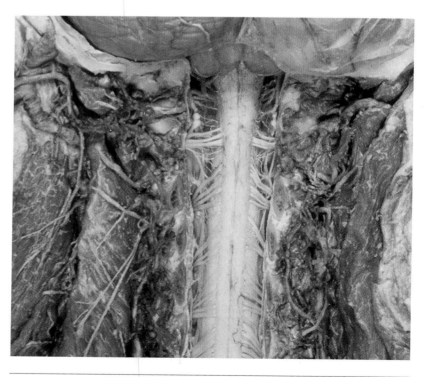

■ **FIGURE 12.8**  Enhanced-color spinal cord.
(Video Surgery/Photo Researchers, Inc.)

Similar to the brain, the spinal cord is also protected by cerebrospinal fluid. The inner core of the spinal cord contains gray matter. This inner core consists of cell bodies and dendrites of peripheral nerves. The outer portion of the spinal cord is myelinated white matter. The white matter is either **ascending tracts** carrying sensory information up to the brain or **descending tracts** carrying motor commands down from the brain to a peripheral nerve.

## Meninges

| | | |
|---|---|---|
| **arachnoid layer** | **pia mater** | **subdural space** |
| **dura mater** | **subarachnoid space** | |

The meninges are three layers of connective tissue membranes that surround the brain and spinal cord (see ■ Figure 12.9). Moving from external to internal, the meninges are

1. **Dura mater** (**DOO** rah **MATE** er): The name means tough mother; it forms a tough, fibrous sac around the CNS.
2. **Subdural** (sub **DOO** ral) **space:** The actual space between the dura mater and arachnoid layers.
3. **Arachnoid** (ah **RAK** noyd) **layer:** The name means spider-like; it is a thin, delicate layer attached to the pia mater by web-like filaments.
4. **Subarachnoid** (sub ah **RAK** noyd) **space:** The space between the arachnoid layer and the pia mater; it contains cerebrospinal fluid.
5. **Pia mater** (**PEE** ah **MATE** er): The name means soft mother; it is the innermost membrane layer and is applied directly to the surface of the brain.

## Peripheral Nervous System

| | | |
|---|---|---|
| **afferent neurons** | **ganglion** | **sensory neurons** |
| **autonomic nervous system** | **motor neurons** | **somatic nerves** |
| **efferent neurons** | **nerve root** | |

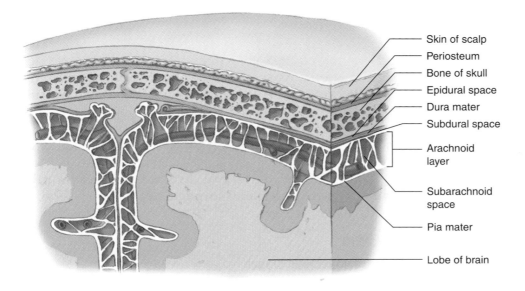

- Skin of scalp
- Periosteum
- Bone of skull
- Epidural space
- Dura mater
- Subdural space
- Arachnoid layer
- Subarachnoid space
- Pia mater
- Lobe of brain

■ **FIGURE 12.9** The meninges of the brain.

## Table 12.1 Cranial Nerves

| Number | Name | Function |
|--------|------|----------|
| I | Olfactory | Transports impulses for sense of smell |
| II | Optic | Carries impulses for sense of sight |
| III | Oculomotor | Motor impulses for eye muscle movement and the pupil of eye |
| IV | Trochlear | Controls oblique muscle of eye on each side |
| V | Trigeminal | Carries sensory facial impulses and controls muscles for chewing; branches into eyes, forehead, upper and lower jaw |
| VI | Abducens | Controls an eyeball muscle to turn eye to side |
| VII | Facial | Controls facial muscles for expression, salivation, and taste on two-thirds of tongue (anterior) |
| VIII | Vestibulocochlear | Responsible for impulses of equilibrium and hearing; also called auditory nerve |
| IX | Glossopharyngeal | Carries sensory impulses from pharynx (swallowing) and taste on one-third of tongue |
| X | Vagus | Supplies most organs in abdominal and thoracic cavities |
| XI | Accessory | Controls the neck and shoulder muscles |
| XII | Hypoglossal | Controls tongue muscles |

The peripheral nervous system (PNS) includes both the 12 pairs of cranial nerves and the 31 pairs of spinal nerves. A nerve is a group or bundle of axon fibers located outside the central nervous system that carries messages between the CNS and the various parts of the body. Whether a nerve is cranial or spinal is determined by where the nerve originates. Cranial nerves arise from the brain, mainly at the medulla oblongata. Spinal nerves split off from the spinal cord, and one pair (a left and a right) exits between each pair of vertebrae. The point where either type of nerve is attached to the CNS is called the **nerve root.** The names of most nerves reflect either the organ the nerve serves or the portion of the body the nerve is traveling through. The entire list of cranial nerves is found in Table 12.1. ■ Figure 12.10 illustrates some of the major spinal nerves in the human body.

Although most nerves carry information to and from the CNS, individual neurons carry information in only one direction. **Afferent (AFF** er ent) **neurons,** also called **sensory neurons,** carry sensory information from a sensory receptor to the CNS. **Efferent (EFF** er ent) **neurons,** also called **motor neurons,** carry activity instructions from the CNS to muscles or glands out in the body. The nerve cell bodies of the neurons forming the nerve are grouped together in a knot-like mass, called a **ganglion (GANG** lee on), located outside the CNS.

The nerves of the PNS are subdivided into two divisions, the **autonomic** (aw toh **NOM** ik) **nervous system** (ANS) and **somatic nerves,** each serving a different area of the body.

### Autonomic Nervous System

**parasympathetic branch**     **sympathetic branch**

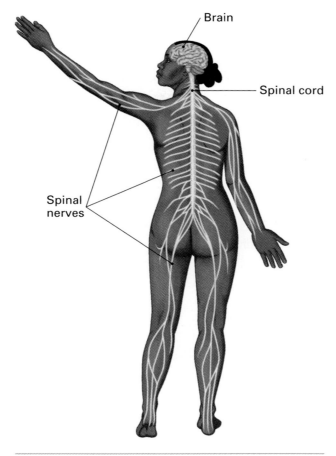

Brain

Spinal cord

Spinal nerves

■ **FIGURE 12.10**  Some of the major spinal nerves found in the human body.

The autonomic nervous system (ANS) is involved with the control of involuntary or unconscious bodily functions. It may increase or decrease the activity of the smooth muscle found in viscera and blood vessels, the cardiac muscle of the heart, and glands. The ANS is divided into two branches: **sympathetic** (sim pah **THET** ik) **branch** and **parasympathetic** (pair ah sim pah **THET** ik) **branch.** The sympathetic nerves stimulate the body in times of stress and crisis. These nerves increase heart rate, dilate airways, increase blood pressure, inhibit digestion, and stimulate the production of adrenaline during a crisis. The parasympathetic nerves serve as a counterbalance for the sympathetic nerves. Therefore, they cause heart rate to slow down, lower blood pressure, and stimulate digestion.

## Somatic Nerves

Somatic nerves serve the skin and skeletal muscles and are mainly involved with the conscious and voluntary activities of the body. The large variety of sensory receptors found in the dermis layer of the skin use somatic nerves to send their information, such as touch, temperature, pressure, and pain, to the brain. These are also the nerves that carry motor commands to skeletal muscles.

# Word Building Relating to the Nervous System

The following list contains examples of medical terms built directly from word parts. The definition for these terms can be determined by a straightforward translation of the word parts.

| Combining Form | Combined With | Medical Term | Definition |
|---|---|---|---|
| cephal/o | -algia | cephalalgia (seff al **AL** jee ah) | head pain (headache) |
| cerebell/o | -ar | cerebellar (ser eh **BELL** ar) | pertaining to the cerebellum |
| | -itis | cerebellitis (ser eh bell **EYE** tis) | cerebellum inflammation |
| cerebr/o | -al | cerebral (seh **REE** bral) | pertaining to the cerebrum |
| | spin/o -al | cerebrospinal (ser eh broh **SPY** nal) | pertaining to the cerebrum and spine |
| encephal/o | electr/o -gram | electroencephalogram (ee lek troh en **SEFF** ah loh gram) (EEG) | record of brain's electricity |
| | -itis | encephalitis (en seff ah **LYE** tis) | brain inflammation |
| | -malacia | encephalomalacia (en seff ah loh mah **LAY** she ah) | brain softening |
| | -sclerosis | encephalosclerosis (en seff ah loh skleh **ROH** sis) | brain hardening |
| mening/o | -cele | meningocele (men **IN** goh seel) | meninges hernia |
| | -itis | meningitis (men in **JYE** tis) | meninges inflammation |
| | myel/o -cele | myelomeningocele (my eh loh meh **NIN** goh seel) | meninges and spinal cord hernia |
| myel/o | -gram | myelogram (**MY** eh loh gram) | record of spinal cord |
| | -itis | myelitis (my eh **LYE** tis) | spinal cord inflammation |
| | -malacia | myelomalacia (my eh loh mah **LAY** she ah) | spinal cord softening |
| | poli/o -itis | poliomyelitis (poh lee oh my ell **EYE** tis) | gray matter of spinal cord inflammation |
| neur/o | -algia | neuralgia (noo **RAL** jee ah) | nerve pain |
| | -ectomy | neurectomy (noo **REK** toh mee) | excision of nerve |
| | -lysis | neurolysis (noo **ROL** ih sis) | nerve destruction |
| | -ologist | neurologist (noo **RAL** oh jist) | specialist in nerves |
| | -ology | neurology (noo **RAL** oh jee) | study of nerves |
| | -oma | neuroma (noo **ROH** mah) | nerve tumor |
| | -otomy | neurotomy (noo **ROT** oh mee) | incision into a nerve |
| | -plasty | neuroplasty (**NOOR** oh plas tee) | surgical repair of nerves |
| | poly- -itis | polyneuritis (pol ee noo **RYE** tis) | inflammation of many nerves |
| | -rrhaphy | neurorrhaphy (noo **ROR** ah fee) | suture of nerve |
| radicul/o | -itis | radiculitis (rah dick yoo **LYE** tis) | nerve root inflammation |

| Suffix | Combined With | Medical Term | Definition |
|--------|---------------|--------------|------------|
| -algesia | an- | analgesia (an al **JEE** zee ah) | absence of pain or sensation |
| -esthesia | an- | anesthesia (an ess **THEE** zee ah) | lack of sensations |
|  | hyper- | hyperesthesia (high per ess **THEE** zee ah) | excessive sensations |
| -kinesia | brady- | bradykinesia (brad ee kin **NEE** see ah) | slow movement |
| -paresis | hemi- | hemiparesis (hem ee par **EE** sis) | weakness of half |
|  | mono- | monoparesis (mon oh pah **REE** sis) | weakness of one |
| -phasia | a- | aphasia (ah **FAY** zee ah) | lack of speech |
|  | dys- | dysphasia (dis **FAY** zee ah) | difficult speech |
| -plegia | hemi- | hemiplegia (hem ee **PLEE** jee ah) | paralysis of half |
|  | mono- | monoplegia (mon oh **PLEE** jee ah) | paralysis of one |
|  | quadri- | quadriplegia (kwod rih **PLEE** jee ah) | paralysis of four |
|  | tetra- | tetraplegia (tet rah **PLEE** jee ah) | paralysis of four |
| -sthenia | a- | asthenia (as **THEE** nee ah) | lack of strength |
|  | my/o a- | myasthenia (my ass **THEE** nee ah) | lack of muscle strength |
| -taxia | a- | ataxia (ah **TAK** see ah) | lack of muscle coordination |

## Vocabulary Relating to the Nervous System

| | |
|---|---|
| **aura (AW ruh)** | Sensations, such as seeing colors or smelling an unusual odor, that occur just prior to an epileptic seizure. |
| **chorea (koh REE ah)** | Involuntary nervous disorder that results in muscular twitching of the limbs or facial muscles. |
| **coma (COH mah)** | Abnormal deep sleep or stupor resulting from an illness or injury. |
| **conscious (KON shus)** | Condition of being awake and aware of surroundings. |
| **convulsion (kon VULL shun)** | Severe involuntary muscle contractions and relaxations. These have a variety of causes, such as epilepsy, fever, and toxic conditions. |
| **delirium (dee LEER ee um)** | An abnormal mental state characterized by confusion, disorientation, and agitation. |
| **dementia (dee MEN she ah)** | Progressive impairment of intellectual function that interferes with performing the activities of daily living. Patients have little awareness of their condition. Found in disorders such as Alzheimer's. |
| **focal (FOE kal) seizure** | A localized epileptic seizure often affecting one limb. |
| **grand mal (GRAND MALL) seizure** | A type of severe epileptic seizure characterized by a loss of consciousness and convulsions. It is also called a *tonic-clonic seizure,* indicating that the seizure alternates between strong continuous muscle spasms (tonic) and rhythmic muscle contraction and relaxation (clonic). |

*continued...*

| | |
|---|---|
| **hemiparesis (hem ee par EE sis)** | Weakness or loss of motion on one side of the body. |
| **hemiplegia (hem ee PLEE jee ah)** | Paralysis on only one side of the body. |
| **intrathecal (in tra THEE kal)** | Pertaining to within the meninges. |
| **lethargy (LETH ar jee)** | Condition of sluggishness or stupor. |
| **neurosurgeon (noo roh SIR jen)** | A physician specialized in treating conditions and diseases of the nervous systems by surgical means. |
| **palsy (PAWL zee)** | Temporary or permanent loss of the ability to control movement. |
| **paralysis (pah RAL ih sis)** | Temporary or permanent loss of function or voluntary movement. |
| **paraplegia (pair ah PLEE jee ah)** | Paralysis of the lower portion of the body and both legs. |
| **paresthesia (par es THEE zee ah)** | An abnormal sensation such as burning or tingling. |
| **petit mal (pet EE MALL) seizure** | A type of epileptic seizure that lasts only a few seconds to half a minute, characterized by a loss of awareness and an absence of activity. It is also called an *absence seizure*. |
| **sciatica (sigh AT ih ka)** | Pain in the low back that radiates down the back of a leg caused by pressure on the sciatic nerve from a herniated nucleus pulposus. |
| **seizure (SEE zyoor)** | Sudden attack of severe muscular contractions associated with a loss of consciousness. This is seen in grand mal epilepsy. |
| **sleep disorder** | Any condition that interferes with sleep other than environmental noises. Can include difficulty sleeping (insomnia), extreme sleepiness (somnolence), nightmares, night terrors, sleepwalking, and apnea. |
| **syncope (SIN koh pee)** | Fainting. |
| **tic (TIK)** | Spasmodic, involuntary muscular contraction involving the head, face, mouth, eyes, neck, and shoulders. |
| **tremor (TREM or)** | Involuntary quivering movement of a part of the body. |
| **unconscious (un KON shus)** | Condition or state of being unaware of surroundings, with the inability to respond to stimuli. |

## Pathology Relating to the Nervous System

| | |
|---|---|
| **Alzheimer's (ALTS high merz) disease** | Chronic, organic mental disorder consisting of dementia, which is more prevalent in adults between 40 and 60. Involves progressive disorientation, apathy, speech and gait disturbances, and loss of memory. Named for Alois Alzheimer, a German neurologist. |
| **amyotrophic lateral sclerosis (ah my oh TROFF ik LAT er al skleh ROH sis) (ALS)** | Disease with muscular weakness and atrophy due to degeneration of motor neurons of the spinal cord. Also called *Lou Gehrig's disease,* after the New York Yankees baseball player who died from the disease. |
| **astrocytoma (ass troh sigh TOH mah)** | Tumor of the brain or spinal cord that is composed of astrocytes, one of the types of neuroglial cells. |
| **Bell's palsy (BELLZ PAWL zee)** | One-sided facial paralysis with an unknown cause. The person cannot control salivation, tearing of the eyes, or expression. The patient will eventually recover. Named for Sir Charles Bell, a Scottish surgeon. |

| | |
|---|---|
| **brain tumor** | Intracranial mass, either benign or malignant. A benign tumor of the brain can still be fatal since it will grow and cause pressure on normal brain tissue (see ■ Figure 12.11). |
| **cerebral aneurysm (AN yoo rizm)** | Localized abnormal dilatation of a blood vessel, usually an artery; the result of a congenital defect or weakness in the wall of the vessel (see ■ Figure 12.12). A ruptured aneurysm is a common cause of a hemorrhagic CVA. |
| **cerebral contusion (kon TOO shun)** | Bruising of the brain from a blow or impact. Symptoms last longer than 24 hours and include unconsciousness, dizziness, vomiting, unequal pupil size, and shock. |
| **cerebral palsy (ser REE bral PAWL zee) (CP)** | Nonprogressive brain damage resulting from a defect or trauma at the time of birth. |
| **cerebrovascular accident (ser eh broh VASS kyoo lar AK sih dent) (CVA)** | Commonly called a *stroke*. The development of an infarct due to loss in the blood supply to an area of the brain. Blood flow can be interrupted by a ruptured blood vessel (hemorrhage), a floating clot (embolus), a stationary clot (thrombosis), or compression (see ■ Figure 12.13). The extent of damage depends on the size and location of the infarct and often includes dysphasia and hemiplegia. |
| **concussion (kon KUSH un)** | Injury to the brain that results from the brain being shaken inside the skull from a blow or impact. Can result in unconsciousness, dizziness, vomiting, unequal pupil size, and shock. Symptoms last 24 hours or less. |
| **encephalocele (en SEFF ah loh seel)** | Congenital gap in the skull with the brain protruding through the gap. |
| **epidural hematoma (ep ih DOO ral hee mah TOH mah)** | Mass of blood in the space outside the dura mater of the brain and spinal cord. |
| **epilepsy (EP ih lep see)** | Recurrent disorder of the brain in which seizures and loss of consciousness occur as a result of uncontrolled electrical activity of the neurons in the brain. |
| **Guillan-Barré (GHEE yan bah RAY) syndrome** | Disease of the nervous system in which nerves lose their myelin covering. May be caused by an autoimmune reaction. Characterized by loss of sensation and/or muscle control in the arms and legs. Symptoms then move toward the trunk and may even result in paralysis of the diaphragm. |
| **Huntington's chorea (HUNT ing tonz koh REE ah)** | Disease of the central nervous system that results in progressive dementia with bizarre involuntary movements of parts of the body. Named for George Huntington, an American physician. |
| **hydrocephalus (high droh SEFF ah lus)** | Accumulation of cerebrospinal fluid within the ventricles of the brain, causing the head to be enlarged. It is treated by creating an artificial shunt for the fluid to leave the brain (see ■ Figure 12.14). |
| **meningioma (meh nin jee OH mah)** | Slow-growing tumor in the meninges of the brain. |
| **meningocele (men IN goh seel)** | Congenital condition in which the meninges protrude through an opening in the vertebral column. See *spina bifida*. |
| **migraine (MY grain)** | A specific type of headache characterized by severe head pain, photophobia, vertigo, and nausea. |
| **multiple sclerosis (MULL tih pl skleh ROH sis) (MS)** | Inflammatory disease of the central nervous system in which there is extreme weakness and numbness due to loss of myelin insulation from nerves. |
| **myasthenia gravis (my ass THEE nee ah GRAV iss)** | Disease with severe muscular weakness and fatigue due to insufficient neurotransmitter at a synapse. |

*continued...*

| | |
|---|---|
| **myelomeningocele** (my eh loh meh NIN goh seel) | Congenital condition in which the meninges and spinal cord protrude through an opening in the vertebral column. See *spina bifida*. |
| **narcolepsy (NAR koh lep see)** | Chronic disorder in which there is an extreme uncontrollable desire to sleep. |
| **Parkinson's disease** (PARK in sons dih ZEEZ) | Chronic disorder of the nervous system with fine tremors, muscular weakness, rigidity, and a shuffling gait. Named for Sir James Parkinson, a British physician. |
| **Reye's syndrome** (RISE SIN drohm) | Combination of symptoms first recognized by R. D. K. Reye, an Australian pathologist, in which there is acute encephalopathy and various organ damage. This occurs in children under 15 years of age who have had a viral infection. For this reason, it's not recommended for children to use aspirin. |
| **shingles (SHING lz)** | Eruption of vesicles on the trunk of the body along a nerve path. Can be painful and generally occurs on only one side of the body. Thought to be caused by the *Herpes zoster* virus (see ▓ Figure 12.15). |
| **spina bifida** (SPY nah BIFF ih dah) | Congenital defect in the walls of the spinal canal in which the laminae of the vertebra do not meet or close. Results in a meningocele or a myelomeningocele—meninges or the spinal cord being pushed through the opening. Can also result in other defects, such as hydrocephalus (see ▓ Figure 12.16). |
| **spinal cord injury (SCI)** | Damage to the spinal cord as a result of trauma. Spinal cord may be bruised or completely severed. |
| **subdural hematoma** (sub DOO ral hee mah TOH mah) | Mass of blood forming beneath the dura mater if the meninges are torn by trauma. May exert fatal pressure on the brain if the hematoma is not drained by surgery (see ▓ Figure 12.17). |
| **tic douloureux** (TIK doo loo ROO) | Painful condition in which the trigeminal nerve is affected by pressure or degeneration. The pain is of a severe stabbing nature and radiates from the jaw and along the face. |
| **transient ischemic** (TRAN shent iss KEM ik) **attack (TIA)** | Temporary interference with blood supply to the brain, causing neurological symptoms such as dizziness, numbness, and hemiparesis. May eventually lead to a full-blown stroke (CVA). |

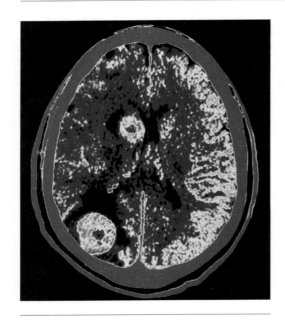

**▓ FIGURE 12.11** Enhanced-color malignant tumor of the brain.
(Scott Camazine/Photo Researchers, Inc.)

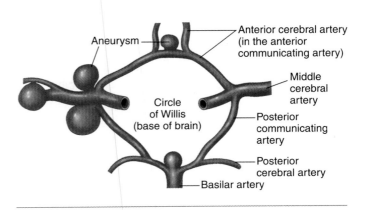

**▓ FIGURE 12.12** Cerebral aneurysms.

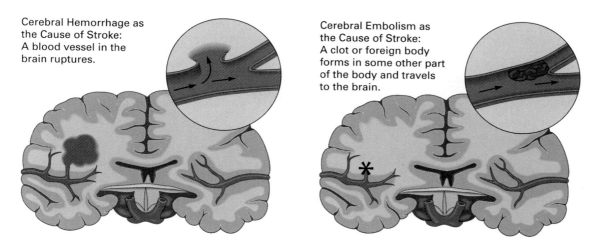

Cerebral Hemorrhage as the Cause of Stroke: A blood vessel in the brain ruptures.

Cerebral Embolism as the Cause of Stroke: A clot or foreign body forms in some other part of the body and travels to the brain.

STROKE

Cerebral Thrombosis as the Cause of Stroke: There is a blood clot in the brain.

Compression as the Cause of Stroke.

**■ FIGURE 12.13** Causes of stroke.

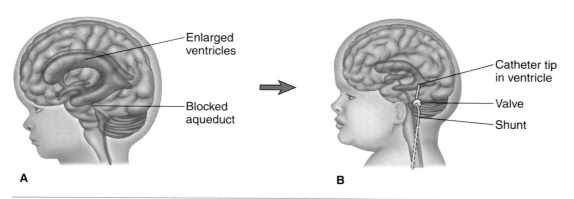

Enlarged ventricles

Blocked aqueduct

Catheter tip in ventricle

Valve

Shunt

A                                    B

**■ FIGURE 12.14** (A) Hydrocephalus; (B) excess cerebrospinal fluid drained by a shunt.

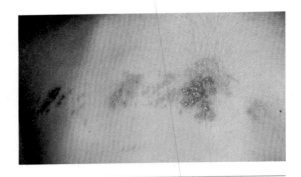

**FIGURE 12.15**  Shingles.

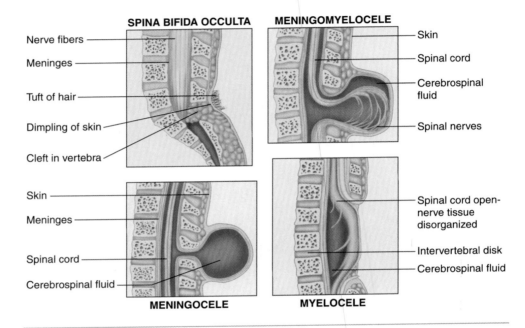

**SPINA BIFIDA OCCULTA**

Nerve fibers

Meninges

Tuft of hair

Dimpling of skin

Cleft in vertebra

**MENINGOMYELOCELE**

Skin

Spinal cord

Cerebrospinal fluid

Spinal nerves

Skin

Meninges

Spinal cord

Cerebrospinal fluid

**MENINGOCELE**

Spinal cord open-nerve tissue disorganized

Intervertebral disk

Cerebrospinal fluid

**MYELOCELE**

**FIGURE 12.16**  Forms of spina bifida.

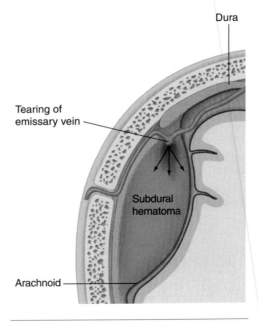

Dura

Tearing of emissary vein

Subdural hematoma

Arachnoid

**FIGURE 12.17**  Subdural hematoma.

# Diagnostic Procedures Relating to the Nervous System

| | |
|---|---|
| **Babinski's (bah BIN skeez) reflex** | Reflex test developed by Joseph Babinski, a French neurologist, to determine lesions and abnormalities in the nervous system. The Babinski reflex is present if the great toe extends instead of flexes when the lateral sole of the foot is stroked. The normal response to this stimulation is flexion of the toe. |
| **brain scan** | Injection of radioactive isotopes into the circulation to determine the function and abnormality of the brain. |
| **cerebral angiography (seh REE bral an jee OG rah fee)** | X-ray of the blood vessels of the brain after the injection of a radiopaque dye. |
| **cerebrospinal fluid analysis (ser eh broh SPY nal FLOO id an NAL ih sis)** | Laboratory examination of the clear, watery, colorless fluid from within the brain and spinal cord. Infections and the abnormal presence of blood can be detected in this test. |
| **echoencephalography (ek oh en SEFF ah log rah fee)** | Recording of the ultrasonic echoes of the brain. Useful in determining abnormal patterns of shifting in the brain. |
| **electroencephalography (ee lek troh en SEFF ah LOG rah fee) (EEG)** | Recording the electrical activity of the brain by placing electrodes at various positions on the scalp. Also used in sleep studies to determine if there is a normal pattern of activity during sleep. |
| **electromyography (ee lek troh my OG rah fee) (EMG)** | Recording of the contraction of muscles as a result of receiving electrical stimulation. |
| **lumbar puncture (LUM bar PUNK chur) (LP)** | Puncture with a needle into the lumbar area (usually the fourth intervertebral space) to withdraw fluid for examination and for the injection of anesthesia (see ▪ Figure 12.18). Also called *spinal puncture* or *spinal tap*. |
| **myelography (my eh LOG rah fee)** | Injection of a radiopaque dye into the spinal canal. An X-ray is then taken to examine the normal and abnormal outlines made by the dye. |
| **pneumoencephalography (noo moh en seff ah LOG rah fee)** | X-ray examination of the brain following withdrawal of cerebrospinal fluid and injection of air or gas via spinal puncture. |
| **positron emission tomography (PAHZ ih tron ee MISH un toh MOG rah fee) (PET)** | Use of positive radionuclides to reconstruct brain sections. Measurement can be taken of oxygen and glucose uptake, cerebral blood flow, and blood volume. The amount of glucose the brain uses indicates how metabolically active the tissue is. |
| **Romberg's (ROM bergs) test** | Test developed by Moritz Romberg, a German physician, that is used to establish neurological function; the person is asked to close his or her eyes and place the feet together. This test for body balance is positive if the patient sways when the eyes are closed. |

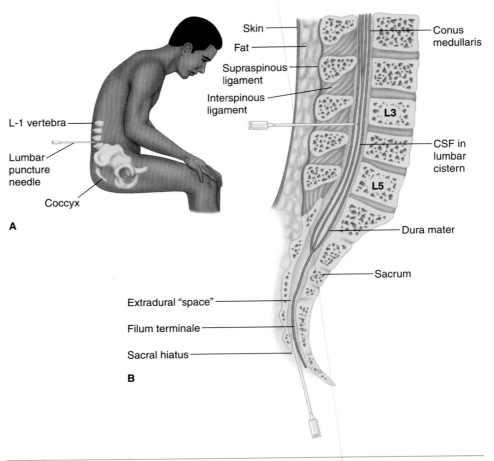

Skin
Fat
Supraspinous ligament
Interspinous ligament

Conus medullaris

L3

CSF in lumbar cistern

L5

L-1 vertebra

Lumbar puncture needle

Coccyx

**A**

Dura mater

Sacrum

Extradural "space"

Filum terminale

Sacral hiatus

**B**

**■ FIGURE 12.18** (A) Lumbar puncture, also known as spinal tap. (B) Section of the vertebral column showing the spinal cord and membranes. A lumbar puncture needle is shown at L3–4 and in the sacral hiatus.

## Therapeutic Procedures Relating to the Nervous System

| | |
|---|---|
| **carotid endarterectomy (kah ROT id end ar ter EK toh mee)** | Surgical procedure for removing an obstruction within the carotid artery, a major artery in the neck that carries oxygenated blood to the brain. Developed to prevent strokes, but is found to be useful only in severe stenosis with TIA. |
| **cerebrospinal fluid (ser eh broh SPY nal FLOO id) shunts** | A surgical procedure in which a bypass is created to drain cerebrospinal fluid. It is used to treat hydrocephalus by draining the excess cerebrospinal fluid from the brain and diverting it to the abdominal cavity. |
| **cordectomy (kor DEK toh me)** | Removal of part of the spinal cord. |
| **cryosurgery (cry oh SER jer ee)** | Use of extreme cold to destroy brain tissue. Used to control bleeding and treat brain tumors. |
| **laminectomy (lam ih NEK toh mee)** | Removal of a portion of a vertebra in order to relieve pressure on the spinal nerve. |
| **nerve block** | Method of regional anesthetic to stop the passage of sensory stimulation along a nerve path. |
| **sympathectomy (sim pah THEK toh mee)** | Excision of a portion of the sympathetic nervous system. Could include a nerve or a ganglion. |
| **trephination (treff ih NAY shun)** | Process of cutting out a piece of bone in the skull to gain entry into the brain or relieve pressure. |

# Pharmacology Relating to the Nervous System

| | |
|---|---|
| **analgesic (an al JEE zik)** | Non-narcotic medication to treat minor to moderate pain. Includes aspirin, acetaminophen, and ibuprofen. |
| **anesthetic (an ess THET ik)** | Drugs that produce a loss of sensation or a loss of consciousness. |
| **anticholinergic (an tih kohl in ER jik)** | Blocks function of the parasympathetic nervous system. Used to treat intestinal, bladder, and bronchial spasms. |
| **anticonvulsant (an tye kon VULL sant)** | Reduces the excitability of neurons and therefore prevents the uncontrolled neuron activity associated with seizures. |
| **barbiturate (bar bi CHUR ate)** | A drug that depresses CNS activity. Used as a sedative and an anticonvulsant. |
| **dopaminergic (dope ah men ER gik) drugs** | Group of medications to treat Parkinson's disease by either replacing the dopamine that is lacking or increasing the strength of the dopamine that is present. |
| **hypnotic (hip NOT tik)** | Drugs that promote sleep. |
| **narcotic (nar KOT tik)** | Morphine and related drugs used to treat severe pain. These drugs have the potential to be habit forming if taken for a prolonged time. Also called *opiates*. |
| **sedative (SED ah tiv)** | A drug that has a relaxing or calming effect. |

# Abbreviations Relating to the Nervous System

| | | | | |
|---|---|---|---|---|
| **ALS** | amyotrophic lateral sclerosis | | **HA** | headache |
| **ANS** | autonomic nervous system | | **ICP** | intracranial pressure |
| **CNS** | central nervous system | | **LP** | lumbar puncture |
| **CP** | cerebral palsy | | **MS** | multiple sclerosis |
| **CSF** | cerebrospinal fluid | | **PET** | positron emission tomography |
| **CVA** | cerebrovascular accident | | **PNS** | peripheral nervous system |
| **CVD** | cerebrovascular disease | | **SAH** | subarachnoid hemorrhage |
| **EEG** | electroencephalogram, electroencephalography | | **SCI** | spinal cord injury |
| **EMG** | electromyogram | | **TIA** | transient ischemic attack |

# Chapter Review

## Pronunciation Practice

 *You will find the pronunciation for each term on the enclosed CD-ROM. Check each one off as you master it.*

- ☐ afferent (**AFF** er ent) neurons
- ☐ Alzheimer's (**ALTS** high merz) disease
- ☐ amyotrophic lateral sclerosis (ah my oh **TROFF** ik **LAT** er al skleh **ROH** sis)
- ☐ analgesia (an al **JEE** zee ah)
- ☐ analgesic (an al **JEE** zik)
- ☐ anesthesia (an ess **THEE** zee ah)
- ☐ anesthetic (an ess **THET** ik)
- ☐ anticholinergic (an tih kohl in **ER** jik)
- ☐ anticonvulsant (an tye kon **VULL** sant)
- ☐ aphasia (ah **FAY** zee ah)
- ☐ arachnoid (ah **RAK** noyd) layer
- ☐ ascending tracts
- ☐ asthenia (as **THEE** nee ah)
- ☐ astrocytoma (ass troh sigh **TOH** mah)
- ☐ ataxia (ah **TAK** see ah)
- ☐ aura (**AW** ruh)
- ☐ autonomic (aw toh **NOM** ik) nervous system
- ☐ axon (**AK** son)
- ☐ Babinski's (bah **BIN** skeez) sign
- ☐ barbiturate (bar bi **CHUR** ate)
- ☐ Bell's palsy (**BELLZ PAWL** zee)
- ☐ bradykinesia (brad ee kin **NEE** see ah)
- ☐ brain
- ☐ brain scan
- ☐ brain stem
- ☐ brain tumor
- ☐ carotid endarterectomy (kah **ROT** id end ar ter **EK** toh mee)
- ☐ central nervous system
- ☐ cephalalgia (seff al **AL** jee ah)
- ☐ cerebellar (ser eh **BELL** ar)
- ☐ cerebellitis (ser eh bell **EYE** tis)
- ☐ cerebellum (ser eh **BELL** um)
- ☐ cerebral (seh **REE** bral)
- ☐ cerebral aneurysm (seh **REE** bral **AN** yoo rizm)

- ☐ cerebral angiography (seh **REE** bral an jee **OG** rah fee)
- ☐ cerebral contusion (seh **REE** bral kon **TOO** shun)
- ☐ cerebral cortex (seh **REE** bral **KOR** teks)
- ☐ cerebral hemispheres (seh **REE** bral **HEM** is feerz)
- ☐ cerebral palsy (ser **REE** bral **PAWL** zee)
- ☐ cerebrospinal (ser eh broh **SPY** nal)
- ☐ cerebrospinal fluid (ser eh broh **SPY** nal **FLOO** id)
- ☐ cerebrospinal fluid analysis (ser eh broh **SPY** nal **FLOO** id an **NAL** ih sis)
- ☐ cerebrospinal fluid (ser eh broh **SPY** nal **FLOO** id) shunts
- ☐ cerebrovascular accident (ser eh broh **VASS** kyoo lar **AK** sih dent)
- ☐ cerebrum (**SER** eh brum)
- ☐ chorea (koh **REE** ah)
- ☐ coma (**COH** mah)
- ☐ concussion (kon **KUSH** un)
- ☐ conscious (**KON** shus)
- ☐ convulsion (kon **VULL** shun)
- ☐ cordectomy (kor **DEK** toh mee)
- ☐ cranial (**KRAY** nee al) nerves
- ☐ cryosurgery (cry oh **SER** jer ee)
- ☐ delirium (dee **LEER** ee um)
- ☐ dementia (dee **MEN** she ah)
- ☐ dendrites (**DEN** drights)
- ☐ descending tracts
- ☐ diencephalon (dye en **SEFF** ah lon)
- ☐ dopaminergic (dope ah men **ER** gik) drugs
- ☐ dura mater (**DOO** rah **MATE** er)
- ☐ dysphasia (dis **FAY** zee ah)
- ☐ echoencephalography (ek oh en **SEFF** ah log rah fee)
- ☐ efferent (**EFF** er ent) neurons
- ☐ electroencephalogram (ee lek troh en **SEFF** ah loh gram)
- ☐ electroencephalography (ee lek troh en seff ah **LOG** rah fee)
- ☐ electromyography (ee lek troh my **OG** rah fee)

- encephalitis (en seff ah **LYE** tis)
- encephalocele (en **SEFF** ah loh seel)
- encephalomalacia (en seff ah loh mah **LAY** she ah)
- encephalosclerosis (en seff ah loh skleh **ROH** sis)
- epidural hematoma (ep ih **DOO** ral hee mah **TOH** mah)
- epilepsy (**EP** ih lep see)
- focal (**FOE** kal) seizure
- frontal lobe
- ganglion (**GANG** lee on)
- glands
- grand mal (**GRAND MALL**) seizure
- gray matter
- Guillan-Barré (**GHEE** yan bah **RAY**) syndrome
- gyri (**JYE** rye)
- hemiparesis (hem ee par **EE** sis)
- hemiplegia (hem ee **PLEE** jee ah)
- Huntington's chorea (**HUNT** ing tonz koh **REE** ah)
- hydrocephalus (high droh **SEFF** ah lus)
- hyperesthesia (high per ess **THEE** zee ah)
- hypnotic (hip **NOT** tik)
- hypothalamus (high poh **THAL** ah mus)
- intrathecal (in tra **THEE** kal)
- laminectomy (lam ih **NEK** toh mee)
- lethargy (**LETH** ar jee)
- lumbar puncture (**LUM** bar **PUNK** chur)
- medulla oblongata (meh **DULL** ah ob long **GAH** tah)
- meninges (men **IN** jeez)
- meningioma (meh nin jee **OH** mah)
- meningitis (men in **JYE** tis)
- meningocele (men **IN** goh seel)
- midbrain
- migraine (**MY** grain)
- monoparesis (mon oh pah **REE** sis)
- monoplegia (mon oh **PLEE** jee ah)
- motor neurons
- multiple sclerosis (**MULL** tih pl skleh **ROH** sis)
- muscles
- myasthenia (my ass **THEE** nee ah)
- myasthenia gravis (my ass **THEE** nee ah **GRAV** iss)
- myelin (**MY** eh lin)
- myelinated (**MY** eh lih nayt ed)
- myelitis (my eh **LYE** tis)
- myelogram (**MY** eh loh gram)

- myelography (my eh **LOG** rah fee)
- myelomalacia (my eh loh mah **LAY** she ah)
- myelomeningocele (my eh loh meh **NIN** goh seel)
- narcolepsy (**NAR** koh lep see)
- narcotic (nar **KOT** tik)
- nerve block
- nerve cell body
- nerve root
- neuralgia (noo **RAL** jee ah)
- neurectomy (noo **REK** toh mee)
- neuroglial (noo **ROH** glee all) cells
- neurologist (noo **RAL** oh jist)
- neurology (noo **RAL** oh jee)
- neurolysis (noo **ROL** ih sis)
- neuroma (noo **ROH** mah)
- neuron (**NOO** ron)
- neuroplasty (**NOOR** oh plas tee)
- neurorrhaphy (noo **ROR** ah fee)
- neurosurgeon (noo roh **SIR** jen)
- neurotomy (noo **ROT** oh mee)
- neurotransmitter (noo roh **TRANS** mit ter)
- occipital (ock **SIP** ih tal) lobe
- palsy (**PAWL** zee)
- paralysis (pah **RAL** ih sis)
- paraplegia (pair ah **PLEE** jee ah)
- parasympathetic (pair ah sim pah **THET** ik) branch
- paresthesia (par es **THEE** zee ah)
- parietal (pah **RYE** eh tal) lobe
- Parkinson's disease (**PARK** in sons dih **ZEEZ**)
- peripheral (per **IF** er al) nervous system
- petit mal (pet **EE MALL**) seizure
- pia mater (**PEE** ah **MATE** er)
- pneumoencephalography (noo moh en seff ah **LOG** rah fee)
- poliomyelitis (poh lee oh my ell **EYE** tis)
- polyneuritis (pol ee noo **RYE** tis)
- pons (**PONZ**)
- positron emission tomography (**PAHZ** ih tron ee **MISH** un toh **MOG** rah fee)
- quadriplegia (kwod rih **PLEE** jee ah)
- radiculitis (rah dick yoo **LYE** tis)
- Reye's syndrome (**RISE SIN** drohm)
- Romberg's (**ROM** bergs) test

- ❑ sciatica (sigh **AT** ih ka)
- ❑ sedative (**SED** ah tiv)
- ❑ seizure (**SEE** zyoor)
- ❑ sensory neurons
- ❑ sensory receptors
- ❑ shingles (**SHING** lz)
- ❑ sleep disorder
- ❑ somatic nerves
- ❑ spina bifida (**SPY** nah **BIFF** ih dah)
- ❑ spinal cavity
- ❑ spinal cord
- ❑ spinal cord injury
- ❑ spinal nerves
- ❑ subarachnoid (sub ah **RAK** noyd) space
- ❑ subdural hematoma (sub **DOO** ral hee mah **TOH** mah)
- ❑ subdural (sub **DOO** ral) space
- ❑ sulci (**SULL** kye)
- ❑ sympathectomy (sim pah **THEK** toh mee)

- ❑ sympathetic (sim pah **THET** ik) branch
- ❑ synapse (sih **NAPSE**)
- ❑ synaptic (sih **NAP** tik) cleft
- ❑ syncope (**SIN** koh pee)
- ❑ temporal (**TEM** por al) lobe
- ❑ tetraplegia (tet rah **PLEE** jee ah)
- ❑ thalamus (**THAL** ah mus)
- ❑ tic (**TIK**)
- ❑ tic douloureux (**TIK** doo loo **ROO**)
- ❑ tract
- ❑ transient ischemic (**TRAN** shent iss **KEM** ik) attack
- ❑ tremor (**TREM** or)
- ❑ trephination (treff ih **NAY** shun)
- ❑ unconscious (un **KON** shus)
- ❑ ventricles (**VEN** trik lz)
- ❑ vertebral (**VER** teh bral) canal
- ❑ vertebral (**VER** teh bral) column
- ❑ white matter

# Case Study

## Discharge Summary

**Admitting Diagnosis:** Paraplegia following motorcycle accident.

**Final Diagnosis:** Comminuted L2 fracture with epidural hematoma and spinal cord damage resulting in complete paraplegia at the L2 level.

**History of Present Illness:** Patient is a 23-year-old male who was involved in a motorcycle accident. He was unconscious for 35 minutes but was fully aware of his surroundings upon regaining consciousness. He was immediately aware of total anesthesia and paralysis below the waist.

**Summary of Hospital Course:** CT scan revealed extensive bone destruction at the fracture site and that the spinal cord was severed. Lumbar puncture revealed sanguinous cerebrospinal fluid. Patient was unable to voluntarily contract any lower extremity muscles and was not able to feel touch or pinpricks. Lumbar laminectomy with spinal fusion was performed to stabilize the fracture and remove the epidural hematoma. The immediate postoperative recovery period proceeded normally with one incidence of pneumonia due to extended bed rest. It responded to antibiotics and respiratory therapy treatments. Patient began intensive rehabilitation with physical therapy and occupational therapy to strengthen upper extremities, as well as transfer and ADL training. After 2 months, X-rays indicated full healing of the spinal fusion and patient was transferred to a rehabilitation institute.

**Discharge Plans:** Patient was transferred to a rehabilitation institute to continue intensive PT and OT. He will require skilled nursing care to evaluate his skin for the development of decubitus ulcers and intermittent urinary catheterization for incontinence. Since spinal cord was severed, it is not expected that this patient will regain muscle function and sensation. However, long-term goals include independent transfers, independent mobility with a wheelchair, and independent ADLs.

### Critical Thinking Questions

1. The final diagnosis of "paraplegia at the L2 level" is not specifically defined by your text. Explain what you believe it to mean in the context of this discharge summary.

2. Is this patient expected to regain use of his muscles? Explain why or why not.

3. The following medical terms are not specifically referred to in this chapter. Using your text as a dictionary, define each term in your own words.

   a. comminuted

   b. sanguinous

   c. decubitus ulcer

   d. catheterization

4. Which of the following is NOT part of this patient's rehabilitation therapy?

   a. arm strengthening

   b. transfer training

   c. instruction in activities of daily living

   d. leg strengthening

5. Describe, in your own words, the patient's long-term goals.

6. Name and describe the complete surgical procedure this patient underwent. Then describe the purpose for this surgery.

# Chart Note Transcription

## Chart Note

The chart note below contains 11 phrases that can be re-worded with a medical term that you learned in this chapter. Each phrase is identified with an underline. Determine the medical term and write your answers in the space provided.

**Current Complaint:** Patient is a 38-year-old female referred to the <u>specialist in the treatment of diseases of the nervous system</u>① by her family physician with complaints of <u>difficulty with speech,</u>② <u>loss of motion on one side of the body,</u>③ and <u>severe involuntary muscle contractions.</u>④

**Past History:** Patient is married and nulliparous. Has been well prior to current symptoms.

**Signs and Symptoms:** Her husband reports he first noted loss of motion on one side of the body when she began to drag her left foot. It has progressed to involve both left upper and lower extremities, with approximately a 50% loss in control of left lower extremity and a 25% loss of control in left upper extremity. Difficulty with speech is mild and mainly with recalling the names of common objects. Severe involuntary muscle contractions appear to be triggered by stress and last approximately 2 minutes. Results of a <u>recording of the electrical activity of the brain</u>⑤ and a <u>puncture with a needle into the low back to withdraw fluid for examination</u>⑥ were normal. However an <u>injection with radioactive isotopes</u>⑦ revealed the presence of a mass in the right <u>outer layer of the largest section of the brain.</u>⑧

**Diagnosis:** <u>Astrocyte tumor</u>⑨ in the right <u>outer layer of the largest section of the brain.</u>⑧

**Treatment:** A right <u>skull incision</u>⑩ was performed to permit <u>the surgical use of extreme cold</u>⑪ to destroy the tumor. Patient experienced moderate improvement in <u>loss of motion on one side of the body</u>③ and <u>severe involuntary muscle contractions,</u>④ but <u>difficulty with speech</u>② was unchanged.

1. _____

2. _____

3. _____

4. _____

5. _____

6. _____

7. _____

8. _____

9. _____

10. _____

11. _____

# Practice Exercises

## A. Complete the following statements.

1. The study of the nervous system is called _____ .

2. The organs of the nervous system are the _____ , _____ , and
   _____ .

3. The two divisions of the nervous system are the _____ and _____ .

4. The neurons that carry impulses away from the brain and spinal cord are called _____
   neurons.

5. The neurons that carry impulses to the brain and spinal cord are called _____ neurons.

6. The disease, caused by a virus, that attacks the gray matter of the spinal cord is _____ .

7. The largest portion of the brain is the _____ .

8. The second largest portion of the brain is the _____ .

9. The occipital lobe controls _____ .

10. The temporal lobe controls _____ and _____ .

11. A CVA on the left side of the brain will affect the _____ side of the patient.

12. The two divisions of the autonomic nervous system are the _____ and
    _____ .

## B. State the described terms using the combining forms provided.

The combining form *neur/o* refers to the nerve. Use it to write a term that means

1. inflammation of the nerve _____

2. specialist in nerves _____

3. pain in the nerve _____

4. inflammation of many nerves _____

5. excision of a nerve _____

6. surgical repair of a nerve _____

7. incision into a nerve _____

8. suture of a nerve _____

The combining form *mening/o* refers to the meninges or membranes. Use it to write a term that means

9. inflammation of the meninges _____

10. protrusion of the meninges _____

11. protrusion of the spinal cord and the meninges _____

The combining form *encephal/o* refers to the brain. Use it to write a term that means

12. X-ray examination of the brain _____

13. disease of the brain _____

14. inflammation of the brain _____

15. protrusion of the brain _____

16. inflammation of brain and spinal cord _____

The combining form *cerebr/o* refers to the cerebrum. Use it to write a term that means

17. pertaining to the cerebrum and spinal cord _____

18. hardening of the cerebrum _____

19. any disease of the cerebrum _____

20. inflammation of the cerebrum and meninges _____

21. pertaining to the cerebrum _____

## C. Match the terms in column A with the definitions in column B.

| A | | B |
|---|---|---|
| 1. _____ chorea | | a. sluggishness or stupor |
| 2. _____ meningitis | | b. bizarre movements |
| 3. _____ palsy | | c. convulsion |
| 4. _____ shingles | | d. congenital hernia of membranes |
| 5. _____ syncope | | e. mild epilepsy |
| 6. _____ lethargy | | f. inflammation of meninges |
| 7. _____ petit mal | | g. shaking, tremors |
| 8. _____ grand mal | | h. painful virus on nerves |
| 9. _____ meningocele | | i. fainting |

## D. Identify the following abbreviations.

1. TIA _____

2. MS _____

3. SCI _____

4. CNS _____

5. PNS _____

6. HA _____

7. CP _____

8. LP _____

9. ALS _____

10. ANS _____

## E. Match the cranial nerves in column A with the functions they control in column B.

| A | | B |
|---|---|---|
| 1. _____ olfactory | | a. carries facial sensory impulses |
| 2. _____ optic | | b. turn eye to side |
| 3. _____ oculomotor | | c. controls tongue muscles |
| 4. _____ trochlear | | d. eye muscles and controls pupils |
| 5. _____ trigeminal | | e. swallowing |
| 6. _____ abducens | | f. controls facial muscles |
| 7. _____ facial | | g. eye muscle movement |
| 8. _____ vestibulocochlear | | h. smell |
| 9. _____ glossopharyngeal | | i. controls neck and shoulder muscles |
| 10. _____ vagus | | j. hearing and equilibrium |
| 11. _____ accessory | | k. vision |
| 12. _____ hypoglossal | | l. organs in lower cavities |

## F. Define the following procedures and tests.

1. myelography _____

2. cerebral angiography _____

3. Babinski's reflex _____

4. Romberg's test _____

5. cerebrospinal fluid analysis _____

6. PET scan _____

7. echoencephalography _____

8. lumbar puncture _____

## G. Define each suffix and provide an example of its use.

| | | Meaning | Example |
|---|---|---|---|
| 1. | -lepsy | _____ | _____ |
| 2. | -plegia | _____ | _____ |
| 3. | -taxia | _____ | _____ |
| 4. | -algesia | _____ | _____ |
| 5. | -sthenia | _____ | _____ |
| 6. | -paresis | _____ | _____ |
| 7. | -phasia | _____ | _____ |
| 8. | -kinesia | _____ | _____ |
| 9. | -esthesia | _____ | _____ |

## H. Define the following combining forms.

1. mening/o _____

2. encephal/o _____

3. cerebell/o _____

4. myel/o _____

5. cephal/o _____

6. thalam/o _____

7. gli/o _____

8. radicul/o _____

9. cerebr/o _____

10. pont/o _____

## I. Define the following terms.

1. glioma _____

2. epilepsy _____

3. anesthesia _____

4. hemiparesis _____

5. neuralgia _____

6. analgesia _____

7. neurasthenia _____

8. quadriplegia _____

9. subdural hematoma _____

10. narcolepsy _____

## J. Match the terms in column A with the definitions in column B.

| A | B |
|---|---|
| 1. _____ neurologist | a. seizures |
| 2. _____ cerebrovascular accident | b. sleep disorder |
| 3. _____ concussion | c. Alzheimer's disease |
| 4. _____ aphasia | d. physician who treats nervous problem |
| 5. _____ narcolepsy | e. stroke |
| 6. _____ epilepsy | f. brain injury from a blow to the head |
| 7. _____ dementia | g. loss of ability to speak |
| 8. _____ hypnotic | h. morphine and related drugs |
| 9. _____ narcotics | i. prevents neuron activity associated with seizures |
| 10. _____ anticonvulsant | j. drug to promote sleep |

# Professional Journal

In this exercise you will now have an opportunity to put the words you have learned into practice. Imagine yourself in the role of an electroneurodiagnostic technologist. If you refer back to the Professional Profile at the beginning of this chapter, you will see that this health care professional conducts diagnostic tests that record the electrical activity of the brain and nervous system. Use the 10 words listed below, or any other new terms from this chapter, to write sentences to describe the patients you saw today.

An example of a sentence is *Dr. Jones ordered an* **EEG** *after her patient came to the emergency room having* **convulsions.**

1.  astrocytoma _____

2.  cerebral hemispheres _____

3.  cerebrovascular accident _____

4.  unconscious _____

5.  encephalomalacia _____

6.  epilepsy _____

7.  hyperesthesia _____

8.  electromyography _____

9.  cranial nerves _____

10. neuralgia _____

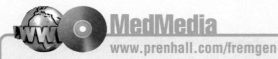

## MedMedia
### www.prenhall.com/fremgen

Use the CD-ROM enclosed with your textbook to gain additional reinforcement through interactive word building exercises, spelling games, labeling activities, and additional quizzes.

Use the above address to access the free, interactive Companion Website created for this textbook. Get hints, instant feedback, and textbook references to chapter-related multiple-choice questions, as well as labeling and matching exercises. In addition, you will find an audio glossary, case studies, and Internet exploration exercises.

***For more information regarding nervous system diseases, visit the following websites:***

Centers for Disease Control and Prevention's Health Topics A to Z at **www.cdc.gov/health/default.htm**

Health Information provided by the National Institutes of Health at **http://health./nih.gov**

Health Information provided by the Stanford Health Library at **http://healthlibrary.stanford.edu**

InteliHealth featuring Harvard Medical School's Consumer Health Information at
   **www.intelihealth.com**

Medical Encyclopedia provided by University of Maryland Medicine at **www.umm.edu/ency**

University of Iowa Health Care's Virtual Hospital at **www.vh.org**

# Chapter 13

# Special Senses:
# The Eye and the Ear

## Learning Objectives

*Upon completion of this chapter, you will be able to:*

- Recognize the combining forms and suffixes introduced in this chapter.
- Gain the ability to pronounce medical terms and major anatomical structures.
- List the major organs of the eye and ear and their functions.
- Describe how we see.
- Describe the path of sound vibration.
- Build eye and ear medical terms from word parts.
- Define vocabulary, pathology, diagnostic, and therapeutic medical terms relating to the eye and ear.
- Recognize types of medications associated with the eye and ear.
- Interpret abbreviations associated with the eye and ear.

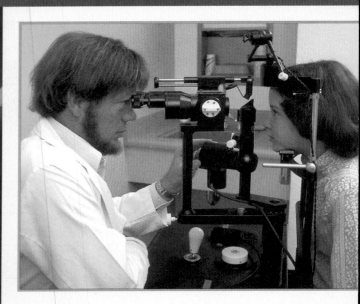

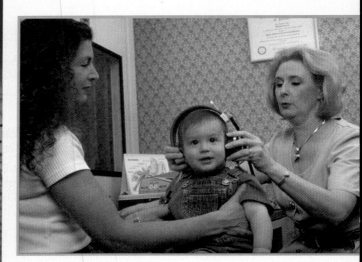

## MedMedia

www.prenhall.com/fremgen

Additional interactive resources and activities for this chapter can be found on the Companion Website. For animations, audio glossary, and review, access the accompanying CD-ROM in this book.

# Professional Profile

## Optometry

Optometry is the professional practice that provides care for the eyes including examining the eyes for diseases, assessing visual acuity, prescribing corrective lenses and eye treatments, and educating patients. Optometry services are found in private offices, acute care facilities, and clinics.

### Doctor of Optometry (OD)

- Also referred to as an optometrist
- Graduates from an accredited 4-year college of optometry after attending at least 3 years of undergraduate college
- May take additional training in pediatric optometry, geriatric optometry, vision therapy, ocular disease, low-vision rehabilitation, or family practice optometry
- Passes written and clinical examinations by the state of employment

### Optician

- Grinds and fits prescription lenses and contacts as prescribed by a physician or optometrist
- Completes a 2- to 4-year apprenticeship
- Licensure required by some states

## Audiology

Audiology is the branch of health care devoted to the study, diagnosis, treatment, and prevention of communication disorders resulting from hearing loss. Audiologists provide a comprehensive array of services related to prevention, diagnosis, and treatment of hearing impairment and its associate communication disorders. Audiologists perform diagnostic hearing tests, fit and dispense hearing aid amplification devices, and rehabilitate persons with hearing loss. Audiology services work with clients of all ages from young children born with hearing impairment to the elderly who experience hearing loss as a part of the aging process. They practice in private offices, hospitals, and schools.

### Doctor of Audiology (AuD)

- Also referred to as an audiologist
- Graduates from an accredited 4-year graduate program in audiology
- Completes an extensive clinical internship in a variety of practice settings
- Passes a national certification examination

*For more information regarding these health careers, visit the following websites:*
American Academy of Audiology at **www.audiology.org**
American Optometric Association at **www.aoanet.org**
National Optometric Association at **www.natoptassoc.org**
Prevent Blindness America at **www.preventblindness.org**

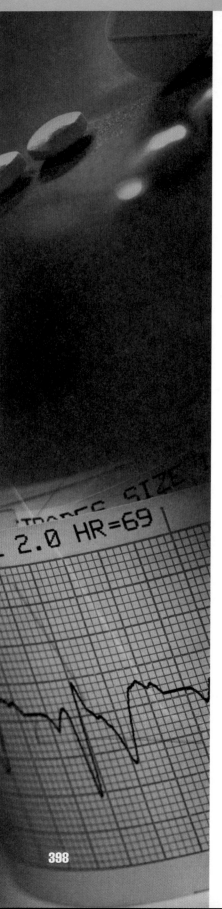

## Part I: The Eye

### Structures Relating to the Eye

| | |
|---|---|
| choroid | iris |
| ciliary body | lacrimal ducts |
| conjunctiva | lacrimal glands |
| cornea | lens |
| eye muscles | pupil |
| eyeball | retina |
| eyelids | sclera |

### Combining Forms Relating to the Eye

| | | | |
|---|---|---|---|
| ambly/o | dull, dim | ocul/o | eye |
| aque/o | water | ophthalm/o | eye |
| blephar/o | eyelid | opt/o | eye, vision |
| conjunctiv/o | conjunctiva | optic/o | eye |
| core/o | pupil | papill/o | optic disk |
| corne/o | cornea | phac/o | lens |
| cycl/o | ciliary muscle | phot/o | light |
| dacry/o | tear, tear duct | presby/o | old age |
| dipl/o | double | pupill/o | pupil |
| glauc/o | gray | retin/o | retina |
| ir/o | iris | scler/o | sclera |
| irid/o | iris | uve/o | vascular |
| kerat/o | cornea | vitre/o | glassy |
| lacrim/o | tears | | |

### Suffixes Relating to the Eye

| Suffix | Meaning | Example |
|---|---|---|
| -chalasis | relaxation | blepharochalasis |
| -opia | vision | hyperopia |
| -tropia | to turn | esotropia |

## Anatomy and Physiology of the Eye

| | | |
|---|---|---|
| conjunctiva | eyelids | ophthalmology |
| eye muscles | lacrimal ducts | optic nerve |
| eyeball | lacrimal glands | |

The study of the eye is known as **ophthalmology** (off thal **MALL** oh gee) (**Ophth.**). The **eyeball** is the incredible organ of sight that transmits an external image by way of the nervous system—the **optic** (**OP** tik) **nerve**—to the brain. The brain then translates these sensory impulses into an image with computer-like accuracy.

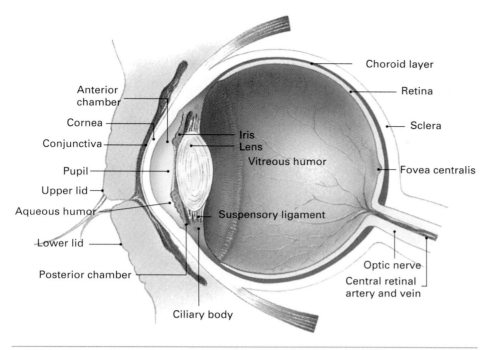

**FIGURE 13.1** Anatomy of the eye.

In addition to the eyeball, several external structures play a role in vision. These are the **eye muscles, eyelids, conjunctiva** (kon **JUNK** tih vah)**, lacrimal** (**LAK** rim al) **glands,** and **lacrimal** (**LAK** rimal) **ducts** (see ▧ Figure 13.1 for anatomy of the eye).

## The Eyeball

**choroid**          **retina**          **sclera**

The actual eyeball is composed of three layers: the **sclera** (**SKLAIR** ah), the **choroid** (**KOR** oyd), and the **retina** (**RET** in ah).

### Sclera

**cornea**

The outer layer, the sclera, provides a tough protective layer for the inner structures of the eye. Another term for the sclera is the *white of the eye.*

The anterior portion of the sclera is called the **cornea** (**COR** nee ah). This is the clear, transparent part of the sclera that allows light to enter the interior of the eye. The cornea, often referred to as the window of the eye, actually bends, or refracts, the light rays.

### Choroid

**ciliary body**       **lens**          **uvea**
**iris**               **pupil**

The second layer or middle layer of the eye is called the choroid. This layer provides the blood supply for the eye and is opaque.

 **MED TERM TIP** The color of the sclera can indicate the presence of disease. For instance, a yellowish cast to the sclera can be present in liver disease and certain anemias.

 **MED TERM TIP** When studying the functions and terminology of the eye, it is helpful to know the meanings of the terms *opaque* and *transparent.* Opaque means that light is unable to pass through. Transparent, however, means that light is permitted through.

The anterior portion of the choroid layer consists of the **iris** (**EYE** ris), **pupil,** and **ciliary** (**SIL** ee ar ee) **body.** The iris is the colored portion of the eye and contains muscle. The pupil is the opening in the center of the iris that allows light rays to enter the eyeball. The iris muscle contracts or relaxes to change the size of the pupil, thereby controlling how much light enters the interior of the eyeball. Behind the iris is the **lens.** The lens is not actually part of the choroid layer, but it is attached to the muscular ciliary body. By pulling on the edge of the lens, these muscles change the shape of the lens so it can focus incoming light onto the retina.

### Retina

| | | |
|---|---|---|
| aqueous humor | macula lutea | rods |
| cones | optic disk | vitreous humor |
| fovea centralis | retinal blood vessels | |

The third and innermost layer of the eyeball is the retina. It contains the sensory receptor cells that respond to light rays, **rods** and **cones.** Rods are active in dim light and help us to see in black and white. Cones are active only in bright light and are responsible for color vision. When the lens projects an image onto the retina, it strikes an area called the **macula lutea** (**MAK** yoo lah loo **TEE** ah), or *yellow spot.* In the center of the macula lutea is a depression called the **fovea centralis** (**FOH** vee ah sen **TRAH** lis), which means *central pit.* This pit contains a high concentration of sensory receptor cells and, therefore, is the point of clearest vision. Also visible on the retina is the **optic disk.** This is the point where the optic nerve leaves the eyeball. There are no sensory receptor cells in the optic disk and therefore it causes a *blind spot* in each eye's field of vision. The interior spaces of the eyeball are not empty. The spaces between the cornea and lens are filled with **aqueous** (**AY** kwee us) **humor,** a watery fluid, and the large open area between the lens and retina contains **vitreous** (**VIT** ree us) **humor,** a semisolid gel. ■ Figure 13.2 is a photo taken through the pupil of the eye. It shows the **retinal** (**RET** in al) **blood vessels.**

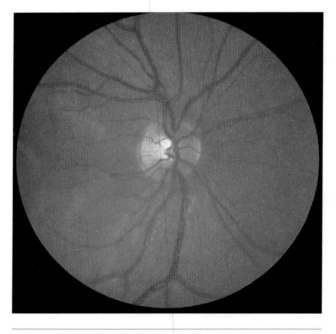

■ **FIGURE 13.2** Retinal blood vessels.

# Muscles of the Eye

**oblique muscles**       **rectus muscles**       **strabismus**

Six muscles connect the actual eyeball to the skull (see ■ Figure 13.3). These muscles change the direction each eye is looking in. In addition, they provide support for the eyeball in the eye socket. Children may be born with a weakness in some of these muscles and may require treatments such as eye exercises or even surgery to correct this problem. This problem is commonly referred to as crossed eyes or **strabismus** (strah **BIZ** mus) (see ■ Figure 13.4). The muscles involved are the four **rectus** (**REK** tus) and two **oblique** (oh **BLEEK**) **muscles**.

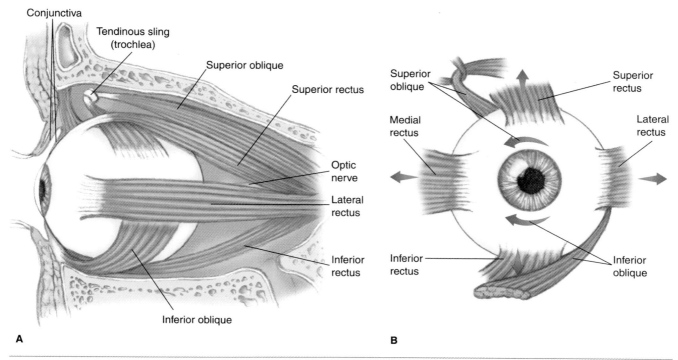

**A**   **B**

■ **FIGURE 13.3**   Eye muscles. (A) Lateral view, left eye; (B) anterior view, left eye.

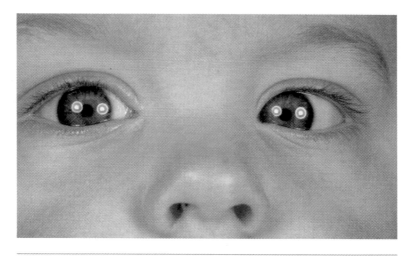

■ **FIGURE 13.4**   Strabismus in young child.
(Barts Medical Library/Phototake NYC)

## The Eyelids

**cilia**                    **eyelashes**                    **sebaceous glands**

A pair of eyelids over each eyeball provides protection from foreign particles, injury from the sun and intense light, and trauma. Both the upper and lower edges of the eyelids have **eyelashes** or **cilia** (**SIL** ee ah) that protect the eye from foreign particles. In addition, **sebaceous** (see **BAY** shus) **glands** are located in the eyelids. These secrete a lubricating oil onto the eyeball.

## Conjunctiva

**mucous membrane**

The conjunctiva of the eye is a **mucous membrane** lining. It forms a continuous covering on the underside of each eyelid and across the anterior surface of each eyeball. This serves as protection for the eye.

## Lacrimal Glands and Ducts

**nasal cavity**                **nasolacrimal duct**                **tears**

The lacrimal gland is located in the outer corner of each eyelid. These glands produce **tears.** Tears serve the important function of washing and lubricating the anterior surface of the eyeball. Lacrimal ducts located in the inner corner of the eye socket then collect the tears and drain them into the **nasolacrimal** (naz oh **LAK** rim al) **duct.** This duct ultimately drains the tears into the **nasal cavity** (see ■ Figure 13.5).

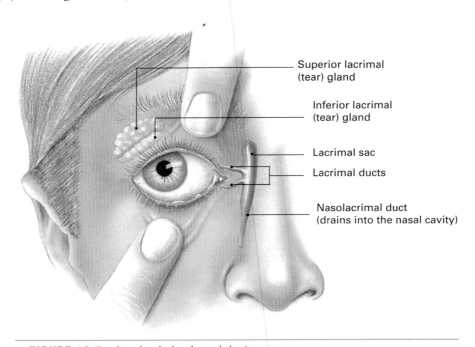

Superior lacrimal (tear) gland

Inferior lacrimal (tear) gland

Lacrimal sac

Lacrimal ducts

Nasolacrimal duct (drains into the nasal cavity)

■ **FIGURE 13.5**   Lacrimal glands and ducts.

# How We See

When light rays strike the eye, they first pass through the cornea, pupil, aqueous humor, lens, and vitreous humor. They then strike the retina and stimulate the rods and cones. When the light rays hit the retina, an upside-down image is sent along nerve impulses to the optic nerve. The optic nerve transmits these impulses to the brain, where the upside-down image is translated into the right-side-up image we are looking at (see ■ Figures 13.6 and 13.7).

Vision requires four mechanisms to be working:

1. Coordination of the external eye muscles so that both eyes move together.
2. The correct amount of light admitted by the pupil.
3. The correct focus of light on the retina by the lens.
4. The optic nerve transmitting sensory images to the brain.

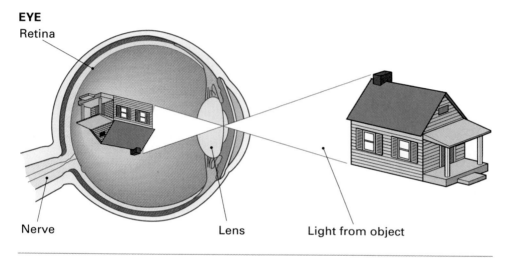

**EYE**

Retina

Nerve

Lens

Light from object

■ **FIGURE 13.6** Image is inverted on the retina. The brain is responsible for righting it.

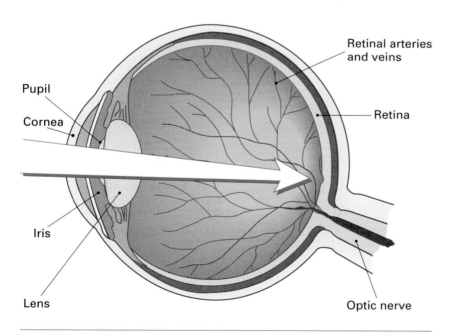

Retinal arteries and veins

Pupil

Cornea

Retina

Iris

Lens

Optic nerve

■ **FIGURE 13.7** Light entering the eye.

# Word Building Relating to the Eye

The following list contains examples of medical terms built directly from word parts. The definitions of these terms can be determined by a straightforward translation of the word parts.

| Combining Form | Combined With | Medical Term | Definition |
|---|---|---|---|
| blephar/o | -itis | blepharitis (blef ah **RYE** tis) | eyelid inflammation |
| | -plasty | blepharoplasty (**BLEF** ah roh plass tee) | surgical repair of eyelid |
| | -ptosis | blepharoptosis (blef ah rop **TOH** sis) | drooping eyelid |
| | -ectomy | blepharectomy (blef ah **REK** toh mee) | excision of the eyelid |
| conjuctiv/o | -itis | conjunctivitis (kon junk tih **VYE** tis) | conjunctiva inflammation |
| | -plasty | conjunctivoplasty (kon junk tih **VOH** plas tee) | surgical repair of the conjunctiva |
| cycl/o | -plegia | cycloplegia (sigh kloh **PLEE** jee ah) | paralysis of the ciliary body |
| dacry/o | cyst/o -itis | dacryocystitis (dak ree oh sis **TYE** tis) | tear bladder inflammation |
| dipl/o | -opia | diplopia (dip **LOH** pee ah) | double vision |
| ir/o | -itis | iritis (ih **RYE** tis) | iris inflammation |
| irid/o | -ectomy | iridectomy (ir id **EK** toh mee) | excision of iris |
| | -plegia | iridoplegia (ir id oh **PLEE** jee ah) | paralysis of iris |
| | scler/o-otomy | iridosclerotomy (ir ih doh skleh **ROT** oh mee) | incision into iris and sclera |
| kerat/o | -itis | keratitis (kair ah **TYE** tis) | cornea inflammation |
| | -plasty | keratoplasty (**KAIR** ah toh plass tee) | surgical repair of cornea |
| | -otomy | keratotomy (kair ah **TOT** oh mee) | incision into the cornea |
| lacrim/o | -al | lacrimal (**LAK** rim al) | pertaining to tears |
| ocul/o | bi- -ar | binocular (bih **NOK** yoo lar) | pertaining to two eyes |
| | intra- -ar | intraocular (in trah **OCK** yoo lar) | pertaining to within the eye |
| | myc/o -osis | oculomycosis (ok yoo loh my **KOH** sis) | abnormal condition of eye fungus |
| ophthalm/o | -algia | ophthalmalgia (off thal **MAL** jee ah) | eye pain |
| | -ic | ophthalmic (off **THAL** mik) | pertaining to the eye |
| | -ologist | ophthalmologist (off thal **MALL** oh jist) | specialist in the eye |
| | -ology | ophthalmology (off thal **MALL** oh jee) | study of the eye |
| | -plegia | ophthalmoplegia (off thal moh **PLEE** jee ah) | eye paralysis |
| | -rrhagia | ophthalmorrhagia (off thal moh **RAH** jee ah) | rapid bleeding from the eye |
| | -scope | ophthalmoscope (off **THAL** moh scope) | instrument to view inside the eye |
| opt/o | -ic | optic (**OP** tik) | pertaining to the eye or vision |
| | -meter | optometer (op **TOM** eh ter) | instrument to measure vision |
| | -metry | optometry (op **TOM** eh tree) | process of measuring vision |
| retin/o | -al | retinal (**RET** in al) | pertaining to the retina |
| | -pathy | retinopathy (ret in **OP** ah thee) | retina disease |
| | -pexy | retinopexy (ret ih noh **PEX** ee) | surgical fixation of the retina |
| scler/o | -malacia | scleromalacia (sklair oh mah **LAY** she ah) | softening of the sclera |
| | -otomy | sclerotomy (skleh **ROT** oh mee) | incision into the sclera |
| | -itis | scleritis (skler **EYE** tis) | inflammation of the sclera |

# Vocabulary Relating to the Eye

| | |
|---|---|
| accommodation (ah kom oh DAY shun) (Acc) | Ability of the eye to adjust to variations in distance. |
| convergence (kon VER jens) | The moving inward of the eyes to see an object close to the face. |
| ectropion (ek TROH pee on) | Term referring to eversion (turning outward) of the eyelid. |
| emmetropia (em eh TROH pee ah) (EM) | State of normal vision. |
| entropion (en TROH pee on) | Term referring to inversion (turning inward) of the eyelid. |
| esotropia (ST) (ess oh TROH pee ah) | Inward turning of the eye. An example of a form of strabismus (muscle weakness of the eye). |
| exophthalmos (eks off THAL mohs) | Abnormal protrusion of the eyeball. Can be due to hyperthyroidism. |
| exotropia (eks oh TROH pee ah) (XT) | Outward turning of the eye. Also an example of strabismus (muscle weakness of the eye). |
| nyctalopia (nik tah LOH pee ah) | Difficulty seeing in dim light. Usually due to damaged rods. |
| optician (op TISH an) | Specialist in grinding corrective lenses. |
| optometrist (op TOM eh trist) | A doctor of optometry specializing in testing visual acuity and prescribing corrective lenses. |
| papilledema (pah pill eh DEEM ah) | Swelling of the optic disk. Often as a result of increased intraocular pressure. Also called *choked disk.* |
| photophobia (foh toh FOH bee ah) | Although the term translates into *fear of light,* it actually means a strong sensitivity to bright light. A person with photophobia has a strong aversion to being in bright light. |
| presbyopia (prez bee OH pee ah) | Visual loss due to old age, resulting in difficulty in focusing for near vision (such as reading). |
| refraction (ree FRAK shun) | Eye examination performed to determine and correct refractive errors in the eye (see ■ Figure 13.8). |
| refractive (ree FRAK tiv) error | Defect in the ability of the eye to accurately focus the image that is hitting it. Occurs in farsightedness and nearsightedness. |
| visual field | The size of the area perceived by one eye when it is stationary. |
| xerophthalmia (zee ROP thal mee ah) | Dry eyes. |

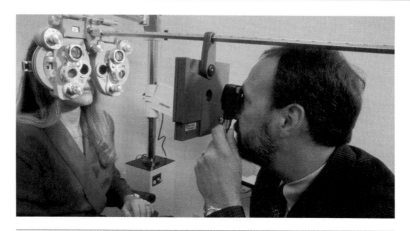

■ **FIGURE 13.8** Ophthalmological examination.
(David Weintraub/Photo Researchers, Inc.)

# Pathology Relating to the Eye

| | |
|---|---|
| **achromatopsia** (ah kroh mah TOP see ah) | Condition of color blindness—unable to perceive one or more colors; more common in males. |
| **amblyopia** (am blee OH pee ah) | Loss of vision not as a result of eye pathology. Usually occurs in patients who see two images. In order to see only one image, the brain will no longer recognize the image being sent to it by one of the eyes. May occur if strabismus is not corrected. This condition is not treatable with a prescription lens. Commonly referred to as *lazy eye.* |
| **astigmatism** (ah STIG mah tizm) (Astigm) | A condition in which light rays are focused unevenly on the retina, which causes a distorted image, due to an abnormal curvature of the cornea. |
| **blepharochalasis** (blef ah roh KAL ah sis) | In this condition, the upper eyelid increases in size due to a loss of elasticity, which is followed by swelling and recurrent edema of the lids. The skin may droop over the edges of the eyes when the eyes are open. |
| **cataract (KAT ah rakt)** | Damage to the lens causing it to become opaque or cloudy, resulting in diminished vision. Treatment is usually surgical removal of the cataract (see ▧ Figure 13.9). |
| **chalazion (kah LAY zee on)** | Small hard tumor or mass, similar to a sebaceous cyst, developing on the eyelids. May require incision and drainage (I & D). |
| **corneal abrasion** | Scraping injury to the cornea. If it does not heal, it may develop into an ulcer. |
| **diabetic retinopathy (dye ah BET ik reh tin OP ah thee)** | These small hemorrhages and edema in the eye develop in the retina as a result of diabetes mellitus. Laser surgery and vitrectomy may be necessary for treatment. |
| **glaucoma (glau KOH mah)** | Increase in intraocular pressure, which, if untreated, may result in atrophy (wasting away) of the optic nerve and blindness. Glaucoma is treated with medication and surgery. There is an increased risk of developing glaucoma in persons over 60 years of age, in people of African ancestry, in persons who have sustained a serious eye injury, and in anyone with a family history of diabetes or glaucoma. |
| **hemianopia** (hem ee ah NOP ee ah) | Loss of vision in half of the visual field. A stroke patient may suffer from this disorder. |
| **hordeolum (hor DEE oh lum)** | Refers to a *stye* (or *sty*), a small purulent inflammatory infection of a sebaceous gland of the eye; treated with hot compresses and surgical incision. |
| **hyperopia** (high per OH pee ah) | With this condition a person can see things in the distance but has trouble reading material at close range (see ▧ Figure 13.10). Also known as *farsightedness.* This condition is corrected with converging or biconvex lenses. |
| **macular (MAK yoo lar) degeneration** | Deterioration of the macular area of the retina of the eye. May be treated with laser surgery to destroy the blood vessels beneath the macula. |
| **monochromatism** (mon oh KROH mah tizm) | Unable to perceive one color. |
| **myopia (my OH pee ah) (MY)** | With this condition a person can see things close up but distance vision is blurred (see ▧ Figure 13.11). Also known as *nearsightedness.* This condition is corrected with diverging or biconcave lenses. |
| **nystagmus (niss TAG mus)** | Jerky-appearing involuntary eye movements, usually left and right. Often an indication of brain injury. |
| **pink eye** | A common term for conjunctivitis. |
| **retinal (RET in al) detachment** | Occurs when the retina becomes separated from the choroid layer. This separation seriously damages blood vessels and nerves, resulting in blindness. |

| retinitis pigmentosa (ret in EYE tis pig men TOH sah) | Progressive disease of the eye that results in the retina becoming hard (sclerosed) and pigmented (colored), and atrophying (wasting away). There is no known cure for this condition. |
|---|---|
| retinoblastoma (RET in noh blast OH mah) | A malignant eye tumor that occurs in children, usually under the age of 3. Requires enucleation. |
| strabismus (strah BIZ mus) | An eye muscle weakness resulting in the eyes looking in different directions at the same time. May be corrected with glasses, eye exercises, and/or surgery. |
| trachoma (tray KOH mah) | Chronic infectious disease of the conjunctiva and cornea caused by bacteria. Occurs more commonly in people living in hot, dry climates. Untreated, it may lead to blindness when the scarring invades the cornea. Trachoma can be treated with antibiotics. |

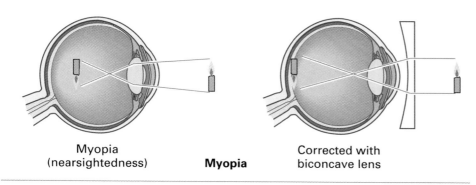

■ **FIGURE 13.9**   Cataract of the right eye.

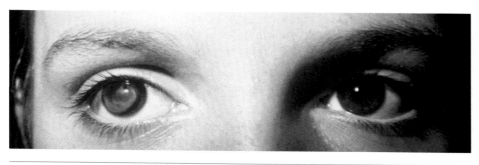

■ **FIGURE 13.10**   How lenses correct visual problems—hyperopia.

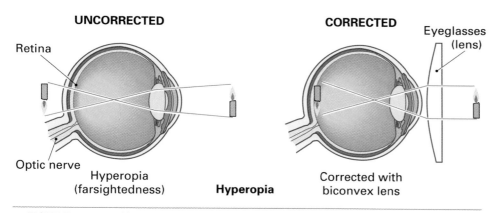

■ **FIGURE 13.11**   How lenses correct visual problems—myopia.

# Diagnostic Procedures Relating to the Eye

| | |
|---|---|
| **color vision tests** | Use of polychromic (multicolored) charts to determine the ability of the patient to recognize color (see ■ Figure 13.12). |
| **fluorescein angiography (floo oh RESS ee in an jee OG rah fee)** | Process of injecting a dye (fluorescein) to observe the movement of blood and detect lesions in the macular area of the retina. Used to determine if there is a detachment of the retina. |
| **fluorescein (floo oh RESS ee in) staining** | Applying dye eyedrops that are a bright green fluorescent color. Used to look for corneal abrasions or ulcers. |
| **gonioscopy (goh nee OSS koh pee)** | Use of an instrument called a gonioscope to examine the anterior chamber of the eye and determine ocular mobility and rotation. |
| **keratometry (kair ah TOM eh tree)** | Measurement of the curvature of the cornea using an instrument called a keratometer. |
| **ophthalmoscopy (off thal MOSS koh pee)** | Examination of the interior of the eyes using an instrument called an ophthalmoscope. The physician dilates the pupil in order to see the cornea, lens, and retina. Used to identify abnormalities in the blood vessels of the eye and some systemic diseases. |
| **slit lamp microscope** | Instrument used in ophthalmology for examining the posterior surface of the cornea. |
| **Snellen's (SNEL enz) chart** | Chart used for testing distance vision named for Hermann Snellen, a Dutch ophthalmologist. It contains letters of varying size and it is administered from a distance of 20 feet. A person who can read at 20 feet what the average person can read at this distance is said to have 20/20 vision. |
| **tonometry (tohn OM eh tree)** | Measurement of the intraocular pressure of the eye using a tonometer to check for the condition of glaucoma. After a local anesthetic is applied, the physician places the tonometer lightly on the eyeball and a pressure measurement is taken. Generally part of a normal eye exam for adults. |
| **visual acuity (VIZH oo al ah KYOO ih tee) (VA) test** | Measurement of the sharpness of a patient's vision. Usually, a Snellen's chart is used for this test in which the patient identifies letters from a distance of 20 feet. |

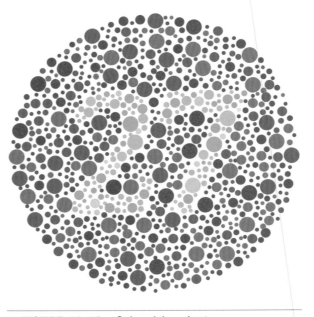

■ **FIGURE 13.12**　Color vision chart.

# Therapeutic Procedures Relating to the Eye

| | |
|---|---|
| **cryoextraction**<br>(cry oh eks TRAK shun) | Procedure in which cataract is lifted from the lens with an extremely cold probe. |
| **cryoretinopexy**<br>(cry oh RET ih noh pek see) | Surgical fixation of the retina by using extreme cold. |
| **enucleation**<br>(ee new klee AH shun) | Surgical removal of an eyeball. |
| **keratoplasty**<br>(KAIR ah toh plass tee) | Surgical repair of the cornea (corneal transplant). |
| **laser-assisted in-situ keratomileusis (in SIH tyoo kair ah toh mih LOO sis) (LASIK)** | Correction of myopia using laser surgery to remove corneal tissue. |
| **laser photocoagulation**<br>(LAY zer foh toh koh ag yoo LAY shun) | The use of a laser beam to destroy very small precise areas of the retina. May be used to treat retinal detachment or macular degeneration. |
| **phacoemulsification** (fak oh ee mull sih fih KAY shun) | Use of high-frequency sound waves to emulsify (liquefy) a lens with a cataract, which is then aspirated (removed by suction) with a needle. |
| **photorefractive keratectomy** (foh toh ree FRAK tiv kair ah TEK toh mee) (PRK) | Use of a laser to reshape the cornea and correct errors of refraction. |
| **radial keratotomy (RAY dee all kair ah TOT oh mee) (RK)** | Spoke-like incisions around the cornea that result in it becoming flatter. A surgical treatment for myopia. |
| **scleral (SKLAIR al) buckling** | Placing a band of silicone around the outside of the sclera, which stabilizes a detaching retina. |
| **strabotomy**<br>(strah BOT oh mee) | Incision into the eye muscles in order to correct strabismus. |

# Pharmacology Relating to the Eye

| | |
|---|---|
| **anesthetic ophthalmic (off THAL mik) solution** | Eyedrops for pain relief associated with eye infections and corneal abrasions. |
| **antibiotic ophthalmic (off THAL mik) solution** | Eyedrops for the treatment of bacterial eye infections. |
| **antiglaucoma (an tye glau KOH mah) medications** | A group of drugs that reduce intraocular pressure by lowering the amount of aqueous humor in the eyeball. May achieve this by either reducing the production of aqueous humor or increasing its outflow. |
| **artificial tears** | Medications, many of them over the counter, to treat dry eyes. |
| **cycloplegic**<br>(sigh kloh PLEE jik) | Drug that paralyzes the ciliary body. Particularly useful during eye examinations and eye surgery. |
| **miotic (my OT ik)** | Any substance that causes the pupil to constrict. |
| **mydriatic (mid ree AT ik)** | Any substance that causes the pupil to dilate. Particularly useful during eye examinations and eye surgery. |

# Abbreviations Relating to the Eye

| | | | |
|---|---|---|---|
| **Acc** | accommodation | **OD** | right eye |
| **ARMD** | age-related macular degeneration | **Ophth.** | ophthalmology |
| **Astigm** | astigmatism | **OS** | left eye |
| **c.gl.** | correction with glasses | **OU** | each eye |
| **cyl. lens** | cylindrical lens | **PERRLA** | pupils equal, round, react to light and accommodation |
| **D** | diopter (lens strength) | | |
| **DVA** | distance visual acuity | **PRK** | photorefractive keratectomy |
| **ECCE** | extracapsular cataract extraction | **REM** | rapid eye movement |
| **EENT** | eye, ear, nose, and throat | **s.gl.** | without correction or glasses |
| **EM** | emmetropia (normal vision) | **SMD** | senile macular degeneration |
| **EOM** | extraocular movement | **ST** | esotropia |
| **ICCE** | intracapsular cataract extraction | **VA** | visual acuity |
| **IOL** | intraocular lens | **VF** | visual field |
| **IOP** | intraocular pressure | **XT** | exotropia |
| **LASIK** | laser-assisted in-situ keratomileusis | | |

**MED TERM TIP**

The abbreviations for right eye (OD) and left eye (OS) are easy to remember when we know their origins. OD stands for *oculus* (eye) *dexter* (right). OS has its origin in *oculus* (eye) *sinister* (left). At one time in history it was considered to be sinister if a person looked at another from only the left side. Hence the term *oculus sinister* (OS) means left eye.

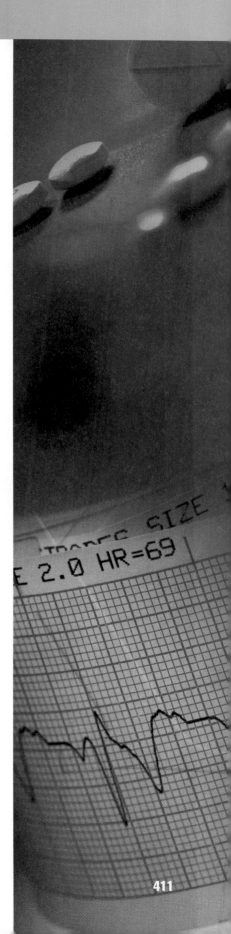

## Part II: The Ear

**Structures Relating to the Ear**

auditory canal
auricle
cochlea
eustachian tube
incus
labyrinth
malleus
oval window
semicircular canals
stapes
tympanic membrane (eardrum)

**Combining Forms Relating to the Ear**

| | | | |
|---|---|---|---|
| acous/o | hearing | labyrinth/o | labyrinth |
| audi/o | hearing | myring/o | eardrum |
| audit/o | hearing | ot/o | ear |
| aur/o | ear | salping/o | eustachian tube |
| auricul/o | ear | staped/o | stapes |
| cochle/o | cochlea | tympan/o | eardrum, middle ear |

**Suffixes Relating to the Ear**

| Suffix | Meaning | Example |
|---|---|---|
| -cusis | hearing | anacusis |
| -otia | ear condition | microtia |

## Anatomy and Physiology of the Ear

| | | |
|---|---|---|
| **audiology** | **hearing** | **vestibular nerve** |
| **cochlear nerve** | **inner ear** | **vestibulocochlear nerve** |
| **equilibrium** | **middle ear** | |
| **external ear** | **otology** | |

The study of the ear is referred to as **otology** (oh **TOL** oh jee) (**Oto**) and the study of hearing disorders is called **audiology** (aw dee **OL** oh jee). There is a large amount of overlap between these two areas, but there are also examples of ear problems that do not affect hearing. The ear is responsible for two senses: **hearing** and **equilibrium** (ee kwih **LIB** ree um), or our sense of balance. Hearing and equilibrium sensory information is carried to the brain by cranial nerve VIII, the **vestibulocochlear** (ves tib yoo loh **KOK** lee ar) **nerve.** This nerve is divided into two major branches. The **cochlear** (**KOK** lee ar) **nerve** carries hearing information and the **vestibular** (ves **TIB** yoo lar) **nerve** carries equilibrium information.

The ear is subdivided into three areas:

1. The **external ear**
2. The **middle ear**
3. The **inner ear**

See ▦ Figure 13.13 for an illustration of the anatomy of the ear.

## The External Ear

| | | |
|---|---|---|
| **auditory canal** | **otoscope** | **pinna** |
| **auricle** | **otoscopy** | **tympanic membrane** |
| **cerumen** | | |

The external ear consists of three parts: the **auricle** (**AW** rih k'l), the **auditory** (**AW** dih tor ee) **canal,** and the **tympanic** (tim **PAN** ik) **membrane.** The auricle or **pinna** (**PIN** ah) is what is commonly referred to as *the ear* because this is the only portion visible. The auricle with its earlobe has a unique shape in each person and functions like a funnel to capture sound waves as they go past the outer ear. The sound then moves along the auditory canal and causes the tympanic membrane (eardrum) to vibrate. The tympanic membrane actually separates the external ear from the middle ear. Ear wax or **cerumen** (seh **ROO** men) is produced in oil glands in the auditory canal. This wax helps to protect and lubricate the ear. It is also just barely liquid at body temperature. This causes cerumen to slowly flow out of the auditory canal, carrying dirt and dust with it. Therefore, the auditory canal is self-cleaning.

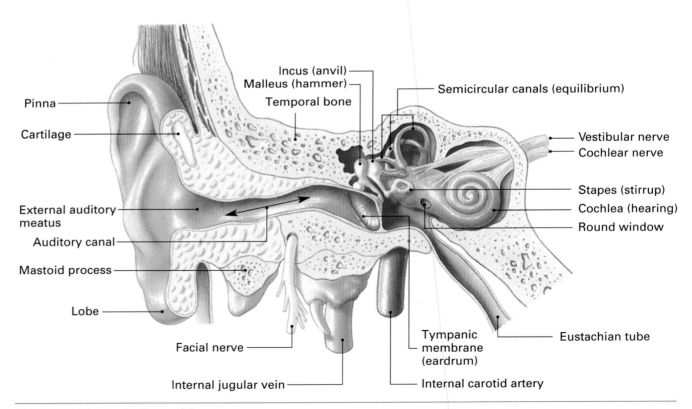

▦ **FIGURE 13.13**  Anatomy of the ear.

Small children are prone to placing objects in their ears. In some cases, as with peas and beans, these become moist in the ear canal and swell, which makes removal difficult. **Otoscopy** (oh **TOSS** koh pee), or the examination of the ear using an **otoscope** (**OH** toh scope), can aid in identifying and removing the cause of hearing loss if it is due to foreign bodies (see ■ Figure 13.14).

## The Middle Ear

| | | |
|---|---|---|
| **auditory tube** | **malleus** | **oval window** |
| **eustachian tube** | **ossicles** | **stapes** |
| **incus** | | |

The middle ear is located in a small cavity in the temporal bone of the skull. This air-filled cavity contains three tiny bones called **ossicles** (**OSS** ih kls). These three bones, the **malleus** (**MAL** ee us), **incus** (**ING** kus), and **stapes** (**STAY** peez), are vital to the hearing process. They amplify the vibrations in the middle ear and transmit them to the inner ear from the malleus to the incus and finally to the stapes. The stapes, the last of the three ossicles, is attached to a very thin membrane that covers the opening to the inner ear called the **oval window.**

The **eustachian** (yoo **STAY** she en) **tube** or **auditory** (**AW** dih tor ee) **tube** connects the nasopharynx with the middle ear. Each time you swallow the eustachian tube opens. This connection allows a person to equalize the pressure between the middle ear cavity and the atmospheric pressure.

The three bones in the middle ear are referred to by terms that are similar to their shape. Thus, the malleus is called the hammer, the incus is the anvil, and the stapes is the stirrup (see ■ Figure 13.15).

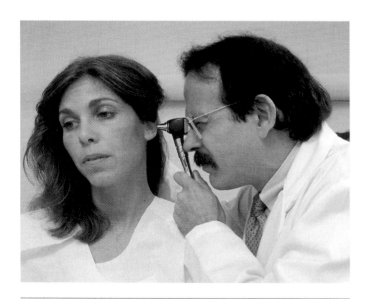

■ **FIGURE 13.14**   Examination of ear using otoscope.

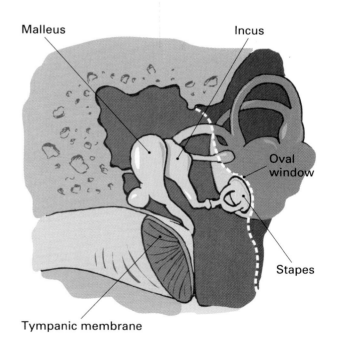

■ **FIGURE 13.15**   Bones in the ear: malleus, stapes, and incus.

Special Senses: The Eye and the Ear   **413**

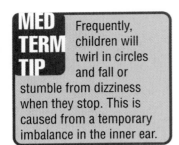

## The Inner Ear

| | | |
|---|---|---|
| **cochlea** | **organs of Corti** | **semicircular canals** |
| **labyrinth** | **saccule** | **utricle** |

The inner ear is also located in a cavity within the temporal bone (refer to Figure 13.13). This fluid-filled cavity is referred to as the **labyrinth** (**LAB** ih rinth) because of its shape. The labyrinth contains the hearing and equilibrium sensory organs: the **cochlea** (**KOK** lee ah) for hearing and the **semicircular canals, utricle** (**YOO** trih k'l), and **saccule** (**SAK** yool) for equilibrium. Each of these organs contains hair cells, the actual sensory receptor cells. In the cochlea, the hair cells are referred to as **organs of Corti** (**KOR** tee).

## How We Hear

**conductive hearing loss**     **sensorineural hearing loss**

■ Figure 13.16 outlines the path of sound through the outer ear and middle ear and into the cochlea of the inner ear. Sound waves traveling down the external auditory canal strike the eardrum, causing it to vibrate. The ossicles conduct these vibrations across the middle ear from the eardrum to the oval window. Oval window movements initiate vibrations in the fluid that fills the cochlea. As the fluid vibrations strike a hair cell it bends the small hairs and stimulates the nerve ending. The nerve ending then sends an electrical impulse to the brain on the cochlear portion of the vestibulocochlear nerve.

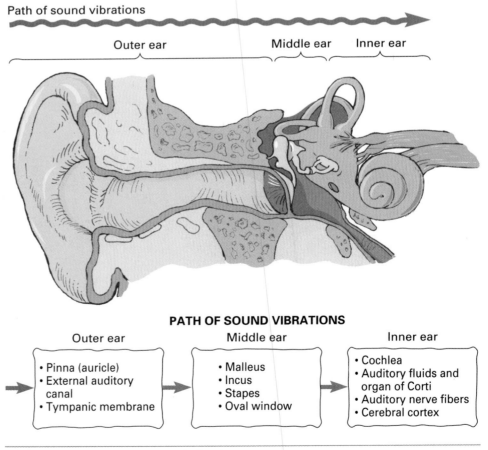

■ **FIGURE 13.16** Path of sound vibrations.

Hearing loss can be divided into two main categories: **conductive** (kon **DUK** tiv) **hearing loss** and **sensorineural** (sen soh ree **NOO** ral) **hearing loss.** Conductive refers to disease or malformation of the outer or middle ear. All sound is weaker and muffled in conductive hearing loss since it is not conducted correctly to the inner ear. Sensorineural hearing loss is the result of damage or malformation of the inner ear (cochlea) or the cochlear nerve. In this hearing loss, some sounds are distorted and heard incorrectly. There can also be a combination of both conductive and sensorineural hearing loss.

**MED TERM TIP**
Hearing impairment is becoming a greater problem for the general population for several reasons. First, people are living longer. Hearing loss can accompany old age, and there are a greater number of people over 50 years of age requiring hearing assistance. In addition, sound technology has produced music quality that was never available before. However, listening to loud music either naturally or through earphones can cause gradual damage to the hearing mechanism.

## Word Building Relating to the Ear

The following list contains examples of medical terms built directly from word parts. The definitions of these terms can be determined by a straightforward translation of the word parts.

| Combining Form | Combined With | Medical Term | Definition |
|---|---|---|---|
| acous/o | -tic | acoustic (ah **KOOS** tik) | pertaining to hearing |
| audi/o | -gram | audiogram (**AW** dee oh gram) | record of hearing |
| | -meter | audiometer (aw dee **OM** eh ter) | instrument to measure hearing |
| | -ologist | audiologist (aw dee **OL** oh jist) | hearing specialist |
| | -ology | audiology (aw dee **OL** oh jee) | study of hearing |
| aur/o | -al | aural (**AW** ral) | pertaining to the ear |
| cochle/o | -ar | cochlear (**KOK** lee ar) | pertaining to the cochlea |
| labyrinth/o | -ectomy | labyrinthectomy (lab ih rin **THEK** toh mee) | excision of the labyrinth |
| | -itis | labyrinthitis (lab ih rin **THIGH** tis) | labyrinth inflammation |
| myring/o | -itis | myringitis (mir ing **JYE** tis) | eardrum inflammation |
| | -ectomy | myringectomy (mir in **GEK** toh mee) | excision of the eardrum |
| | -otomy | myringotomy (mir in **GOT** oh mee) | incision into eardrum |
| | -plasty | myringoplasty (mir **IN** goh plass tee) | surgical repair of eardrum |
| ot/o | -algia | otalgia (oh **TAL** jee ah) | ear pain |
| | -ic | otic (**OH** tik) | pertaining to the ear |
| | -itis | otitis (oh **TYE** tis) | ear inflammation |
| | myc/o -osis | otomycosis (oh toh my **KOH** sis) | abnormal condition of ear fungus |
| | -ologist | otologist (oh **TOL** oh jist) | ear specialist |
| | -ology | otology (oh **TOL** oh jee) | study of the ear |

*continued...*

| Combining Form | Combined With | Medical Term | Definition |
|---|---|---|---|
| | py/o -rrhea | otopyorrhea (oh toh pye oh **REE** ah) | pus discharge from ear |
| | -scope | otoscope (**OH** toh scope) | instrument to view inside the ear |
| | -scopy | otoscopy (oh **TOSS** koh pee) | process of viewing the ear |
| | -plasty | otoplasty (**OH** toh plas tee) | surgical repair of the (external) ear |
| salping/o | -itis | salpingitis (sal pin **JIH** tis) | eustachian tube inflammation |
| | -otomy | salpingotomy (sal pin **GOT** oh mee) | incision into eustachian tube |
| tympan/o | -ic | tympanic (tim **PAN** ik) | pertaining to the eardrum |
| | -itis | tympanitis (tim pan **EYE** tis) | eardrum inflammation |
| | -meter | tympanometer (tim pah **NOM** eh ter) | instrument to measure eardrum |
| | -plasty | tympanoplasty (tim pan oh **PLASS** tee) | surgical repair of eardrum |
| | -rrhexis | tympanorrhexis (tim pan oh **REK** sis) | eardrum rupture |
| | -otomy | tympanotomy (tim pan **OT** oh mee) | incision into the eardrum |
| | -ectomy | tympanectomy (tim pan **EK** toh mee) | excision of the eardrum |

| Suffix | Combined With | Medical Term | Definition |
|---|---|---|---|
| -otia | micro- | microtia (my **KROH** she ah) | (abnormally) small ears |
| | macro- | macrotia (mah **KROH** she ah) | (abnormally) large ears |

## Vocabulary Relating to the Ear

| | |
|---|---|
| **American Sign Language (ASL)** | Nonverbal method of communicating in which the hands and fingers are used to indicate words and concepts. Used by both persons who are deaf and persons with speech impairments (see ▪ Figure 13.17). |
| **binaural (bin AW rall)** | Referring to both ears. |
| **decibel (DES ih bel) (dB)** | Measures the intensity or loudness of a sound. Zero decibels is the quietest sound measured and 120 dB is the loudest sound commonly measured. |
| **fingerspelling** | Use of various hand and finger shapes and positions that represent the written alphabet. These positions can be strung together to form words. |
| **hertz (Hz)** | Measurement of the frequency or pitch of sound. The lowest pitch on an audiogram is 250 Hz. The measurement can go as high as 8000 Hz, which is the highest pitch measured. |
| **interpreter** | Person with training in areas such as sign language, fingerspelling, and speech, who can transmit verbal or written messages to people with hearing impairments. |
| **monaural (mon AW rall)** | Referring to one ear. |
| **otorhinolaryngologist (oh toh rye noh lair in GOL oh jist)** | A physician who specializes in the treatment of diseases of the ear, nose, and throat. |
| **otorhinolaryngology (oh toh rye rye noh lair in GOL oh jee) (ENT)** | Branch of medicine that treats diseases of the ear, nose, and throat. Also referred to as *ENT*. |

| | |
|---|---|
| **presbycusis (pres bih KOO sis)** | Normal loss of hearing that can accompany the aging process. |
| **residual (rih ZID yoo al) hearing** | Amount of hearing that is still present after damage has occurred to the auditory mechanism. |
| **Signing Exact English (SEE–2)** | Translation of English into signs. American Sign Language (ASL) is used in combination with other sign languages and fingerspelling to correspond exactly to the spoken English. |
| **speechreading** | Ability to watch a person's mouth and word formation during speaking to interpret what they are saying. Also referred to as *lipreading*. |
| **tinnitus (tin EYE tus)** | Ringing in the ears. |
| **vertigo (VER tih goh)** | Dizziness. |

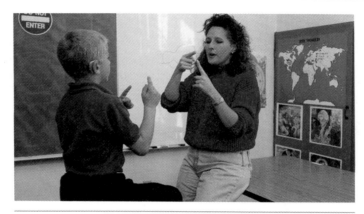

■ **FIGURE 13.17** Sign-language teacher with child who has a hearing impairment and is wearing a behind-the-ear hearing aid. (Trevon Baker/About Faces)

## Pathology Relating to the Ear

| | |
|---|---|
| **acoustic neuroma (ah KOOS tik noor OH mah)** | Benign tumor of the eighth cranial nerve sheath. The pressure causes symptoms such as tinnitus, headache, dizziness, and progressive hearing loss. |
| **anacusis (an ah KOO sis)** | Total absence of hearing; inability to perceive sound. Also called *deafness*. |
| **deafness** | The inability to hear or having some degree of hearing impairment. |
| **hearing impairment** | Loss of hearing sufficient to interfere with a person's ability to communicate. |
| **labyrinthitis (lab ih rin THIGH tis)** | Also referred to as an *inner ear infection*. May affect both the hearing and equilibrium portions of the inner ear. |
| **Ménière's disease (may nee ARZ dih ZEEZ)** | Abnormal condition within the labyrinth of the inner ear that can lead to a progressive loss of hearing. The symptoms are dizziness or vertigo, hearing loss, and tinnitus (ringing in the ears). Named for Prosper Ménière, a French physician. |
| **otitis externa (oh TYE tis ex TERN ah) (OE)** | External ear infection. Most commonly caused by fungus. Also called *otomycosis* and commonly referred to as *swimmer's ear*. |
| **otitis media (oh TYE tis MEE dee ah) (OM)** | Commonly referred to as a *middle ear infection;* seen frequently in children. Often preceded by an upper respiratory infection. Fluid accumulates in the middle ear cavity. The fluid may be watery, *serous otitis media,* or full of pus, *purulent otitis media.* |
| **otosclerosis (oh toh sklair OH sis)** | Loss of mobility of the stapes bone, leading to progressive hearing loss. |

# Diagnostic Procedures Relating to the Ear

| audiometry (aw dee OM eh tree) | Test of hearing ability by determining the lowest and highest intensity (decibels) and frequencies (hertz) that a person can distinguish. The patient may sit in a soundproof booth and receive sounds through earphones as the technician decreases the sound or lowers the tones (see ▓ Figure 13.18). |
| --- | --- |
| falling test | Test used to observe balance and equilibrium. The patient is observed balancing on one foot, then with one foot in front of the other, and then walking forward with eyes open. The same test is conducted with the patient's eyes closed. Swaying and falling with the eyes closed can indicate an ear and equilibrium malfunction. |
| hearing level | Audiometer reading in decibels (dB) corresponding to the listener's hearing threshold ratio that corresponds to the softest sound the listener can hear. |
| otoscopy (oh TOSS koh pee) | Use of a lighted otoscope to examine the auditory canal and middle ear (see ▓ Figure 13.19). |
| Rinne (RIN eh) and Weber tuning-fork tests | The physician holds a tuning fork, which is an instrument that produces a constant pitch when it is struck, against or near the bones on the side of the head. These tests assess both nerve and bone conduction of sound. Friedrich Rinne was a German otologist, and Ernst Weber was a German physiologist. |
| tympanometry (tim pah NOM eh tree) | Measurement of the movement of the tympanic membrane. Can indicate the presence of pressure in the middle ear. |

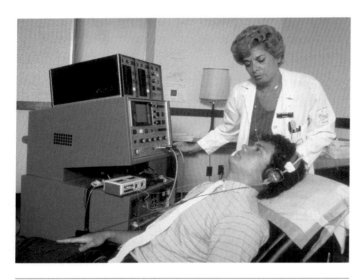

▓ **FIGURE 13.18** Audiologist performing a hearing test with audiometer.
(Ann Chwatsky/Phototake NYC)

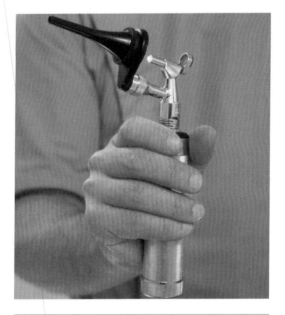

▓ **FIGURE 13.19** Otoscope.
(Richard Hutchings/Photo Researchers, Inc.)

# Therapeutic Procedures Relating to the Ear

| | |
|---|---|
| **amplification**<br>**(am plih fih KAY shun) device** | Used to increase certain sounds for people with hearing impairments. Also known as *hearing aid.* |
| **cochlear (KOK lee ar) implant** | Mechanical device surgically placed under the skin behind the outer ear (pinna) that converts sound signals into magnetic impulses to stimulate the auditory nerve. Can be beneficial for those with profound sensorineural hearing loss. |
| **hearing aid** | Apparatus or mechanical device used by persons with impaired hearing to amplify sound. Same as *amplification device* (see ▣ Figure 13.20). |
| **myringotomy**<br>**(mir in GOT oh mee)** | Surgical puncture of the eardrum with removal of fluid and pus from the middle ear to eliminate a persistent ear infection and excessive pressure on the tympanic membrane. A polyethylene tube is placed in the tympanic membrane to allow for drainage of the middle ear cavity. |
| **otoplasty (OH toh plass tee)** | Corrective surgery to change the size of the external ear or pinna. The surgery can either enlarge or decrease the size of the pinna. |
| **otoscopy (oh TOSS koh pee)** | Examination of the ear canal, eardrum, and outer ear using the otoscope. Foreign material can be removed from the ear canal with this procedure (refer to Figure 13.19). |
| **polyethylene**<br>**(pol ee ETH ih leen) tube**<br>**(PE tube)** | Small tube surgically placed in a child's eardrum to assist in drainage of infection. |
| **stapedectomy**<br>**(stay pee DEK toh mee)** | Removal of the stapes bone to treat otosclerosis (hardening of the bone). A prosthesis or artificial stapes may be implanted. |
| **tympanoplasty**<br>**(tim pan oh PLASS tee)** | Another term for the surgical reconstruction of the eardrum. Also called *myringoplasty.* |

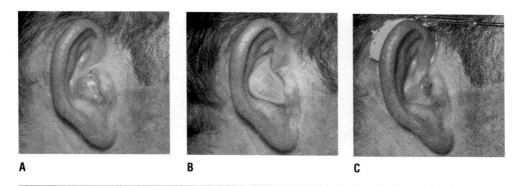

A          B          C

▣ **FIGURE 13.20**  (A) Small hearing aid in ear canal, (B) large hearing aid in ear canal, (C) hearing aid attached to glasses.
(Jane Schemilt/Science Photo Library/Photo Researchers, Inc.)

# Pharmacology Relating to the Ear

| | |
|---|---|
| **antibiotic otic (OH tik) solution** | Eardrops to treat otitis externa. |
| **antihistamines (an tye HISS tah meens)** | Some types of antihistamine medications are effective in treating the nausea associated with vertigo. |
| **anti-inflammatory otic (OH tik) solution** | Reduces inflammation, itching, and edema associated with otitis externa. |
| **oral antibiotics** | Oral antibiotics are required to treat otitis media and labyrinthitis because the tympanic membrane prevents eardrops from reaching the middle ear cavity. |

# Abbreviations Relating to the Ear

| | | | | |
|---|---|---|---|---|
| **AD** | right ear | **Hz** | hertz |
| **AS** | left ear | **OM** | otitis media |
| **ASL** | American Sign Language | **Oto** | otology |
| **AU** | both ears | **PE tube** | polyethylene tube placed in the eardrum |
| **BC** | bone conduction | **PORP** | partial ossicular replacement prosthesis |
| **dB** | decibel | **SEE–2** | Signing Exact English |
| **EENT** | eyes, ears, nose, throat | **SOM** | serous otitis media |
| **ENT** | ear, nose, and throat | **TORP** | total ossicular replacement prosthesis |
| **HEENT** | head, ears, eyes, nose, throat | | |

# Chapter Review

## Pronunciation Practice

 *You will find the pronunciation for each term on the enclosed CD-ROM. Check each one off as you master it.*

- ❑ accommodation (ah kom oh **DAY** shun)
- ❑ achromatopsia (ah kroh mah **TOP** see ah)
- ❑ acoustic (ah **KOOS** tik)
- ❑ acoustic neuroma (ah **KOOS** tik noor **OH** mah)
- ❑ amblyopia (am blee **OH** pee ah)
- ❑ American Sign Language
- ❑ amplification (am plih fih **KAY** shun) device
- ❑ anacusis (an ah **KOO** sis)
- ❑ anesthetic ophthalmic (off **THAL** mik) solutions
- ❑ antibiotic ophthalmic (off **THAL** mik) solution
- ❑ antibiotic otic (**OH** tik) solution
- ❑ antiglaucoma (an tye glau **KOH** mah) medications
- ❑ antihistamines (an tye **HISS** tah meens)
- ❑ anti-inflammatory otic (**OH** tik) solution
- ❑ aqueous (**AY** kwee us) humor
- ❑ artificial tears
- ❑ astigmatism (ah **STIG** mah tizm)
- ❑ audiogram (**AW** dee oh gram)
- ❑ audiologist (aw dee **OL** oh jist)
- ❑ audiology (aw dee **OL** oh jee)
- ❑ audiometer (aw dee **OM** eh ter)
- ❑ audiometry (aw dee **OM** eh tree)
- ❑ auditory (**AW** dih tor ee) canal
- ❑ auditory (**AW** dih tor ee) tube
- ❑ aural (**AW** ral)
- ❑ auricle (**AW** rih k'l)
- ❑ binaural (bin **AW** rall)
- ❑ binocular (bih **NOK** yoo lar)
- ❑ blepharectomy (blef ah **REK** toh mee)
- ❑ blepharitis (blef ah **RYE** tis)
- ❑ blepharochalasis (blef ah roh **KAL** ah sis)
- ❑ blepharoplasty (**BLEF** ah roh plass tee)
- ❑ blepharoptosis (blef ah rop **TOH** sis)
- ❑ cataract (**KAT** ah rakt)
- ❑ cerumen (seh **ROO** men)

- ❑ chalazion (kah **LAY** zee on)
- ❑ choroid (**KOR** oyd)
- ❑ cilia (**SIL** ee ah)
- ❑ ciliary (**SIL** ee ar ee) body
- ❑ cochlea (**KOK** lee ah)
- ❑ cochlear (**KOK** lee ar)
- ❑ cochlear (**KOK** lee ar) implant
- ❑ cochlear (**KOK** lee ar) nerve
- ❑ color vision tests
- ❑ conductive (kon **DUK** tiv) hearing loss
- ❑ cones
- ❑ conjunctiva (kon **JUNK** tih vah)
- ❑ conjunctivitis (kon junk tih **VYE** tis)
- ❑ conjunctivoplasty (kon junk tih **VOH** plas tee)
- ❑ convergence (kon **VER** jens)
- ❑ cornea (**COR** nee ah)
- ❑ corneal abrasion
- ❑ cryoextraction (cry oh eks **TRAK** shun)
- ❑ cryoretinopexy (cry oh **RET** ih noh pek see)
- ❑ cycloplegia (sigh kloh **PLEE** jee ah)
- ❑ cycloplegic (sigh kloh **PLEE** jik)
- ❑ dacryocystitis (dak ree oh sis **TYE** tis)
- ❑ deafness
- ❑ decibel (**DES** ih bel)
- ❑ diabetic retinopathy (dye ah **BET** ik reh tin **OP** ah thee)
- ❑ diplopia (dip **LOH** pee ah)
- ❑ ectropion (ek **TROH** pee on)
- ❑ emmetropia (em eh **TROH** pee ah)
- ❑ entropion (en **TROH** pee on)
- ❑ enucleation (ee new klee **AH** shun)
- ❑ equilibrium (ee kwih **LIB** ree um)
- ❑ esotropia (ess oh **TROH** pee ah)
- ❑ eustachian (yoo **STAY** she en) tube
- ❑ exophthalmos (eks off **THAL** mohs)
- ❑ exotropia (eks oh **TROH** pee ah)

- external ear
- eye muscles
- eyeball
- eyelashes
- eyelids
- falling test
- fingerspelling
- fluorescein angiography (floo oh **RESS** ee in an jee **OG** rah fee)
- fluorescein (floo oh **RESS** ee in) staining
- fovea centralis (**FOH** vee ah sen **TRAH** lis)
- glaucoma (glau **KOH** mah)
- gonioscopy (goh nee **OSS** koh pee)
- hearing
- hearing aid
- hearing impairment
- hearing level
- hemianopia (hem ee ah **NOP** ee ah)
- hertz
- hordeolum (hor **DEE** oh lum)
- hyperopia (high per **OH** pee ah)
- incus (**ING** kus)
- inner ear
- interpreter
- intraocular (in trah **OCK** yoo lar)
- iridectomy (ir id **EK** toh mee)
- iridoplegia (ir id oh **PLEE** jee ah)
- iridosclerotomy (ir ih doh skleh **ROT** oh mee)
- iris (**EYE** ris)
- iritis (ih **RYE** tis)
- keratitis (kair ah **TYE** tis)
- keratometry (kair ah **TOM** eh tree)
- keratoplasty (**KAIR** ah toh plass tee)
- keratotomy (kair ah **TOT** oh mee)
- labyrinth (**LAB** ih rinth)
- labyrinthectomy (lab ih rin **THEK** toh mee)
- labyrinthitis (lab ih rin **THIGH** tis)
- lacrimal (**LAK** rim al)
- lacrimal (**LAK** rim al) ducts
- lacrimal (**LAK** rim al) glands
- laser-assisted in-situ keratomileusis (in **SIH** tyoo kair ah toh mih **LOO** sis)
- laser photocoagulation (**LAY** zer foh toh koh ag yoo **LAY** shun)
- lens
- macrotia (mah **KROH** she ah)
- macula lutea (**MAK** yoo lah loo **TEE** ah)
- macular (**MAK** yoo lar) degeneration
- malleus (**MAL** ee us)
- Ménière's disease (may nee **ARZ** dih **ZEEZ**)
- microtia (my **KROH** she ah)
- middle ear
- miotic (my **OT** ik)
- monaural (mon **AW** rall)
- monochromatism (mon oh **KROH** mah tizm)
- mucous membrane
- mydriatic (mid ree **AT** ik)
- myopia (my **OH** pee ah)
- myringectomy (mir in **GEK** toh mee)
- myringitis (mir ing **JYE** tis)
- myringoplasty (mir **IN** goh plass tee)
- myringotomy (mir in **GOT** oh mee)
- nasal cavity
- nasolacrimal (naz oh **LAK** rim al) duct
- nyctalopia (nik tah **LOH** pee ah)
- nystagmus (niss **TAG** mus)
- oblique (oh **BLEEK**) muscle
- oculomycosis (ok yoo loh my **KOH** sis)
- ophthalmalgia (off thal **MAL** jee ah)
- ophthalmic (off **THAL** mik)
- ophthalmologist (off thal **MALL** oh jist)
- ophthalmology (off thal **MALL** oh jee)
- ophthalmoplegia (off thal moh **PLEE** jee ah)
- ophthalmorrhagia (off thal moh **RAH** jee ah)
- ophthalmoscope (off **THAL** moh scope)
- ophthalmoscopy (off thal **MOSS** koh pee)
- optic (**OP** tik)
- optic (**OP** tik) disk
- optic (**OP** tik) nerve
- optician (op **TISH** an)
- optometer (op **TOM** eh ter)
- optometrist (op **TOM** eh trist)
- optometry (op **TOM** eh tree)
- oral antibiotics
- organs of Corti (**KOR** tee)
- ossicles (**OSS** ih kls)
- otalgia (oh **TAL** jee ah)

- otic (**OH** tik)
- otitis (oh **TYE** tis)
- otitis externa (oh **TYE** tis ex **TERN** ah)
- otitis media (oh **TYE** tis **MEE** dee ah)
- otologist (oh **TOL** oh jist)
- otology (oh **TOL** oh jee)
- otomycosis (oh toh my **KOH** sis)
- otoplasty (**OH** toh plass tee)
- otopyorrhea (oh toh pye oh **REE** ah)
- otorhinolaryngologist (oh toh rye noh lair in **GOL** oh jist)
- otorhinolaryngology (oh toh rye noh lair in **GOL** oh jee)
- otosclerosis (oh toh sklair **OH** sis)
- otoscope (**OH** toh scope)
- otoscopy (oh **TOSS** koh pee)
- oval window
- papilledema (pah pill eh **DEEM** ah)
- phacoemulsification (fak oh ee mull sih fih **KAY** shun)
- photorefractive keratectomy (foh toh ree **FRAK** tiv kair ah **TEK** toh mee)
- photophobia (foh toh **FOH** bee ah)
- pink eye
- pinna (**PIN** ah)
- polyethylene (pol ee **ETH** ih leen) tube
- presbycusis (pres bih **KOO** sis)
- presbyopia (prez bee **OH** pee ah)
- pupil
- radial keratotomy (**RAY** dee all kair ah **TOT** oh mee)
- rectus (**REK** tus) muscle
- refraction (ree **FRAK** shun)
- refractive (ree **FRAK** tiv) error
- residual (rih **ZID** yoo al) hearing
- retina (**RET** in ah)
- retinal (**RET** in al)
- retinal (**RET** in al) blood vessels
- retinal (**RET** in al) detachment
- retinitis pigmentosa (ret in **EYE** tis pig men **TOH** sah)
- retinoblastoma (**RET** in noh blast **OH** mah)
- retinopathy (ret in **OP** ah thee)
- retinopexy (ret ih noh **PEX** ee)
- Rinne (**RIN** eh) and Weber tuning-fork test
- rods
- saccule (**SAK** yool)
- salpingitis (sal pin **JIH** tis)
- salpingotomy (sal pin **GOT** oh mee)
- sclera (**SKLAIR** ah)
- scleral (**SKLAIR** al) buckling
- scleritis (skler **EYE** tis)
- scleromalacia (sklair oh mah **LAY** she ah)
- sclerotomy (skleh **ROT** oh mee)
- sebaceous (see **BAY** shus) glands
- semicircular canals
- sensorineural (sen soh ree **NOO** ral) hearing loss
- Signing Exact English
- slit lamp microscope
- Snellen's (**SNEL** enz) chart
- speechreading
- stapedectomy (stay pee **DEK** toh mee)
- stapes (**STAY** peez)
- strabismus (strah **BIZ** mus)
- strabotomy (strah **BOT** oh mee)
- tears
- tinnitus (tin **EYE** tus)
- tonometry (tohn **OM** eh tree)
- trachoma (tray **KOH** mah)
- tympanectomy (tim pan **EK** toh mee)
- tympanic (tim **PAN** ik)
- tympanic (tim **PAN** ik) membrane
- tympanitis (tim pan **EYE** tis)
- tympanometer (tim pah **NOM** eh ter)
- tympanometry (tim pah **NOM** eh tree)
- tympanoplasty (tim pan oh **PLASS** tee)
- tympanorrhexis (tim pan oh **REK** sis)
- tympanotomy (tim pan **OT** oh mee)
- uvea (**YOO** vee ah)
- utricle (**YOO** trih k'l)
- vertigo (**VER** tih goh)
- vestibular (ves **TIB** yoo lar) nerve
- vestibulocochlear (ves tib yoo loh **KOK** lee ar) nerve
- visual acuity (**VIZH** oo al ah **KYOO** ih tee) test
- visual field
- vitreous (**VIT** ree us) humor
- xerophthalmia (zee **ROP** thal mee ah)

# Case Study

## Ophthalmology Consultation Report

**Reason for Consultation:** Evaluation of progressive loss of vision in right eye.

**History of Present Illness:** Patient has noted gradual deterioration of vision and increasing photophobia during the past 1 year, particularly in the right eye. She states that it feels like there is a film over her right eye. She denies any change in vision in her left eye.

**Past Medical History:** Patient has used corrective lenses her entire adult life to correct hyperopia. She is not married and is nulligravida. Past medical history includes left breast cancer successfully treated with left breast mastectomy 10 years ago and cholelithiasis necessitating a cholecystectomy 2 years ago. She has no history of cardiac problems or hypertension.

**Results of Physical Examination:** Visual acuity test showed no change in this patient's long-standing hyperopia. The eye muscles function properly and there is no evidence of conjunctivitis or nystagmus. The pupils react properly to light. Intraocular pressure is normal. Ophthalmoscopy after application of mydriatic drops revealed presence of large opaque cataract in lens of right eye. There is a very small cataract forming in the left eye. There is no evidence of retinopathy, macular degeneration, or keratitis.

**Assessment:** Diminished vision in OD secondary to cataract.

**Recommendations:** Phacoemulsification of cataract followed by aspiration of lens and prosthetic lens implant.

## Critical Thinking Questions

1. The results of the physical exam state that the patient's pupils react properly to light. What does this mean? How do pupils react in bright and dim light? Why is this important?

2. Carefully read the results of the physical examination and list the eye structures that do not have any problems.

3. Briefly describe the pathologies that form the patient's past medical history that required surgery, and the surgeries.

4. The ophthalmologist placed mydriatic drops in her eyes. For what purpose? What is the general name for drops with the opposite effect?

5. This patient wears corrective lenses for which condition?
   a. farsightedness
   b. nearsightedness
   c. abnormal curvature of the cornea

6. Her cataract was removed by phacoemulsification. Using your text as a reference, what other procedure could have been used to remove a cataract?

# Chart Note Transcription

## Chart Note

The chart note below contains 10 phrases that can be reworded with a medical term that you learned in this chapter. Each phrase is identified with an underline. Determine the medical term and write your answers in the space provided.

**Current Complaint:** An 8-year-old female was referred to the specialist in the treatment of diseases of the ear, nose, and throat① by her pediatrician for evaluation of chronic left middle ear infection.②

**Past History:** Patient's mother reports that her daughter began to experience recurrent ear infections at approximately 6 months of age. Frequency of the infections has increased during the past 2 years and she is missing school. Mother also reports the child's teacher feels she is having difficulty hearing in the classroom.

**Signs and Symptoms:** Both ears③ visual examination of the external ear canal and eardrum④ revealed that the membrane between the external ear canal and middle ear⑤ is normal on the right and bulging on the left. An excessive amount of ear wax⑥ was noted in both ears.③ Measurement of the movement of the eardrum⑦ indicates that there is a buildup of fluid in the left middle ear. Tests of hearing ability⑧ report normal hearing on the right and loss of hearing as a result of the blocking of sound transmission in the middle ear⑨ on the left. Patient also noted to have acute pharyngitis with purulent drainage at time of evaluation.

**Diagnosis:** Hearing loss secondary to chronic left middle ear infection.

**Treatment:** Left eardrum incision⑩ with placement of polyethylene tube for drainage.

1. _____
2. _____
3. _____
4. _____
5. _____
6. _____
7. _____
8. _____
9. _____
10. _____

# Practice Exercises

## A. Complete the following statements.

1. The study of the eye is _____ .

2. The external structures of the eye consist of the _____ , _____ , _____ , _____ , and _____ .

3. Another term for eyelashes is _____ .

4. The glands responsible for tears are called _____ glands.

5. The clear, transparent portion of the sclera is called the _____ .

6. The innermost layer of the eye, which is composed of sensory receptors, is the _____ .

7. The pupil of the eye is actually a hole in the _____ .

8. The ability of the eye to adjust to variations in distance vision is called _____ .

9. The three bones in the middle ear are the _____ , _____ , and _____ .

10. The study of the ear is called _____ .

11. Another term for the eardrum is _____ .

12. _____ is produced in the oil glands in the auditory canal.

13. The _____ tube connects the nasopharynx with the middle ear.

14. The inner ear is located in a cavity within the _____ bone.

15. The _____ is responsible for conducting impulses from the ear to the brain.

16. _____ hearing loss is the result of blocking sound transmission in the middle ear.

## B. State the terms described using the combining forms provided.

The combining form *blephar/o* refers to the eyelid. Use it to write a term that means

1. inflammation of the eyelid _____

2. surgical repair of the eyelid _____

3. relaxation of the upper eyelid _____

The combining form *retin/o* refers to the retina. Use it to write a term that means

4. a disease of the retina _____

5. surgical fixation of the retina _____

The combining form *ophthalm/o* refers to the eye. Use it to write a term that means

6. the study of the eye _____

7. pertaining to the eye _____

8. an eye examination using a scope _____

The combining form *irid/o* refers to the iris. Use it to write a term that means

9. iris paralysis _____

10. excision of the iris _____

11. iris softening _____

The combining form *ot/o* refers to the ear. Write a word that means

12. ear surgical repair _____

13. pus flow from the ear _____

14. pain in the ear _____

15. inflammation of the ear _____

16. hardening of the ear _____

17. study of the ear _____

The combining form *audi/o* refers to hearing. Write a word that means

18. record of hearing _____

19. instrument to measure hearing _____

20. study of hearing _____

## C. Write the suffix for each expression and provide an example of its use.

| | | Suffix | Example |
|---|---|---|---|
| 1. | to turn | _____ | _____ |
| 2. | vision | _____ | _____ |
| 3. | inflammation of | _____ | _____ |
| 4. | the study of | _____ | _____ |
| 5. | incision into | _____ | _____ |
| 6. | surgical repair | _____ | _____ |
| 7. | surgical fixation | _____ | _____ |
| 8. | abnormal narrowing | _____ | _____ |
| 9. | ear condition | _____ | _____ |
| 10. | hearing | _____ | _____ |

## D. Define the following combining forms.

1. dacry/o _____

2. uve/o _____

3. aque/o _____

4. phot/o _____

5. kerat/o _____

6. vitre/o _____

7. dipl/o _____

8. glauc/o _____

9. presby/o _____

10. ambly/o _____

11. aur/o _____

12. staped/o _____

13. acous/o _____

14. salping/o _____

15. myring/o _____

## E. Define the following terms.

1. amblyopia _____
2. diplopia _____
3. mydriatic _____
4. miotic _____
5. presbyopia _____
6. tinnitus _____
7. stapes _____
8. tympanometry _____
9. eustachian tube _____
10. labyrinth _____
11. audiogram _____
12. otitis media _____

## F. Match the terms in column A with the definitions in column B.

| A | B |
|---|---|
| 1. _____ accommodation | a. opacity of the lens |
| 2. _____ sclera | b. muscle regulating size of pupil |
| 3. _____ cataract | c. nearsightedness |
| 4. _____ conjunctiva | d. protective membrane of eye |
| 5. _____ iris | e. blind spot |
| 6. _____ refraction | f. involuntary movements of eye |
| 7. _____ myopia | g. white of eye |
| 8. _____ nystagmus | h. eye changes for near and far vision |
| 9. _____ optic disk | i. bend light rays |
| 10. _____ vitreous humor | j. material filling eyeball |
| 11. _____ emmetropia | k. normal refraction of eye |
| 12. _____ myringotomy | l. decreases amount of aqueous humor inside eye |
| 13. _____ tympanoplasty | m. removal of stapes bone |
| 14. _____ otoplasty | n. reconstruction of eardrum |
| 15. _____ stapedectomy | o. surgical puncture of eardrum |
| 16. _____ antiglaucoma drugs | p. change size of pinna |

## G. Identify the following abbreviations.

1. OS _____
2. OU _____
3. REM _____
4. Acc _____
5. SMD _____
6. PERRLA _____

7. IOP _____

8. XT _____

9. OD _____

10. VF _____

11. PE tube _____

12. EENT _____

13. BC _____

14. AU _____

15. OM _____

**H. Use the following terms in the sentences that follow. There are more terms than you will need to complete the exercise.**

emmetropia          hyperopia          cataract          strabismus

exophthalmos        conjunctivitis     tonometry         Ménière's disease

entropion           chalazion          presbycusis       inner ear

otorhinolaryngologist   hordeolum       myopia            acoustic neuroma

1. Cheri is having a regular eye checkup. The pressure reading test that the physician will do to detect glaucoma is _____ .

2. Gracibel has developed a painful, hard mass/tumor on her eyelid. This is called a(n) _____ .

3. Carlos's ophthalmologist tells him that he has normal vision. This is called _____ .

4. Ana has been given an antibiotic eye ointment for pink eye. The medical term for this condition is _____ .

5. Adrian is nearsighted and cannot read signs in the distance. This is called _____ .

6. Ivan is scheduled to have surgery to have the opaque lens of his right eye removed. This condition is a(n) _____ .

7. Roberto has developed a sty on the corner of his left eye. He has been told to treat it with hot compresses. This condition is called a(n) _____ .

8. Lorenzo has an uncomfortable disorder in which his eyelashes are rubbing his cornea, due to inversion of his eyelid. This condition is called _____ .

9. Judith has twin boys with crossed eyes that will require surgical correction. The medical term for this condition is _____ .

10. Beth is farsighted and has difficulty reading textbooks. Her eyeglass correction will be for _____ .

11. Tina suffered from a lack of iodine in her diet and developed a thyroid problem. After her thyroid problem was corrected, she still had protruding eyeballs. This is called _____ .

12. Grace was told by her physician that her hearing loss was a part of the aging process. The term for this is _____ .

13. Stacey is having frequent middle ear infections and wishes to be treated by a specialist. She would go to a(n) _____ .

14. Warren was told that his dizziness may be caused by a problem in the _____ area.

15. Shantel is suffering from an abnormal condition of the inner ear, vertigo, and tinnitus. She may have _____ .

16. Keisha was told that her tumor of the eighth cranial nerve was benign, but she still experienced a hearing loss as a result of the tumor. This tumor is called a(n) _____ .

# Professional Journal

In this exercise you will now have an opportunity to put the words you have learned into practice. Imagine yourself in the role of an optometrist. If you refer back to the Professional Profile at the beginning of this chapter, you will see that this health care professional is responsible for examining eyes for diseases, assessing visual acuity, prescribing corrective lenses and eye treatments, and educating patients. Use the 10 words listed below, or any other new terms from this chapter, to write sentences to describe the patients you saw today.

An example of a sentence is *The patient's increased* **intraocular** *pressure and* **glaucoma** *eventually resulted in her blindness.*

1. blepharectomy _____

2. cataract _____

3. conjunctivitis _____

4. myopia _____

5. fluorescein angiography _____

6. macular degeneration _____

7. miotic drops _____

8. radial keratotomy _____

9. cornea _____

10. photophobia _____

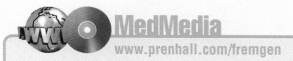

**MedMedia**
www.prenhall.com/fremgen

Use the CD-ROM enclosed with your textbook to gain additional reinforcement through interactive word building exercises, spelling games, labeling activities, and additional quizzes.

Use the above address to access the free, interactive Companion Website created for this textbook. Get hints, instant feedback, and textbook references to chapter-related multiple-choice questions, as well as labeling and matching exercises. In addition, you will find an audio glossary, case studies, and Internet exploration exercises.

*For more information regarding eye or ear diseases, visit the following websites:*

Centers for Disease Control and Prevention's Health Topics A to Z at **www.cdc.gov/health/default.htm**

Health Information provided by the National Institutes of Health at **http://health./nih.gov**

Health Information provided by the Stanford Health Library at **http://healthlibrary.stanford.edu**

InteliHealth featuring Harvard Medical School"s Consumer Health Information at **www.intelihealth.com**

Medical Encyclopedia provided by University of Maryland Medicine at **www.umm.edu/ency**

University of Iowa Health Care's Virtual Hospital at **www.vh.org**

# Chapter 14
# Special Topics

## Learning Objectives

*Upon completion of this chapter, you will be able to:*

- Recognize the combining forms and suffixes for the medical fields introduced in this chapter.

- Gain the ability to pronounce medical terms.

- Discuss pertinent information relating to each special topic covered in this chapter.

- Build medical terms relating to the topics.

- Define vocabulary, pathology, diagnostic, and therapeutic medical terms relating to the topics.

- Interpret abbreviations associated with the topics.

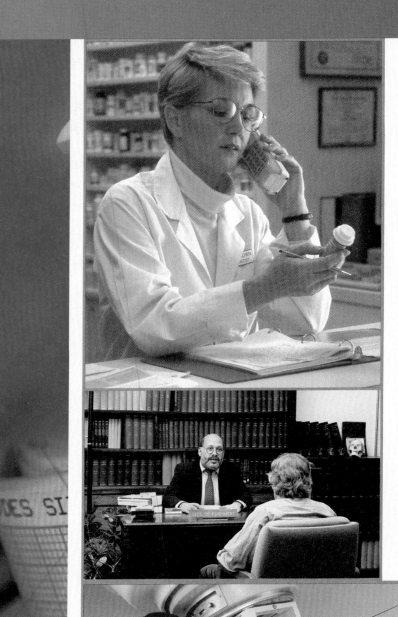

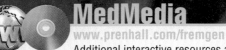

## MedMedia
www.prenhall.com/fremgen
Additional interactive resources and activities for this chapter can be found on the Companion Website. For animations, audio glossary, and review, access the accompanying CD-ROM in this book.

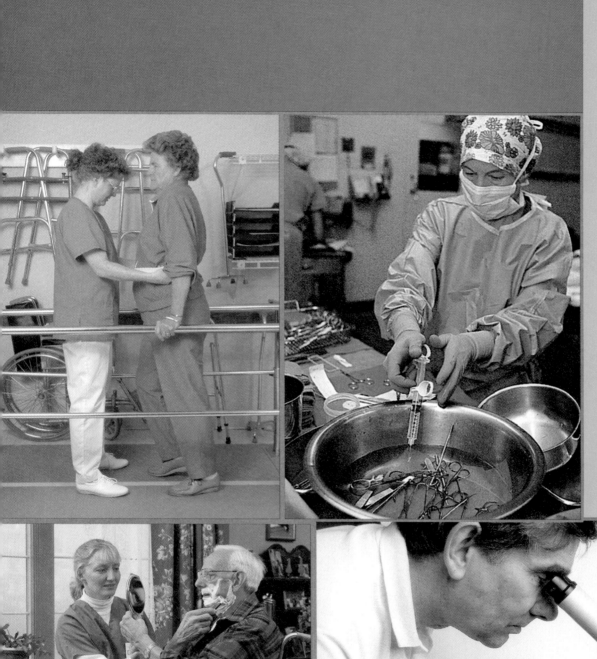

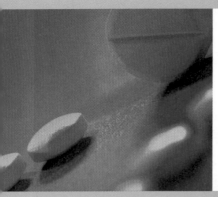

# Introduction

There are many specialized areas within medicine and each has medical terms relating to that field. This chapter presents medical terminology from six of these fields:

1. Pharmacology
2. Mental health
3. Diagnostic imaging
4. Rehabilitation services
5. Surgery
6. Oncology

# Part I: Pharmacology

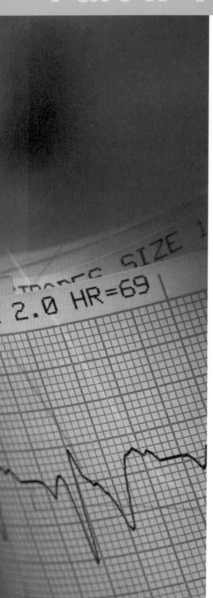

## Professional Profile

### Pharmacy

Pharmacists prepare and dispense drugs. The pharmacist receives drug requests made by physicians and also gathers pertinent information that would affect the dispensing of certain drugs, such as allergies, previous drug interactions, and patient history. They also review patients' medications for drug interactions, provide health care workers with information regarding drugs, and educate the public concerning their drugs. Pharmacy workers are found in acute and long-term care facilities, clinics, community-based pharmacies, health departments, and pharmaceutical companies.

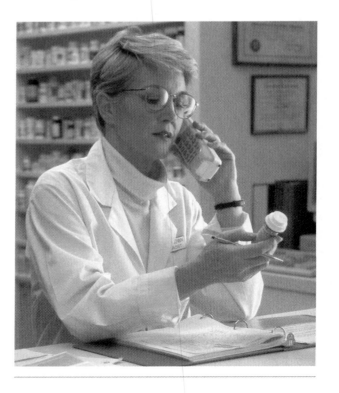

## Pharmacist (RPh or PharmD)

- Fills prescriptions as written by physicians, dentists, and other doctors
- Graduates from an accredited 5-year baccalaureate or 6-year graduate pharmacy program
- Completes an internship
- Passes an examination

## Pharmacy Technician

- Works under the supervision of a pharmacist
- Performs computer order entry, generates prescription labels, and keeps electronic patient profiles
- Completes a 1- to 2-year associate's degree program
- Some states offer certification

*For more information regarding these health careers, visit the following websites:*
American Association of Colleges of Pharmacy at **www.aacp.org**
American Association of Pharmacy Technicians at
**www.pharmacytechnician.com**
American Pharmaceutical Association at **www.aphanet.org**

# Overview

## Combining Forms Relating to Pharmacology

| | | | |
|---|---|---|---|
| aer/o | air | or/o | mouth |
| bucc/o | cheek | pharmac/o | drug |
| chem/o | drug | rect/o | rectum |
| cutane/o | skin | toxic/o | poison |
| derm/o | skin | vagin/o | vagina |
| lingu/o | tongue | ven/o | vein |
| muscul/o | muscle | | |

## Prefixes Relating to Pharmacology

| Prefix | Meaning | Example |
|---|---|---|
| intra- | within | intravenous |
| sub- | under | sublingual |
| trans- | across | transdermal |

# Pharmacology

**Pharmacology** (far ma **KALL** oh jee) is the study of the origin, characteristics, and effects of drugs. Drugs are obtained from many different sources. Some drugs, such as vitamins, are found naturally in the foods we eat. Others, such as hormones, are obtained from animals. Penicillin and some of the other antibiotics are developed from mold, which is a fungus. Plants have been the source of many of today's drugs. Many drugs, such as those used in chemotherapy, are synthetic, which means they are developed by artificial means in the laboratory.

**MED TERM TIP** The terms *drug* and *medication* have the same meaning. However, the general public often uses the term *drug* to refer to a narcotic type of medication. The term can also mean illegal chemical substances. For purposes of medical terminology, use of the word *drug* means medication.

## Drug Names

Every drug has three different names:

1. **Chemical** (**KEM** ih cal) **name**
2. **Generic**, or **nonproprietary, name**
3. **Brand, trade,** or **proprietary** (proh **PRYE** ah tair ee) **name**

All drugs are chemicals. The chemical name describes the chemical formula or molecular structure of a particular drug. For example, the chemical name for ibuprofen, an over-the-counter pain medication, is 2-*p*-isobutylphenyl propionic acid. Just as in this case, chemical names are usually very long, so a shorter name is given to the drug. This name is the generic or nonproprietary name, and it is recognized and accepted as the official name for a drug.

Each drug has only one generic name, such as ibuprofen, and this name is not subject to trademark, so any **pharmaceutical** (far mih **SOO** tih kal) manufacturer may use it. However, the pharmaceutical company that originally developed the drug has exclusive rights to produce it for 17 years. After that time, any manufacturer may produce and sell the drug. When a company manufactures a drug for sale, it must choose a brand, or proprietary, name for its product. This is the company's trademark for the drug. For example, ibuprofen is known by several brand names, including Motrin™, Advil™, and Nuprin™. All three are the same ibuprofen; they are just marketed by different pharmaceutical companies. (See Table 14.1 for examples of different drug names.)

Generic drugs are usually priced lower than brand name drugs. A physician can indicate on the prescription if the **pharmacist** (**FAR** mah sist) may substitute a generic drug for a brand name. The physician may prefer that a particular brand name drug be used if he or she believes it to be more effective than the generic drug.

**MED TERM TIP** It is critical that patients receive the correct drug, but it is not possible to list or remember all the drug names. You must acquire the habit of looking up any drug name you do not recognize in the *Physician's Desk Reference (PDR)*. Every medical office or medical facility should have a copy of this book.

| Table 14.1 | Examples of Different Drug Names | |
|---|---|---|
| **Chemical Name** | **Generic Name** | **Brand Names** |
| 2-*p*-isobutylphenyl propionic acid | Ibuprofen | Motrin™ |
| | | Advil™ |
| | | Nuprin™ |
| Acetylsalicylic acid | Aspirin | Anacin™ |
| | | Bufferin™ |
| | | Excedrin™ |
| *S*-2-[1-(methylamino) ethyl] benzenemethanol hydrochloride | Pseudoephedrine hydrochloride | Sudafed™ Actifed™ |
| | | Nucofed™ |

# Legal Classification of Drugs

A **prescription** (prih **SKRIP** shun) **drug** can only be ordered by a licensed physician, dentist, or veterinarian. These drugs must include the words "Caution: Federal law prohibits dispensing without prescription" on their labels. Antibiotics, such as penicillin, and heart medications, such as digoxin, are available only by prescription. A **prescription** (prih **SKRIP** shun) is the written explanation to the pharmacist regarding the name of the medication, the dosage, and the times of administration. A licensed physician can also give a prescription order orally to the pharmacist.

A drug that does not require a prescription is referred to as an **over-the-counter** (OTC) **drug.** Many medications or drugs can be purchased without a prescription, for example, aspirin, antacids, and antidiarrheal medications. However, taking aspirin along with an anticoagulant, such as coumadin, can cause internal bleeding in some people, and OTC antacids interfere with the absorption of the prescription drug tetracycline into the body. It is better for the physician or pharmacist to advise the patient on the proper OTC drugs to use with prescription drugs.

Certain drugs are **controlled substances** if they have a potential for being addictive (habit forming) or can be abused. The **Drug Enforcement Agency** (DEA) enforces the control of these drugs. Some of the more commonly prescribed controlled substances are:

- anabolic steroids
- butabarbital
- chloral hydrate
- cocaine
- codeine
- diazepam
- heroin
- LSD
- marijuana
- morphine
- opium
- phenobarbital
- secobarbital

Controlled drugs are classified as Schedule I through Schedule V, which indicates their potential for abuse. The differences between each schedule are listed in Table 14.2.

| Table 14.2 | Schedule for Controlled Substances |
|---|---|
| **Classification** | **Meaning** |
| Schedule I | Drugs with the highest potential for addiction and abuse. They are not accepted for medical use. Examples are heroin and LSD. |
| Schedule II | Drugs with a high potential for addiction and abuse accepted for medical use in the United States. Examples are codeine, cocaine, morphine, opium, and secobarbital. |
| Schedule III | Drugs with a moderate to low potential for addiction and abuse. Examples are butabarbital, anabolic steroids, and acetaminophen with codeine. |
| Schedule IV | Drugs with a lower potential for addiction and abuse than Schedule III drugs. Examples are chloral hydrate, phenobarbital, and diazepam. |
| Schedule V | Drugs with a low potential for addiction and abuse. An example is low-strength codeine combined with other drugs to suppress coughing. |

```
┌─────────────────────────────────────────────────────────┐
│                                                         │
│   Melvin A. Brown, M.D.                                 │
│   Chicago, IL 60000                                     │
│                                                         │
│   DEA# 123456789     Phone# 123-0000                   │
│   NAME  (patient name here)   AGE _____              │
│   ADDRESS _____   DATE _____        │
│   Rx      Estrace 1 mg.                                 │
│           dtd C                                         │
│           Sig: 1 q am                                   │
│   [x]  LABEL                                            │
│   REFILL   3   TIMES                                    │
│   [ ] MAY SUBSTITUTE                                    │
│   [x] MAY NOT SUBSTITUTE       (physician signature here) M.D. │
│                                                         │
│   _____                │
│                                                         │
└─────────────────────────────────────────────────────────┘
```

**FIGURE 14.1**   Sample prescription.

## How to Read a Prescription

A prescription is not difficult to read once you understand the symbols that are used. Symbols and abbreviations based on Latin and Greek words are used to save time for the physician. For example, the abbreviation po, meaning to be taken by mouth, comes from the Latin term *per os,* which means by mouth.

See ▪ Figure 14.1 for an example of a prescription. In this example, the prescription is for the patient to take (Rx) the medication Estrace™, which is a form of the hormone estrogen. The pharmacist is instructed to give the patient (dtd) 100 (C) tablets of the 1 mg size. The instructions on the label are to say (Sig) to take 1 tablet every morning (1 q am). The instructions conclude by informing the pharmacist to refill the prescription three times and not to substitute with another (generic) medication.

On some prescriptions the physician will give a prn refill order, meaning that the prescription can be refilled as needed. The physician will fill in the name, address, age of the patient, and date. He or she must also sign his or her name at the bottom of the prescription. A blank prescription cannot be handed to a patient.

The physician's instruction to the patient will be placed on the label. The pharmacist will also include instructions about the medication and alert the patient to side effects that may need to be reported to the physician. In addition, any special instructions regarding the medication (i.e., take with meals, do not take along with dairy products) will also be supplied by the pharmacist.

## Routes and Methods of Drug Administration

The method by which a drug is introduced into the body is referred to as the *route of administration.* To be effective, drugs must be administered by a particular route. In some cases, there may be a variety of routes by which a drug can be administered. For instance, the female hormone estrogen can be administered orally in pill form or on a patch applied to the skin. In general, the routes of administration are as follows:

**Oral** (**OR** al): This method includes all drugs that are given by mouth. The advantages are ease of administration and a slow rate of absorption via stomach and intestinal wall. The disadvantages include slowness of absorption and destruction of some chemical compounds by gastric juices. In addition, some medications, such as aspirin, can have a corrosive action on the stomach lining.

**Sublingual** (sub **LING** gwal): These are drugs that are held under the tongue and not swallowed. The medication is absorbed by the blood vessels on the underside of the tongue as the saliva dissolves it. The rate of absorption is quicker than the oral route. Nitroglycerin to treat angina or chest pain is administered by this route (see ▨ Figure 14.2).

**Inhalation** (in hah **LAY** shun): Includes drugs that are inhaled directly into the nose and mouth. **Aerosol** (**AIR** oh sol) sprays are administered by this route (see ▨ Figure 14.3).

**Parenteral** (par **EN** ter al): This is an invasive method of administering drugs since it requires the skin to be punctured by a needle. The needle with syringe attached is introduced either under the skin or into a muscle, vein, or body cavity. See Table 14.3 for a description of the methods for parenteral administration.

**Transdermal** (tranz **DER** mal): The medication coats the underside of a patch, which is applied to the skin. The medication is then absorbed across the skin. Examples include birth control patches and nicotine patches.

**Rectal** (**REK** tal): This medication is introduced directly into the rectal cavity in the form of **suppositories** (suh **POZ** ih tor ees) or solution. Drugs may have to be administered by this route if the patient is unable to take them by mouth due to nausea, vomiting, or surgery.

**Topical** (**TOP** ih kal): This medication is applied directly to the skin or mucous membranes. They are distributed in ointment, cream, or lotion form, and are used to treat skin infections and eruptions.

**Vaginal** (**VAJ** in al): Tablets and suppositories may be inserted vaginally to treat vaginal yeast infections and other irritations.

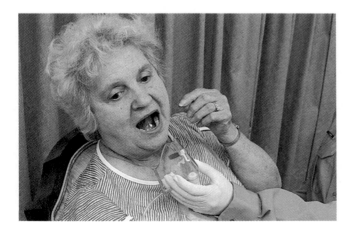

▨ **FIGURE 14.2** Patient taking a nitroglycerine tablet sublingually.

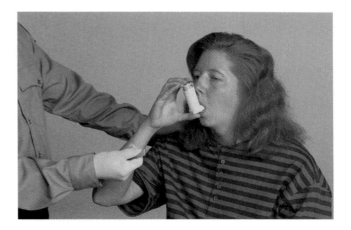

▨ **FIGURE 14.3** A prescribed inhaler may help a patient who has respiratory problems.

**Eyedrops:** These drops are used during eye examinations to dilate the pupil of the eye for better examination of the interior of the eye. They are also placed into the eye to control eye pressure in glaucoma and treat infections.

**Eardrops:** These drops are placed directly into the ear canal for the purpose of relieving pain or treating infection.

**Buccal (BUCK al):** Drugs that are placed under the lip or between the cheek and gum.

| Table 14.3 | Methods for Parenteral Administration of Drugs |
|---|---|
| **Method** | **Description** |
| **intracavitary (in trah KAV ih tair ee)** | Injection into a body cavity such as the peritoneal and chest cavity. |
| **intradermal (in trah DER mal) (ID)** | Very shallow injection just under the top layer of skin. Commonly used in skin testing for allergies (see ■ Figure 14.4). |
| **intramuscular (in trah MUSS kyoo lar) (IM)** | Injection directly into the muscle of the buttocks, thigh, or upper arm. They are used when there is a large amount of medication or it is irritating (see ■ Figures 14.4 and 14.5). |
| **intrathecal (in trah THEE kal)** | Injection into the meningeal space surrounding the brain and spinal cord. |
| **intravenous (in trah VEE nus) (IV)** | Injection into the veins. This route can be set up so that there is a continuous administration of medication (see Figure 14.4). |
| **subcutaneous (sub kyoo TAY nee us) (SC)** | Injection into the subcutaneous layer of the skin, usually the upper, outer arm (see Figure 14.4). |

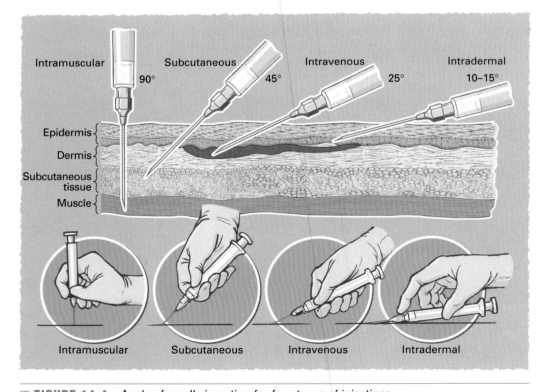

■ **FIGURE 14.4** Angle of needle insertion for four types of injections.

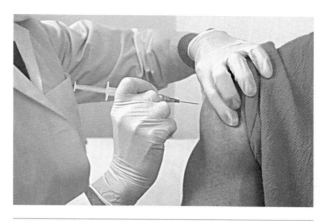

**FIGURE 14.5**   Intramuscular injections.

# Vocabulary Relating to Pharmacology

| | |
|---|---|
| addiction (ah DICK shun) | Acquired dependence on a drug. |
| additive | The sum of the action of two (or more) drugs given. In this case, the total strength of the medications is equal to the sum of the strength of each individual drug. |
| antidote (AN tih doht) | Substance that will neutralize poisons or their side effects. |
| broad spectrum | Ability of a drug to be effective against a wide range of microorganisms. |
| contraindication (kon trah in dih KAY shun) | Condition in which a particular drug should not be used. |
| cumulative action | Action that occurs in the body when a drug is allowed to accumulate or stay in the body. |
| dilute | To weaken the strength of a substance by adding something else. |
| drug interaction | Occurs when the effect of one drug is altered because it was taken at the same time as another drug. |
| drug tolerance | Decrease in susceptibility to a drug after continued use of the drug. |
| habituation (hah bich yoo AY shun) | Development of an emotional dependence on a drug due to repeated use. |
| iatrogenic (eye ah troh JEN ik) | Usually an unfavorable response that results from taking a medication. |
| idiosyncrasy (id ee oh SIN krah see) | Unusual or abnormal response to a drug or food. |
| placebo (plah SEE boh) | Inactive, harmless substance used to satisfy a patient's desire for medication. This is also used in research when given to a control group of patients in a study in which another group receives a drug. The effect of the placebo versus the drug is then observed. |
| potentiation (poe ten chee A shun) | Giving a patient a second drug to boost (potentiate) the effect of another drug. The total strength of the drugs is greater than the sum of the strength of the individual drugs. |
| prophylaxis (proh fih LAK sis) | Prevention of disease. For example, an antibiotic can be used to prevent the occurrence of a disease. |
| side effect | Response to a drug other than the effect desired. Also called an *adverse reaction*. |
| tolerance (TAHL er ans) | Development of a capacity for withstanding a large amount of a substance, such as foods, drugs, or poison, without any adverse effect. A decreased sensitivity to further doses will develop. |
| toxicity (tok SISS ih tee) | Extent or degree to which a substance is poisonous. |
| unit dose | Drug dosage system that provides prepackaged, prelabeled, individual medications that are ready for immediate use by the patient. |

# Abbreviations Relating to Pharmacology

| | | | |
|---|---|---|---|
| @ | at | ii | two |
| ā | before | iii | three |
| ac | before meals | IM | intramuscular |
| AD | right ear | inj | injection |
| ad lib | as desired | IU | international unit |
| am, AM | morning | IV | intravenous |
| amt | amount | kg | kilogram |
| ante | before | L | liter |
| APAP | acetaminophen (Tylenol™) | liq | liquid |
| aq | aqueous (water) | mcg | microgram |
| ASA | aspirin | mEq | milliequivalent |
| bid | twice a day | mg | milligram |
| C | 100 | mL | milliliter |
| c̄ | with | noc | night |
| cap(s) | capsule(s) | no sub | no substitute |
| cc | cubic centimeter | non rep | do not repeat |
| d | day | NPO | nothing by mouth |
| d/c, DISC | discontinue | NS | normal saline |
| DC, disc | discontinue | od | overdose |
| DEA | Drug Enforcement Agency | oint | ointment |
| dil | dilute | OTC | over the counter |
| disp | dispense | oz | ounce |
| dr | dram | p̄ | after |
| dtd | give of such a dose | pc | after meals |
| Dx | diagnosis | PCA | patient-controlled administration |
| elix | elixir | PDR | *Physician's Desk Reference* |
| emul | emulsion | per | with |
| et | and | PM, pm | evening |
| FDA | Federal Drug Administration | PO | phone order |
| fl | fluid | po | by mouth |
| gm | gram | prn | as needed |
| gr | grain | pt | pint, patient |
| gt | drop | q | every |
| gtt | drops | qam | every morning |
| hs | at bedtime | qd | once a day/every day |
| ī | one | qh | every hour |
| ID | intradermal | qhs | at bedtime |

| | | | |
|---|---|---|---|
| qid | four times a day | syr | syrup |
| qod | every other day | T, tbsp | tablespoon |
| qs | quantity sufficient | t, tsp | teaspoon |
| Rx | take | tab | tablet |
| s̄ | without | tid | three times a day |
| SC | subcutaneous | tinc, tr | tincture |
| Sig | label as follows/directions | TO | telephone order |
| sl | under the tongue | top | apply topically |
| sol | solution | u | unit |
| s̄s̄ | one-half | ung | ointment |
| stat | at once/immediately | VO | verbal order |
| Subc, SubQ | subcutaneous | wt | weight |
| suppos, supp. | suppository | x | times |
| susp | suspension | | |

**MED TERM TIP**

Many abbreviations have multiple meanings, such as od, which can mean overdose (od) or right eye (OD), depending on whether the letters are lowercase or capitalized. Care must be taken when reading abbreviations since some may be written too quickly, making them difficult to decipher. Never create your own abbreviations. Some of the most common abbreviations are listed above.

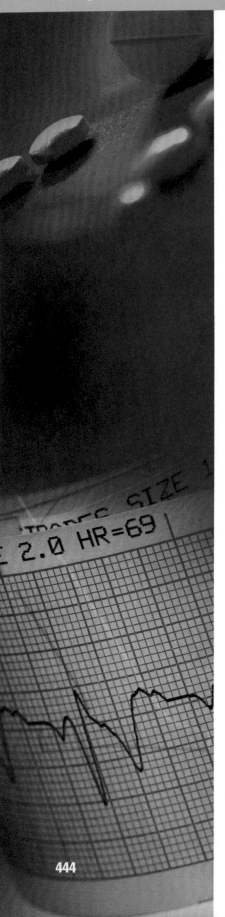

## Professional Profile

### Mental Health

Mental health workers work together to diagnose and treat clients with mental and emotional disorders, counsel persons with substance abuse problems, and assist in resolving family conflicts. They work in hospitals, mental health facilities, rehabilitation facilities, and in private practices.

### Psychiatrists (MD or DO)

- A physician with specialized training in diagnosing and treating mental disorders
- Prescribes medication and conducts counseling

### Clinical Psychologist (PhD)

- Diagnoses and treats mental disorders
- Specializes in using individual and group counseling to treat patients
- Completes a PhD degree in clinical or counseling psychology
- Completes a 2-year supervised clinical internship

### Psychiatric Mental Health Technician

- Works under the supervision of physicians, psychologists, and nurses
- Also known as psychiatric aides
- May also assist with nursing and personal care tasks
- Receives on-the-job training

*For more information regarding these health careers, visit the following websites:*
American Psychiatric Association at **www.psych.org**
American Psychological Association at **www.apa.org**

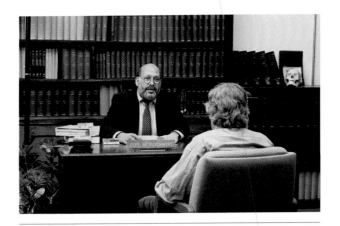

# Overview

## Combining Forms Relating to Mental Health

| | |
|---|---|
| anxi/o | anxiety |
| ment/o | mind |
| phren/o | mind |
| psych/o | mind |
| schiz/o | divided |
| somat/o | body |
| somn/o | sleep |

## Suffixes Relating to Mental Health

| Suffix | Meaning | Example |
|---|---|---|
| -iatrist | physician | psychiatrist |
| -mania | excessive preoccupation | pyromania |
| -philia | affinity for, craving for | pedophilia |
| -phobia | irrational fear | photophobia |

# Mental Health Disciplines

## Psychology

**Psychology** (sigh **KALL** oh jee) is the study of human behavior and thought process. This behavioral science is primarily concerned with understanding how human beings interact with their physical environment and with each other. Behavior can be divided into two categories, normal and abnormal. The study of **normal psychology** includes how the personality develops, how people handle stress, and the stages of mental development. In contrast, **abnormal psychology** studies and treats behaviors that are outside of normal and that are detrimental to the person or society. These maladaptive behaviors range from occasional difficulty coping with stress, to bizarre actions and beliefs, to total withdrawal. A **clinical psychologist** (sigh **KALL** oh jist) is a specialist in evaluating and treating persons with mental and emotional disorders.

 **MED TERM TIP** All social interactions pose some problems for some people. These problems are not necessarily abnormal. One means of judging if behavior is abnormal is to compare one person's behavior with others in the community. Also, if a person's behavior interferes with the activities of daily living it is often considered abnormal.

## Psychiatry

**Psychiatry** (sigh **KIGH** ah tree) is the branch of medicine that deals with the diagnosis, treatment, and prevention of mental disorders. A **psychiatrist** (sigh **KIGH** ah trist) is a medical physician specializing in the care of patients with mental, emotional, and behavioral disorders. Other health professions also have specialty areas in caring for clients with mental illness. Good examples are **psychiatric** (sigh kee **AT** rik) **nurses** and **psychiatric social workers.**

# Pathology Relating to Mental Health

The legal definition of mental disorder is "impaired judgment and lack of self-control." The guide for terminology and classifications relating to psychiatric disorders is the *Diagnostic and Statistical Manual of Mental Disorders* (DSM-IV, 1994), which is published by the American Psychiatric Association. The DSM organizes mental disorders into 14 major diagnostic categories of mental disorders.

| | |
|---|---|
| **Anxiety disorders** | Characterized by persistent worry and apprehension; includes:<br>• **panic attacks**<br>• **anxiety** (ang **ZY** eh tee)<br>• **phobias** (**FOH** bee ahs)—irrational fear, such as **photophobia** (foh toh **FOH** bee ah), or fear of light<br>• **obsessive-compulsive disorder** (ob **SESS** iv kom **PUHL** siv) (OCD)—performing repetitive rituals to reduce anxiety |
| **Cognitive disorders** | Deterioration of mental functions due to temporary brain or permanent brain dysfunction; also called **organic mental disease;** includes:<br>• **dementia** (dee **MEN** she ah)—progressive confusion and disorientation<br>• degenerative disorders such as **Alzheimer's disease** (**ALTS** high merz dih **ZEEZ**) |
| **Disorders diagnosed in infancy and childhood** | Mental disorders associated with childhood; includes:<br>• **mental retardation**<br>• **attention deficit disorder** (**DEFF** ih sit dis **OR** der) (ADD)<br>• **autism** (**AW** tizm)—extreme withdrawal |
| **Dissociative disorders** | Disorders in which severe emotional conflict is so repressed that a split in the personality occurs; includes:<br>• **amnesia** (am **NEE** zee ah)—loss of memory<br>• **multiple personality disorder** (**MULL** tih pl per son **AL** ih tee dis **OR** der) |
| **Eating disorders** | Abnormal behaviors related to eating; includes:<br>• **anorexia nervosa** (an oh **REK** see ah ner **VOH** sah)—refusal to eat (see ■ Figure 14.6)<br>• **bulimia** (boo **LIM** ee ah)—binge eating and intentional vomiting |
| **Factitious disorders** | Intentionally feigning illness symptoms in order to gain attention; includes:<br>• **malingering**—pretending illness or injury |
| **Impulse control disorders** | Inability to resist an impulse to perform some act that is harmful to the individual or others; includes:<br>• **kleptomania** (klep toh **MAY** nee ah)—stealing<br>• **pyromania** (pie roh **MAY** nee ah)—setting fires<br>• **explosive disorder** (ek **SPLOH** siv dis **OR** der)—violent rages<br>• **pathological** (path ah **LOJ** ih kal) **gambling** |
| **Mood disorders** | Characterized by instability in mood; includes:<br>• **major depression** with suicide potential<br>• **mania** (**MAY** nee ah)—extreme elation<br>• **bipolar disorder** (by **POHL** ar dis **OR** der) (BPD)—alternation between periods of deep depression and mania |
| **Personality disorders** | Inflexible or maladaptive behavior patterns that affect person's ability to function in society; includes:<br>• **paranoid personality disorder** (**PAIR** ah noyd per son **AL** ih tee dis **OR** der)—exaggerated feelings of persecution<br>• **narcissistic personality disorder** (nar sis **SIST** ik per son **AL** ih tee dis **OR** der)—abnormal sense of self-importance<br>• **antisocial personality disorder** (an tih **SOH** shal per son **AL** ih tee dis **OR** der)—behaviors that are against legal or social norms<br>• **passive aggressive personality** (**PASS** iv ah **GRESS** iv per son **AL** ih tee)—indirect expression of hostility or anger |

| Schizophrenia | Mental disorders characterized by distortions of reality such as:<br>• **delusions** (dee **LOO** zhuns)—a false belief held even in the face of contrary evidence<br>• **hallucinations** (hah loo sih **NAY** shuns)—perceiving something that is not there |
| --- | --- |
| Sexual disorders | Disorders include aberrant sexual activity and sexual dysfunction; includes:<br>• **pedophilia** (pee doh **FILL** ee ah)—sexual interest in children<br>• **masochism** (**MAS** oh kizm)—gratification derived from being hurt or abused<br>• **voyeurism** (**VOY** er izm)—gratification derived from observing others engaged in sexual acts<br>• **low sex drive**<br>• **premature ejaculation** (ee jak yoo **LAY** shun) |
| Sleeping disorders | Disorders relating to sleeping; includes:<br>• **insomnia** (in **SOM** nee ah)—inability to sleep<br>• **sleepwalking** |
| Somatoform disorders | Patient has physical symptoms for which no physical disease can be determined; includes:<br>• **hypochondria** (high poh **KON** dree ah)—a preoccupation with health concerns<br>• **conversion reaction**—anxiety is transformed into physical symptoms such as heart palpitations, paralysis, or blindness |
| Substance-related disorders | Overindulgence or dependence on chemical substances including alcohol, illegal drugs, and prescription drugs |

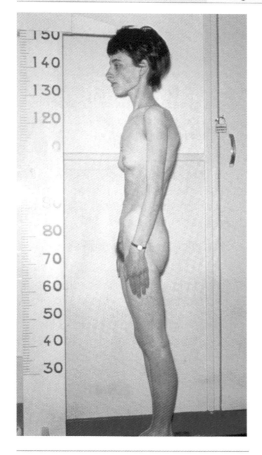

■ **FIGURE 14.6** Anorexia nervosa in a young woman.
(CNRI/Phototake NYC)

**MED TERM TIP**

Mental disorders are sometimes more simply characterized by whether they are a **neurosis** (noo **ROH** sis) or a **psychosis** (sigh **KOH** sis). Neuroses are inappropriate coping mechanisms to handle stress, such as phobias and panic attacks. Psychoses involve extreme distortions of reality and disorganization of a person's thinking, including bizarre behaviors, hallucinations, and delusions. Schizophrenia is an example of a psychosis.

# Therapeutic Procedures Relating to Mental Health

Treatments for mental disorders include a variety of methods such as **psychotherapy** (sigh koh **THAIR** ah pee), **psychopharmacology** (sigh koh far mah **KALL** oh jee), and **electroconvulsive therapy** (ee lek troh kon **VULL** siv **THAIR** ah pee) (ECT).

| | |
|---|---|
| **PSYCHOTHERAPY** | A method of treating mental disorders by mental rather than chemical or physical means. It includes psychoanalysis, humanistic therapies, and family and group therapy. |
| **Psychoanalysis** | A method of obtaining a detailed account of the past and present emotional and mental experiences from the patient to determine the source of the problem and eliminate the effects. It is a system developed by Sigmund Freud that encourages the patient to discuss repressed, painful, or hidden experiences with the hope of eliminating or minimizing the problem. |
| **Humanistic psychotherapy** | The therapist does not delve into the patients' past when using these methods. Instead, it is believed that patients can learn how to use their own internal resources to deal with their problems. The therapist creates a therapeutic atmosphere, which builds patients' self-esteem and encourages them to discuss their problems, thereby gaining insight in how to handle them. Also called *client-centered* or *nondirective psychotherapy*. |
| **Family and group psychotherapy** | Often described as solution focused, the therapist places minimal emphasis on patients' past history and strong emphasis on having patients state and discuss their goals and then find a way to achieve them. |
| **PSYCHOPHARMACOLOGY** | The study of the effects of drugs on the mind and particularly the use of drugs in treating mental disorders. The main classes of drugs for the treatment of mental disorders are antipsychotic drugs, antidepressant drugs, minor tranquilizers, and lithium. |
| **Antipsychotic drugs** | The major tranquilizers include chlorpromazine (Thorazine™), haloperidol (Haldol™), clozapine (Clozaril™), and risperidone. These drugs have transformed the treatment of patients with psychoses and schizophrenia by reducing patient agitation and panic and shortening schizophrenic episodes. One of the side effects of these drugs is involuntary muscle movements, which approximately one-fourth of all adults who take the drugs develop. |
| **Antidepressant drugs** | These drugs are classified as stimulants and alter the patient's mood by affecting levels of neurotransmitters in the brain. Antidepressants, such as monoamine oxidase (MAO) inhibitors, are nonaddictive but they can produce unpleasant side effects such as dry mouth, weight gain, blurred vision, and nausea. |
| **Minor tranquilizers** | Include Valium™ and Xanax™. These are also classified as CNS depressants and are prescribed for anxiety. |
| **Lithium** | A special category of drug. It is used successfully to calm patients who suffer from bipolar disorder (depression alternating with manic excitement). |
| **ELECTROCONVULSIVE THERAPY (ECT)** | A procedure occasionally used for cases of prolonged major depression. This is a controversial treatment in which an electrode is placed on one or both sides of the patient's head and a current is turned on briefly causing a convulsive seizure. A low level of voltage is used in modern ECT, and the patient is administered a muscle relaxant and anthesia. Advocates of this treatment state that it is a more effective way to treat severe depression than using drugs. It is not effective with disorders other than depression, such as schizophrenia and alcoholism. |

## Abbreviations Relating to Mental Health

| | | | |
|---|---|---|---|
| **AD** | Alzheimer's disease | **ECT** | electroconvulsive therapy |
| **ADD** | attention deficit disorder | **MA** | mental age |
| **ADHD** | attention-deficit/hyperactivity disorder | **MAO** | monoamine oxidase |
| **BPD** | bipolar disorder | **MMPI** | Minnesota Multiphasic Personality Inventory |
| **CA** | chronological age | | |
| **DSM** | *Diagnostic and Statistical Manual of Mental Disorders* | **OCD** | obsessive-compulsive disorder |
| | | **SAD** | seasonal affective disorder |

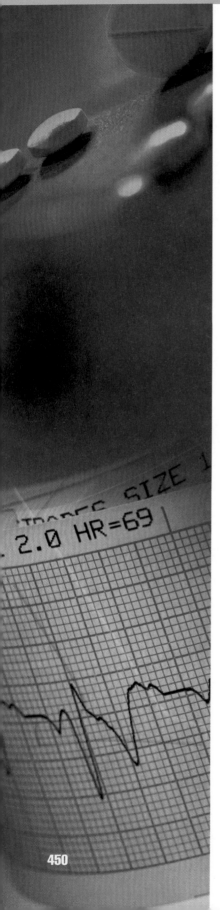

# Part III: Diagnostic Imaging

## Professional Profile

### Diagnostic Imaging

Diagnostic imaging services produce images of internal body parts through the use of X-ray, ultrasound, magnetic resonance imaging (MRI), or radionuclide slides. These images are then used by physicians and other health care personnel in diagnosing and planning patient treatment. Diagnostic imaging services are found in acute care facilities, clinics, physicians' offices, and private imaging services.

### Registered Radiologic Technologist (RRT)

- Performs imaging procedures as ordered by a physician including X-rays, computed tomography (CT), MRI, and fluoroscopy
- Operates at least two different types of imaging equipment
- Graduates from an accredited 1-year certificate, 2-year associate's degree, or 4-year bachelor's degree radiologic program
- Passes registration examination

### Diagnostic Medical Sonographer

- Performs ultrasound procedures as ordered by a physician
- Completes an accredited 1-year certificate program, a 2-year associate's degree, or a 4-year bachelor's degree

### Nuclear Medicine Technologist

- Performs nuclear medicine scans as ordered by a physician
- Completes an accredited 1-year certificate program, a 2-year associate's degree, or a 4-year bachelor's degree
- Some states require licensure

*For more information regarding these health careers, visit the following websites:*
American Registry of Radiologic Technologists at **www.arrt.org**
Society of Diagnostic Medical Sonographers at **www.sdms.org**
Society of Nuclear Medicine at **www.snm.org**

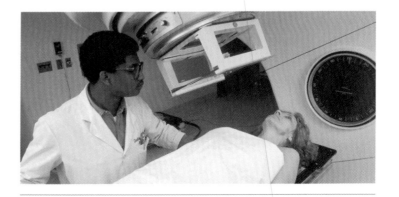

# Overview

## Combining Forms Relating to Diagnostic Imaging

| | |
|---|---|
| fluor/o | fluorescence, luminous |
| radi/o | X-ray |
| roentgen/o | X-ray |
| son/o | sound |
| tom/o | to cut |

## Suffixes Relating to Diagnostic Imaging

| Suffix | Meaning | Example |
|---|---|---|
| -gram | record | myelogram |
| -graphy | recording | mammography |
| -lucent | to shine through | radiolucent |
| -opaque | nontransparent | radiopaque |

# Diagnostic Imaging

Diagnostic imaging is the medical specialty that uses a variety of methods to produce images of the internal structures of the body. These images are then used to diagnose disease. This area of medicine began as **roentgenology** (rent gen **ALL** oh jee), named after Wilhelm Roentgen, a German physicist, who discovered roentgen rays in 1895. This discovery, now commonly known as **X-rays,** revolutionized the diagnosis of disease.

## Vocabulary Relating to Diagnostic Imaging

| | |
|---|---|
| **anteroposterior view (AP view)** | Positioning the patient so that the X-rays pass through the body from the anterior side to the posterior side. |
| **barium (BAH ree um) (Ba)** | Soft metallic element from the earth used as a radiopaque X-ray dye. |
| **cyclotron (SIGH kloh tron)** | Equipment consisting of a particle accelerator in which the particles are rotated between magnets. |
| **electron (ee LEK tron)** | Minute particle with a negative electrical charge that is emitted from radioactive substances. These are called rays. |
| **film** | Thin sheet of cellulose material coated with a light-sensitive substance that is used in taking photographs. There is a special photographic film that is sensitive to X-rays. |
| **film badge** | Badge containing film that is sensitive to X-rays. This is worn by all personnel in radiology to measure the amount of X-rays to which they are exposed. |
| **Geiger (GYE ger) counter** | Instrument used for detecting radiation. |
| **lateral view** | Positioning the patient so that the side of the body faces the X-ray machine. |
| **oblique (oh BLEEK) view** | Positioning the patient so that the X-rays pass through the body on an angle. |
| **posteroanterior view (PA view)** | Positioning the patient so that the X-rays pass through the body from the posterior side to the anterior side. |
| **radioactive (ray dee oh AK tiv)** | Substance capable of emitting or sending out radiant energy. |

*continued...*

| | |
|---|---|
| **radiography**<br>**(ray dee OG rah fee)** | Making of X-ray pictures. |
| **radioisotope**<br>**(ray dee oh EYE soh tohp)** | Radioactive form of an element. |
| **radiologist**<br>**(ray dee ALL oh jist)** | Physician who practices diagnosis and treatment by using radiant energy. He or she is responsible for interpreting X-ray films. |
| **radiolucent**<br>**(ray dee oh LOO cent)** | Structures that allow X-rays to pass through; exposes the photographic plate and appears as a black area on the X-ray. |
| **radiopaque (ray dee oh PAYK)** | Structures that are impenetrable to X-rays, appearing as a light area on the radiograph (X-ray). |
| **roentgen (RENT gen)** | Unit for describing an exposure dose of radiation. |
| **scan** | Recording on a photographic plate the emission of radioactive waves after a substance has been injected into the body (see ▨ Figure 14.7). |
| **shield** | Protective device used to protect against radiation. |
| **tagging** | Attaching a radioactive material to a chemical, and tracing it as it moves through the body. |
| **uptake** | Absorption of radioactive material and medicines into an organ or tissue. |
| **X-ray** | High-energy wave that can penetrate most solid matter and present the image on photographic film (see ▨ Figure 14.8). |

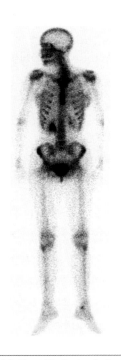

**▨ FIGURE 14.7**  Whole-body bone scan.

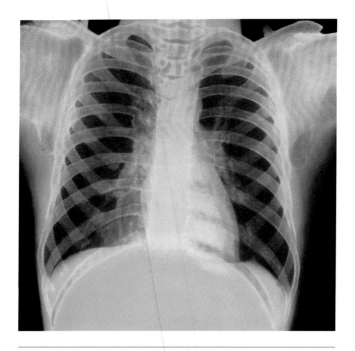

**▨ FIGURE 14.8**  Enhanced color X-ray of normal chest in an 11-year-old boy.
(Science Photo Library/Photo Researchers, Inc.)

# Diagnostic Imaging Procedures

| | |
|---|---|
| **computed tomography (toh MOG rah fee) scan (CT scan)** | An imaging technique that is able to produce a cross-sectional view of the body. X-ray pictures are taken at multiple angles through the body. A computer then uses all these images to construct a composite cross-section. Refer back to Figure 12.11 in Chapter 12 for an example of a CT scan showing a brain tumor. |
| **contrast studies** | A radiopaque substance is injected or swallowed. X-rays are then taken that will outline the body structure containing the radiopaque substance. For example, angiograms and myelograms. |
| **Doppler ultrasound** | Use of ultrasound to record the velocity of blood flowing through blood vessels. Used to detect blood clots and blood vessel obstructions. |
| **fluoroscopy (floo or OS koh pee)** | X-rays strike a fluorescing screen rather than a photographic plate, causing it to glow. The glowing screen changes from minute to minute, therefore movement, such as the heart beating or the digestive tract moving, can be seen. |
| **magnetic resonance (REZ oh nence) imaging (MRI)** | Use of electromagnetic energy to produce an image of soft tissues in any plane of the body. Atoms behave differently when placed in a strong magnetic field. When the body is exposed to this magnetic field the nuclei of the body's atoms emit radio-frequency signals that can be used to create an image (see ■ Figures 14.9 and 14.10). |
| **nuclear medicine** | Use of radioactive substances to diagnose diseases. A radioactive substance known to accumulate in certain body tissues is injected or inhaled. After waiting for the substance to travel to the body area of interest, the radioactivity level is recorded. Commonly referred to as a *scan*. See Table 14.4 for examples of the radioactive substances used in nuclear medicine. |
| **positron emission tomography (POS ih tron eh MIS shun toh MOG rah fee) (PET)** | Image is produced following the injection of radioactive glucose. The glucose will accumulate in areas of high metabolic activity. Therefore this process will highlight areas that are consuming a large quantity of glucose. This may show an active area of the brain or a tumor (see ■ Figure 14.11). |
| **radiology (ray dee ALL oh jee)** | The use of high-energy radiation, X-rays, to expose a photographic plate. The image is a black-and-white picture with radiopaque structures such as bone appearing white and radiolucent tissue such as muscles appearing dark. |
| **ultrasound (ULL trah sound) (US)** | The use of high-frequency sound waves to produce an image. Sound waves directed into the body from a transducer will bounce off internal structures and echo back to the transducer. The speed of the echo is dependent on the density of the tissue. A computer is able to correlate speed of echo with density and produce an image. Used to visualize internal organs, heart valves, and fetuses (see ■ Figure 14.12). |

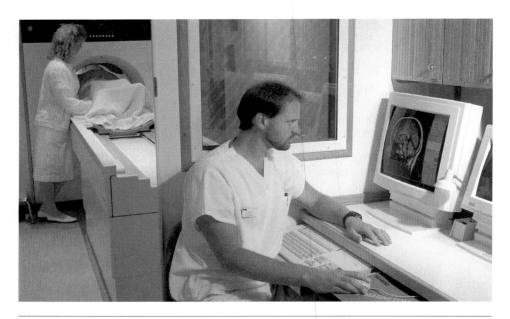

**■ FIGURE 14.9** MRI lab.
(Will and Demi McIntyre/Photo Researchers, Inc.)

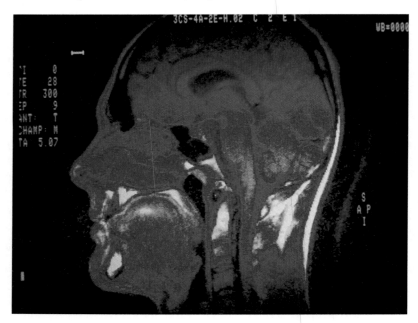

**■ FIGURE 14.10** Enhanced color MRI of midsagittal of head and brain.
(Philippe Plailly/Science Photo Library/Photo Researchers, Inc.)

| Table 14.4 | Substances Used to Visualize Various Body Organs in Nuclear Medicine |
|---|---|
| **Organ** | **Substance** |
| bone | technetium ($^{99m}$Tc) labeled phosphate |
| tumors | gallium ($^{67}$Ga) |
| lungs | xenon ($^{133}$Xe) |
| liver | technetium ($^{99m}$Tc) labeled sulfur |
| heart | thallium ($^{201}$Tl) |
| thyroid | iodine ($^{131}$I) |

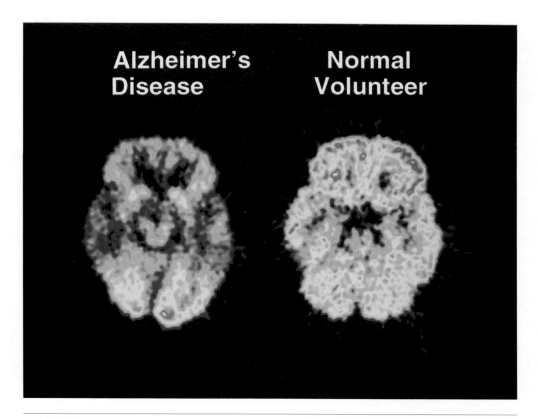

**FIGURE 14.11** PET scan comparing the metabolic activity levels of a normal brain and the brain of an Alzheimer's sufferer. Red and yellow colors indicate high activity levels; while blue colors represent low activity levels.

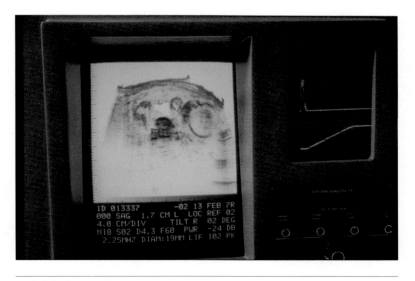

**FIGURE 14.12** A human fetus is displayed on an ultrasound monitor.

| | | | | |
|---|---|---|---|---|
| $^{67}$Ga | radioactive gallium | | IVC | intravenous cholangiogram |
| $^{99m}$Tc | radioactive technetium | | IVP | intravenous pyelogram |
| $^{131}$I | radioactive iodine | | KUB | kidneys, ureters, bladder |
| $^{201}$Tl | radioactive thallium | | LAT | lateral |
| $^{133}$Xe | radioactive xenon | | LGI | lower gastrointestinal series |
| ACAT | automated computerized axial tomography | | LL | left lateral |
| Angio | angiography | | mA | milliampere |
| AP | anteroposterior | | mCi | millicurie |
| Ba | barium | | MRA | magnetic resonance angiography |
| BaE | barium enema | | MRI | magnetic resonance imaging |
| CAT | computerized axial tomography | | NMR | nuclear magnetic resonance |
| Ci | curie | | PA | posteroanterior |
| CT | computerized tomography | | PET | positive emission tomography |
| CXR | chest X-ray | | PTC | percutaneous transhepatic cholangiography |
| decub | lying down | | R | roentgen |
| DI | diagnostic imaging | | Ra | radium |
| DSA | digital subtraction angiography | | rad | radiation absorbed dose |
| ERCP | endoscopic retrograde cholangiopancreatography | | RL | right lateral |
| | | | RRT | registered radiologic technologist |
| Fx | fracture | | UGI | upper gastrointestinal series |
| GB | gallbladder X-ray | | US | ultrasound |

# Part IV: Rehabilitation Services

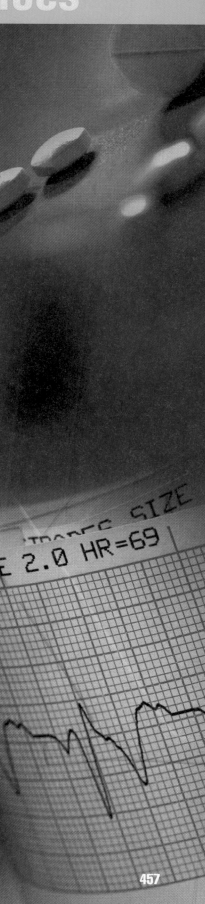

## Professional Profile

### Physical Therapy and Occupational Therapy

Rehabilitation services consist of physical therapy and occupational therapy. These allied health personnel plan and carry out treatment programs to develop, restore, or maintain function. Rehabilitation services are found in acute and long-term facilities, rehabilitation centers, health maintenance organizations, schools, home health agencies, private practices, clinics, and mental health facilities.

### Physical Therapy

Physical therapy specializes in programs for movement dysfunction and physical disabilities resulting from muscle, bone, joint, and nerve injuries or disease. They work with patients/clients to help them overcome these barriers to mobility.

### Physical Therapist (PT or DPT)

- Graduates from an accredited 4-year bachelor's or 5-year graduate program in physical therapy
- Completes a 4-month clinical internship
- Passes a national licensing examination

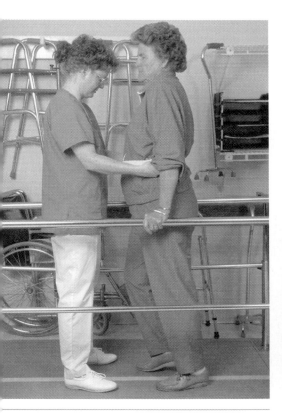

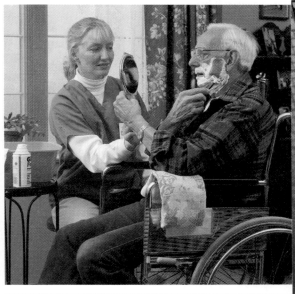

### Physical Therapy Assistant (PTA)

- Works under the supervision of a physical therapist
- Graduates from an accredited 2-year associate's degree physical therapy assistant program
- Passes a national licensing examination

### Occupational Therapy

Occupational therapists specialize in rehabilitating patients/clients to perform activities that are essential for daily living. They develop a treatment plan and programs to restore personal care skills to persons with physical, mental, emotional, and/or developmental problems.

### Occupational Therapist (OTR)

- Graduates from an approved 4-year college or university occupational therapy program
- Completes 6 months of clinical experience
- Passes a national certification examination

### Certified Occupational Therapy Assistant (COTA)

- Works under the supervision of an occupational therapist
- Graduates from a 2-year approved occupational therapy assistant program
- Completes supervised clinical fieldwork
- Passes a national certification examination

*For more information regarding these health careers, visit the following websites:*
American Occupational Therapy Association at **www.aota.org**
American Physical Therapy Association at **www.apta.org**

## Overview

### Combining Forms Relating to Rehabilitation Services

| | |
|---|---|
| cry/o | cold |
| electr/o | electric current |
| erg/o | work |
| hydr/o | water |
| my/o | muscle |
| orth/o | straight, correct |
| phon/o | sound |
| prosth/o | addition |
| therm/o | heat |

### Suffixes Relating to Rehabilitation Services

| Suffix | Meaning | Example |
|---|---|---|
| -phoresis | carrying | phonophoresis |
| -therapy | treatment | hydrotherapy |

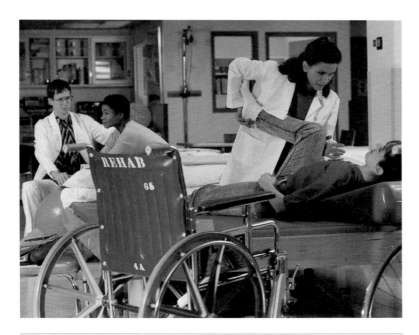

■ **FIGURE 14.13**  Physical therapy department.
(Yoav Levy/Phototake NYC)

# Rehabilitation Services

The goal of rehabilitation is to prevent disability and restore as much function as possible following disease, illness, or injury. Rehabilitation services include the medical specialties of **physical therapy** (PT) and **occupational therapy** (OT).

## Physical Therapy

The medical specialty of physical therapy (PT) involves treating disorders using physical means and methods. Physical therapy personnel assess joint motion, muscle strength and endurance, function of heart and lungs, and performance of activities required in daily living, and carry out other responsibilities (see ■ Figure 14.13). Physical therapy treatment includes gait training, therapeutic exercise, massage, joint and soft tissue mobilization, thermal and cryotherapy, electrical stimulation, ultrasound, and hydrotherapy. These methods strengthen muscles, improve motion and circulation, reduce pain, and increase function.

## Occupational Therapy

The medical specialty of occupational therapy (OT) assists patients to regain, develop, and improve skills that are important for independent functioning. Occupational therapy personnel work with people who, because of illness, injury, or developmental or psychological impairments, require specialized training in skills that will enable them to lead independent, productive, and satisfying lives. Occupational therapists instruct patients in the use of adaptive equipment and techniques, body mechanics, and energy conservation. They also employ modalities such as heat, cold, and therapeutic exercise.

## Vocabulary Relating to Rehabilitation Services

| | |
|---|---|
| **activities of daily living (ADL)** | The activities usually performed in the course of a normal day, such as eating, dressing, and washing. |
| **adaptive equipment** | Modification of equipment or devices to improve the function and independence of a person with a disability (see ■ Figure 14.14). |
| **body mechanics** | Use of good posture and position while performing activities of daily living to prevent injury and stress on body parts. |
| **ergonomics (er goh NOM iks)** | The study of human work including how the requirements for performing work and the work environment affect the musculoskeletal and nervous systems. |
| **fine motor skills** | The use of precise and coordinated movements in such activities such as writing, buttoning, and cutting. |
| **gait (GAYT)** | Manner of walking. |
| **gross motor skills** | The use of large muscle groups that coordinate body movements such as walking, running, jumping, and balance. |
| **lower extremity (LE)** | The leg. |
| **mobility** | State of having normal movement of all body parts. |
| **orthotics (or THOT iks)** | The use of equipment, such as splints and braces, to support a paralyzed muscle, promote a specific motion, or correct musculoskeletal deformities. |
| **physiatrist (fiz ee AT rist)** | Physician who specializes in physical medicine. |
| **physical medicine** | Use of natural methods, including physical therapy, to cure diseases and disorders. |
| **prosthetics (pros THET iks)** | Artificial devices, such as limbs and joints, that replace a missing body part (see ■ Figure 14.15). |
| **range of motion (ROM)** | The range of movement of a joint, from maximum flexion through maximum extension. It is measured as degrees of a circle. |
| **rehabilitation (ree hah bill ih TAY shun)** | Process of treatment and exercise that can help a person with a disability attain maximum function and well-being. |
| **upper extremity (UE)** | The arm. |

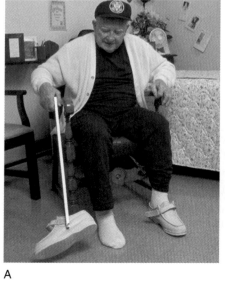
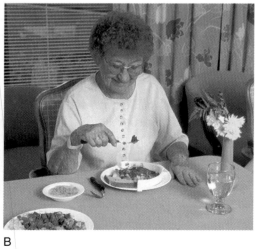

A       B

■ **FIGURE 14.14** (A) Using adaptive equipment to assist in putting on shoes. (B) Nursing home resident dining with adaptive edge on plate.

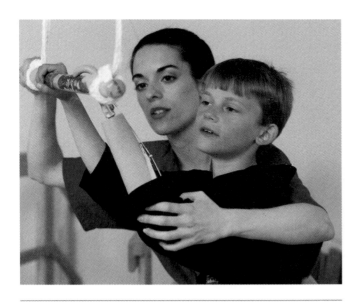

■ **FIGURE 14.15**  Occupational therapist assisting child in use of prosthetic arm.
(Yoav Levy/Phototake NYC)

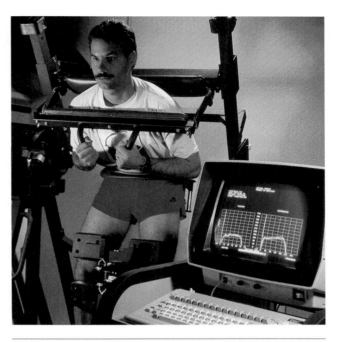

■ **FIGURE 14.16**  Measuring active-resistive exercise.
(Stevie Grand/Science Photo Library/Photo Researchers, Inc.)

# Therapeutic Procedures Relating to Rehabilitation Services

| | |
|---|---|
| **active exercises** | Exercises that a patient performs without assistance. |
| **active range of motion (AROM)** | Range of motion for joints that a patient is able to perform without assistance from someone else. |
| **active-resistive exercises** | Exercises in which the patient works against an artificial resistance applied to a muscle, such as a weight. Used to increase strength (see ■ Figure 14.16). |
| **cryotherapy (cry oh THAIR ah pee)** | Using cold for therapeutic purposes. |
| **debridement (day breed MON)** | Removal of dead or damaged tissue from a wound. Commonly performed for burn therapy. |
| **electromyogram (ee lek troh MY oh gram) (EMG)** | Graphic recording of the contraction of a muscle. The result of applying an electrical stimulation to the muscle. |
| **hydrotherapy (high droh THAIR ah pee)** | Application of warm water as a therapeutic treatment. Can be done in baths, swimming pools, and whirlpools. |
| **ice packs** | Using ice in a bag or container to treat localized conditions. |
| **massage (mah SAHZH)** | Kneading or applying pressure by hands to a part of the patient's body to promote muscle relaxation and reduce tension. |
| **moist hot packs** | Applying moist warmth to a body part to produce the slight dilation of blood vessels in the skin. Causes muscle relaxation in the deeper regions of the body and increases circulation, which aids healing. |
| **nerve conduction velocity** | A test to determine if nerves have been damaged by recording the rate at which an electrical impulse travels along a nerve. If the nerve is damaged, the velocity will be decreased. |

*continued...*

| | |
|---|---|
| pain control | Managing pain through a variety of means, including medications, biofeedback, and mechanical devices. |
| passive range of motion (PROM) | Therapist putting a patient's joints through a full range of motion without assistance from the patient. |
| percussion (per KUH shun) | Use of the fingertips to tap the body lightly and sharply. Aids in determining the size, position, and consistency of the underlying body part. |
| phonophoresis (foh noh foh REE sis) | The use of ultrasound waves to introduce medication across the skin and into the subcutaneous tissues. |
| postural drainage with clapping | Draining secretions from the bronchi or a lung cavity by having the patient lie so that gravity allows drainage to occur. Clapping is using the hand in a cupped position to perform percussion on the chest. Assists in loosening secretions and mucus. |
| therapeutic (thair ah PEW tik) exercise | Exercise planned and carried out to achieve a specific physical benefit, such as improved range of motion, muscle strength, or cardiovascular function. |
| thermotherapy (ther moh THAIR ah pee) | Applying heat to the body for therapeutic purposes. |
| traction (TRAK shun) | Process of pulling or drawing, usually with a mechanical device. Used in treating orthopedic (bone and joint) problems and injuries. |
| transcutaneous electrical nerve stimulation (tranz kyoo TAY nee us ee LEK trih kl nerve stim yoo LAY shun) (TENS) | The application of an electric current to a peripheral nerve to relieve pain. |
| ultrasound (ULL trah sound) (US) | The use of high-frequency sound waves to create heat in soft tissues under the skin. It is particularly useful for treating injuries to muscles, tendons, and ligaments, as well as muscle spasms. |
| whirlpool | Bath in which there are continuous jets of hot water reaching the body surfaces. |

# Abbreviations Relating to Rehabilitation Services

| | | | |
|---|---|---|---|
| ADL | activities of daily living | PROM | passive range of motion |
| AROM | active range of motion | PT | physical therapy |
| EMG | electromyogram | ROM | range of motion |
| e-stim | electrical stimulation | TENS | transcutaneous electrical stimulation |
| LE | lower extremity | UE | upper extremity |
| OT | occupational therapy | US | ultrasound |

## Professional Profile

### Surgical Technology

Surgical technologists are members of the surgery team. Their duties include preparing the operating room and instruments, preparing the patient for surgery, assisting the surgical team during the procedure, and carrying out postsurgical duties. A scrub technologist is responsible for handing instruments to the surgeon. The circulating technologist assists by remaining unsterile during the procedure in order to manage the operating room, check supplies, and keep records. The surgical first assistant has advanced training in order to assist the surgeon directly with exposing the incision and controlling bleeding.

### Certified Surgical Technologist (CST)

- Assists physicians and other health care workers before, during, and after surgery
- Completes an accredited 9-month certification program or a 2-year associate's degree
- Voluntary certification is available

*For more information regarding these health careers, visit the following website:* Association of Surgical Technologists at **www.ast.sorg**

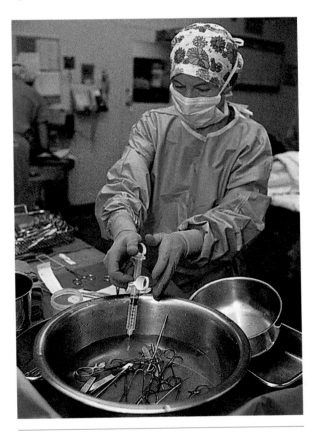

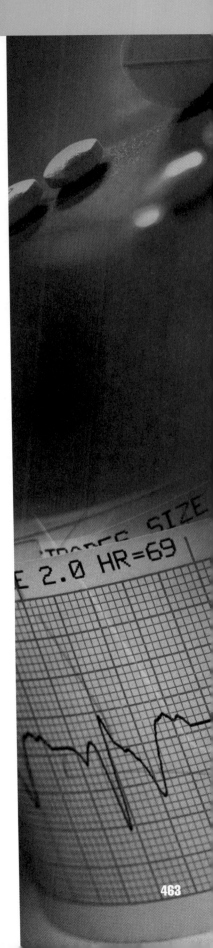

# Overview

## Combining Forms Relating to Surgery

| cis/o | to cut | esthesi/o | sensation, feeling |
|-------|--------|-----------|--------------------|
| cry/o | cold | sect/o | cut |
| electr/o | electricity | | |

## Suffixes Relating to Surgery

| Suffix | Meaning | Example |
|--------|---------|---------|
| -ectomy | excision | gastrectomy |
| -otomy | incision | thoracotomy |
| -plasty | surgical repair | dermatoplasty |
| -scopic | to view inside | endoscopic |

# Surgery

**Surgery** is the branch of medicine dealing with operative procedures to correct deformities and defects, repair injuries, and diagnose and cure diseases. A **surgeon** is a physician who has completed additional training of 5 years or more in a surgical specialty area. These specialty areas include orthopedics; neurosurgery; gynecology; ophthalmology; urology; and thoracic, vascular, cardiac, plastic, and general surgery. The surgeon must complete an **operative report** for every procedure that he or she performs. This is a detailed description that includes the following:

- preoperative diagnosis
- indication for the procedure
- name of the procedure
- surgical techniques employed
- findings during surgery
- postoperative diagnosis
- name of the surgeon

This report also includes information pertaining to the patient such as name, address, age, patient number, and date of the procedure.

Surgical terminology includes terms related to anesthesiology, surgical instruments, surgical procedures, incisions, and suture materials. Specific surgical procedures are frequently named by using the combining form for the body part being operated on and adding a suffix that describes the procedure. For example, an incision into the chest is a **thoracotomy** (thor ah **KOT** oh mee), removal of the stomach is **gastrectomy** (gas **TREK** toh mee), and surgical repair of the skin is **dermatoplasty** (**DER** mah toh plas tee). A list of the most frequently used surgical suffixes is found in Chapter 1 and common surgical procedures are defined in each system chapter.

## Anesthesia

An **anesthesiologist** (an es thee zee **OL** oh jist) is a physician who specializes in the practice of administering anesthetics (see ■ Figure 14.17). A **nurse anesthetist** (ah **NES** the tist) is a registered nurse who has received additional training and education in the administration of anesthetic medications. **Anesthesia** (an ess **THEE** zee ah) results in the loss of feeling or sensation. The most common types of anesthesia are general, regional, local, and topical anesthesia.

- **General anesthesia** (GA) produces a loss of consciousness including an absence of pain sensation. It is administered to a patient by either an **intravenous** (in trah **VEE** nus) (IV) or **inhalation** (in hah **LAY** shun)

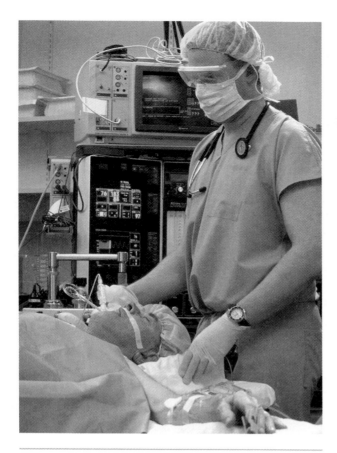

**■ FIGURE 14.17**   Anesthesiologist.
(Tom Stewart/The Stock Market)

method. The patient's vital signs (VS) (heart rate, breathing rate, pulse, and blood pressure) are carefully monitored when using a general anesthetic.

- **Regional anesthesia** is also referred to as a *nerve block*. This anesthetic interrupts a patient's pain sensation in a particular region of the body. The anesthetic is injected near the nerve that will be blocked from sensation. The patient usually remains conscious.

- **Local anesthesia** produces a loss of sensation in one localized part of the body. The patient remains conscious. The anesthetic is administered either topically or via a **subcutaneous** (sub kyoo **TAY** nee us) route.

- **Topical anesthesia** uses an anesthetic liquid or gel placed directly into a specific area. The patient remains conscious. This type of anesthetic is used on the skin, the cornea, and the mucous membranes in dental work.

## Surgical Instruments

Physicians have developed surgical instruments since the time of the early Egyptians. Instruments include surgical knives, saws, clamps, drills, and needles. Some of the more commonly used surgical instruments are listed in Table 14.5.

## Surgical Positions

Patients are placed in specific positions so the surgeon is able to reach the area that is to be operated on. Table 14.6 describes and ■ Figure 14.18 illustrates some common surgical positions.

### Table 14.5  Common Surgical Instruments

| Instrument | Use |
|---|---|
| aspirator (**AS** pih ray tor) | suctions fluid |
| clamp | grasps tissue; controls bleeding |
| curette (kyoo **RET**) | scrapes and removes tissue |
| dilator (dye **LAY** tor) | enlarges an opening by stretching |
| forceps (**FOR** seps) | grasps tissue |
| hemostat (**HEE** moh stat) | forceps to grasp blood vessel to control bleeding |
| probe | explores tissue |
| scalpel | cuts and separates tissue |
| speculum (**SPEK** yoo lum) | spreads apart walls of a cavity |
| tenaculum (teh **NAK** yoo lum) | long handled clamp |
| trephine (treh **FINE**) | saw that removes disk-shaped piece of tissue or bone |

### Table 14.6  Common Surgical Positions

| Surgical Position | Description |
|---|---|
| Fowler | sitting with back positioned at a 45° angle |
| Lateral recumbent (**LAT** er al ree **KUM** bent) | lying on either the left or right side |
| Lithotomy (lith **OT** oh mee) | lying face up with hips and knees bent at 90° angles |
| Prone (**PROHN**) | lying horizontal with face down |
| Supine (soo **PINE**) | lying horizontal and face up; also called dorsal recumbent |
| Trendelenburg (**TREN** dee len berg) | lying face up and on an incline with head lower than legs |

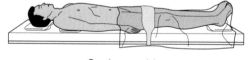

Supine position

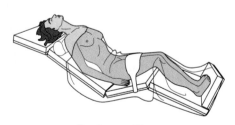

Fowler position

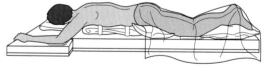

Prone position

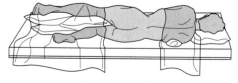

Lateral position

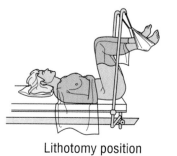

Lithotomy position

■ **FIGURE 14.18**  Common surgical positions.

# Vocabulary Relating to Surgery

| | |
|---|---|
| **analgesic (an al JEE zik)** | Medication to relieve pain. |
| **anesthetic (an ess THET ik)** | Medication to produce partial to complete loss of sensation. |
| **cauterization (kaw ter ih ZAY shun)** | Using heat, cold, electricity, or chemicals to scar, burn, or cut tissues. |
| **circulating nurse** | Nurse who assists the surgeon and scrub nurse by providing needed materials during the procedure and by handling the surgical specimen. This person does not wear sterile clothing and may enter and leave the operating room during the procedure. |
| **cryosurgery (cry oh SER jer ee)** | Using extreme cold to destroy tissue. |
| **day surgery** | A type of outpatient surgery in which the patient is discharged on the same day he or she is admitted; also called *ambulatory surgery.* |
| **dissection (dih SEK shun)** | The surgical cutting of parts for separation and study. |
| **draping** | Process of covering the patient with sterile cloths that allow only the operative site to be exposed to the surgeon. |
| **electrocautery (ee lek troh KAW ter ee)** | Use of an electric current to stop bleeding by coagulating blood vessels. |
| **endoscopic (en doh SKOP ik) surgery** | Use of a lighted instrument to examine the interior of a cavity. |
| **hemostasis (hee moh STAY sis)** | Stopping the flow of blood using instruments, pressure, and/or medication. |
| **laser surgery** | Use of a controlled beam of light for cutting, hemostasis, or tissue destruction. |
| **perioperative (per ee OP er ah tiv)** | The period of time that includes before, during, and after a surgical procedure. |
| **postoperative (post OP er ah tiv)** | The period of time immediately following the surgery. |
| **preoperative (pree OP er ah tiv) (preop, pre-op)** | The period of time preceding surgery. |
| **resection (ree SEK shun)** | To surgically cut out; excision. |
| **scrub nurse** | Surgical assistant who hands instruments to the surgeon. This person wears sterile clothing and maintains the sterile operative field. |
| **suture (SOO cher) material** | Used to close a wound or incision. Examples are catgut, silk thread, or staples. They may or may not be removed when the wound heals, depending on the type of material that is used. |

# Abbreviations Relating to Surgery

| | | | | |
|---|---|---|---|---|
| **D & C** | dilation and curettage | | **PARR** | postanesthetic recovery room |
| **EAU** | exam under anesthesia | | **preop, pre-op** | preoperative |
| **Endo** | endoscopy | | **prep** | preparation, prepared |
| **GA** | general anesthesia | | **T & A** | tonsillectomy and adenoidectomy |
| **I & D** | incision and drainage | | **TAH** | total abdominal hysterectomy |
| **MUA** | manipulation under anesthesia | | **TURP** | transurethral resection of prostate |
| **OR** | operating room | | | |

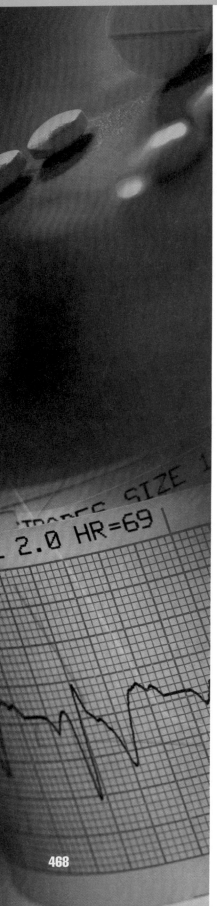

## Professional Profile

### Cytotechnology

Cytotechnologists are laboratory professionals who use microscopes to analyze slides of cell specimens for abnormalities. By looking at the nucleus and other cellular structures, they identify signs of cancer and other diseases. Cytotechnologists usually work closely with pathologists in hospitals and private laboratories.

### Cytotechnologist (CT)

- Works in a laboratory under supervision of a pathologist
- Completes an accredited program after 2 or 3 years of undergraduate courses
- Passes certification exam

*For more information regarding these health careers, visit the following websites:*
American Society of Cytopathology at **www.cytopathology.org**
American Society for Cytotechnology at **www.asct.com**

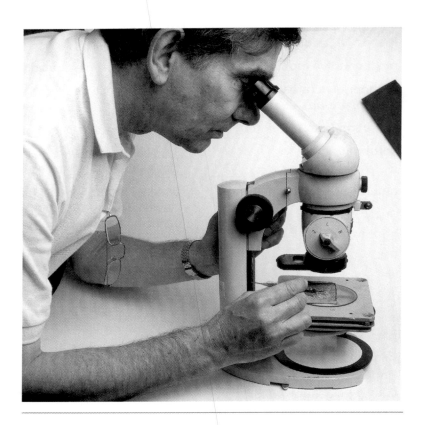

# Overview

## Combining Forms Relating to Oncology

| | |
|---|---|
| blast/o | primitive cell |
| carcin/o | cancerous |
| chem/o | chemical |
| mut/a | genetic change, mutation |
| onc/o | tumor |
| path/o | disease |
| tox/o | toxic |

## Suffixes Relating to Oncology

| Suffix | Meaning | Example |
|---|---|---|
| -gen | producing | carcinogen |
| -oma | tumor, mass | adenoma |
| -plasia | growth, formation | hyperplasia |
| -plasm | growth, formation | neoplasm |
| -therapy | treatment | chemotherapy |

# Oncology

**Oncology** (ong **KALL** oh jee) is the branch of medicine dealing with **tumors** (**TOO** mors). A tumor can be classified as **benign** (bee **NINE**) or **malignant** (mah **LIG** nant). A benign tumor is one that is generally not progressive or re-curring. Generally, a benign tumor will have the suffix *-oma* at the end of the term. However, a malignant tumor indicates that there is a cancerous growth present (see  Figure 14.19). These terms will usually have the word **carcinoma** (kar sin **NOH** mah) added. The medical specialty of oncology pri-marily treats patients who have cancer.

> **MED TERM TIP**
> Carcinoma or cancer (Ca) can affect almost every organ in the body. The medical term reflects the area of the body affected as well as the type of tumor cell. For example, there can be an esophageal carcinoma, gastric adenocarcinoma, or adenocarcinoma of the uterus.

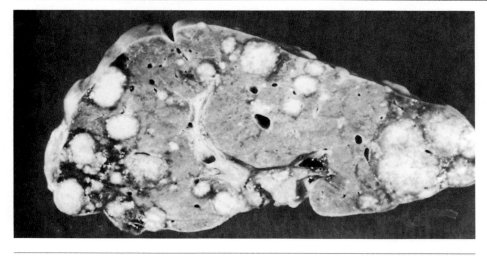

■ **FIGURE 14.19**  Malignant tumors of the liver that have metastasized from other sites. (Courtesy of Dr. David R. Duffell)

The treatment for cancer can consist of a variety or a combination of treatments. The **protocol** (**PROH** toh kall) (prot) for a particular patient will consist of the actual plan of care, including the medications, surgeries, and treatments. Often, the entire health care team, including the physician, oncologist, radiologist, nurse, and patient, will assist in designing the treatment plan (see ▓ Figure 14.20).

## Staging Tumors

The process of classifying tumors based on their degree of tissue invasion and the potential response to therapy is referred to as **staging.** The TNM staging system is frequently used. The *T* refers to the tumor's size and invasion, the *N* refers to lymph node involvement, and the *M* refers to the presence of **metastases** (mets) (meh **TASS** tah seez) of the tumor cells.

In addition, a tumor can be graded from grade I through grade IV. The **grade** is based on the microscopic appearance of the tumor cells. The **pathologist** (path **ALL** oh jist) rates or grades the cells based on whether the tumor resembles the normal tissue. The classification system is illustrated in Table 14.7. A grade I tumor is well differentiated and is easier to treat than the more advanced grades.

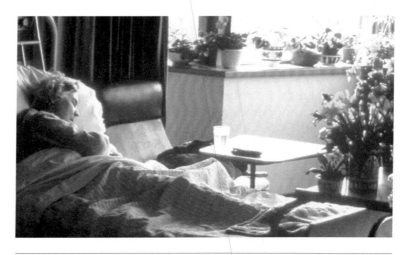

▓ **FIGURE 14.20**   Elderly patient in a hospice setting. Hospice is an interdisciplinary program of care and supportive services.
(John Moss/Science Source/Photo Researchers, Inc.)

| Table 14.7 | Tumor Grade Classification |
|---|---|
| **Grade** | **Meaning** |
| GX | The grade cannot be determined. |
| GI | The cells are well differentiated. |
| GII | The cells are moderately differentiated. |
| GIII | The cells are poorly differentiated. |
| GIV | The cells are undifferentiated. |

# Vocabulary Relating to Oncology

| | |
|---|---|
| **carcinogen (kar SIN oh jen)** | Substance or chemical agent that produces or increases the risk of developing cancer. For example, cigarette smoke and insecticides are considered to be carcinogens. |
| **carcinoma (kar sin NOH mah), in situ (CIS)** | Malignant tumor that has not extended beyond the original site. |
| **encapsulated (en CAP soo lay ted)** | Growth enclosed in a sheath of tissue that prevents tumor cells from invading surrounding tissue. |
| **hyperplasia (high per PLAY zee ah)** | Excessive development of normal cells within an organ. |
| **invasive (in VAY siv) disease** | Tendency of a malignant tumor to spread to immediately surrounding tissue and organs. |
| **metastasis (meh TASS tah sis) (mets)** | Movement and spread of cancer cells from one part of the body to another. Metastases is plural (see ■ Figure 14.21). |
| **morbidity (mor BID ih tee)** | Number that represents the number of sick persons in a particular population. |
| **mortality (mor TAL ih tee)** | Number that represents the number of deaths in a particular population. |
| **mutation (mew TAY shun)** | Change or transformation from the original. |
| **neoplasm (NEE oh plazm)** | New and abnormal growth or tumor. These can be benign or malignant. |
| **oncogenic (ong koh JEN ik)** | Cancer causing. |
| **primary site** | Term that is used to designate where a malignant tumor first appeared. |
| **protocol (PROH toh kall) (prot)** | Plan of treatment for cancer patients developed by examining all the options available, including radiation therapy, chemotherapy, removal of entire organ with the tumor, removal of only the tumor, removal of surrounding lymph nodes, and others. |
| **remission (rih MISH un)** | Period during which the symptoms of a disease or disorder leave. Can be temporary. |

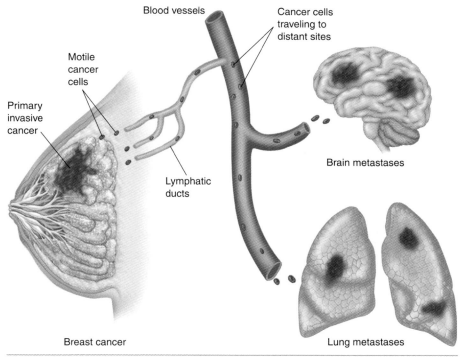

Blood vessels

Cancer cells traveling to distant sites

Motile cancer cells

Primary invasive cancer

Lymphatic ducts

Brain metastases

Breast cancer

Lung metastases

■ **FIGURE 14.21** Primary breast tumor metastasizes through the lymph vessels and bloodstream to secondary sites in the brain and lungs.

## Diagnostic Procedures Relating to Oncology

| | |
|---|---|
| **biopsy (BYE op see) (bx)** | Excision of a small piece of tissue for microscopic examination to assist in determining a diagnosis. |
| **bone marrow biopsy (BYE op see)** | Removal of a small amount of bone marrow for microscopic examination to determine the presence of malignant tumor cells. |
| **cytologic (sigh toh LAH jik) testing** | Examination of cells to determine their structure and origin. PAP smears are considered a form of cytologic testing. |
| **exploratory surgery (ek SPLOR ah tor ee SER jer ee)** | Surgery performed for the purpose of determining if cancer is present or if a known cancer has spread. Biopsies are generally performed. |
| **lumbar puncture (LUM bar PUNK chur)** | Puncture made by placing a needle into the fourth intervertebral space of the lumbar area to remove spinal fluid for analysis. |
| **needle biopsy (BYE op see)** | Core of tissue is removed using a needle. The tissue cells are then tested for the abnormal cellular growth of cancer. |
| **staging laparotomy (lap ah ROT oh mee)** | Surgical procedure in which the abdomen is entered to determine the extent and staging of a tumor. |

## Therapeutic Procedures Relating to Oncology

| | |
|---|---|
| **chemotherapy (kee moh THAIR ah pee) (chemo)** | Treating disease by using chemicals that have a toxic effect on the body, especially cancerous tissue. |
| **cryosurgery (cry oh SER jer ee)** | Technique of exposing tissues to extreme cold to produce cell injury and destruction. Used in the treatment of malignant tumors to control pain and bleeding. |
| **hormone therapy (HOR mohn THAIR ah pee)** | Treatment of cancer with natural hormones or with chemicals that produce hormone-like effects. |
| **immunotherapy (im yoo noh THAIR ah pee)** | The production or strengthening of immunity. |
| **palliative therapy (PAL ee ah tiv THAIR ah pee)** | Treatment designed to reduce the intensity of painful symptoms, but does not produce a cure. |
| **radiation therapy (ray dee AY shun THAIR ah pee)** | Exposing tumors and surrounding tissues to X-rays or gamma rays to interfere with their ability to multiply. |
| **radical surgery** | Extensive surgery to remove as much tissue associated with a tumor as possible. |
| **radioactive (ray dee oh AK tiv) implant** | Embedding a radioactive source directly into tissue to provide a highly localized radiation dosage to damage nearby cancerous cells. Also called *brachytherapy*. |

## Abbreviations Relating to Oncology

| | | | | |
|---|---|---|---|---|
| **Ba** | barium | | **MTX** | methotrexate |
| **bx** | biopsy | | **NPDL** | nodular, poorly differentiated lymphocytes |
| **Ca** | cancer | | **PAP** | Papanicolaou test |
| **chemo** | chemotherapy | | **prot** | protocol |
| **CIS** | carcinoma in situ | | **PSA** | prostate-specific antigen |
| **5-FU** | 5-fluorouracil | | **st** | stage |
| **GA** | gallium | | **TNM** | tumor, nodes, metastases |
| **mets** | metastases | | | |

# Chapter Review

## Pronunciation Practice

 *You will find the pronunciation for each term on the enclosed CD-ROM. Check each one off as you master it.*

- [ ] abnormal psychology
- [ ] active exercises
- [ ] active range of motion
- [ ] active-resistive exercises
- [ ] activities of daily living
- [ ] adaptive equipment
- [ ] addiction (ah **DICK** shun)
- [ ] additive
- [ ] aerosol (**AIR** oh sol)
- [ ] Alzheimer's disease (**ALTS** high merz dih **ZEEZ**)
- [ ] amnesia (am **NEE** zee ah)
- [ ] analgesic (an al **JEE** zik)
- [ ] anesthesia (an ess **THEE** zee ah)
- [ ] anesthesiologist (an es thee zee **OL** oh jist)
- [ ] anesthetic (an ess **THET** ik)
- [ ] anorexia nervosa (an oh **REK** see ah ner **VOH** sah)
- [ ] anteroposterior view
- [ ] antidote (**AN** tih doht)
- [ ] antisocial personality disorder (an tih **SOH** shal per son **AL** ih tee dis **OR** der)
- [ ] anxiety (ang **ZY** eh tee)
- [ ] anxiety (ang **ZY** eh tee) disorders
- [ ] aspirator (**AS** pih ray tor)
- [ ] attention deficit disorder (**DEFF** ih sit dis **OR** der)
- [ ] autism (**AW** tizm)
- [ ] barium (**BAH** ree um)
- [ ] benign (bee **NINE**)
- [ ] biopsy (**BYE** op see)
- [ ] bipolar disorder (by **POHL** ar dis **OR** der)
- [ ] body mechanics
- [ ] bone marrow biopsy (**BYE** op see)
- [ ] brand name
- [ ] broad spectrum
- [ ] buccal (**BUCK** al)
- [ ] bulimia (boo **LIM** ee ah)

- [ ] carcinogen (kar **SIN** oh jen)
- [ ] carcinoma (kar sin **NOH** mah)
- [ ] carcinoma (kar sin **NOH** mah) in situ
- [ ] cauterization (kaw ter ih **ZAY** shun)
- [ ] chemical (**KEM** ih cal) name
- [ ] chemotherapy (kee moh **THAIR** ah pee)
- [ ] circulating nurse
- [ ] clamp
- [ ] clinical psychologist (sigh **KALL** oh jist)
- [ ] cognitive disorders
- [ ] computed tomography (toh **MOG** rah fee) scan
- [ ] contraindication (kon trah in dih **KAY** shun)
- [ ] contrast studies
- [ ] controlled substances
- [ ] conversion reaction
- [ ] cryosurgery (cry oh **SER** jer ee)
- [ ] cryotherapy (cry oh **THAIR** ah pee)
- [ ] cumulative action
- [ ] curette (kyoo **RET**)
- [ ] cyclotron (**SIGH** kloh tron)
- [ ] cytologic (sigh toh **LAH** jik) testing
- [ ] day surgery
- [ ] debridement (day breed **MON**)
- [ ] delusions (dee **LOO** zhuns)
- [ ] dementia (dee **MEN** she ah)
- [ ] dermatoplasty (**DER** mah toh plas tee)
- [ ] *Diagnostic and Statistical Manual of Mental Disorders*
- [ ] dilator (dye **LAY** tor)
- [ ] dilute
- [ ] disorders diagnosed in infancy and childhood
- [ ] dissection (dih **SEK** shun)
- [ ] dissociative disorders
- [ ] Doppler ultrasound
- [ ] draping

- Drug Enforcement Agency
- drug interaction
- drug tolerance (**TAHL** er ans)
- eardrops
- eating disorders
- electrocautery (ee lek troh **KAW** ter ee)
- electroconvulsive therapy (ee lek troh kon **VULL** siv **THAIR** ah pee)
- electromyogram (ee lek troh **MY** oh gram)
- electron (ee **LEK** tron)
- encapsulated (en **CAP** soo lay ted)
- endoscopic (en doh **SKOP** ik) surgery
- ergonomics (er goh **NOM** iks)
- exploratory surgery (ek **SPLOR** ah tor ee **SER** jer ee)
- explosive disorder (ek **SPLOH** siv dis **OR** der)
- eyedrops
- factitious disorders
- film
- film badge
- fine motor skills
- fluoroscopy (floo or **OS** koh pee)
- forceps (**FOR** seps)
- Fowler
- gait (**GAYT**)
- gastrectomy (gas **TREK** toh mee)
- Geiger (**GYE** ger) counter
- general anesthesia
- generic name
- grade
- gross motor skills
- habituation (hah bich yoo **AY** shun)
- hallucinations (hah loo sih **NAY** shuns)
- hemostasis (hee moh **STAY** sis)
- hemostat (**HEE** moh stat)
- hormone therapy (**HOR** mohn **THAIR** ah pee)
- hydrotherapy (high droh **THAIR** ah pee)
- hyperplasia (high per **PLAY** zee ah)
- hypochondria (high poh **KON** dree ah)
- iatrogenic (eye ah troh **JEN** ik)
- ice packs
- idiosyncrasy (id ee oh **SIN** krah see)
- immunotherapy (im yoo noh **THAIR** ah pee)
- impulse control disorders

- inhalation (in hah **LAY** shun)
- insomnia (in **SOM** nee ah)
- intracavitary (in trah **KAV** ih tair ee)
- intradermal (in trah **DER** mal)
- intramuscular (in trah **MUSS** kyoo lar)
- intrathecal (in trah **THEE** kal)
- intravenous (in trah **VEE** nus)
- invasive (in **VAY** siv) disease
- kleptomania (klep toh **MAY** nee ah)
- laser surgery
- lateral recumbent (**LAT** er al ree **KUM** bent)
- lateral (**LAT** er al) view
- lithotomy (lith **OT** oh mee)
- local anesthesia
- low sex drive
- lower extremity
- lumbar puncture (**LUM** bar **PUNK** chur)
- magnetic resonance (**REZ** oh nence) imaging
- major depression
- malignant (mah **LIG** nant)
- malingering
- mania (**MAY** nee ah)
- masochism (**MAS** oh kizm)
- massage (mah **SAHZH**)
- mental retardation
- metastases (meh **TASS** tah seez)
- metastasis (meh **TASS** tah sis)
- mobility
- moist hot packs
- mood disorders
- morbidity (mor **BID** ih tee)
- mortality (mor **TAL** ih tee)
- multiple personality disorder (**MULL** tih pl per son **AL** ih tee dis **OR** der)
- mutation (mew **TAY** shun)
- narcissistic personality disorder (nar sis **SIST** ik per son **AL** ih tee dis **OR** der)
- needle biopsy (**BYE** op see)
- neoplasm (**NEE** oh plazm)
- nerve conduction velocity
- neurosis (noo **ROH** sis)
- nonprescription drug
- nonproprietary name

- ❏ normal psychology
- ❏ nuclear medicine
- ❏ nurse anesthetist (ah **NES** the tist)
- ❏ oblique (oh **BLEEK**) view
- ❏ obsessive-compulsive disorder (ob **SESS** iv kom **PUHL** siv dis **OR** der)
- ❏ occupational therapy
- ❏ oncogenic (ong koh **JEN** ik)
- ❏ oncology (ong **KALL** oh jee)
- ❏ operative report
- ❏ oral (**OR** al)
- ❏ organic mental disease
- ❏ orthotics (or **THOT** iks)
- ❏ over-the-counter (OTC) drug
- ❏ pain control
- ❏ palliative therapy (**PAL** ee ah tiv **THAIR** ah pee)
- ❏ panic attacks
- ❏ paranoid personality disorder (**PAIR** ah noyd per son **AL** ih tee dis **OR** der)
- ❏ parenteral (par **EN** ter al)
- ❏ passive aggressive personality (**PASS** iv ah **GRESS** iv per son **AL** ih tee)
- ❏ passive range of motion
- ❏ pathological (path ah **LOJ** ih kal) gambling
- ❏ pathologist (path **ALL** oh jist)
- ❏ pedophilia (pee doh **FILL** ee ah)
- ❏ percussion (per **KUH** shun)
- ❏ perioperative (per ee **OP** er ah tiv)
- ❏ personality disorder (per son **AL** ih tee dis **OR** der)
- ❏ pharmaceutical (far mih **SOO** tih kal)
- ❏ pharmacist (**FAR** mah sist)
- ❏ pharmacology (far mah **KALL** oh jee)
- ❏ phobias (**FOH** bee ahs)
- ❏ phonophoresis (foh noh foh **REE** sis)
- ❏ photophobia (foh toh **FOH** bee ah)
- ❏ physiatrist (fiz ee **AT** rist)
- ❏ physical medicine
- ❏ physical therapy
- ❏ *Physician's Desk Reference*
- ❏ placebo (plah **SEE** boh)
- ❏ positron emission tomography (**POS** ih tron eh **MIS** shun toh **MOG** rah fee)
- ❏ posteroanterior view
- ❏ postoperative (post **OP** er ah tiv)

- ❏ postural drainage with clapping
- ❏ potentiation (poe ten chee **A** shun)
- ❏ premature ejaculation (ee jak yoo **LAY** shun)
- ❏ preoperative (pree **OP** er ah tiv)
- ❏ prescription (prih **SKRIP** shun)
- ❏ prescription (prih **SKRIP** shun) drug
- ❏ primary site
- ❏ probe
- ❏ prone (**PROHN**)
- ❏ prophylaxis (proh fih **LAK** sis)
- ❏ proprietary (proh **PRYE** ah tair ee) name
- ❏ prosthetics (pros **THET** iks)
- ❏ protocol (**PROH** toh kall)
- ❏ psychiatric (sigh kee **AT** rik) nurses
- ❏ psychiatric (sigh kee **AT** rik) social workers
- ❏ psychiatrist (sigh **KIGH** ah trist)
- ❏ psychiatry (sigh **KIGH** ah tree)
- ❏ psychology (sigh **KALL** oh jee)
- ❏ psychopharmacology (sigh koh far mah **KALL** oh jee)
- ❏ psychosis (sigh **KOH** sis)
- ❏ psychotherapy (sigh koh **THAIR** ah pee)
- ❏ pyromania (pie roh **MAY** nee ah)
- ❏ radiation therapy (ray dee **AY** shun **THAIR** ah pee)
- ❏ radical surgery
- ❏ radioactive (ray dee oh **AK** tiv)
- ❏ radioactive (ray dee oh **AK** tiv) implant
- ❏ radiography (ray dee **OG** rah fee)
- ❏ radioisotope (ray dee oh **EYE** soh tohp)
- ❏ radiologist (ray dee **ALL** oh jist)
- ❏ radiology (ray dee **ALL** oh jee)
- ❏ radiolucent (ray dee oh **LOO** cent)
- ❏ radiopaque (ray dee oh **PAYK**)
- ❏ range of motion
- ❏ rectal (**REK** tal)
- ❏ regional anesthesia
- ❏ rehabilitation (ree hah bill ih **TAY** shun)
- ❏ remission (rih **MISH** un)
- ❏ resection (ree **SEK** shun)
- ❏ roentgen (**RENT** gen)
- ❏ roentgenology (rent gen **ALL** oh jee)
- ❏ scalpel
- ❏ scan
- ❏ schizophrenia

- scrub nurse
- sexual disorders
- shield
- side effect
- sleeping disorders
- sleepwalking
- somatoform disorders
- speculum (**SPEK** yoo lum)
- staging
- staging laparotomy (lap ah **ROT** oh mee)
- subcutaneous (sub kyoo **TAY** nee us)
- sublingual (sub **LING** gwal)
- substance-related disorders
- supine (soo **PINE**)
- suppositories (suh **POZ** ih tor ees)
- surgeon
- surgery
- suture (**SOO** cher) material
- tagging
- tenaculum (teh **NAK** yoo lum)
- therapeutic (thair ah **PEW** tik) exercise
- thermotherapy (ther moh **THAIR** ah pee)

- thoracotomy (thor ah **KOT** oh mee)
- tolerance (**TAHL** er ans)
- topical (**TOP** ih kal)
- topical (**TOP** ih kal) anesthesia
- toxicity (tok **SISS** ih tee)
- traction (**TRAK** shun)
- trade name
- transcutaneous electrical nerve stimulation (tranz kyoo **TAY** nee us ee **LEK** trih kl nerve stim yoo **LAY** shun)
- transdermal (tranz **DER** mal)
- Trendelenburg (**TREN** dee len berg)
- trephine (treh **FINE**)
- tumors (**TOO** mors)
- ultrasound (**ULL** trah sound)
- unit dose
- upper extremity
- uptake
- vaginal (**VAJ** in al)
- voyeurism (**VOY** er izm)
- whirlpool
- X-rays

# Case Study

## Oncology Consultation Report

**Current Complaint:** Patient is a 72-year-old female complaining of increasing level of dyspnea with activity during the past 6 months. She now has a frequent harsh cough producing thick sputum and occasional hemoptysis.

**History:** Patient has had hysterectomy for endometriosis at age 45, cholecystectomy for cholelithiasis at age 62, and recent compression fracture of lumbar spine secondary to osteoporosis. Her only current medication is a calcium supplement for osteoporosis.

**Physical Examination:** Patient is thin and short of stature. She has mild kyphosis. She is alert and answers all questions appropriately. She is not SOB sitting in examination room. Auscultation of chest reveals marked rales, but no rhonchi. She has a persistent cough and sputum was collected for a sputum culture and sensitivity and a sputum cytologic testing.

**Diagnostic Test Results:** Chest radiograph revealed a suspicious cloudy area in right lung. Follow-up with CT scan of the bronchial tree confirmed the presence of a mass in the right lung. Sputum specimen was negative for the presence of bacteria. Sputum cytologic testing revealed malignant cells, indicating presence of cancerous tumor in the lungs.

**Diagnosis:** Bronchogenic carcinoma.

**Treatment Plan:** Patient will be referred to thoracic surgeon for consultation regarding thoracotomy and lobectomy. Following recovery from this surgery she is to return to oncology clinic for chemotherapy and to determine if the tumor has metastasized.

## Critical Thinking Questions

1. The patient had three complaints. List the three complaints and describe each in your own words.

    a.

    b.

    c.

2. This patient had two surgical procedures. Name them and explain why each is necessary.

    a.

    b.

3. The patient has had mild kyphosis. What is kyphosis and which system is this pathology associated with?

4. What do the two abbreviations used in this case study stand for?

    a. SOB

    b. CT scan

5. The patient will have a surgical procedure before chemotherapy that is described by two words. List them and describe what each means.

    a.

    b.

6. What does the term *metastasized* mean?

## Chart Note

The chart note below contains 11 phrases that can be re-worded with a medical term that you learned in this chapter. Each phrase is identified with an underline. Determine the medical term and write your answers in the space provided.

**Current Complaint:** A 56-year-old male was referred to a specialist in the treatment of cancer① for treatment of a suspicious right kidney mass discovered by his internist on a CT scan.

**Past History:** Patient had been aware of right side pain, difficulty urinating, and weight loss during the past 6 months.

**Signs and Symptoms:** A surgery performed to determine if cancer is present② was performed and small samples of tissue removed for examination under a microscope③ were taken from the suspicious right kidney mass. After it was determined to be cancerous with a tendency to grow worse,④ a right nephrectomy was performed. Reports indicate that the new and abnormal growth⑤ was graded to be moderately differentiated⑥ and well enclosed in a sheath of tissue⑦ with no signs of spreading to another part of the body.⑧

**Diagnosis:** Cancerous tumor of the right kidney.⑨

**Treatment:** Post surgery the patient began a plan of treatment⑩ of the use of chemical agents with a specific toxic effect.⑪

1. _____
2. _____
3. _____
4. _____
5. _____
6. _____
7. _____
8. _____
9. _____
10. _____
11. _____

# Practice Exercises

## A. Complete the following statements:

1. The reference book containing important information regarding medications is the _____ .
2. A person specializing in the dispensing of medications is a _____ .
3. The accepted official name for a drug is the _____ name.
4. The trade name for a drug is the _____ name.
5. What does the chemical name represent? _____
6. What federal agency enforces controls over the use of drugs causing dependency? _____

## B. Name the route of drug administration for the following descriptions.

1. under the tongue _____
2. into the anus or rectum _____
3. applied to the skin _____
4. injected under the first layer of skin _____
5. injected into a muscle _____
6. injected into a vein _____
7. by mouth _____

## C. Define the following terms in the space provided.

1. idiosyncrasy _____
2. parenteral _____
3. placebo _____
4. toxicity _____
5. side effect _____
6. unit dose _____
7. habituation _____
8. antidote _____
9. contraindication _____
10. prophylaxis _____

## D. Give the meaning of the following abbreviations in the space provided.

1. gr _____
2. bid _____
3. tid _____
4. ad lib _____
5. prn _____
6. ante _____
7. OTC _____
8. gt _____

9. Sig _____

10. stat _____

11. tinc _____

12. qd _____

13. noc _____

14. NPO _____

15. hs _____

16. ung _____

17. TO _____

18. gtt _____

19. C _____

20. d/c _____

## E. Write out the following prescription instructions in the space provided.

1. Pravachol, 20 mg., Sig. i qd @ noc, 30, refill 3x, no sub. _____

2. Lanoxin 0.125 mg., Sig. iii stat, then ii q AM, C, refills prn. _____

3. Synthroid 0.075 mg., Sig. i qd, C, refill x4. _____

4. Norvasc 5 mg., i q am, 60, refillable. _____

## F. Match the mental disorder category with the correct example.

### A

_____ 1. cognitive disorders

_____ 2. factitious disorders

_____ 3. dissociative disorders

_____ 4. eating disorders

_____ 5. sleeping disorders

_____ 6. mood disorders

_____ 7. impulse control disorders

_____ 8. somatoform disorders

_____ 9. personality disorders

_____ 10. sexual disorders

_____ 11. anxiety disorders

### B

a. hypochondria

b. kleptomania

c. masochism

d. narcissistic personality

e. insomnia

f. bipolar disease

g. panic attacks

h. amnesia

i. dementia

j. anorexia nervosa

k. malingering

## G. Identify each mental health treatment from its description.

1. depressant drugs prescribed for anxiety _____

2. client-centered psychotherapy _____

3. drug used to calm patients with bipolar disorder _____

4. reduces patient agitation and panic and shortens schizophrenic episodes _____

5. obtains a detailed account of the past and present emotional and mental experiences _____

6. stimulants that alter the patient's mood by affecting neurotransmitter levels _____

## H. Identify the following abbreviations.

1. MRI _____
2. Ba _____
3. AP _____
4. CT _____
5. RL _____
6. PA _____
7. LL _____
8. PET _____
9. UGI _____
10. KUB _____

## I. Match the terms in column A with the definitions in column B.

| A | B |
|---|---|
| _____ 1. ultrasound | a. radiopaque substances used to outline hollow structures |
| _____ 2. MRI | b. records velocity of blood flowing through vessels |
| _____ 3. Doppler US | c. image created by electromagnetic energy |
| _____ 4. nuclear medicine scan | d. glowing screen shows movement |
| _____ 5. CT scan | e. making an X-ray |
| _____ 6. contrast study | f. multiple-angle X-rays compiled into a cross-section |
| _____ 7. fluoroscopy | g. uses radioactive substances |
| _____ 8. radiography | h. image of internal organs using sound waves |
| _____ 9. PET scan | i. indicates metabolic activity |

## J. Identify the following abbreviations.

1. ROM _____
2. OT _____
3. ADL _____
4. LE _____
5. EMG _____
6. TENS _____
7. PT _____
8. PROM _____
9. e-stim _____
10. US _____

## K. Identify the rehabilitation procedure described by each phrase.

1. kneading or applying pressure by hands _____
2. removal of dead and damaged tissue from a wound _____
3. using water for treatment purposes _____

4. drainage of secretions from the bronchi _____

5. exercises performed by a patient without resistance _____

6. medication introduced by ultrasound waves _____

7. use of cold for therapeutic purposes _____

8. pulling with a mechanical device _____

## L. Match each term with its definition.

| A | B |
|---|---|
| _____ 1. forceps | a. scrapes and removes tissue |
| _____ 2. tenaculum | b. cuts and separates tissue |
| _____ 3. Trendelenburg | c. lying horizontal and face up |
| _____ 4. lithotomy | d. lying on either the left or right side |
| _____ 5. curette | e. long handled clamp |
| _____ 6. aspirator | f. explores tissue |
| _____ 7. supine | g. lying face up with hips and knees bent at 90° angle |
| _____ 8. probe | h. grasps tissue |
| _____ 9. scalpel | i. suctions fluid |
| _____ 10. lateral recumbent | j. lying face up on an incline, head lower than legs |

## M. Identify the type of anesthesia for each description.

1. produces loss of consciousness and absence of pain _____

2. produces loss of sensation in one localized part of the body _____

3. anesthetic applied directly onto a specific skin area _____

4. also referred to as a nerve block _____

## N. Match the following terms to their definitions:

| A | B |
|---|---|
| _____ 1. oncogenic | a. examine cells to determine their structure and origin |
| _____ 2. benign | b. the plan for care for any individual patient |
| _____ 3. encapsulated | c. biopsy |
| _____ 4. PAP | d. growth that is not recurrent or progressive |
| _____ 5. primary site | e. placing a radioactive substance directly into the tissue |
| _____ 6. protocol | f. where the malignant tumor first appeared |
| _____ 7. staging laparotomy | g. growth is enclosed in a tissue sheath |
| _____ 8. cytologic testing | h. cancer causing |
| _____ 9. radioactive implant | i. abdominal surgery to determine extent of tumor |
| _____ 10. bx | j. Papanicolaou test |

# Professional Journal

In this exercise you will now have an opportunity to put the words you have learned into practice. Many new medical professionals have been introduced in the Professional Profiles throughout this chapter: pharmacist, psychiatrist, psychologist, radiologic technologist, sonographer, nuclear medicine technologist, physical therapist, occupational therapist, surgery technologist, and cytotechnologist. Imagine yourself in the role of three different professionals from this chapter. Review the terms associated with each profession and write three to four sentences for each to describe the patients you saw today.

An example of a sentence for a physical therapist is *My first patient this afternoon suffered from severe muscle spasms in his low back, which got much better after I gave him an ultrasound treatment.*

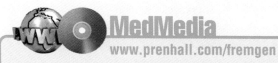

www.prenhall.com/fremgen

Use the CD-ROM enclosed with your textbook to gain additional reinforcement through interactive word building exercises, spelling games, labeling activities, and additional quizzes.

Use the above address to access the free, interactive Companion Website created for this textbook. Get hints, instant feedback, and textbook references to chapter-related multiple-choice questions, as well as labeling and matching exercises. In addition, you will find an audio glossary, case studies, and Internet exploration exercises.

***For more information regarding general disease information, visit the following websites:***

Centers for Disease Control and Prevention's Health Topics A to Z at
   **www.cdc.gov/health/default.htm**

Health Information provided by the National Institutes of Health at **http://health/nih.gov**

Health Information provided by the Stanford Health Library at **http://healthlibrary.stanford.edu**

InteliHealth featuring Harvard Medical School's Consumer Health Information at
   **www.intelihealth.com**

Medical Encyclopedia provided by University of Maryland Medicine at **www.umm.edu/ency**

University of Iowa Health Care's Virtual Hospital at **www.vh.org**

# Appendix

## Abbreviations

| Abbreviation | Meaning |
|---|---|
| @ | at |
| 5-FU | 5-fluorouracil |
| $^{67}$Ga | radioactive gallium |
| $^{99m}$Tc | radioactive technetium |
| $^{131}$I | radioactive iodine |
| $^{133}$Xe | radioactive xenon |
| $^{201}$TI | radioactive thallium |
| ā | before |
| AB | abortion |
| ABGs | arterial blood gases |
| ac | before meals |
| ACAT | automated computerized axial tomography |
| Acc | accommodation |
| ACL | anterior cruciate ligament |
| ACTH | adrenocorticotropic hormone |
| AD | right ear, Alzheimer's disease |
| ad lib | as desired |
| ADD | attention deficit disorder |
| ADH | antidiuretic hormone |
| ADHD | attention-deficit-hyperactivity disorder |
| ADL | activities of daily living |
| AE | above elbow |
| AF | atrial fibrillation |
| AGN | acute glomerulonephritis |
| AHF | antihemophilic factor |
| AI | artificial insemination |
| AIDS | acquired immunodeficiency syndrome |
| AK | above knee |
| ALL | acute lymphocytic leukemia |
| ALS | amyotropic lateral sclerosis |
| ALT | alanine transaminase |
| am, AM | morning |
| AMI | acute myocardial infarction |
| AML | acute myelogenous leukemia |
| amt | amount |
| Angio | angiography |
| ANS | autonomic nervous system |
| ante | before |

| Abbreviation | Meaning |
|---|---|
| AP | anteroposterior |
| APAP | acetaminophen (Tylenol™) |
| aq | aqueous (water) |
| ARC | AIDS-related complex |
| ARD | acute respiratory disease |
| ARDS | adult respiratory distress syndrome |
| ARF | acute respiratory failure, acute renal failure |
| ARMD | age-related macular degeneration |
| AROM | active range of motion |
| AS | aortic stenosis, arteriosclerosis, left ear |
| ASA | aspirin |
| ASCVD | arteriosclerotic cardiovascular disease |
| ASD | atrial septal defect |
| ASHD | arteriosclerotic heart disease |
| ASL | American Sign Language |
| AST | aspartate transaminase |
| Astigm. | astigmatism |
| ATN | acute tubulor necrosis |
| AU | both ears |
| AuD | doctor of audiology |
| AV, A-V | atrioventricular |
| Ba | barium |
| BaE | barium enema |
| basos | basophil |
| BBB | bundle branch block (L for left; R for right) |
| BC | bone conduction |
| BCC | basal cell carcinoma |
| BDT | bone density testing |
| BE | barium enema, below elbow |
| bid | twice a day |
| BK | below knee |
| BM | bowel movement |
| BMR | basal metabolic rate |
| BMT | bone marrow transplant |
| BNO | bladder neck obstruction |
| BP | blood pressure |
| BPD | bipolar disorder |
| BPH | benign prostatic hypertrophy |

| Abbreviation | Meaning |
|---|---|
| bpm | beats per minute |
| Bronch | bronchoscopy |
| BS | bowel sounds |
| BSE | breast self-examination |
| BSN | bachelor of science in nursing |
| BUN | blood urea nitrogen |
| BX, bx | biopsy |
| c̄ | with |
| C | 100 |
| C1, C2, etc. | first cervical vertebra, second cervical vertebra, etc. |
| $Ca^{2+}$ | calcium |
| CA | cancer, chronological age |
| CABG | coronary artery bypass graft |
| CAD | coronary artery disease |
| cap(s) | capsule(s) |
| CAPD | continuous ambulatory peritoneal dialysis |
| CAT | computerized axial tomography |
| cath | catheterization |
| CBC | complete blood count |
| CBD | common bile duct |
| cc | cubic centimeter |
| CC | clean catch urine specimen cardiac catheterization chief complaint |
| CCC | speech-language pathologist |
| CCS | certified coding specialist |
| CCU | cardiac care unit, coronary care unit |
| CD4 | protein on T-cell helper lymphocyte |
| CDH | congenital dislocation of the hip |
| c.gl. | correction with glasses |
| CGL | chronic granulocytic leukemia |
| chemo | chemotherapy |
| CHF | congestive heart failure |
| chol | cholesterol |
| Ci | curie |
| CIS | carcinoma in situ |
| $Cl^-$ | chloride |
| CLL | chronic lymphocytic leukemia |
| CLS | clinical laboratory scientist |
| CLT | clinical laboratory technician |
| CMA | certified medical assistant |
| CML | chronic myelogenous leukemia |
| CNA | certified nurse aide |

| Abbreviation | Meaning |
|---|---|
| CNIM | certification in neurophysiologic intraoperative monitoring |
| CNS | central nervous system |
| $CO_2$ | carbon dioxide |
| CoA | coarctation of the aorta |
| COLD | chronic obstructive lung disease |
| COPD | chronic obstructive pulmonary disease |
| COTA | certified occupational therapy assistant |
| CP | cerebral palsy, chest pain |
| CPD | cephalopelvic disproportion |
| CPK | creatine phosphokinase |
| CPR | cardiopulmonary resuscitation |
| CRF | chronic renal failure |
| crit | hematocrit |
| CRT | certified respiratory therapist |
| C & S | culture and sensitivity test |
| CS, CS-section | cesarean section |
| CSD | congenital septal defect |
| CSF | cerebrospinal fluid |
| CT | computerized tomography, cytotechnologist |
| CTA | clear to auscultation |
| CTS | carpal tunnel syndrome |
| CUC | chronic ulcerative colitis |
| CV | cardiovascular |
| CVA | cerebrovascular accident |
| CVD | cerebrovascular disease |
| CVS | chorionic villus biopsy |
| Cx | cervix |
| CXR | chest X-ray |
| cyl lens | cylindrical lens |
| cysto | cystoscopic exam |
| d | day |
| D | diopter (lens strength) |
| D & C | dilation and curettage |
| D/C, d/c | discontinue |
| dB | decibel |
| DC | doctor of chiropractic |
| DDM | doctor of dental medicine |
| DDS | doctor of dental surgery |
| DEA | Drug Enforcement Agency |
| decub | lying down, decubitus ulcer |
| Derm, derm | dermatology |
| DI | diabetes insipidus, diagnostic imaging |

| Abbreviation | Meaning |
|---|---|
| diff | differential |
| dil | dilute |
| disc | discontinue |
| disp | dispense |
| DJD | degenerative joint disease |
| DM | diabetes mellitus |
| DO | doctor of osteopathy |
| DOB | date of birth |
| DOE | dyspnea on exertion |
| DPT | diphtheria, pertussis, tetanus; doctor of physical therapy |
| dr | dram |
| DRE | digital rectal exam |
| DSA | digital subtraction angiography |
| DSM-IV | *Diagnostic and Statistical Manual for Mental Disorders,* Fourth edition |
| DTR | deep tendon reflex; dietetic technician, registered |
| DUB | dysfunctional uterine bleeding |
| DVA | distance visual acuity |
| DVT | deep vein thrombosis |
| Dx | diagnosis |
| E. coli | *Escherichia coli* |
| EAU | exam under anesthesia |
| EBV | Epstein–Barr virus |
| ECC | endocervical curettage, extracorporeal circulation |
| ECCE | extracapsular cataract extraction |
| ECG | electrocardiogram |
| Echo | echocardiogram |
| ECT | electroconvulsive therapy |
| ED | erectile dysfunction |
| EDC | estimated date of confinement |
| EEG | electroencephalogram, electroencephalography |
| EENT | eyes, ears, nose, throat |
| EGD | esophagogastroduodenoscopy |
| EKG | electrocardiogram |
| ELISA | enzyme-linked immunosorbent assay |
| elix | elixir |
| EM | emmetropia (normal vision) |
| EMB | endometrial biopsy |
| EMG | electromyogram |
| EMT-B | emergency medical technician–basic |
| EMT-I | emergency medical technician–intermediate |
| EMT-P | emergency medical technician–paramedic |

| Abbreviation | Meaning |
|---|---|
| emul | emulsion |
| Endo | endoscopy |
| ENT | ear, nose, and throat |
| EOM | extraocular movement |
| eosins, eos | eosinophil |
| ER | emergency room |
| ERCP | endoscopic retrograde cholangiopancreatography |
| ERT | estrogen replacement therapy |
| ERV | expiratory reserve volume |
| ESR | erythrocyte sedimentation rate |
| ESRD | end-stage renal disease |
| e-stim | electrical stimulation |
| ESWL | extracorporeal shock-wave lithotripsy |
| et | and |
| ET | endotracheal |
| FBS | fasting blood sugar |
| FDA | Federal Drug Administration |
| Fe | iron |
| FEF | forced expiratory flow |
| FEKG | fetal electrocardiogram |
| FEV | forced expiratory volume |
| FHR | fetal heart rate |
| FHT | fetal heart tone |
| fl | fluid |
| FOBT | fecal occult blood test |
| FRC | functional residual capacity |
| FS | frozen section |
| FSH | follicle-stimulating hormone |
| FTND | full-term normal delivery |
| FVC | forced vital capacity |
| Fx, FX | fracture |
| GI | first pregnancy |
| Ga | gallium |
| GA | general anesthesia |
| GB | gallbladder |
| GC | gonorrhea |
| GERD | gastroesophageal reflux disease |
| GH | growth hormone |
| GI | gastrointestinal |
| gm | gram |
| GOT | glutamic oxaloacetic transaminase |
| gr | grain |
| grav I | first pregnancy |

| Abbreviation | Meaning |
|---|---|
| gt | drop |
| gtt | drops |
| GTT | glucose tolerance test |
| GU | genitourinary |
| GVHD | graft vs. host disease |
| GYN, gyn | gynecology |
| H$_2$O | water |
| HA | headache |
| HAV | hepatitis A virus |
| Hb | hemoglobin |
| HBOT | hyperbaric oxygen therapy |
| HBV | hepatitis B virus |
| HCG, hCG | human chorionic gonadotropin |
| HCO$_3^-$ | bicarbonate |
| HCT, Hct | hematocrit |
| HCV | hepatitis C virus |
| HD | Hodgkin's disease |
| HDL | high-density lipoproteins |
| HDN | hemolytic disease of the newborn |
| HEENT | head, ears, eyes, nose, throat |
| Hgb, HGB | hemoglobin |
| HIV | human immunodeficieny virus |
| HMD | hyaline membrane disease |
| HNP | herniated nucleus pulposus |
| HPV | human papilloma virus |
| HRT | hormone replacement therapy |
| hs | hour of sleep |
| HSG | hysterosalpingography |
| HSV | *Herpes simplex* virus |
| HTN | hypertension |
| Hz | Hertz |
| i̅ | one |
| IBD | inflammatory bowel disease |
| IBS | irritable bowel syndrome |
| IC | inspiratory capacity |
| ICCE | intracapsular cataract cryoextraction |
| ICP | intracranial pressure |
| ICU | intensive care unit |
| I & D | incision and drainage |
| ID | intradermal |
| IDDM | insulin-dependent diabetes mellitus |
| Ig | immunoglobins (IgA, IgD, IgE, IgG, IgM) |
| ii̅ | two |

| Abbreviation | Meaning |
|---|---|
| iii̅ | three |
| IM | intramuscular |
| inj | injection |
| I & O | intake and output |
| IOL | intraocular lens |
| IOP | intraocular pressure |
| IPD | intermittent peritoneal dialysis |
| IPPB | intermittent positive pressure breathing |
| IRDS | infant respiratory distress syndrome |
| IRV | inspiratory reserve volume |
| IU | international unit |
| IUD | intrauterine device |
| IV | intravenous |
| IVC | intravenous cholangiogram |
| IVF | *in vitro* fertilization |
| IVP | intravenous pyelogram |
| JRA | juvenile rheumatoid arthritis |
| JVP | jugular venous pulse |
| K$^+$ | potassium |
| kg | kilogram |
| KS | Kaposi's sarcoma |
| KUB | kidney, ureter, bladder |
| L | left, liter |
| L1, L2, etc. | first lumbar vertebra, second lumbar vertebra, etc. |
| LASIK | laser-assisted in-situ keratomileusis |
| LAT, lat | lateral |
| LAVH | laparoscopic-assisted vaginal hysterectomy |
| LBW | low birth weight |
| LDH | lactate dehydrogenase |
| LDL | low-density lipoproteins |
| LE | lower extremity |
| LGI | lower gastrointestinal series |
| LH | luteinizing hormone |
| liq | liquid |
| LL | left lateral |
| LLE | left lower extremity |
| LLL | left lower lobe |
| LLQ | left lower quadrant |
| LMP | last menstrual period |
| LP | lumbar puncture |
| LPN | licensed practical nurse |
| LUE | left upper extremity |

| Abbreviation | Meaning |
|---|---|
| LUL | left upper lobe |
| LUQ | left upper quadrant |
| LVAD | left ventricular assist device |
| LVH | left ventricular hypertrophy |
| lymphs | lymphocyte |
| LVN | licensed vocational nurse |
| mA | milliampere |
| MA | mental age |
| MAO | monoamine oxidase |
| mcg | microgram |
| mCi | millicurie |
| MCV | mean corpuscular volume |
| MD | doctor of medicine, muscular dystrophy |
| mEq | milliequivalent |
| mets | metastases |
| mg | milligram |
| MH | marital history |
| MI | myocardial infarction, mitral insufficiency |
| mL | milliliter |
| MLT | medical laboratory technician |
| mm | millimeter |
| MM | malignant melanoma |
| mm Hg | millimeters of mercury |
| MMPI | Minnesota Multiphasic Personality Inventory |
| Mono | mononucleosis |
| monos | monocyte |
| MR | mitral regurgitation |
| MRA | magnetic resonance angiography |
| MRI | magnetic resonance imaging |
| MS | mitral stenosis, multiple sclerosis, musculoskeletal |
| MSH | melanocyte-stimulating hormone |
| MSN | master of science in nursing |
| MT | medical technologist |
| MTX | methotrexate |
| MUA | manipulation under anesthesia |
| MV | minute volume |
| MVP | mitral valve prolapse |
| n & v | nausea and vomiting |
| Na$^+$ | sodium |
| NB | newborn |
| NG | nasogastric (tube) |
| NGU | nongonococcal urethritis |

| Abbreviation | Meaning |
|---|---|
| NHL | non-Hodgkin's lymphoma |
| NIDDM | non–insulin-dependent diabetes mellitus |
| NK | natural killer cells |
| NMR | nuclear magnetic resonance |
| no sub | no substitute |
| noc | night |
| non rep | do not repeat |
| NP | nurse practitioner |
| NPDL | nodular, poorly differentiated lymphocytes |
| NPH | neutral protamine Hagedorn (insulin) |
| NPO | nothing by mouth |
| NS | normal saline |
| NSAID | nonsteroidal anti-inflammatory drug |
| NSR | normal sinus rhythm |
| O$_2$ | oxygen |
| OA | osteoarthritis |
| OB | obstetrics |
| OCD | obsessive-compulsive disorder |
| OCPs | oral contraceptive pills |
| OD | overdose, right eye, doctor of optometry |
| oint. | ointment |
| OM | otitis media |
| O & P | ova and parasites |
| Ophth. | ophthalmology |
| OR | operating room |
| ORIF | open reduction–internal fixation |
| Orth, ortho | orthopedics |
| OS | left eye |
| OT | occupational therapy |
| OTC | over the counter |
| Oto | otology |
| OTR | occupational therapist |
| OU | each eye |
| oz | ounce |
| p̄ | after |
| P | pulse |
| PI | first delivery |
| PA | posteroanterior, physician assistant, pernicious anemia |
| PAC | premature atrial contraction |
| PAP | Papanicolaou test, pulmonary arterial pressure |
| para I | first delivery |

| Abbreviation | Meaning |
|---|---|
| PARR | postanesthetic recovery room |
| PBI | protein-bound iodine |
| pc | after meals |
| PCA | patient-controlled administration |
| PCP | *Pneumocystis carinii* pneumonia |
| PCV | packed cell volume |
| PDA | patent ductus arteriosus |
| PDR | *Physician's Desk Reference* |
| PE tube | polyethylene tube placed in the eardrum |
| PEG | pneumoencephalogram, percutaneous endoscopic gastrostomy |
| per | with |
| PERRLA | pupils equal, round, react to light and accommodation |
| PET | positron emission tomography |
| PFT | pulmonary function test |
| pH | acidity or alkalinity of urine |
| PharmD | doctor of pharmacy |
| PID | pelvic inflammatory disease |
| PKU | phenylketonuria |
| PM, pm | evening |
| PMNs | polymorphonuclear neutrophil |
| PMP | previous menstrual period |
| PMS | premenstrual syndrome |
| PND | paroxysmal nocturnal dyspnea, postnasal drip |
| PNS | peripheral nervous system |
| PO, po | phone order, by mouth |
| polys | polymorphonuclear neutrophil |
| PORP | partial ossicular replacement prosthesis |
| pp | postprandial (after meals) |
| PPD | purified protein derivative (tuberculin test) |
| preop, pre-op | preoperative |
| prep | preparation, prepared |
| PRK | photo refractive keratectomy |
| PRL | prolactin |
| prn | as needed |
| Pro-time | prothrombin time |
| PROM | passive range of motion |
| prot | protocol |
| PSA | prostate specific antigen |
| pt | pint |
| PT | prothrombin time, physical therapy, physical therapist |

| Abbreviation | Meaning |
|---|---|
| PTA | physical therapy assistant |
| PTC | percutaneous transhepatic cholangiography |
| PTCA | percutaneous transluminal coronary angioplasty |
| PTH | parathyroid hormone |
| PUD | peptic ulcer disease |
| PVC | premature ventricular contraction |
| q̄ | every |
| qam | every morning |
| qd | once a day, every day |
| qh | every hour |
| qhs | every night |
| qid | four times a day |
| qod | every other day |
| qs | quantity sufficient |
| R | respiration, right, roentgen |
| Ra | radium |
| RA | rheumatoid arthritis |
| rad | radiation absorbed dose |
| RAI | radioactive iodine |
| RAIU | radioactive iodine uptake |
| RBC | red blood cell |
| RD | respiratory disease, registered dietitian |
| RDA | recommended daily allowance |
| RDH | registered dental hygienist |
| RDS | respiratory distress syndrome |
| REEGT | registered electroencephalography technologist |
| REM | rapid eye movement |
| REPT | registered evoked potential technologist |
| Rh− | Rh-negative |
| Rh+ | Rh-positive |
| RHIA | registered health information administrator |
| RHIT | registered health information technician |
| RIA | radioimmunoassay |
| RL | right lateral |
| RLE | right lower extremity |
| RLL | right lower lobe |
| RLQ | right lower quadrant |
| RML | right mediolateral, right middle lobe |
| RN | registered nurse |
| ROM | range of motion |
| RP | retrograde pyelogram |
| RPh | registered pharmacist |
| RPR | rapid plasma reagin (test for syphilis) |

| Abbreviation | Meaning |
|---|---|
| RPSGT | registered polysomnographic technologist |
| RRT | registered radiologic technologist, registered respiratory therapist |
| RUE | right upper extremity |
| RUL | right upper lobe |
| RUQ | right upper quadrant |
| RV | reserve volume |
| Rx | take |
| s̄ | without |
| S1 | first heart sound |
| S2 | second heart sound |
| SA, S-A | sinoatrial |
| SAD | seasonal affective disorder |
| SAH | subarachnoid hemorrhage |
| SBFT | small bowel follow-through |
| SC, sc | subcutaneous |
| SCC | squamous cell carcinoma |
| SCI | spinal cord injury |
| SCIDS | severe combined immunodeficiency syndrome |
| Sed-rate | erythrocyte sedimentation rate |
| SEE-2 | Signing Exact English |
| SG | skin graft, specific gravity |
| s.gl. | without correction or glasses |
| SGOT | serum glutamic oxaloacetic transaminase |
| SIDS | sudden infant death syndrome |
| Sig | label as follows/directions |
| SK | streptokinase |
| sl | under the tongue |
| SLE | systemic lupus erythematosus |
| SMAC | sequential multiple analyzer computer |
| SMD | senile macular degeneration |
| SOB | shortness of breath |
| sol | solution |
| SOM | serous otitis media |
| SPP | suprapubic prostatectomy |
| SR | erythrocyte sedimentation rate |
| ss | one-half |
| st | stage |
| ST | skin test, esotropia |
| stat, STAT | at once, immediately |
| STD | skin test done, sexually transmitted disease |
| STSG | split-thickness skin graft |
| subcu | subcutaneous |

| Abbreviation | Meaning |
|---|---|
| subq | subcutaneous |
| supp. | suppository |
| suppos | suppository |
| susp | suspension |
| syr | syrup |
| T | tablespoon |
| t | teaspoon |
| T & A | tonsillectomy and adenoidectomy |
| T1, T2, etc. | first thoracic vertebra, second thoracic vertebra, etc. |
| $T_3$ | triiodothyronine |
| $T_4$ | thyroxine |
| $T_7$ | free thyroxine index |
| tab | tablet |
| TAH-BSO | total abdominal hysterectomy–bilateral salpingo-ophorectomy |
| TB | tuberculosis |
| tbsp | tablespoon |
| TENS | transcutaneous electrical nerve stimulation |
| TFT | thyroid function test |
| THA | total hip arthroplasty |
| THR | total hip replacement |
| TIA | transient ischemic attack |
| tid | three times a day |
| tinc | tincture |
| TKA | total knee arthroplasty |
| TKR | total knee replacement |
| TLC | total lung capacity |
| TMJ | temporomandibular joint |
| TNM | tumor, nodes, metastases |
| TO | telephone order |
| top | apply topically |
| TORP | total ossicular replacement prosthesis |
| tPA | tissue-type plasminogen activator |
| TPN | total parenteral nutrition |
| TPR | temperature, pulse, and respiration |
| tr | tincture |
| TSH | thyroid-stimulating hormone |
| tsp | teaspoon |
| TSS | toxic shock syndrome |
| TUR | transurethral resection |
| TURP | transurethral resection of prostate |
| TV | tidal volume |

| Abbreviation | Meaning | Abbreviation | Meaning |
|---|---|---|---|
| TX, Tx | traction, treatment | VCUG | voiding cystourethrography |
| u | unit | VD | venereal disease |
| U/A, UA | urinalysis | VF | visual field |
| UC | uterine contractions, urine culture | VFib | ventricular fibrillation |
| UE | upper extremity | VLDL | very low density lipoproteins |
| UGI | upper gastrointestinal, upper gastrointestinal series | VO | verbal order |
| ung | ointment | VS | vital signs |
| URI | upper respiratory infection | VSD | ventricular septal defect |
| US | ultrasound | VT | ventricular tachycardia |
| UTI | urinary tract infection | WBC | white blood cell |
| UV | ultraviolet | wt | weight |
| VA | visual acuity | x | times |
| VC | vital capacity | XT | exotropia |

# Combining Forms

| Combining Form | Meaning |
|---|---|
| abdomin/o | abdomen |
| acous/o | hearing |
| acr/o | extremities |
| aden/o | gland |
| adenoid/o | adenoids |
| adip/o | fat |
| adren/o | adrenal glands |
| adrenal/o | adrenal glands |
| aer/o | air |
| agglutin/o | clumping |
| albin/o | white |
| albumin/o | albumin |
| alveol/o | alveolus; air sac |
| ambly/o | dull or dim |
| amni/o | amnion |
| an/o | anus |
| andr/o | male |
| angi/o | vessel |
| ankyl/o | stiff joint |
| anter/o | front |
| anthrac/o | coal |
| anxi/o | anxiety |
| aort/o | aorta |
| append/o | appendix |
| appendic/o | appendix |
| aque/o | water |
| arteri/o | artery |
| arthr/o | joint |
| articul/o | joint |
| atel/o | incomplete |
| ather/o | fatty substance, plaque |
| atri/o | atrium |
| audi/o | hearing |
| audit/o | hearing |
| aur/o | ear |
| auricul/o | ear |
| azot/o | nitrogenous waste |
| bacteri/o | bacteria |
| balan/o | glans penis |
| bi/o | life |
| blast/o | primitive cell |
| blephar/o | eyelid |
| bronch/o | bronchus |

| Combining Form | Meaning |
|---|---|
| bronchus/o | bronchiole |
| bronchiol/o | bronchiole |
| bucc/o | cheek |
| burs/o | sac |
| calc/o | calcium |
| carcin/o | cancer |
| cardi/o | heart |
| carp/o | wrist |
| caud/o | tail |
| cec/o | cecum |
| cephal/o | head |
| cerebell/o | cerebellum |
| cerebr/o | cerebrum |
| cervic/o | neck, cervix |
| cheil/o | lip |
| chem/o | chemical, drug |
| chol/e | bile, gall |
| cholangi/o | bile duct |
| cholecyst/o | gallbladder |
| choledoch/o | common bile duct |
| chondr/o | cartilage |
| chori/o | chorion |
| chrom/o | color |
| cis/o | to cut |
| clavicul/o | clavicle, collar bone |
| coagul/o | clotting |
| coccyg/o | coccyx, tailbone |
| cochle/o | cochlea |
| col/o | colon |
| colon/o | colon |
| colp/o | vagina |
| coni/o | dust |
| conjunctiv/o | conjunctiva |
| core/o | pupil |
| corne/o | cornea |
| coron/o | heart |
| cost/o | rib |
| crani/o | skull |
| crin/o | secrete |
| cry/o | cold |
| crypt/o | hidden |
| culd/o | cul-de-sac |
| cutane/o | skin |
| cyan/o | blue |

| Combining Form | Meaning | Combining Form | Meaning |
|---|---|---|---|
| cycl/o | ciliary muscle | hem/o | blood |
| cyst/o | bladder | hemangi/o | blood vessel |
| cyt/o | cell | hemat/o | blood |
| dacry/o | tear; tear duct | hepat/o | liver |
| dent/o | tooth | hidr/o | sweat |
| derm/o | skin | hist/o | tissue |
| dermat/o | skin | home/o | sameness |
| diaphor/o | profuse sweating | humer/o | humerus, upper arm bone |
| diaphragmat/o | diaphragm | hydr/o | water |
| dipl/o | double | hymen/o | hymen |
| dist/o | away from | hyster/o | uterus |
| dors/o | back of body | ichthy/o | scaly, dry |
| duoden/o | duodenum | ile/o | ileum |
| electr/o | electricity | ili/o | ilium |
| embry/o | embryo | immun/o | immune, protection |
| encephal/o | brain | infer/o | below |
| enter/o | small intestines | ir/o | iris |
| epididym/o | epididymis | irid/o | iris |
| epiglott/o | epiglottis | ischi/o | ischium |
| episi/o | vulva | jejun/o | jejunum |
| epitheli/o | epithelium | kal/i | potassium |
| erg/o | work | kerat/o | cornea, hard, horny |
| erythr/o | red | keton/o | ketone |
| esophag/o | esophagus | kyph/o | hump |
| esthesi/o | feeling, sensation | labi/o | lip |
| estr/o | female | labyrinth/o | labyrinth |
| fasci/o | fibrous band | lacrim/o | tears |
| femor/o | femur, thigh bone | lact/o | milk |
| fet/o | fetus | lamin/o | lamina |
| fibr/o | fibers | lapar/o | abdomen |
| fibrin/o | fibers, fibrous | laryng/o | larynx, voice box |
| fibul/o | fibula | later/o | side |
| fluor/o | fluorescence, luminous | leiomy/o | smooth muscle |
| gastr/o | stomach | leuk/o | white |
| gingiv/o | gums | lingu/o | tongue |
| glauc/o | gray | lip/o | fat |
| gli/o | glue | lith/o | stone |
| glomerul/o | glomerulus | lob/o | lobe |
| gloss/o | tongue | lord/o | swayback, curve |
| glyc/o | sugar | lumb/o | loin, lower back |
| glycos/o | sugar, glucose | lymph/o | lymph |
| gonad/o | sex glands | lymphaden/o | lymph node |
| granul/o | granules | lymphangi/o | lymph vessel |
| gynec/o | female | mamm/o | breast |

| Combining Form | Meaning | | Combining Form | Meaning |
|---|---|---|---|---|
| mandibul/o | mandible, lower jawbone | | organ/o | organ |
| mast/o | breast | | orth/o | straight, upright |
| maxill/o | maxilla, upper jaw bone | | oste/o | bone |
| meat/o | meatus | | ot/o | ear |
| medi/o | middle | | ov/o | egg |
| medull/o | medulla | | ovari/o | ovary |
| melan/o | black | | ox/i | oxygen |
| men/o | menses, menstruation | | ox/o | oxygen |
| mening/o | meninges | | pachy/o | thick |
| meningi/o | meninges | | palat/o | palate |
| ment/o | mind | | pancreat/o | pancreas |
| metacarp/o | metacarpus, hand bones | | papill/o | optic disk |
| metatars/o | metatarsals, foot bones | | parathyroid/o | parathyroid gland |
| metr/o | uterus | | part/o | childbirth |
| morph/o | shape | | patell/o | patella, knee cap |
| muscul/o | muscle | | path/o | disease |
| mut/a | genetic change, mutation | | ped/o | foot, child |
| my/o | muscle | | pelv/o | pelvis |
| myc/o | fungus | | pericardi/o | pericardium |
| myel/o | spinal cord, bone marrow | | perine/o | perineum |
| myocardi/o | heart muscle | | phac/o | lens |
| myos/o | muscle | | phag/o | eat, swallow |
| myring/o | eardrum | | phalang/o | phalanges, bones of fingers and toes |
| narc/o | stupor | | pharmac/o | drug |
| nas/o | nose | | pharyng/o | throat, pharynx |
| nat/o | birth | | phas/o | speech |
| natr/o | sodium | | phleb/o | vein |
| necr/o | death | | phon/o | sound |
| nephr/o | kidney | | phot/o | light |
| neur/o | nerve | | phren/o | diaphragm, mind |
| noct/i | night | | pil/o | hair |
| o/o | egg | | pineal/o | pineal gland |
| ocul/o | eye | | pituitar/o | pituitary gland |
| odont/o | tooth | | plant/o | sole of the foot |
| olig/o | scanty | | pleur/o | pleura |
| omphal/o | navel, umbilicus | | pneum/o | lung, air |
| onc/o | tumor | | pneumon/o | lung, air |
| onych/o | nail | | poli/o | gray matter |
| oophor/o | ovary | | pont/o | pons |
| ophthalm/o | eye | | poster/o | back |
| opt/o | eye, vision | | presby/o | old age |
| optic/o | eye | | proct/o | anus and rectum |
| or/o | mouth | | prostat/o | prostate |
| orch/o | testes | | prosth/o | addition |
| orchi/o | testes | | proxim/o | near |
| orchid/o | testes | | psych/o | mind |

| Combining Form | Meaning | Combining Form | Meaning |
|---|---|---|---|
| **pub/o** | pubis | **ten/o** | tendon |
| **pulmon/o** | lung | **tend/o** | tendon |
| **pupill/o** | pupil | **tendin/o** | tendon |
| **py/o** | pus | **test/o** | testes |
| **pyel/o** | renal pelvis | **testicul/o** | testes |
| **pylor/o** | pylorus | **thalam/o** | thalamus |
| **radi/o** | radiation, X-ray, radius, forearm bone | **therm/o** | heat |
| **radicul/o** | nerve root | **thorac/o** | chest |
| **rect/o** | rectum | **thromb/o** | clot |
| **ren/o** | kidney | **thym/o** | thymus |
| **retin/o** | retina | **thyr/o** | thyroid gland |
| **rhabdomy/o** | skeletal muscle | **thyroid/o** | thyroid gland |
| **rhin/o** | nose | **tibi/o** | tibia, shin bone |
| **rhytid/o** | wrinkle | **tom/o** | to cut |
| **roentgen/o** | X-ray | **tonsill/o** | tonsils |
| **sacr/o** | sacrum | **tox/o** | toxic, poison |
| **salping/o** | fallopian tubes, uterine tubes, eustachian tubes | **toxic/o** | toxic, poison |
| **sanguin/o** | blood | **trache/o** | trachea, windpipe |
| **scapul/o** | scapula, shoulder blade | **trich/o** | hair |
| **schiz/o** | divided | **tympan/o** | eardrum |
| **scler/o** | hard, sclera | **uln/o** | ulna, forearm bone |
| **scoli/o** | crooked, bent | **ungu/o** | nail |
| **seb/o** | sebum, oil | **ur/o** | urine, urinary tract |
| **sect/o** | cut | **ureter/o** | ureter, urinary tube |
| **sial/o** | saliva | **urethr/o** | urethra |
| **sialaden/o** | salivary gland | **urin/o** | urine |
| **sigmoid/o** | sigmoid colon | **uter/o** | uterus |
| **sinus/o** | sinus, cavity | **uve/o** | vascular |
| **somat/o** | body | **vagin/o** | vagina |
| **somn/o** | sleep | **valv/o** | valve |
| **son/o** | sound | **valvul/o** | valve |
| **spermat/o** | sperm | **varic/o** | varicose veins |
| **sphygm/o** | pulse | **vas/o** | vas deferens |
| **spin/o** | spine, backbone | **ven/o** | vein |
| **spir/o** | breathing | **ventr/o** | belly |
| **splen/o** | spleen | **ventricul/o** | ventricle |
| **spondyl/o** | vertebrae, backbone | **vertebr/o** | vertebra, backbone |
| **staped/o** | stapes | **vesic/o** | bladder |
| **stern/o** | sternum, breast bone | **vesicul/o** | seminal vesicle |
| **steth/o** | chest | **viscer/o** | internal organ |
| **stomat/o** | mouth | **vitre/o** | glassy |
| **super/o** | above | **vulv/o** | vulva |
| **synovi/o** | synovial membrane | **xanth/o** | yellow |
| **system/o** | system | **xer/o** | dry |
| **tars/o** | ankle | | |

# Prefixes

| Prefix | Meaning | Prefix | Meaning |
|--------|---------|--------|---------|
| **a-** | without, away from | **micro-** | small |
| **ab-** | away from | **mono-** | one |
| **ad-** | towards | **multi-** | many |
| **an-** | without | **neo-** | new |
| **ante-** | before, in front of | **nulli-** | none |
| **anti-** | against | **pan-** | all |
| **auto-** | self | **para-** | beside, beyond, near |
| **bi-** | two | **per-** | through |
| **brady-** | slow | **peri-** | around or about |
| **circum-** | around | **poly-** | many |
| **di-** | two | **post-** | behind or after |
| **dys-** | painful, difficult | **pre-** | before, in front of |
| **endo-** | within, inner | **pseudo-** | false |
| **epi-** | upon, over, above | **quad-** | four |
| **eu-** | normal, good | **retro-** | backward, behind |
| **hemi-** | half | **semi-** | partial, half |
| **hetero-** | different | **sub-** | below, under |
| **homo-** | same | **super-** | above, excess |
| **hydro-** | water | **supra-** | above |
| **hyper-** | over, above | **tachy-** | rapid, fast |
| **hypo-** | under, below | **trans-** | through, across |
| **infra-** | under, beneath, below | **tri-** | three |
| **inter-** | among, between | **ultra-** | beyond, excess |
| **intra-** | within, inside | **uni-** | one |
| **macro-** | large | | |

## Suffixes

| Suffix | Meaning | Suffix | Meaning |
|--------|---------|--------|---------|
| -ac | pertaining to | -gravida | pregnancy |
| -al | pertaining to | -ia | state, condition |
| -algesia | pain, sensitivity | -iac | pertaining to |
| -algia | pain | -iasis | abnormal condition |
| -an | pertaining to | -iatrist | physician |
| -apheresis | removal, carry away | -ic | pertaining to |
| -ar | pertaining to | -ical | pertaining to |
| -arche | beginning | -ile | pertaining to |
| -ary | pertaining to | -ior | pertaining to |
| -asthenia | weakness | -ism | state of |
| -blast | immature, embryonic | -itis | inflammation |
| -capnia | carbon dioxide | -kinesia | movement |
| -cele | hernia, protrusion | -lepsy | seizure |
| -centesis | puncture to withdraw fluid | -listhesis | slipping |
| -chalasis | relaxation | -lith | stone |
| -cise | cut | -lithiasis | condition of stones |
| -clasia | to surgically break | -logist | one who studies |
| -crine | to secrete | -logy | study of |
| -cusis | hearing | -lucent | to shine through |
| -cyesis | state of pregnancy | -lysis | destruction |
| -cyte | cell | -malacia | softening |
| -cytosis | more than the normal number of cells | -mania | excessive excitement |
| -derma | skin | -manometer | instrument to measure pressure |
| -desis | stabilize, fuse | -megaly | enlargement, large |
| -dipsia | thirst | -meter | instrument for measuring |
| -dynia | pain | -metry | process of measuring |
| -eal | pertaining to | -ole | small |
| -ectasia | dilation | -oma | tumor, mass |
| -ectasis | dilatation, expansion | -opaque | nontransparent |
| -ectomy | surgical removal, excision | -opia | vision |
| -ectopia | displacement | -opsy | view of |
| -emesis | vomit | -orexia | appetite |
| -emia | blood condition | -ory | pertaining to |
| -esthesia | feeling, sensation | -ose | pertaining to |
| -gen | that which produces | -osis | abnormal condition |
| -genesis | produces, generates | -osmia | smell |
| -genic | producing | -ostomy | surgically create an opening |
| -globin | protein | -otia | ear condition |
| -globulin | protein | -otomy | cutting into, incision |
| -gram | record, picture | -ous | pertaining to |
| -graph | instrument for recording | -para | to bear (offspring) |
| -graphy | process of recording | -paresis | weakness |

| Suffix | Meaning | Suffix | Meaning |
|--------|---------|--------|---------|
| **-pathy** | disease | **-rrhea** | discharge, flow |
| **-penia** | abnormal decrease, too few | **-rrhexis** | rupture |
| **-pepsia** | digestion | **-salpinx** | fallopian tube |
| **-pexy** | surgical fixation | **-sclerosis** | hardening |
| **-phage** | eat, swallow | **-scope** | instrument for viewing |
| **-phagia** | eat, swallow | **-scopic** | to view inside |
| **-phasia** | speech | **-scopy** | process of visually examining |
| **-philia** | to have an attraction for | **-spermia** | condition of sperm |
| **-phobia** | irrational fear | **-stasis** | standing still |
| **-phonia** | voice | **-stenosis** | narrowing |
| **-phoresis** | carrying | **-sthenia** | strength |
| **-plakia** | plate | **-taxia** | muscular coordination |
| **-plasia** | growth, formation, development | **-tension** | pressure |
| **-plasm** | growth, formation, development | **-therapy** | treatment |
| **-plasty** | surgical repair | **-thorax** | chest |
| **-plegia** | paralysis | **-tic** | pertaining to |
| **-pnea** | breathing | **-tocia** | labor, childbirth |
| **-poiesis** | formation | **-tome** | instrument used to cut |
| **-porosis** | porous | **-tripsy** | surgical crushing |
| **-prandial** | pertaining to a meal | **-trophy** | nourishment, development |
| **-ptosis** | drooping | **-tropia** | to turn |
| **-ptysis** | spitting | **-tropin** | stimulate |
| **-rrhage** | excessive, abnormal flow | **-ule** | small |
| **-rrhaphy** | suture | **-uria** | condition of the urine |

# Chapter Review Answers

## Chapter 1 Answers

### Practice Exercises

**A.** 1. combining form 2. o 3. suffix 4. prefix 5. spelling 6. word root, combining vowel, prefix, suffix

**B.** 1. gland 2. cancer 3. heart 4. chemical 5. to cut 6. skin 7. small intestines 8. stomach 9. female 10. blood 11. water 12. immune 13. voice box 14. shape 15. kidney 16. nerve 17. eye 18. ear 19. lung 20. nose 21. urine, urinary tract

**C.** 1. surgical repair 2. narrowing 3. inflammation of 4. pertaining to 5. pain 6. cutting into 7. enlargement 8. surgical removal of 9. excessive, abnormal flow 10. puncture to remove fluid 11. record or picture 12. pertaining to 13. abnormal softening 14. state of 15. to suture 16. surgical creation of opening 17. surgical fixation 18. discharge or flow 19. process of visually examining 20. tumor, mass

**D.** 1. pulmonology 2. neuralgia 3. rhinorrhea 4. nephromalacia 5. cardiomegaly 6. gastrotomy 7. dermatitis 8. laryngectomy 9. arthritis 10. adenopathy

**E.** 1. intra-/endo- 2. macro- 3. pre-/ante- 4. peri- 5. neo- 6. a-/an- 7. hemi-/semi- 8. dys- 9. supra-/super-/hyper- 10. hyper-/ super- 11. poly-/multi- 12. brady- 13. auto- 14. trans- 15. bi-/di-

**F.** 1. tachy-, fast 2. pseudo-, false 3. hypo-, under/below 4. inter-, among/between 5. eu-, normal/good 6. post-, after 7. mono-, one 8. sub-, below/under

**G.** 1. metastases 2. ova 3. diverticula 4. atria 5. diagnoses 6. vertebrae

**H.** 1. cardiology 2. gastrology 3. dermatology 4. ophthalmology 5. urology 6. nephrology 7. hematology 8. gynecology 9. neurology

**I.** 1. cardiomalacia 2. gastrostomy 3. rhinorrhea 4. hypertrophy 5. pathology 6. adenoma 7. gastroenterology 8. otitis 9. hydrotherapy 10. carcinogen

### Professional Journal

1. gastrectomy 2. correct 3. correct 4. intrapulmonary 5. rhinoplasty 6. correct 7. nephrorrhaphy 8. correct 9. tachycardia 10. ophthalmologist

## Chapter 2 Answers

### Practice Exercises

**A.** 1. histology 2. epithelial 3. anatomical position 4. sagittal 5. right lower 6. cranial, spinal 7. nine 8. right iliac 9. left hypochondriac

**B.** 1. c 2. a 3. b

**C.** 1. n 2. f 3. k 4. d 5. a 6. e 7. m 8. i 9. b 10. j 11. h 12. l 13. c 14. g

**D.** 1. epi-; above 2. inter-; between 3. intra-; within 4. peri-; around or about 5. post-; behind or after 6. retro-; behind or backward 7. sub-; under or below 8. trans-; through or across

**E.** 1. dorsal 2. thoracic 3. superior 4. caudal 5. visceral 6. lateral 7. distal 8. neural 9. systemic 10. muscular 11. ventral 12. anterior 13. cephalic 14. medial

**F.** 1. MS 2. lat 3. RUQ 4. CV 5. GI 6. AP 7. GU 8. LLQ

**G.** 1. internal organ 2. back 3. abdomen 4. chest 5. middle 6. belly 7. front 8. tissues 9. epithelium 10. skull 11. body 12. near to 13. head

**H.** 1. otorhinolaryngology 2. cardiology 3. gynecology 4. orthopedics 5. ophthalmology

## Chapter 3 Answers

### Case Study (Critical Thinking Questions)

1. c—intense itching (urticaria) 2. translated into student's own words: size of 10 × 14 mm; left cheek 20 mm anterior to the ear; erythema; poorly defined borders, depigmentation, vesicles 3. wear sunscreen and a hat 4. congestive heart failure; CHF; dyspnea, lower extremity edema, cyanosis 5. biopsy 6. excision; dermatoplasty

### Chart Note Transcription

1. ulcer—open sore 2. dermatologist—specialist in treating diseases of the skin 3. pruritus—severe itching 4. erythema— redness of the skin 5. pustules—raised spots containing pus 6. dermis—middle skin layer 7. necrosis—tissue death 8. culture and sensitivity—sample was grown in the lab to identify the microorganism and determine the best antibiotic 9. cellulitis— inflammation of skin cells and tissue 10. debridement—removal of damaged tissue

### Practice Exercises

**A.** 1. dermatitis 2. dermatosis 3. dermatome 4. dermatologist 5. dermatoplasty 6. dermatology 7. melanoma 8. melanocyte 9. rhytidectomy 10. rhytidoplasty 11. trichomycosis 12. onychomalacia 13. paronychia 14. onychophagia 15. onychectomy

**B.** 1. cold 2. skin 3. profuse sweating 4. pus 5. blue 6. nail 7. fat 8. horny/hard

**C.** 1. skin 2. black pigment 3. oil 4. skin 5. outer layer of skin 6. hard protein in epidermis, hair, and nails 7. soft tissue covering nail root 8. hair shaft grows inside it

**D.** 1. redness involving superficial layer of skin 2. burn damage through epidermis and into dermis causing vesicles 3. burn damage to full thickness of epidermis and dermis

**E.** 1. e 2. g 3. j 4. k 5. a 6. c 7. m 8. f 9. h 10. l 11. i 12. d 13. b

**F.** 1. h 2. i 3. d 4. e 5. c 6. a 7. f 8. g 9. b

**G.** 1. FS 2. I & D 3. ID 4. subq, subcu, SC, sc 5. UV 6. ung 7. BX, bx

**H.** 1. dermis 2. shingles 3. xeroderma 4. petechiae 5. tinea 6. scabies 7. paronychia 8. Kaposi's sarcoma 9. malignant melanoma 10. impetigo 11. pustule 12. macule 13. polyp 14. papule 15. fissure

**I.** 1. hypodermic, or subcutaneous 2. intradermal 3. epidermis

## Chapter 4 Answers

### Case Study (Critical Thinking Questions)

1. rehabilitation specialist; Motrin (a nonsteroidal anti-inflammatory medication), physical therapy for range of motion and strengthening exercises, and low-fat, low-calorie diet 2. arthroscopy; torn lateral meniscus and chondromalacia; arthroscopic meniscectomy 3. a—nonsurgical treatments, such as medicine and therapy; b—a patient who has not been admitted to the hospital 4. physical therapy for lower extremity ROM and strengthening exercises, and gait training with a walker; occupational therapy for ADL instruction, especially dressing and personal care 5. patient was able to bend knee to 90° but lacked 5° of being able to straighten it back out

### Chart Note Transcription

1. Colles' fracture (fx)—wrist broken bone 2. cast—immobilization by solid material 3. fracture—broken bone 4. orthopedist—physician who specializes in treating bone conditions 5. osteoporosis—porous bones 6. computerized axial tomography (CT or CAT scan)—computer-assisted X-ray 7. flexion—a bent position 8. extension—movement toward a straight position 9. comminuted fracture (fx)—shattered broken bone 10. femur—thigh bone 11. total hip replacement (THR)—implantation of an artificial hip joint

### Practice Exercises

**A.** 1. axial, appendicular 2. cervical, thoracic, lumbar, sacrum, coccyx 3. frame, protect vital organs, work with muscles for movement, store minerals, red blood cell production 4. femur 5. patella 6. periosteum 7. wrist 8. 400 9. 206 10. skeletal, smooth, cardiac 11. orthopedist 12. podiatrist

**B.** 1. osteocyte 2. osteoblast 3. osteoporosis 4. osteoplasty 5. osteotomy 6. osteotome 7. osteomyelitis 8. osteomalacia 9. osteochondroma 10. myopathy 11. myoplasty 12. myorrhaphy 13. rhabdomyoma 14. rhabdomyolysis 15. tenodynia 16. tenomyopathy 17. arthrodesis 18. arthroplasty 19. arthrotomy 20. arthritis 21. arthrochondritis 22. arthralgia 23. craniotomy 24. cranioplasty 25. intracranial

**C.** 1. -desis 2. -asthenia 3. -malacia 4. -clasia 5. -kinesia 6. -porosis

**D.** 1. femoral 2. sternal 3. clavicular 4. coccygeal 5. maxillary 6. tibial 7. patellar 8. phalangeal 9. humeral 10. pubic

**E.** 1. lamina, part of vertebra 2. stiff joint 3. cartilage 4. vertebrae, backbone 5. muscle 6. straight 7. hump 8. tendon 9. bone marrow 10. joint

**F.** 1. surgical repair of cartilage 2. slow movement 3. porous bone 4. abnormal condition of swayback 5. lack of development/nourishment 6. bone marrow tumor 7. finger bones, toe bones 8. tail bone 9. puncture of a joint to withdraw fluid 10. stone in a bursa

**G.** 1. cervical, 7 2. thoracic, 12 3. lumbar, 5 4. sacrum, 1 (5 fused) 5. coccyx, 1 (3–5 fused)

**H.** 1. S = -scopy; visual examination of inside of a joint 2. P = inter-, S = -al; pertaining to between vertebrae 3. S = -malacia; softening of cartilage 4. S = -ectomy; surgical removal of disk 5. S = -rrhaphy; suturing of a muscle 6. P = sub-, -ar = pertaining to; pertaining to under the scapula

**I.** 1. e 2. d 3. b 4. c 5. a 6. h 7. g 8. f

**J.** 1. c 2. h 3. f 4. g 5. d 6. e 7. a 8. b

**K.** 1. medical doctor who treats musculoskeletal system 2. uses manipulation of vertebral column 3. specialist in treating disorders of feet 4. fitting of braces and splints 5. fabricates and fits artificial limbs

**L.** 1. degenerative joint disease 2. electromyography 3. first cervical vertebra 4. sixth thoracic vertebra 5. intramuscular 6. range of motion 7. juvenile rheumatoid arthritis 8. left lower extremity 9. orthopedics 10. carpal tunnel syndrome

**M.** 1. CDH 2. TKR 3. HNP 4. DTR 5. UE 6. L5 7. BDT 8. AK 9. fx/FX 10. NSAID

**N.** 1. osteoporosis 2. rickets 3. lateral epicondylitis 4. whiplash 5. osteogenic sarcoma 6. scoliosis 7. pseudotrophic muscular dystrophy 8. systemic lupus erythematosus

## Chapter 5 Answers

### Case Study (Critical Thinking Questions)

1. Lopressor to control blood pressure, Norpace to slow down the heart rate, Valium to reduce anxiety, Lasix to reduce swelling 2. EKG, cardiac enzymes blood test; myocardial infarction 3. patient developed dyspnea and cyanosis 4. b—dizziness 5. mitral valve replacement 6. compare: both conditions allow blood to flow backwards; contrast: prolapse—too floppy, valve droops down, and stenosis—too stiff, preventing it from opening all the way or closing all the way

### Chart Note Transcription

1. angina pectoris—severe pain around the heart 2. bradycardia—abnormally slow heartbeat 3. hypertension—high blood pressure 4. myocardial infarction (MI)—death of heart muscle 5. electrocardiogram (EKG, ECG)—record of the heart's electrical activity 6. cardiac enzymes—blood test to determine the amount of heart damage 7. coronary thrombosis—blood clot in a coronary vessel 8. cardiac catheterization—passing a thin tube through a blood vessel into the heart to detect abnormalities 9. stress test (treadmill test)—evaluate heart fitness by having

patient exercise on a treadmill 10. percutaneous transluminal coronary angioplasty (PTCA)—inflating a balloon catheter to dilate a narrow vessel 11. coronary artery bypass graft (CABG)—open-heart surgery to create a shunt around a blocked vessel

## Practice Exercises

**A.** 1. cardiology 2. endocardium, myocardium, epicardium 3. sinoatrial node 4. pulmonary artery 5. tricuspid, pulmonary, mitral (bicuspid), aortic 6. atria, ventricles

**B.** 1. cardiodynia 2. cardiomyopathy 3. cardiomegaly 4. tachycardia 5. bradycardia 6. carditis 7. phlebitis 8. phlebotomy 9. phleborrhaphy 10. arterial 11. arteriosclerosis

**C.** 1. endocarditis 2. epicarditis 3. myocarditis

**D.** 1. heart 2. valve 3. chest 4. artery 5. vein 6. vessel 7. ventricle 8. clot 9. atrium 10. fatty substance

**E.** 1. venous 2. tachycardia 3. cardiologist 4. electrocardiography 5. hypertension 6. hypotension 7. endocarditis 8. cyanosis 9. thrombolysis 10. arteriostenosis

**F.** 1. -tension 2. -stenosis 3. -manometer 4. -ule, -ole 5. -sclerosis

**G.** 1. blood pressure 2. congestive heart failure 3. myocardial infarction 4. coronary care unit 5. premature ventricular contraction 6. cardiopulmonary resuscitation 7. coronary artery disease 8. chest pain 9. electrocardiogram 10. first heart sound

**H.** 1. MVP 2. VSD 3. PTCA 4. Vfib 5. DVT 6. LDH 7. CoA 8. tPA 9. CV 10. ECC

**I.** 1. f 2. h 3. d 4. g 5. b 6. i 7. a 8. c 9. e 10. j

**J.** 1. murmur 2. defibrillation 3. hypertension 4. pacemaker 5. varicose veins 6. angina pectoris 7. CCU 8. MI 9. angiography 10. echocardiogram 11. angioma 12. Holter monitor 13. CHF

## Chapter 6 Answers

### Case Study (Critical Thinking Questions)

1. feeling "run down," intermittent diarrhea, weight loss, dry cough 2. negative means absence; there was no evidence of pneumonia in the X-ray 3. a—the original or critical reaction; b—contained within a capsule; c—fluid collecting within the abdominal cavity; d—spread to a distant site 4. ultrasound 5. d—an enlarged spleen (splenomegaly) 6. magnetic resonance image (MRI); brain, liver 7. resolved: ascites, diarrhea; persisted: dry cough

### Chart Note Transcription

1. hematologist—specialist in treating blood disorders 2. ELISA—immunoassay test for AIDS 3. prothrombin time—measure of the blood's coagulation abilities 4. complete blood count (CBC)—blood test to count all the blood cells 5. erythropenia—too few red blood cells 6. thrombocytopenia—too few clotting cells 7. leukocytosis—too many white blood cells 8. bone marrow aspiration—sample of bone marrow obtained for microscopic examination 9. leukemia—cancer of the white blood cell forming bone marrow 10. homologous transfusion—replacement blood from another person

## Practice Exercises

**A.** 1. hematology 2. spleen, tonsils, thymus 3. thoracic duct, right lymphatic duct 4. axillary, cervical, mediastinal, inguinal 5. phagocytosis 6. erythrocytes (red blood cells), leukocytes (white blood cells), platelets (thrombocytes) 7. plasma

**B.** 1. splenomegaly 2. splenectomy 3. splenorrhaphy 4. splenotomy 5. splenoma 6. splenomalacia 7. lymphocytes 8. lymphoma 9. lymphadenopathy 10. lymphadenoma 11. lymphadenitis 12. immunologist 13. immunoglobulin 14. immunology 15. hematocytopenia 16. hematic 17. hematoma 18. hematopoiesis 19. hemostasis 20. hemolysis

**C.** 1. leukocytopenia 2. erythropenia 3. thrombocytopenia 4. lymphocytopenia 5. leukocytosis 6. erythrocytosis 7. thrombocytosis 8. hemoglobin 9. immunoglobulin 10. erythrocyte 11. leukocyte 12. lymphocyte

**D.** 1. myel/o 2. thromb/o 3. sanguin/o, hem/o, hemat/o 4. aden/o 5. tox/o 6. phag/o 7. lymphangi/o 8. tonsill/o 9. splen/o 10. lymph/o

**E.** 1. basophil 2. complete blood count 3. hemoglobin 4. prothrombin time 5. graft vs. host disease 6. red blood count/red blood cell 7. packed cell volume 8. erythrocyte sedimentation rate 9. differential 10. lymphocyte 11. acquired immunodeficiency syndrome 12. AIDS-related complex 13. human immunodeficiency virus 14. acute lymphocytic leukemia 15. bone marrow transplant 16. mononucleosis 17. Kaposi's sarcoma

**F.** 1. e 2. i 3. f 4. a 5. h 6. d 7. c 8. g 9. b

**G.** 1. f 2. h 3. d 4. a 5. i 6. b 7. g 8. c 9. j 10. e

**H.** 1. polycythemia vera 2. mononucleosis 3. anaphylactic shock 4. HIV 5. Kaposi's sarcoma 6. AIDS 7. Hodgkin's disease 8. *Pneumocystis carinii* 9. peritonsillar abscess

## Chapter 7 Answers

### Case Study (Critical Thinking Questions)

1. sudden attack 2. intravenous, immediately, arterial blood gases 3. steroid to reduce inflammation; Alupent to relax bronchospasms 4. what triggers his attacks; referred patient to an allergist 5. hacking and producing thick, nonpurulent phlegm 6. a—crackling lung sounds

### Chart Note Transcription

1. dyspnea—painful and labored breathing 2. tachypnea—rapid breathing 3. arterial blood gases (ABGs)—a blood test to measure the levels of oxygen in the blood 4. hypoxemia—low level of oxygen in the blood 5. auscultation—process of listening to body sounds 6. rales—abnormal crackling sounds 7. purulent—pus-filled 8. sputum—mucus coughed up from the respiratory tract 9. CXR—chest X-ray 10. pneumonia—inflammatory condition of the lungs caused by bacterial infection 11. endotracheal intubation—a tube placed through the mouth to create an airway

## Practice Exercises

**A.** 1. exchange of $O_2$ and $CO_2$ 2. ventilation 3. exchange of $O_2$ and $CO_2$ in the lungs 4. exchange of $O_2$ and $CO_2$ at cellular level 5. nose, pharynx, larynx, trachea, bronchial tubes, lungs 6. pharynx 7. epiglottis 8. filter out dust 9. diaphragm 10. 12–20 11. 30–60 12. 3/2 13. alveoli 14. pleura 15. palate 16. bronchioles

**B.** 1. rhinitis 2. rhinorrhagia 3. rhinorrhea 4. rhinoplasty 5. laryngitis 6. laryngospasm 7. laryngoscopy 8. laryngeal 9. laryngotomy 10. laryngectomy 11. laryngoplasty 12. laryngoplegia 13. bronchorrhagia 14. bronchitis 15. bronchoscopy 16. bronchopathy 17. bronchospasm 18. thoracoplasty 19. thoracotomy 20. thoracalgia 21. thoracoscopy 22. tracheotomy 23. tracheoplasty 24. tracheostenosis 25. tracheopathy 26. tracheorrhaphy 27. tracheitis 28. tracheostomy

**C.** 1. trachea or windpipe 2. larynx 3. bronchus 4. breathing 5. lung or air 6. nose 7. pus 8. pleura 9. epiglottis 10. alveolus or air sac 11. lung 12. tonsil 13. sinus 14. lobe 15. nose

**D.** 1. dilation 2. carbon dioxide 3. voice 4. chest 5. breathing 6. spitting 7. smell

**E.** 1. eupnea 2. dyspnea 3. tachypnea 4. orthopnea 5. apnea

**F.** 1. volume of air in the lungs after a maximal inhalation or inspiration 2. amount of air entering lungs in a single inspiration or leaving air in single expiration of quiet breathing 3. air remaining in the lungs after a forced expiration

**G.** 1. inhalation or inspiration 2. hemoptysis 3. pulmonary emboli 4. sinusitis 5. pharyngitis 6. pneumothorax 7. bronchoplegia 8. pleurotomy 9. pleurisy 10. diaphragmatocele

**H.** 1. URI 2. PFT 3. LLL 4. $O_2$ 5. $CO_2$ 6. IPPB 7. COLD 8. Bronch 9. TLC 10. TB 11. PND

**I.** 1. chest X-ray 2. tidal volume 3. temperature, pulse, respirations 4. arterial blood gases 5. respiratory disease 6. right upper lobe 7. sudden infant death syndrome 8. total lung capacity 9. adult respiratory distress syndrome 10. hyperbaric oxygen therapy 11. clear to auscultation 12. tonsillectomy and adenoidectomy

# Chapter 8 Answers

## Case Study (Critical Thinking Questions)

1. left upper quadrant, stomach, spleen 2. complete blood count (CBC), occult blood test 3. gastroscopy; a deep ulcer 1.5 cm in diameter, evidence of bleeding 4. gastric carcinoma 5. d—a blood transfusion 6. tonsillectomy, compound fracture, BPH, and TUR

## Chart Note Transcription

1. gastroenterologist—physician who specializes in the treatment of the gastrointestinal tract 2. constipation—difficulty with having a bowel movement 3. cholelithiasis—the presence of gallstones 4. cholecystectomy—surgical removal of the gallbladder 5. gastroesophageal reflux disease—acid backing up from the stomach into the esophagus 6. ascites—fluid collecting in the abdominal cavity 7. barium enema—X-ray of the colon

after inserting barium dye with an enema 8. polyposis—presence of multiple small tumors growing on a stalk 9. colonoscopy—visual examination of the colon by a fiberscope inserted through the rectum 10. sigmoid colon—section of colon between the descending colon and the rectum 11. colectomy—surgical removal of the colon 12. colostomy—the surgical creation of an opening of the colon through the abdominal wall

## Practice Exercises

**A.** 1. esophagus 2. liver 3. ileum 4. anus and rectum 5. tongue 6. lip 7. jejunum 8. sigmoid colon 9. rectum 10. gum 11. gallbladder 12. duodenum 13. anus 14. small intestine 15. teeth

**B.** 1. gastritis 2. gastroenterology 3. gastrectomy 4. gastroscopy 5. gastrorrhaphy 6. gastromegaly 7. gastrotomy 8. esophagitis 9. esophagoscopy 10. esophagoplasty 11. esophageal 12. esophagectomy 13. proctostenosis 14. proctoptosis 15. proctitis 16. proctodynia, proctalgia 17. cholecystectomy 18. cholecystolithiasis 19. cholecystolithotripsy 20. cholecystitis 21. laparoscope 22. laparotomy 23. laparoscopy 24. hepatoma 25. hepatomegaly 26. hepatic 27. hepatitis 28. pancreatitis 29. pancreatic 30. colostomy 31. colitis

**C.** 1. postprandial 2. cholelithiasis 3. anorexia 4. dysphagia 5. hematemesis 6. bradypepsia

**D.** 1. bowel movement 2. upper gastrointestinal series 3. barium enema 4. bowel sounds 5. recommended daily allowance 6. ova and parasites 7. by mouth 8. common bile duct 9. nothing by mouth 10. postprandial 11. nasogastric 12. gastrointestinal 13. hepatitis B virus 14. fecal occult blood test 15. inflammatory bowel disease

**E.** 1. cholangi/o = bile duct, pacreat/o = pancreas 2. -graphy = process of recording 3. process of making an X-ray recording of bile duct and pancreas

**F.** 1. h 2. i 3. f 4. c 5. a 6. j 7. l 8. e 9. b 10. k 11. d 12. g

**G.** 1. liver biopsy 2. colostomy 3. barium swallow 4. lower GI series 5. colectomy 6. fecal occult blood test 7. lithotripsy 8. anastomosis 9. gastrectomy 10. cholangiography 11. colonoscopy 12. ileostomy

**H.** 1. d 2. g 3. h 4. e 5. f 6. b 7. c 8. a

# Chapter 9 Answers

## Case Study (Critical Thinking Questions)

1. bladder neck obstruction 2. severe right side pain, unable to stand fully erect, 101°F temperature, sweaty and flushed skin 3. large enough to be visible with the naked eye 4. a—present from birth b—of long duration c—disease-causing d—by mouth 5. a—protein 6. alike: both are infections of kidney tissue; different: glomerulonephritis—infection is in the glomerulus and it allows protein to leak into the urine; pyelonephritis—infection is in the renal pelvis portion of the kidney, more common, often caused by bladder infection moving up the ureters to the kidney

## Chart Note Transcription

1. urologist—specialist in the treatment of diseases of the urinary system 2. hematuria—blood in the urine 3. cystitis—bladder infection 4. clean-catch specimen—technique used to obtain an uncontaminated urine sample 5. urinalysis (U/A, UA)—laboratory analysis of the urine 6. pyuria—pus in the urine 7. retrograde pyelogram—a kidney X-ray made after inserting dye into the bladder 8. ureter—tube between the kidney and bladder 9. ureterolith—stone in the tube between the kidney and the bladder 10. extracorporeal shockwave lithotripsy (ESWL)—use of ultrasound waves to break up stones 11. calculi—kidney stones

## Practice Exercises

**A.** 1. nephropexy 2. nephrogram 3. nephrolithiasis 4. nephrectomy 5. nephritis 6. nephropathy 7. nephrosclerosis 8. cystitis 9. cystorrhagia 10. cystoplasty 11. cystoscope 12. cystalgia 13. pyeloplasty 14. pyelitis 15. pyelogram 16. ureterolith 17. ureteroplasty 18. ureterectomy 19. urethroplasty 20. urethrostomy

**B.** 1. urination, voiding 2. increases urine production 3. pain associated with kidney stone 4. inserting a tube through urethra into the bladder 5. inflammation of renal pelvis 6. inflammation of kidney and renal pelvis 7. incision to remove stone 8. bedwetting 9. enlargement of uretheral opening 10. damage to glomerulus secondary to diabetes mellitus 11. lab test of chemical composition of urine 12. decrease in force of urine stream

**C.** 1. anuria 2. hematuria 3. calculus/nephrolith 4. lithotripsy 5. urethritis 6. pyuria 7. bacteriuria 8. dysuria 9. ketonuria 10. albuminuria 11. polyuria

**D.** 1. $K^+$ 2. Na+ 3. UA 4. BUN 5. SG 6. IVP 7. BNO 8. I & O 9. ATN 10. ESRD

**E.** 1. kidneys, ureters, bladder 2. catheter/catheterization 3. cystoscopy 4. genitourinary 5. extracorporeal shockwave lithotripsy 6. urinary tract infection 7. urine culture 8. retrograde pyelogram 9. acute renal failure 10. blood urea nitrogen 11. chronic renal failure 12. water

**F.** 1. c 2. g 3. h 4. i 5. f 6. e 7. d 8. b 9. a 10. j

**G.** 1. renal transplant 2. nephropexy 3. urinary tract infection 4. pyelolithectomy 5. renal biopsy 6. ureterectomy 7. cystostomy 8. cystoscopy 9. IVP

## Chapter 10 Answers

### Case Study (Critical Thinking Questions)

1. oophorectomy and chemotherapy; full body CT scan 2. menarche at 13, menorrhagia with chronic anemia 3. c—nullipara and d—multigravida 4. pelvic ultrasound; because the placenta overlies the cervix, it will detach before the baby can physically be born 5. size consistent with 25 weeks of gestation, turned head down, umbilical cord is not around the neck, fetal heart tones are strong, male, no evidence of developmental or genetic disorders 6. a—a greater than normal level of risk of problems developing or fetal death with this pregnancy; b—she looks like she is 8 months pregnant (her abdomen is not too small or too large)

## Chart Note Transcription

1. ejaculation—release of semen from the urethra 2. cryptorchidism—failure of the testes to descend into the scrotum 3. orchidopexy—surgical fixation of the testes 4. vasectomy—removal of a segment of the vas deferens 5. sexual intercourse—the process of sexual relations 6. digital rectal exam (DRE)—palpation of the prostate gland through the rectum 7. prostate cancer—slow-growing cancer that frequently affects males over age 50 8. prostate-specific antigen (PSA)—blood test for prostate cancer 9. benign prostatic hypertrophy (BPH)—noncancerous enlargement of prostate gland 10. transurethral resection (TUR)—surgical removal of prostate tissue through the urethra

## Practice Exercises

**A.** 1. gynecology 2. gynecologist 3. genitalia 4. gestation 5. menopause 6. ovum 7. endometrium 8. uterus 9. fallopian tubes 10. total abdominal hysterectomy–bilateral salpingo-oophorectomy

**B.** 1. colposcopy 2. colposcope 3. colporrhaphy 4. cervicitis 5. cervical 6. hysteropathy 7. hysteropexy 8. hysterectomy 9. hysterorrhexis 10. hysterorrhaphy 11. oophoritis 12. oophorectomy 13. multigravida 14. nulligravida 15. primigravida 16. nullipara 17. multipara 18. primipara

**C.** 1. cervix 2. last menstrual period 3. marital history 4. pelvic inflammatory disease 5. date of birth 6. cesarean section 7. newborn 8. premenstrual syndrome 9. toxic shock syndrome 10. low birth weight

**D.** 1. PKU 2. AI 3. UC 4. FTND 5. IUD 6. D & C 7. DUB 8. gyn/GYN 9. AB 10. OCPs

**E.** 1. uterus 2. uterus 3. female 4. vulva 5. ovary 6. ovary 7. fallopian tube 8. menstruation or menses 9. vagina 10. breast

**F.** 1. b 2. e 3. h 4. c 5. i 6. j 7. d 8. n 9. l 10. f 11. o 12. g 13. k 14. m 15. a

**G.** 1. conization 2. stillbirth 3. puberty 4. premenstrual syndrome 5. laparoscopy 6. fibroid tumor 7. D & C 8. eclampsia 9. endometriosis 10. cesarean section

**H.** 1. e 2. i 3. h 4. c 5. a 6. d 7. g 8. b 9. f

**I.** 1. urinary, reproductive 2. scrotum, penis, testes, epididymis 3. foreskin 4. testes 5. bulbourethral glands 6. testosterone 7. perineum

**J.** 1. prostatectomy 2. prostatic 3. prostatitis 4. prostatorrhea 5. orchiectomy 6. orchioplasty 7. orchiotomy 8. orchiopathy 9. vesiculopathy 10. vesiculitis

**K.** 1. suprapubic prostatectomy 2. transurethral resection 3. genitourinary 4. benign prostatic hypertrophy 5. digital rectal exam 6. prostate-specific antigen

**L.** 1. the formation of mature sperm 2. accumulation of fluid within the testes 3. surgical removal of the prostate gland by inserting a device through the urethra and removing prostate tissue 4. failure to produce sperm 5. surgical removal of the testes. 6. surgical removal of part or all of the vas deferens 7. destruction of tissue with an electric current, caustic agent, hot iron, or by freezing

## Chapter 11 Answers

### Case Study (Critical Thinking Questions)

1. hyperglycemia; ketoacidosis; glycosuria 2. student answers will vary 3. a—damage to the retina as a result of diabetes b—a therapeutic plan c—state of profound unconsciousness d—twice a day 4. fasting blood sugar, serum glucose level, 2-hour postprandial glucose tolerance test 5. abdominal X-ray, pancreas CT scan 6. 2,000-calorie ADA diet with three meals and two snacks, may engage in any activity, return to school next Monday, check serum glucose level b.i.d., and call office for insulin dosage

### Chart Note Transcription

1. endocrinologist—specialist in the treatment of diseases of the endocrine glands 2. obesity—an abnormal amount of fat in the body 3. hirsutism—excessive amount of hair for a female 4. radioimmunoassay (RIA)—test to measure the hormone levels in blood plasma 5. cortisol—steroid hormone that regulates carbohydrates in the body 6. adenoma—gland tumor 7. adrenal cortex—outer layer of the adrenal gland 8. Cushing's syndrome—a group of symptoms associated with hypersecretion of the adrenal cortex 9. adenoma—gland tumor 10. adrenal cortex—outer layer of the adrenal gland 11. adrenalectomy—surgical removal of the adrenal gland

### Practice Exercises

**A.** 1. endocrinology 2. pituitary 3. gonads 4. corticosteroids 5. testosterone 6. estrogen, progesterone 7. antidiuretic hormone (ADH) 8. $T_4$ 9. exophthalmos 10. adenocarcinoma

**B.** 1. thyroidectomy 2. thyroiditis 3. euthyroid 4. thyroidotomy 5. pancreatitis 6. pancreatectomy 7. pancreatotomy 8. adrenalectomy 9. adrenalitis 10. thymoma 11. thymectomy

**C.** 1. b 2. a 3. e 4. k 5. h 6. j 7. i 8. f 9. g 10. c 11. d

**D.** 1. protein-bound iodine 2. potassium 3. thyroxine 4. glucose tolerance test 5. diabetes mellitus 6. basal metabolic rate 7. sodium 8. antidiuretic hormone

**E.** 1. NIDDM 2. IDDM 3. ACTH 4. PTH 5. $T_3$ 6. TSH 7. FBS 8. PRL

**F.** 1. glycosuria 2. endocrine 3. polyuria 4. hypercalcemia 5. polydipsia

**G.** 1. hormone obtained from cortex of adrenal gland 2. having excessive hair 3. a nervous condition characterized with spasms of extremities; can occur from imbalance of pH and calcium or disorder of parathyroid gland 4. disorder of the retina occurring with diabetes 5. increase of blood sugar in diabetes 6. decrease of blood sugar 7. another term for epinephrine; produced by inner portion of adrenal gland. 8. hormone produced by pancreas; essential for metabolism of blood sugar 9. toxic condition due to hyperactivity of thyroid gland 10. four small glands located near thyroid; assist in regulating amount of calcium in blood

## Chapter 12 Answers

### Case Study (Critical Thinking Questions)

1. the muscles that receive nerve supply from or below the 2nd lumbar vertebra are paralyzed 2. no, the spinal cord was completely severed 3. a—comminuted—shattered bone; b—sanguinous—bloody; c—decubitus ulcer—pressure sore; d—catheterization—thin, flexible tube inserted into the bladder 4. d—leg strengthening 5. independent transfers, independent wheelchair mobility, independent ADLs. 6. lumbar laminectomy with spinal fusion; stabilize the fracture and remove the epidural hematoma

### Chart Note Transcription

1. neurologist—specialist in the treatment of diseases of the nervous system 2. dysphasia—difficulty with speech 3. hemiparesis—loss of motion on one side of the body 4. convulsions—severe involuntary muscle contractions 5. electroencephalography (EEG)—recording of the electrical activity of the brain 6. lumbar puncture (LP)—puncture with a needle into the low back to withdraw fluid for examination 7. brain scan—injection of radioactive isotopes 8. cerebral cortex—outer layer of the largest section of the brain 9. astrocytoma—astrocyte tumor 10. craniotomy—skull incision 11. cryosurgery—the use of extreme cold to destroy

### Practice Exercises

**A.** 1. neurology 2. brain, spinal cord, nerves 3. peripheral nervous system, central nervous system 4. efferent or motor 5. afferent or sensory 6. poliomyelitis 7. cerebrum 8. cerebellum 9. eyesight 10. hearing, smell 11. right 12. parasympathetic, sympathetic

**B.** 1. neuritis 2. neurologist 3. neuralgia 4. polyneuritis 5. neurectomy 6. neuroplasty 7. neurotomy 8. neurorrhaphy 9. meningitis 10. meningocele 11. myelomeningocele 12. encephalography 13. encephalopathy 14. encephalitis 15. encephalocele 16. encephalomyelitis 17. cerebrospinal 18. cerebrosclerosis 19. cerebropathy 20. cerebromeningitis 21. cerebral

**C.** 1. b 2. f 3. g 4. h 5. i 6. a 7. e 8. c 9. d

**D.** 1. transient ischemic attack 2. multiple sclerosis 3. spinal cord injury 4. central nervous system 5. peripheral nervous system 6. headache 7. cerebral palsy 8. lumbar puncture 9. amyotrophic lateral sclerosis 10. autonomic nervous system

**E.** 1. h 2. k 3. d 4. g 5. a 6. b 7. f 8. j 9. e 10. l 11. i 12. c

**F.** 1. injecting radiopaque dye into spinal canal to examine under X-ray the outlines made by the dye 2. X-ray of the blood vessels of the brain after the injection of radiopaque dye 3. reflex test on bottom of foot to detect lesion and abnormalities of nervous system 4. test of balance to determine neurological function 5. laboratory examination of fluid taken from the brain and spinal cord 6. positron emission tomography to measure cerebral blood flow, blood volume, oxygen, and glucose uptake 7. recording the ultrasonic echoes of the brain 8. needle puncture into the spinal cavity to withdraw fluid

**G.** 1. seizures 2. paralysis 3. muscular coordination 4. pain, sensitivity 5. strength 6. weakness 7. speech 8. movement 9. feeling, sensation

**H.** 1. meninges 2. brain 3. cerebellum 4. spinal cord 5. head 6. thalamus 7. glue 8. nerve root 9. cerebrum 10. pons

**I.** 1. tumor of glial cells 2. seizure 3. without sensation 4. paralysis of one-half of body 5. nerve pain 6. without pain sensitivity 7. lack of nervous strength 8. paralysis of all four limbs 9. accumulation of blood in the subdural space 10. extreme uncontrollable desire to sleep

**J.** 1. d 2. e 3. f 4. g 5. b 6. a 7. c 8. j 9. h 10. i

## Chapter 13 Answers

### Case Study (Critical Thinking Questions)

1. pupils open and close correctly when the physician shines a light into the eye; pupils become smaller in bright light and larger in dim light; it is important to prevent too much light from reaching the inside of the eyeball 2. eye muscles, conjunctiva, iris/pupil, retina, macular area of the retina, cornea 3. breast cancer with a mastectomy, cholelithiasis with a cholecystectomy 4. dilate the pupil, miotic drops 5. a—farsightedness (hyperopia) 6. cryoextraction

### Chart Note Transcription

1. otorhinolaryngologist (ENT)—specialist in the treatment of diseases of the ear, nose, and throat 2. otitis media (OM)—middle ear infection 3. AU, binaural—both ears 4. otoscopy—visual examination of the external ear canal and eardrum 5. tympanic membrane—membrane between the outer and middle ear 6. cerumen—ear wax 7. tympanometry—measurement of the movement of the eardrum 8. audiometric test—test of hearing ability 9. conductive hearing loss—loss of hearing as the result of the blocking of sound transmission in the middle ear 10. myringotomy—eardrum incision

### Practice Exercises

**A.** 1. ophthalmology 2. eye muscles, eyelids, conjunctiva, lacrimal gland, and ducts 3. cilia 4. lacrimal 5. cornea 6. retina 7. iris 8. accommodation 9. malleus, incus, stapes 10. otology 11. tympanic membrane 12. cerumen 13. eustachian or auditory 14. temporal 15. vestibulocochlear nerve 16. conductive

**B.** 1. blepharitis 2. blepharoplasty 3. blepharochalasis 4. retinopathy 5. retinopexy 6. ophthalmology 7. ophthalmic

8. ophthalmoscopy 9. iridoplegia 10. iridectomy 11. iridomalacia 12. otoplasty 13. otopyorrhea 14. otalgia 15. otitis 16. otosclerosis 17. otology 18. audiogram 19. audiometer 20. audiology

**C.** 1. -tropia 2. -opia 3. -itis 4. -logy 5. -otomy 6. -plasty 7. -pexy 8. -stenosis 9. -otia 10. -cusis

**D.** 1. tear or tear duct 2. vascular 3. water 4. light 5. cornea 6. glassy 7. double 8. gray 9. old age 10. dull or dim 11. ear 12. stapes 13. hearing 14. eustachian or auditory tube 15. eardrum or tympanic membrane

**E.** 1. dull/dim vision 2. double vision 3. enlarge or widen pupil 4. constrict pupil 5. diminished vision of old age 6. ringing in the ears 7. middle ear bone 8. measure movement in eardrum 9. auditory tube 10. inner ear 11. results of hearing test 12. middle ear infection

**F.** 1. h 2. g 3. a 4. d 5. b 6. i 7. c 8. f 9. e 10. j 11. k 12. o 13. n 14. p 15. m 16. l

**G.** 1. left eye 2. both eyes 3. rapid eye movement 4. accommodation 5. senile macular degeneration 6. pupils equal, round, react to light and accommodation 7. intraocular pressure 8. exotropia 9. right eye 10. visual field 11. polyethylene tube 12. eyes, ears, nose, throat 13. bone conduction 14. both ears 15. otitis media

**H.** 1. tonometry 2. chalazion 3. emmetropia 4. conjunctivitis 5. myopia 6. cataract 7. hordeolum 8. entropion 9. strabismus 10. hyperopia 11. exophthalmos 12. presbycusis 13. otorhinolaryngologist 14. inner ear 15. Ménière's disease 16. acoustic neuroma

## Chapter 14 Answers

### Case Study (Critical Thinking Questions)

1. a—dyspnea—difficulty breathing b—cough producing thick sputum—coughing up thick mucus material c—hemoptysis—coughing blood 2. a—uterus surgically removed due to endometrium becoming displaced in the pelvic cavity b—gallbladder removed due to gallstones 3. increased thoracic curvature, musculoskeletal system 4. a—shortness of breath b—computed tomography scan 5. a—incision into the chest b—removal of a lobe of the lung 6. the tumor has spread to other areas of the body

### Chart Note Transcription

1. oncologist—specialist in the treatment of cancer 2. exploratory surgery—surgery performed to determine if cancer is present 3. biopsies—small samples of tissue removed for examination under a microscope 4. malignant—cancerous with a tendency to grow worse 5. neoplasm—new and abnormal growth 6. Grade II—graded to be moderately differentiated 7. encapsulated—enclosed in a sheath of tissue 8. metastases—spreading to another part of the body 9. nephrocarcinoma—cancerous tumor of the kidney 10. protocol—plan of treatment 11. chemotherapy—use of chemical agents with a specific toxic effect

## Practice Exercises

**A.** 1. *Physician's Desk Reference* (PDR) 2. pharmacist 3. generic or nonproprietary 4. brand or proprietary 5. the chemical formula 6. Drug Enforcement Agency

**B.** 1. sublingual 2. rectal 3. topical 4. intradermal 5. intramuscular 6. intravenous 7. oral

**C.** 1. unusual or abnormal response to a drug 2. administration of a drug through a needle and syringe under the skin, or into a muscle, vein, or body cavity. 3. harmless substance to satisfy patient's desire for medication 4. extent to which a substance is poisonous 5. response to drug other than the expected response 6. prepackaged and prelabeled method of medication distribution 7. emotional dependence on a drug 8. substance that neutralizes poisons 9. condition under which a particular drug should not be used 10. prevention of disease

**D.** 1. grain 2. two times a day 3. three times a day 4. as desired 5. as needed 6. before 7. over the counter 8. drop 9. label as follows/directions 10. immediately 11. tincture 12. every day 13. night 14. nothing by mouth 15. at bedtime 16. ointment 17. telephone order 18. drops 19. 100 20. discontinue

**E.** 1. Pravachol, 20 milligrams each, take one every day at bedtime, supply with 30, refill three times with no substitutions. 2. Lanoxin, 0.125 milligram each, take three now and then 2 every morning, supply with 100 and may refill as needed.

3. Synthroid, 0.075 milligram each, take 1 every day, supply with 100 and may refill four times. 4. Norvasc, 5 milligram each, take 1 every morning, supply with 60 and may refill

**F.** 1. i 2. k 3. h 4. j 5. e 6. f 7. b 8. a 9. d 10. c 11. g

**G.** 1. minor tranquilizers 2. humanistic psychotherapy 3. lithium 4. antipsychotic drugs 5. psychoanalysis 6. antidepressant drugs

**H.** 1. magnetic resonance imaging 2. barium 3. anteroposterior 4. computerized tomography 5. right lateral 6. posteroanterior 7. left lateral 8. positive emission tomography 9. upper gastrointestinal series 10. kidneys, ureters, bladder

**I.** 1. h 2. c 3. b 4. g 5. f 6. a 7. d 8. e 9. i

**J.** 1. range of motion 2. occupational therapy 3. activities of daily living 4. lower extremity 5. electromyogram 6. transcutaneous electrical nerve stimulation 7. physical therapy 8. passive range of motion 9. electrical stimulation 10. ultrasound

**K.** 1. massage 2. debridement 3. hydrotherapy 4. postural drainage with clapping 5. active exercises 6. phonophoresis 7. cryotherapy 8. traction

**L.** 1. h 2. e 3. j 4. g 5. a 6. i 7. c 8. f 9. b 10. d

**M.** 1. general anesthesia 2. local anesthesia 3. topical anesthesia 4. regional anesthesia

**N.** 1. h 2. d 3. g 4. j 5. f 6. b 7. i 8. a 9. e 10. c

# Glossary

**abdominal**   Pertaining to the abdomen.

**abdominal cavity**   The superior portion of the abdominopelvic cavity.

**abdominal ultrasonography**   Using ultrasound equipment to produce sound waves that create an image of the abdominal organs.

**abdominopelvic cavity**   A ventral cavity consisting of the abdominal and pelvic cavities. It contains digestive, urinary, and reproductive organs.

**abduction**   Directional term meaning to move away from the median or middle line of the body.

**abnormal psychology**   The study and treatment of behaviors that are outside of normal and are detrimental to the person or society. These maladaptive behaviors range from occasional difficulty coping with stress, to bizarre actions and beliefs, to total withdrawal.

**ABO system**   The major system of blood typing.

**abortion (AB)**   Termination of a pregnancy before the fetus reaches a viable point in development.

**abrasion**   Scraping away a portion of the surface of the skin. Performed to remove acne scars, tattoos, and scar tissue.

**abruptio placentae**   Emergency condition in which the placenta tears away from the uterine wall before the 20th week of pregnancy. Requires immediate delivery of the baby.

**abscess**   Swelling of soft tissues of the jaw as a result of infection.

**acapnia**   Lack of carbon dioxide.

**accessory organs**   The accessory organs to the digestive system consist of the organs that are part of the system, but not part of the continuous tube from mouth to anus. The accessory organs are the liver, pancreas, gallbladder, and salivary glands.

**accommodation (Acc)**   Ability of the eye to adjust to variations in distance.

**achromatopsia**   Condition of color blindness; more common in males.

**acidosis**   Excessive acidity of body fluids due to the accumulation of acids, as in diabetic acidosis.

**acne**   Inflammatory disease of the sebaceous glands and hair follicles that results in papules and pustules.

**acne rosacea**   Hypertrophy of sebaceous glands causing thickened skin generally on the nose, forehead, and cheeks.

**acne vulgaris**   A common form of acne occurring in adolescence from an oversecretion of the oil glands. It is characterized by papules, pustules, blackheads, and whiteheads.

**acoustic**   Pertaining to hearing.

**acoustic neuroma**   Benign tumor of the eighth cranial nerve sheath, which can cause symptoms from pressure being exerted on tissues.

**acquired immunity**   The protective response of the body to a specific pathogen.

**acquired immunodeficiency syndrome (AIDS)**   Disease that involves a defect in the cell-mediated immunity system. A syndrome of opportunistic infections that occur in the final stages of infection with the human immunodeficiency virus (HIV). This virus attacks T4 lymphocytes and destroys them, which reduces the person's ability to fight infection.

**acromegaly**   Chronic disease of adults that results in an elongation and enlargement of the bones of the head and extremities. There can also be mood changes.

**action**   The type of movement a muscle produces.

**active acquired immunity**   Immunity developing after direct exposure to a pathogen.

**active exercises**   Exercises that a patient performs without assistance.

**active range of motion (AROM)**   Range of motion for joints that a patient is able to perform without the assistance of someone else.

**active-resistive exercises**   Exercises in which the patient will work against an artificial resistance applied to a muscle, such as a weight. Used to increase strength.

**activities of daily living (ADL)**   The activities usually performed in the course of a normal day, such as eating, dressing, and washing.

**acute care hospital**   Hospitals that typically provide services to diagnose (laboratory, diagnostic imaging) and treat (surgery, medications, therapy) diseases for a short period of time. In addition, they usually provide emergency and obstetrical care. Also called general hospital.

**acute tubular necrosis (ATN)**   Damage to the renal tubules due to presence of toxins in the urine or to ischemia; results in oliguria.

**adaptive equipment**   Equipment used by the elderly that has been structured to aid them in mobility, eating, and managing the other activities of daily living. This equipment includes special walkers and spoons for the stroke patient.

**addiction**   Acquired dependence on a drug.

**Addison's disease**   Disease named for Thomas Addison, a British physician, that results from a deficiency in adrenocortical hormones. There may be an increased pigmentation of the skin, generalized weakness, and weight loss.

**additive**   The sum of the action of two (or more) drugs given; in this case, the total strength of the medications is equal to the sum of the strength of each individual drug.

**adduction**   Directional term meaning to move toward the median or middle line of the body.

**adductor longus**   A leg muscle named for the direction the fibers pull. This muscle contracts to adduct or pull the leg in toward the midline.

**adenocarcinoma**   Malignant adenoma in a glandular organ.

**adenoidectomy**   Excision of the adenoids.

**adenoiditis**   Inflammation of the adenoid tissue.

**adenoids**   Another term for pharyngeal tonsils. The tonsils are a collection of lymphatic tissue found in the nasopharynx to combat microorganisms entering the body through the nose.

**adenoma**   Neoplasm or tumor of a gland.

**adhesion**  Scar tissue forming in the fascia surrounding a muscle making it difficult to stretch the muscle.

**adipectomy**  Surgical removal of fat.

**adipose tissue**  A type of connective tissue. Also called fat. It stores energy and provides protective padding for underlying structures.

**adrenal cortex**  The outer portion of the adrenal glands; secretes several families of hormones: mineralocorticoids, glucocorticoids, and steroid sex hormones.

**adrenal feminization**  Development of female secondary sexual characteristics (such as breasts) in a male; often as a result of increased estrogen secretion by the adrenal cortex.

**adrenal glands**  A pair of glands in the endocrine system located just above each kidney. These glands are composed of two sections, the cortex and the medulla, that function independently of each other. The cortex secretes steroids, such as aldosterone, cortisol, androgens, estrogens, and progestins. The medulla secretes epinephrine and norepinephrine. The adrenal glands are regulated by adrenocorticotropic hormone, which is secreted by the pituitary gland.

**adrenal medulla**  The inner portion of the adrenal gland. It secretes epinephrine and norepinephrine.

**adrenal virilism**  Development of male secondary sexual characteristics (such as deeper voice and facial hair) in a female; often as a result of increased androgen secretion by the adrenal cortex.

**adrenalectomy**  Excision of the adrenal gland.

**adrenaline**  A hormone produced by the adrenal medulla. Also known as epinephrine. Some of its actions include increasing heart rate and force of contraction, bronchodilation, and relaxation of intestinal muscles.

**adrenalitis**  Inflammation of an adrenal gland.

**adrenocorticotropic hormone (ACTH)**  A hormone secreted by anterior pituitary. It regulates function of the adrenal gland cortex.

**adrenomegaly**  Enlarged adrenal gland.

**adrenopathy**  Adrenal gland disease.

**adult respiratory distress syndrome (ARDS)**  Acute respiratory failure in adults characterized by tachypnea, dyspnea, cyanosis, tachycardia, and hypoxemia.

**aerosol**  Drugs inhaled directly into the nose and mouth.

**afferent arteriole**  Arteriole that carries blood into the glomerulus.

**afferent neurons**  Nerve that carries impulses to the brain and spinal cord from the skin and sense organs. Also called sensory neurons.

**afterbirth**  Another name for the placenta.

**agglutinate**  Clumping together to form small clusters. Platelets agglutinate to start the clotting process.

**agranulocyte**  Nongranular leukocyte. This is one of the two types of leukocytes found in plasma that are classified as either monocytes or lymphocytes.

**AIDS-related complex (ARC)**  Early stage of AIDS. There is a positive test for the virus but only mild symptoms of weight loss, fatigue, skin rash, and anorexia.

**alanine transaminase (ALT)**  An enzyme normally present in the blood. Blood levels are increased in persons with liver disease.

**albino**  A person not able to produce melanin. An albino person has white hair and skin and the pupils of the eye are red.

**albumin**  A protein that is normally found circulating in the bloodstream. It is abnormal for albumin to be in the urine.

**albuminuria**  Albumin (protein) in the urine.

**aldosterone**  A hormone produced by the adrenal cortex. It regulates the levels of sodium and potassium in the body and as a side effect the volume of water lost in urine.

**alimentary canal**  Also known as the gastrointestinal system or digestive system. This system covers the area between the mouth and the anus and includes 30 feet of intestinal tubing. It has a wide range of functions. This system serves to store and digest food, absorb nutrients, and eliminate waste. The major organs of this system are the mouth, pharynx, esophagus, stomach, small intestine, colon, rectum, and anus.

**allergen**  Antigen capable of causing a hypersensitivity or allergy in the body.

**allergist**  A physician who specializes in testing for and treating allergies.

**allergy**  Hypersensitivity to a substance in the environment or a medication.

**allograft**  Skin graft from one person to another; donor is usually a cadaver.

**alopecia**  Absence or loss of hair, especially of the head.

**alveoli**  The tiny air sacs at the end of each bronchiole. The alveoli are surrounded by a capillary network. Gas exchange takes place as oxygen and carbon dioxide diffuse across the alveolar and capillary walls.

**Alzheimer's disease**  Chronic, organic mental disorder consisting of dementia that is more prevalent in adults between 40 and 60. Involves progressive disorientation, apathy, speech and gait disturbances, and loss of memory.

**amblyopia**  Loss of vision not as a result of eye pathology; usually occurs in patients who see two images. In order to see only one image, the brain will no longer recognize the image being sent to it by one of the eyes; may occur if strabismus is not corrected; commonly referred to as lazy eye.

**ambulatory care center**  A facility that provides services that do not require overnight hospitalization. The services range from simple surgeries, to diagnostic testing, to therapy. Also called a surgical center or an outpatient clinic.

**amenorrhea**  Absence of menstruation, which can be the result of many factors, including pregnancy, menopause, and dieting.

**American Sign Language (ASL)**  Nonverbal method of communicating in which the hands and fingers are used to indicate words and concepts. Used by people who are deaf and speech impaired.

**amino acids**  An organic substance found in plasma. It is used by cells to build proteins.

**amnesia**  Loss of memory in which people forget their identity as a result of a head injury or disorder, such as epilepsy, senility, and alcoholism. Can be either temporary or permanent.

**amniocentesis**  Puncturing of the amniotic sac using a needle and syringe for the purpose of withdrawing amniotic fluid for testing. Can assist in determining fetal maturity, development, and genetic disorders.

**amnion**  The inner of two membranous sacs surrounding the fetus. The amniotic sac contains amniotic fluid in which the baby floats.

**amniorrhea**  Discharge of amniotic fluid.

**amniotic fluid**  The fluid inside the amniotic sac.

**amniotomy**  Incision into the amniotic sac.

**amplification device**  Used to increase certain sounds for people with hearing impairments. Also known as hearing aid.

**amputation**  Partial or complete removal of a limb for a variety of reasons, including tumors, gangrene, intractable pain, crushing injury, or uncontrollable infection.

**amylase**  Digestive enzyme found in saliva that begins the digestion of carbohydrates.

**amyotrophic lateral sclerosis (ALS)**  Disease with muscular weakness and atrophy due to degeneration of motor neurons of the spinal cord. Also called Lou Gehrig's disease, after the New York Yankees' baseball player who died from the disease.

**anacusis**  Total absence of hearing; unable to perceive sound. Also called deafness.

**anal fissure**  Crack-like split in the rectum or anal canal.

**anal fistula**  Abnormal tube-like passage from the surface around the anal opening directly into the rectum.

**anal sphincter**  Ring of muscle that controls anal opening.

**analgesia**  A reduction in the perception of pain or sensation due to a neurological condition or medication.

**analgesic**  Relieves pain without the loss of consciousness. May be either narcotic or non-narcotic. Narcotic drugs are derived from the opium poppy and act on the brain to cause pain relief and drowsiness.

**anaphylactic shock**  Life-threatening condition resulting from the ingestion of food or medications that produce a severe allergic response. There are circulatory and respiratory problems that occur, including respiratory distress, hypotension, edema, tachycardia, and convulsions.

**anaphylaxis**  Severe reaction to an antigen.

**anastomosis**  Creating a passageway or opening between two organs or vessels.

**anatomical position**  Used to describe the positions and relationships of a structure in the human body. For descriptive purposes the assumption is always that the person is in the anatomical position. The body is standing erect with the arms at the side of the body, the palms of the hands facing forward, and the eyes looking straight ahead. The legs are parallel with the feet and toes pointing forward.

**ancillary report**  Report in a patient's medical record from various treatments and therapies the patient has received, such as rehabilitation, social services, respiratory therapy, or from the dietician.

**androgen**  A class of steroid hormones secreted by the adrenal cortex. These hormones, such as testosterone, produce a masculinizing effect.

**androgen therapy**  Replacement male hormones to treat patients who produce insufficient hormone naturally.

**andropathy**  Male disease.

**anemia**  Reduction in the number of red blood cells (RBCs) or amount of hemoglobin in the blood; results in less oxygen reaching the tissues.

**anesthesia**  Partial or complete loss of sensation with or without a loss of consciousness as a result of a drug, disease, or injury.

**anesthesiologist**  A physician who has a specialization in the practice of administering anesthetics.

**anesthesiologist's report**  A medical record document that relates the details regarding the drugs given to a patient and the patient's response to anesthesia and vital signs during surgery.

**anesthetic**  Produces a lack of feeling that may be of local or general effect, depending on the type of administration.

**anesthetic ophthalmic solutions**  Eyedrops for pain relief associated with eye infections and corneal abrasions.

**aneurysm**  Weakness in the wall of an artery that results in localized widening of the artery.

**aneurysmectomy**  Surgical removal of the sac of an aneurysm.

**angina pectoris**  Severe chest pain with a sensation of constriction around the heart. Caused by a deficiency of oxygen to the heart muscle.

**angiocarditis**  Inflammation of the heart and blood vessels.

**angiography**  Process of taking an X-ray of blood or lymphatic vessels after injection of a radiopaque substance.

**angioma**  Tumor, usually benign, consisting of blood vessels.

**angioplasty**  Surgical repair of blood vessels.

**angiorrhaphy**  Suturing a vessel.

**angiospasm**  Involuntary muscle contraction of a vessel.

**angiostenosis**  Narrowing of a vessel.

**anhidrosis**  Abnormal condition of no sweat.

**ankylosing spondylitis**  Inflammatory spinal condition that resembles rheumatoid arthritis; results in gradual stiffening and fusion of the vertebrae; more common in men than women.

**anorchism**  Congenital absence of one or both testes.

**anorexia**  Loss of appetite that can accompany other conditions such as a gastrointestinal (GI) upset.

**anorexia nervosa**  A type of eating disorder characterized by severe disturbance in body image and marked refusal to eat.

**anorexiant**  Treats obesity by suppressing appetite.

**anosmia**  Loss of the sense of smell.

**anoxia**  Lack of oxygen.

**antacid**  Neutralizes acid in the stomach.

**antagonistic pairs**  Pair of muscles arranged around a joint that produce opposite actions.

**anteflexion**  While the uterus is normally in this position, an exaggeration of the forward bend of the uterus is abnormal. The forward bend is near the neck of the uterus. The position of cervix, or opening of the uterus, remains normal.

**antepartum**  Before birth.

**anterior**  Directional term meaning near or on the front or belly side of the body.

**anterior lobe**  The anterior portion of the pituitary gland. It secretes adrenocorticotropic hormone, follicle-stimulating hormone, growth hormone, luteinizing hormone, melanocyte-stimulating hormone, prolactin, and thyroid-stimulating hormone.

**anteroposterior (AP) view**  Positioning the patient so that the X-rays pass through the body from the anterior side to the posterior side.

**anthracosis** A type of pneumoconiosis that develops from the collection of coal dust in the lung. Also called black lung or miner's lung.

**antiarrhythmic** Controls cardiac arrhythmias by altering nerve impulses within the heart.

**antibiotic** Destroys or prohibits the growth of microorganisms. Used to treat bacterial infections. Have not been found to be effective in treating viral infections. To be effective, it must be taken regularly for a specified period.

**antibiotic ophthalmic solution** Eyedrops for the treatment of bacterial eye infections.

**antibiotic otic solution** Eardrops to treat otitis externa.

**antibody** Protein material produced in the body as a response to the invasion of a foreign substance.

**antibody-mediated immunity** The production of antibodies by B cells in response to an antigen. Also called humoral immunity.

**anticholinergic** Blocks the function of the parasympathetic nervous system. Used to treat intestinal, bladder, and bronchial spasms.

**anticoagulant** Substance that prevents or delays the clotting or coagulation of blood.

**anticonvulsant** Prevents or relieves convulsions. Drugs such as phenobarbital reduce excessive stimulation in the brain to control seizures and other symptoms of epilepsy.

**antidiarrheal** Prevents or relieves diarrhea.

**antidiuretic hormone (ADH)** A hormone secreted by the posterior pituitary. It promotes water reabsorption by the kidney tubules.

**antidote** Substance that will neutralize poisons or their side effects.

**antiemetic** Controls nausea and vomiting.

**antifungal** Kills fungi infecting the skin.

**antigen** Substance that is capable of inducing the formation of an antibody. The antibody then intereacts with the antigen in the antigen–antibody reaction.

**antigen–antibody reaction** Combination of the antigen with its specific antibody to increase susceptibility to phagocytosis and immunity.

**antiglaucoma medications** A group of drugs that reduce intraocular pressure by lowering the amount of aqueous humor in the eyeball; may achieve this by either reducing the production of aqueous humor or increasing its outflow.

**antihemorrhagic** Substance that prevents or stops hemorrhaging.

**antihistamine** Acts to control allergic symptoms by counteracting histamine, which exists naturally in the body, and which is released in allergic reactions.

**antihypertensive** Prevents or controls high blood pressure. Some of these drugs act to block nerve impulses that cause arteries to constict and thus increase the blood pressure. Other drugs slow the heart rate and decrease its force of contraction. Still others may reduce the amount of the hormone aldosterone in the blood that is causing the blood pressure to rise.

**anti-inflammatory** Acts to counteract inflammation.

**anti-inflammatory drug** Reduces skin inflammation or itching.

**anti-inflammatory otic solution** Reduces inflammation, itching, and edema associated with otitis externa.

**antilipidemic** Reduces amount of cholesterol and lipids in the bloodstream; treats hyperlipidemia.

**antiparasitic** Kills mites or lice.

**antiplatelet agent** Interferes with the action of platelets; prolongs bleeding time; commonly referred to as blood thinner.

**antiprostatic agent** Medication to treat early cases of benign prostatic hypertrophy; may prevent surgery for mild cases.

**antipruritic** Reduces severe itching.

**antiseptic** Used to kill bacteria in skin cuts and wounds or at a surgical site.

**antisocial personality** A personality disorder in which the patient engages in behaviors that are illegal or outside of social norms.

**antispasmodic** Medication to prevent or reduce bladder muscle spasms.

**antitussive** Controls or relieves coughing. Codeine is an ingredient in many prescription cough medicines that acts upon the brain to control coughing.

**antiviral** Weakens a viral infection in the body, often by interfering with the virus's ability to replicate.

**antrum** The tapered distal end of the stomach.

**anuria** Complete suppression of urine formed by the kidneys and a complete lack of urine excretion.

**anus** The terminal opening of the digestive tube.

**anxiety** A feeling of apprehension or worry.

**anxiety disorders** Characterized by persistent worry and apprehension; includes panic attacks, anxiety, phobias, and obsessive-compulsive disorder.

**aorta** The largest artery in the body. It is located in the mediastinum and carries oxygenated blood away from the left side of the heart.

**aortic** Pertaining to the aorta.

**aortic stenosis** Narrowing of the aorta.

**aortic valve** The semilunar valve between the left ventricle of the heart and the aorta in the heart. It prevents blood from flowing backwards into the ventricle.

**aortogram** X-ray record of the aorta after a radiopaque dye has been inserted.

**apex** Directional term meaning tip or summit.

**Apgar score** Evaluation of a neonate's adjustment to the outside world; observes color, heart rate, muscle tone, respiratory rate, and response to stimulus.

**aphagia** Not eating.

**aphasia** Inability to communicate through speech. Often an aftereffect of a stroke (CVA).

**aphonia** No voice.

**aplastic anemia** Severe form of anemia that develops as a consequence of loss of functioning red bone marrow; results in a decrease in the number of all the formed elements; treatment may eventually require a bone marrow transplant.

**apnea** The condition of not breathing.

**apocrine gland** Type of sweat gland that opens into hair follicles located in the pubic, anal, and mammary areas. These glands secrete a substance that can produce an odor when it comes into contact with bacteria on the skin causing what is commonly referred to as body odor.

**appendectomy**  Surgical removal of the appendix.

**appendicitis**  Inflammation of the appendix.

**appendicular skeleton**  The appendicular skeleton consists of the bones of the upper and lower extremities, shoulder, and pelvis.

**appendix**  A small outgrowth at the end of the cecum. Its function or purpose is unknown.

**aqueous humor**  A watery fluid filling the spaces between the cornea and lens.

**arachnoid layer**  The delicate middle layer of the meninges.

**areola**  The pigmented area around the nipple of the breast.

**arrhythmia**  Irregularity in the heartbeat or action.

**arterial**  Pertaining to the artery.

**arterial anastomosis**  Surgical joining together of two arteries; performed if an artery is severed or if a damaged section of an artery is removed.

**arterial blood gases (ABG)**  Lab test that measures the amount of oxygen, carbon dioxide, and nitrogen in the blood, and the pH.

**arteries**  The blood vessels that carry blood away from the heart.

**arterioles**  The smallest branches of the arteries. They carry blood to the capillaries.

**arteriorrhexis**  A ruptured artery.

**arteriosclerosis**  Condition with thickening, hardening, and loss of elasticity of the walls of the arteries.

**arteriosclerotic heart disease (ASHD)**  Chronic heart disorder caused by a hardening of the walls of the coronary arteries.

**arthralgia**  Pain in a joint.

**arthritis**  Inflammation of a joint that is usually accompanied by pain and swelling. A chronic disease.

**arthrocentesis**  Removal of synovial fluid with a needle from a joint space, such as in the knee, for examination.

**arthroclasia**  Surgically breaking loose a stiffened joint.

**arthrodesis**  Surgical fusion or stiffening of a joint to provide stability. This is sometimes done to relieve the pain of arthritis.

**arthrography**  Visualization of a joint by radiographic study after injection of a contrast medium into the joint space.

**arthroscopic surgery**  Use of an arthroscope to facilitate performing surgery on a joint.

**arthroscopy**  Examination of the interior of a joint by entering the joint with an arthroscope. The arthroscope contains a small television camera that allows the physician to view the interior of the joint on a monitor during the procedure.

**arthrotomy**  Surgically cutting into a joint.

**articular cartilage**  Layer of cartilage covering the ends of bones forming a synovial joint.

**articulation**  Another term for a joint, the point where two bones meet.

**artificial tears**  Medications, many of them over the counter, to treat dry eyes.

**asbestosis**  A type of pneumoconiosis that develops from collection of asbestos fibers in the lungs; may lead to the development of lung cancer.

**ascending colon**  The section of the colon following the cecum. It ascends the right side of the abdomen.

**ascending tracts**  Nerve tracts carrying sensory information up the spinal cord to the brain.

**ascites**  Collection or accumulation of fluid in the peritoneal cavity.

**aspartate transaminase (AST)**  An enzyme normally present in the blood. Blood levels are increased in persons with liver disease.

**aspermia**  Lack of, or failure to ejaculate, sperm.

**asphyxia**  Lack of oxygen that can lead to unconsciousness and death if not corrected immediately. Some of the common causes are drowning, foreign body in the respiratory tract, poisoning, and electric shock.

**aspirator**  A surgical instrument used to suction fluids.

**asthenia**  Lack or loss of strength, causing extreme weakness.

**asthma**  Disease caused by various conditions, such as allergens, and resulting in constriction of the bronchial airways and labored respirations. Can cause violent spasms of the bronchi (bronchospasms) but is generally not a life-threatening condition. Medication can be very effective.

**astigmatism (Astigm)**  A condition in which light rays are focused unevenly on the eye, which causes a distorted image due to an abnormal curvature of the cornea.

**astrocytoma**  Tumor of the brain or spinal cord that is composed of astrocytes.

**ataxia**  Having a lack of muscle coordination as a result of a disorder or disease.

**atelectasis**  Condition in which lung tissue collapses, which prevents the respiratory exchange of oxygen and carbon dioxide. Can be caused by a variety of conditions, including pressure upon the lung from a tumor or other object.

**atherectomy**  Excision of fatty substance.

**atherosclerosis**  The most common form of arteriosclerosis. Caused by the formation of yellowish plaques of cholesterol buildup on the inner walls of the arteries.

**atresia**  Congenital lack of a normal body opening.

**atria**  The two upper chambers of the heart. The left atrium receives blood returning from the lungs, and the right atrium receives blood returning from the body.

**atrial**  Pertaining to the atrium.

**atrioventricular node**  This area at the junction of the right atrium and ventricle receives the stimulus from the sinoatrial node and sends the impulse to the ventricles through the bundle of His.

**atrioventricular valve (AV)**  The heart valves located between an atria and a ventricle. Includes the tricuspid valve in the right side of the heart and the bicuspid or mitral valve in the left side of the heart.

**atrophy**  Lack or loss of normal development.

**attention deficit disorder**  A type of mental disorder diagnosed in childhood characterized by poor attention and inability to control behavior. The child may or may not be hyperactive.

**atypical**  Abnormal.

**audiogram**  Chart that shows the faintest sounds a patient can hear during audiometry testing.

**audiologist (AuD)**  Provides a comprehensive array of services related to prevention, diagnosis, and treatment of hearing impairment and its associated communication disorders.

**audiology**  Study of hearing.

**audiometer**  Instrument to measure hearing.

**audiometry**  Process of measuring hearing.

**auditory canal**   The canal that leads from the external opening of the ear to the eardrum.

**auditory tube**   Another name for the eustachian tube connecting the middle ear and pharynx.

**aura**   Sensations, such as seeing colors or smelling an unusual odor, that occur just prior to an epileptic seizure.

**aural**   Pertaining to the ear.

**auricle**   Also called the pinna. The external ear. It functions to capture sound waves as they go past the outer ear.

**auscultation**   Listening to the sounds within the body by using a stethoscope.

**autism**   A type of mental disorder diagnosed in childhood in which the child exhibits an extreme degree of withdrawal from all social contacts.

**autograft**   Skin graft from a person's own body.

**autoimmune disease**   A disease that results from the body's immune system attacking its own cells as if they were pathogens; examples include systemic lupus erythematosus, rheumatoid arthritis, and multiple sclerosis.

**autologous transfusion**   Procedure for collecting and storing a patient's own blood several weeks prior to the actual need. It can then be used to replace blood lost during a surgical procedure.

**autonomic nervous system**   The portion of the nervous system that consists of nerves to the internal organs that function involuntarily. It regulates the functions of glands (especially the salivary, gastric, and sweat glands), the adrenal medulla, heart, and smooth muscle tissue. This system is divided into two parts: sympathetic and parasympathetic.

**axial skeleton**   The axial skeleton includes the bones in the head, spine, chest, and trunk.

**axillary**   Commonly referred to as the armpit. There is a collection of lymph nodes in this area that drains each arm.

**axon**   Single projection of a neuron that conducts impulse away from nerve cell body.

**azoturia**   Nitrogenous waste in the urine.

**B cells**   Common name for B lymphocytes, responds to foreign antigens by producing protective antibodies.

**B lymphocytes**   The humoral immunity cells, which respond to foreign antigens by producing protective antibodies. Simply referred to as B cells.

**Babinski's sign**   Reflex test to determine lesions and abnormalities in the nervous system. The Babinski reflex is present if the great toe extends instead of flexes when the lateral sole of the foot is stroked. The normal response to this stimulation would be a flexion, or upward movement, of the toe.

**bacteria**   Primitive, single-celled microorganisms that are present everywhere. Some are capable of causing disease in humans.

**bacteriuria**   Bacteria in the urine.

**balanitis**   Inflammation of the skin covering the glans penis.

**balanoplasty**   Surgical repair of the glans penis.

**balanorrhea**   Discharge from the glans penis.

**ball and socket**   A type of freely moving synovial joint. The two main examples in humans are the shoulder and hip joints.

**barbiturate**   A drug that depresses CNS activity; used as a sedative and an anticonvulsant.

**barium (Ba)**   Soft metallic element from the earth used as a radiopaque X-ray dye.

**barium enema (BE, lower GI series)**   Radiographic examination of the small intestine, large intestine, or colon in which an enema containing barium (Ba) is administered to the patient while the X-ray pictures are taken.

**barium swallow (upper GI series)**   A barium (Ba) mixture swallowed while X-ray pictures are taken of the esophagus, stomach, and duodenum used to visualize the upper gastrointestinal tract (upper GI).

**barrier contraception**   Prevention of a pregnancy using a device to prevent sperm from meeting an ovum; examples include condoms, diaphragms, and cervical caps.

**Bartholin's glands**   Glands located on either side of the vaginal opening that secrete mucus for vaginal lubrication.

**basal cell carcinoma**   Tumor of the basal cell layer of the epidermis. A frequent type of skin cancer that rarely metastasizes or spreads. These cancers can arise on sun-exposed skin.

**basal layer**   The deepest layer of the epidermis. This living layer constantly multiplies and divides to supply cells to replace the cells that are sloughed off the skin surface.

**basal metabolic rate (BMR)**   Somewhat outdated test to measure the energy used when the body is in a state of rest.

**base**   Directional term meaning bottom or lower part.

**basophils**   A granulocyte white blood cell that releases histamine and heparin in damaged tissues.

**Bell's palsy**   One-sided facial paralysis with an unknown cause. The person cannot control salivation, tearing of the eyes, or expression. The patient will eventually recover.

**benign**   A tumor that is not cancerous. A benign tumor is generally not progressive or recurring.

**benign prostatic hypertrophy (BPH)**   Enlargement of the prostate gland commonly seen in males over 50.

**bicarbonate (HCO$_3^-$)**   An electrolyte and blood buffer whose level in the body is regulated by excretion by the kidney.

**biceps**   An arm muscle named for the number of attachment points. *Bi-* means two and biceps have two heads attached to the bone.

**bicuspid valve**   A valve between the left atrium and ventricle. It prevents blood from flowing backwards into the atrium. It has two cusps or flaps. It is also called the mitral valve.

**bicuspids**   Premolar permanent teeth having two cusps or projections that assist in grinding food. Humans have eight bicuspids.

**bile**   Substance produced by the liver and stored in the gallbladder. It is added to the chyme in the duodenum and functions to emulsify fats so they can be digested and absorbed. Cholesterol is essential to bile production.

**bilirubin**   Waste product produced from destruction of worn-out red blood cells; disposed of by the liver.

**binaural**   Referring to both ears.

**binocular**   Pertaining to two eyes.

**biopsy (BX, bx)** A piece of tissue is removed by syringe and needle, knife, punch, or brush to examine under a microscope. Used to aid in diagnosis.

**bipolar disorder** A mental disorder in which the patient has alternating periods of depression and mania.

**bite-wing X-ray** X-ray taken with part of the film holder held between the teeth, and the film held parallel to the teeth.

**bladder neck obstruction** Blockage of the bladder outlet into the urethra.

**bleeding time** Test to measure the amount of time needed for the blood to coagulate.

**blepharectomy** Excision of the eyelid.

**blepharitis** Inflammatory condition of the eyelash follicles and glands of the eyelids that results in swelling, redness, and crusts of dried mucus on the lids. Can be the result of allergy or infection.

**blepharochalasis** In this condition the upper eyelid increases in size due to a loss of elasticity, which is followed by swelling and recurrent edema of the lids. The skin may droop over the edges of the eyes when the eyes are open.

**blepharoplasty** Surgical repair of the eyelid.

**blepharoptosis** Drooping eyelid.

**blood** The major component of the hematic system. It consists of watery plasma, red blood cells, and white blood cells.

**blood clot** The hard collection of fibrin, blood cells, and tissue debris that is the end result of hemostasis or the blood clotting process.

**blood culture and sensitivity (C&S)** Sample of blood is incubated in the laboratory to check for bacterial growth; if bacteria are present, they are identified and tested to determine which antibiotics they are sensitive to.

**blood pressure (BP)** Measurement of the pressure that is exerted by blood against the walls of a blood vessel.

**blood serum test** Blood test to measure the level of substances such as calcium, electrolytes, testosterone, insulin, and glucose. Used to assist in determining the function of various endocrine glands.

**blood sinuses** Spread-out blood vessels within the spleen that result in slow-moving blood flow.

**blood transfusion** Artificial transfer of blood into the bloodstream.

**blood typing** The blood of one person is different from another's due to the presence of antigens on the surface of the erythrocytes. The major method of typing blood is the ABO system and includes types A, B, O, and AB. The other major method of typing blood is the Rh factor, consisting of the two types, Rh+ and Rh−.

**blood urea nitrogen (BUN)** Blood test to measure kidney function by the level of nitrogenous waste, or urea, that is in the blood.

**blood vessels** The closed system of tubes that conducts blood throughout the body. It consists of arteries, veins, and capillaries.

**body** The main portion of the stomach.

**body mechanics** Use of good posture and position while performing activities of daily living to prevent injury and stress on body parts.

**bolus** Chewed up morsel of food ready to be swallowed.

**bone** A type of connective tissue and an organ of the musculoskeletal system. They provide support for the body and serve as sites of muscle attachments.

**bone graft** Piece of bone taken from the patient and used to replace a removed bone or a bony defect at another site.

**bone marrow** Soft tissue found inside cavities in bones; produces blood cells.

**bone marrow aspiration** Removing a sample of bone marrow by syringe for microscopic examination. Useful for diagnosing such diseases as leukemia. For example, a proliferation (massive increase) of a white blood cells cloud confirm the diagnosis of acute leukemia.

**bone marrow biopsy** Removal of a small amount of bone marrow for microscopic examination to determine the presence of malignant tumor cells.

**bone marrow transplant (BMT)** Patient receives red bone marrow from a donor after the patient's own bone marrow has been destroyed by radiation or chemotherapy.

**bone reabsorption inhibitors** Conditions that result in weak and fragile bones, such as osteoporosis and Paget's disease, are improved by medications that reduce the reabsorption of bones.

**bone scan** Patient is given a radioactive dye and then scanning equipment is used to visualize bones. It is especially useful in observing the progress of treatment for osteomyelitis and cancer metastases to the bone.

**borborygmus** Rumbling and gurgling bowel sounds.

**Bowman's capsule** Also called the glomerular capsule. Part of the renal corpuscle. It is a double-walled cup-like structure that encircles the glomerulus. In the filtration stage of urine production, waste products filtered from the blood enter Bowman's capsule as the glomerular filtrate.

**bradycardia** Abonormally slow heart rate, below 60 bpm.

**bradykinesia** Slow movement, commonly seen with the rigidity of Parkinson's disease.

**bradypepsia** Slow digestion rate.

**bradypnea** Slow breathing.

**brain** The brain is one of the largest organs in the body and coordinates most body activities. It is the center for all thought, memory, judgment, and emotion. Each part of the brain is responsible for controlling different body functions, such as temperature regulation and breathing. The four sections to the brain are the cerebrum, cerebellum, diencephalon, and brain stem.

**brain scan** Injection of radioactive isotopes into the circulation to determine the function and abnormality of the brain.

**brain stem** This area of the brain has three components: medulla oblongata, pons, and the midbrain. The brain stem is a pathway for impulses to be conducted between the brain and the spinal cord. It also contains the centers that control respiration, heart rate, and blood pressure. In addition, the 12 pairs of cranial nerves begin in the brain stem.

**brain tumor** Intracranial mass, either benign or malignant. A benign tumor of the brain can be fatal since it will grow and cause pressure on normal brain tissue. The most malignant brain tumors in children are gliomas.

**brand name**  The name a pharmaceutical company chooses as the trademark or market name for its drug. Also called proprietary or trade name.

**breast cancer**  Malignant tumor of the breast; usually forms in the milk-producing gland tissue or the lining of the milk ducts.

**breasts**  Milk-producing glands to provide nutrition for newborn. Also called mammary glands.

**breech presentation**  Placement of the fetus in which the buttocks or feet are presented first for delivery rather than the head.

**bridge**  Dental appliance that is attached to adjacent teeth for support to replace missing teeth.

**broad spectrum**  Ability of a drug to be effective against a wide range of microorganisms.

**bronchial tubes**  An organ of the respiratory system that carries air into each lung.

**bronchiectasis**  Results from a dilation of a bronchus or the bronchi that can be the result of infection. This abnormal stretching can be irreversible and result in destruction of the bronchial walls. The major symptom is a large amount of purulent (pus-filled) sputum. Rales (bubbling chest sound) and hemoptysis may be present.

**bronchioles**  The narrowest air tubes in the lungs. Each bronchiole terminates in tiny air sacs called alveoli.

**bronchitis**  An acute or chronic inflammation of the lower respiratory tract that often occurs after other childhood infections such as measles.

**bronchodilator**  Dilates or opens the bronchi (airways in the lungs) to improve breathing.

**bronchogenic carcinoma**  Malignant lung tumor that originates in the bronchi. Usually associated with a history of cigarette smoking.

**bronchogram**  An X-ray record of the lungs and bronchial tubes.

**bronchography**  Process of taking an X-ray of the lung after a radiopaque substance has been placed into the trachea or bronchial tree.

**bronchoplasty**  Surgical repair of a bronchial defect.

**bronchoscope**  An instrument to view inside a bronchus.

**bronchoscopy (Broncho)**  Using the bronchoscope to visualize the bronchi. The instrument can also be used to obtain tissue for biopsy and to remove foreign objects.

**bronchospasm**  An involuntary muscle spasm in the bronchi.

**bronchus**  The distal end of the trachea splits into a left and right main bronchi as it enters each lung. Each main bronchus is subdivided into smaller branches. The smallest bronchi are the bronchioles. Each bronchiole ends in tiny air sacs called alveoli.

**bruit**  Term used interchangeably with the word *murmur*. A gentle, blowing sound that is heard during auscultation.

**bruxism**  Clinching and grinding teeth, often during sleep.

**buccal**  Drugs that are placed under the lip or between the cheek and gum.

**buccolabial**  Pertaining to cheeks and lips.

**bulbourethral gland**  Also called Cowper's gland. These two small male reproductive system glands are located on either side of the urethra just distal to the prostate. The secretion from these glands neutralizes the acidity in the urethra and the vagina.

**bulimia**  Eating disorder that is characterized by recurrent binge eating and then purging of the food with laxatives and vomiting.

**bundle branches**  Part of the conduction system of the heart; the electrical signal travels down the interventricular septum.

**bundle of His**  The bundle of His is located in the interventricular septum. It receives the electrical impulse from the atrioventricular node and distributes it through the ventricular walls causing them to contract simultaneously.

**bunion**  Inflammation of the bursa of the great toe.

**bunionectomy**  Removal of the bursa at the joint of the great toe.

**burn**  A full-thickness burn exists when all the layers are burned; also called a third-degree burn. A partial-thickness burn exists when the first layer of skin, the epidermis, is burned, and the second layer of skin, dermis, is damaged; also called a second-degree burn.

**burn, first degree**  Damage to the epidermis layer of the skin; characterized by hyperemia, but no blisters or scars.

**burn, second degree**  Damage extends through the epidermis and into the dermis, causing vesicles to form; scarring may occur; also called partial-thickness burn.

**burn, third degree**  Damage to full thickness of skin and into underlying tissues; infection is a major concern with third-degree burns, and fluid loss can be life threatening; grafts are usually required and scarring will occur; also called full-thickness burn.

**bursa**  A sac-like connective tissue structure found in some joints. It protects moving parts from friction. Some common bursa locations are the elbow, knee, and shoulder joints.

**bursectomy**  Excision of a bursa.

**bursitis**  Inflammation of a bursa between bony prominences and muscles or tendons. Common in the shoulder and knee.

**bursolith**  A stone in a bursa.

**calcitonin**  A hormone secreted by the thyroid gland. It stimulates deposition of calcium into bone.

**calcium**  An inorganic substance found in plasma. It is important for bones, muscles, and nerves.

**calcium supplements**  Maintaining high blood levels of calcium in association with vitamin D helps maintain bone density and treats osteomalacia, osteoporosis, and rickets.

**calculus**  A stone formed within an organ by an accumulation of mineral salts. Found in the kidney, renal plural is calculi.

**callus**  The mass of bone tissue that forms at a fracture site during its healing.

**calyx**  A duct that connects the renal papilla to the renal pelvis. Urine flows from the collecting tubule through the calyx and into the renal pelvis.

**cancellous bone**  The bony tissue found inside a bone. It contains cavities that hold red bone marrow. Also called spongy bone.

**cancerous tumor**  Malignant growths in the body.

**candidiasis**  Yeast-like infection of the skin and mucous membranes that can result in white plaques on the tongue and vagina.

**canines**  Also called the cuspid teeth or eyeteeth. Permanent teeth located between the incisors and the biscuspids that assist in biting and cutting food. Humans have four canine teeth.

**capillaries**  The smallest blood or lymphatic vessels. Blood capillaries are very thin to allow gas, nutrient, and waste exchange between the blood and the tissues. Lymph capillaries collect lymph fluid from the tissues and carry it to the larger lymph vessels.

**capillary bed**  The network of capillaries found in a given tissue or organ.

**carbon dioxide**  A waste product of cellular energy production. It is removed from the cells by the blood and eliminated from the body by the lungs.

**carbuncle**  Inflammation and infection of the skin and hair follicle that may result from several untreated boils. Most commonly found on neck, upper back, or head.

**carcinogen**  substance or chemical agent that produces cancer or increases the risk of developing it. For example, cigarette smoke and insecticides are considered to be carcinogens.

**carcinoma**  New growth or malignant tumor that occurs in epithelial tissue. Can spread to other organs through the blood or direct extension from the organ.

**carcinoma in situ (CIS)**  Malignant tumor that has not extended beyond the original site.

**cardiac**  Pertaining to the heart.

**cardiac arrest**  When the heart stops beating and circulation ceases.

**cardiac catheterization**  Passage of a thin tube (catheter) through an arm vein and the blood vessel leading into the heart. Done to detect abnormalities, to collect cardiac blood samples, and to determine the pressure within the cardiac area.

**cardiac enzymes**  Complex protein molecules found only in heart muscle. Cardiac enzymes are taken by blood sample to determine the amount of the heart disease or damage.

**cardiac muscle**  The involuntary muscle found in the heart.

**cardiac scan**  Patient is given radioactive thallium intravenously and then scanning equipment is used to visualize the heart; it is especially useful in determining myocardial damage.

**cardiac sonographer**  Uses ultrasound to produce a moving image of the heart for diagnostic purposes.

**cardiac sphincter**  Also called the lower esophageal sphincter. Prevents food and gastric juices from backing up into the esophagus.

**cardiodynia**  Heart pain.

**cardiologist**  A physician specializing in treating diseases and conditions of the cardiovascular system.

**cardiology**  The branch of medicine specializing in conditions of the cardiovascular system.

**cardiology technologist**  Assists with invasive heart procedures including cardiac catheterizations and angioplasty procedures.

**cardiomegaly**  Abnormally enlarged heart.

**cardiomyopathy**  General term for a disease of the myocardium that may be caused by alcohol abuse, parasites, viral infection, and congestive heart failure.

**cardiopulmonary resuscitation (CPR)**  Emergency treatment provided by persons trained in CPR and given to patients when their respirations and heart stop. CPR provides oxygen to the brain, heart, and other vital organs until medical treatment can restore a normal heart and pulmonary function.

**cardiorrhaphy**  Surgical suturing of the heart.

**cardiotonic**  Strengthens the heart muscle.

**cardiovascular system (CV)**  System that transports blood to all areas of the body. Organs of the cardiovascular system include the heart and blood vessels (arteries, veins, and capillaries). Also called the circulatory system.

**caries**  Gradual decay and disintegration of teeth that can result in inflamed tissue and abscessed teeth.

**carotid endarterectomy**  Surgical procedure for removing an obstruction within the carotid artery, a major artery in the neck that carries oxygenated blood to the brain. Developed to prevent strokes but found to be useful only in severe stenosis with TIA.

**carpal tunnel release**  Surgical cutting of the ligament in the wrist to relieve nerve pressure caused by carpal tunnel disease, which can be caused by repetitive motion such as typing.

**carpal tunnel syndrome**  A painful disorder of the wrist and hand, induced by compression of the median nerve as it passes under ligaments on the palm side of the wrist. Symptoms include weakness, pain, burning, tingling, and aching in the forearm, wrist, and hand.

**carpals**  The wrist bones in the upper extremity.

**cartilage**  Strong, flexible connective tissue found in several locations in the body, such as covering the ends of bones in a synovial joint, nasal septum, external ear, eustachian tube, larynx, trachea, bronchi, and the intervertebral discs.

**cartilaginous joint**  A joint that allows slight movement but holds bones firmly in place by a solid piece of cartilage. The public symphysis is an example of a cartilaginous joint. The fetal skeleton is composed of cartilaginous tissue.

**cast**  Application of a solid material to immobilize an extremity or portion of the body as a result of a fracture, dislocation, or severe injury. It is most often made of plaster of paris.

**castration**  Excision of the testicles in the male or the ovaries in the female.

**cataract**  Diminished vision resulting from the lens of the eye becoming opaque or cloudy. Treatment is usually surgical removal of the cataract.

**catheterization**  Insertion of a tube through the urethra and into the urinary bladder for the purpose of withdrawing urine or inserting dye.

**caudal**  Directional term meaning toward the feet or tail, or below.

**cauterization**  Destruction of tissue using an electric current, a caustic product, or a hot iron, or by freezing.

**cecum**  First portion of the colon. It is a blind pouch off the beginning of the large intestine. The appendix grows out of the end of the cecum.

**cell**  The basic unit of all living things. All tissues and organs in the body are composed of cells. They perform survival functions such as reproduction, respiration, metabolism, and excretion. Some cells are also able to carry on specialized functions, such as contraction by muscle cells and electrical impulse transmission by nerve cells.

**cell-mediated immunity**  Immunity that results from the activation of sensitized T lymphocytes. The immune response causes antigens to be destroyed by the direct action of cells. Also called cellular immunity.

**cellular immunity** Also called cell-mediated immunity. This process results in the production of T cells and natural killer, NK, cells that directly attach to foreign cells. This immune response fights invasion by viruses, bacteria, fungi, and cancer.

**cellulitis** Inflammation of the cellular or connective tissues.

**central nervous system** The portion of the nervous system that consists of the brain and spinal cord. It receives impulses from all over the body, processes this information, and then responds with an action. It consists of both gray matter and white matter.

**cephalalgia** A headache.

**cephalic** Directional term meaning toward the head, or above.

**cerebellar** Pertaining to the cerebellum.

**cerebellitis** Inflammation of the cerebellum.

**cerebellum** The second largest portion of the brain, located beneath the posterior portion of the cerebrum. This part of the brain aids in coordinating voluntary body movements and maintaining balance and equilibrium. It is attached to the brain stem by the pons. The cerebellum refines the muscular movement that is initiated in the cerebrum.

**cerebral** Pertaining to the cerebrum.

**cerebral aneurysm** Localized abnormal dilatation of a blood vessel, usually an artery; the result of a congenital defect or weakness in the wall of the vessel; a ruptured aneurysm is a common cause for a hemorrhagic CVA.

**cerebral angiography** X-ray of the blood vessels of the brain after the injection of a radiopaque dye.

**cerebral contusion** Bruising of the brain from a blow or impact; symptoms last longer than 24 hours and include unconsciousness, dizziness, vomiting, unequal pupil size, and shock.

**cerebral cortex** The outer layer of the cerebrum. It is composed of folds of gray matter called gyri, which are separated by sulci.

**cerebral hemispheres** The division of the cerebrum into right and left halves.

**cerebral palsy (CP)** A group of disabilities caused by injury to the brain either before or during birth or very early in infancy. This is the most common permanent disability in childhood.

**cerebrospinal** Pertaining to the cerebrum and spine.

**cerebrospinal fluid** Watery, clear fluid found in the ventricles of the brain. It provides protection from shock or sudden motion to the brain.

**cerebrospinal fluid (CSF) analysis** Laboratory examination of the clear, watery, colorless fluid from within the brain and spinal cord. Infections and the abnormal presence of blood can be detected in this test.

**cerebrospinal fluid shunts** A surgical procedure in which a bypass is created to drain cerebrospinal fluid. It is used to treat hydrocephalus by draining the excess cerebrospinal fluid from the brain and diverting it to the abdominal cavity.

**cerebrovascular accident (CVA)** Also called a stroke. The development of an infarct due to loss in the blood supply to an area of the brain. Blood flow can interrupted by a ruptured blood vessel (hemorrhage), a floating clot (embolus), a stationary clot (thrombosis), or compression. The extent of damage depends on the size and location of the infarct and often includes speech problems and muscle paralysis.

**cerebrum** The largest section of the brain. It is located in the upper portion and is the area that possesses our thoughts, judgment, memory, and association skills, and the ability to discriminate between items. The outer layer of the cerebrum is the cerebral cortex, which is composed of folds of gray matter. The elevated portions of the cerebrum, or convolutions, are called gyri and are separated by fissures or sulci. The cerebrum has both a left and right division or hemisphere. Each hemisphere has four lobes: frontal, parietal, occipital, and temporal.

**certified coding specialist (CCS)** Classifies medical information using an established coding system for billing and insurance purposes.

**certified medical assistant (CMA)** Performs various duties in the physician's office including front office management and assisting with medical duties.

**certified nurse aide** Trained in basic patient care such as taking vital signs, bathing, and feeding.

**certified respiratory therapist** Performs general respiratory care procedures.

**cerumen** Also called ear wax. A thick, waxy substance produced by oil glands in the auditory canal. This wax helps to protect and lubricate the ear.

**cervical** Pertaining to the neck.

**cervical biopsy** Taking a sample of tissue from the cervix to test for the presence of cancer cells.

**cervical cancer** Malignant growth in the cervix. An especially difficult type of cancer to treat, it causes 5% of the cancer deaths in women. PAP tests have helped to detect early cervical cancer.

**cervical vertebrae** The seven vertebrae in the neck region.

**cervicectomy** Excision of the cervix.

**cervix** The narrow, distal portion of the uterus that joins to the vagina.

**cesarean section (CS, C-section)** Surgical delivery of a baby through an incision into the abdominal and uterine walls. Legend has it that the Roman emperor Julius Caesar was the first person born by this method.

**chalazion** Small, hard tumor or mass, similar to a sebaceous cyst, developing on the eyelids. May require incision and drainage (I & D).

**chancroid** Highly infectious nonsyphilitic venereal ulcer.

**cheeks** Form the lateral walls of the oral cavity.

**cheilitis** Lip inflammation.

**cheilorrhaphy** Suture of the lip.

**chemabrasion** Abrasion using chemicals; also called a chemical peel.

**chemical name** The name for a drug based on its chemical formula or molecular structure.

**chemical thyroidectomy** Large dose of radioactive iodine is given in order to kill thyroid gland cells without having to actually do surgery.

**chemotherapy (chemo)** Treating disease by using chemicals that have a toxic effect on the body, especially cancerous tissue.

**chest X-ray (CXR)**   Taking a radiograhic picture of the lungs and heart from the back and sides.

**Cheyne–Stokes respiration**   Abnormal breathing pattern in which there are long periods (10 to 60 seconds) of apnea followed by deeper, more rapid breathing.

**chiropractor**   Utilize manipulation, especially of the spinal column, to correct skeletal alignment problems in order to alleviate stresses that may be affecting other body systems.

**chlamydia**   Parasitic microorganism causing genital infections in males and females; can lead to pelvic inflammatory disease in females and eventual infertility.

**chloride (Cl⁻)**   An electrolyte, a small biologically important molecule, regulated by excretion by the kidney.

**cholecystectomy**   Surgical excision of the gallbladder. Removal of the gallbladder through the laparoscope is a newer procedure with fewer complications than the more invasive abdominal surgery. The laparoscope requires a small incision into the abdominal cavity.

**cholecystitis**   Inflammation of the gallbladder.

**cholecystogram**   Dye given orally to the patient is absorbed and enters the gallbladder. An X-ray is then taken.

**cholecystography**   The patient swallows a radiopaque dye so X-ray pictures can be taken that allow visualization of the gallbladder and its components.

**choledocholithotomy**   Removal of a gallstone through an incision into the bile duct.

**choledocholithotripsy**   Crushing of a gallstone in the common bile duct.

**cholelithiasis**   Formation or presence of stones or calculi in the gallbladder or common bile duct.

**cholesterol**   An organic substance found in plasma. It is used by cells to build cell membranes and by the liver to produce bile. Too much cholesterol is associated with blocked arteries.

**chondrectomy**   Excision of cartilage.

**chondromalacia**   Softening of cartilage.

**chondroplasty**   Surgical repair of cartilage.

**chorea**   Involuntary nervous disorder that results in muscular twitching of the limbs or facial muscles.

**choriocarcinoma**   Rare type of cancer of the uterus. May occur following a normal pregnancy or abortion.

**chorion**   The outer of two membranous sacs surrounding the fetus. It helps to form the placenta.

**chorionic villus sampling (CVS)**   Removal of a small piece of the chorion for genetic analysis; may be done at an earlier stage of pregnancy than amniocentesis.

**choroid**   The middle layer of the eyeball. This layer provides the blood supply for the eye.

**chronic obstructive pulmonary disease (COPD)**   Progressive, chronic, and usually irreversible condition in which the lungs have a diminished capacity for inspiration (inhalation) and expiration (exhalation). The person may have difficulty breathing on exertion (dyspnea) and a cough. Also called chronic obstructive lung disease (COLD).

**chyme**   Semisoft mixture of food and digestive fluids that pass from the stomach into the small intestines.

**cicatrix**   A scar.

**cilia**   A term for eyelashes that protect the eye from foreign particles or for nasal hairs that help filter dust and bacteria out of inhaled air.

**ciliary body**   The intraocular eye muscles that change the shape of the lens.

**circadian rhythm**   The 24-hour clock that governs our periods of wakefulness and sleepiness.

**circulating nurse**   Nurse who assists the surgeon and scrub nurse by providing needed materials during the procedure and by handling the surgical specimen. This person does not wear sterile clothing and may enter and leave the operating room during the procedure.

**circulatory system**   System that transports blood to all areas of the body. The organs of the circulatory system include the heart and blood vessels (arteries, veins, and capillaries). Also called the cardiovascular system.

**circumcision**   Surgical removal of the end of the prepuce or foreskin of the penis. Generally performed on the newborn male at the request of the parents. The primary reason is for ease of hygiene. Circumcision is also a ritual practice in some religions.

**circumduction**   Movement in a circular direction from a central point.

**cirrhosis**   Chronic disease of the liver.

**clamp**   A surgical instrument used to grasp tissue and control bleeding.

**clavicle**   Also called the collar bone. A bone of the pectoral girdle.

**clavicular**   Pertaining to the clavicle or collar bone.

**clean catch specimen (CG)**   Urine sample obtained after cleaning off the urinary opening and catching or collecting a sample in midstream (halfway through the urination process) to minimize contamination from the genitalia.

**cleft lip**   Congenital anomaly in which the upper lip fails to come together. Often seen along with a cleft palate. Corrected with surgery.

**cleft palate**   Congenital anomaly in which the roof of the mouth has a split or fissure. Corrected with surgery.

**clinical laboratory scientist (CLS)**   Performs laboratory tests as ordered by a physician.

**clinical laboratory technician (CLT)**   Performs laboratory tests under the supervision of a clinical laboratory scientist.

**clinical psychologist (PhD)**   Diagnoses and treats mental disorders; specializes in using individual and group counseling to treat patients with mental and emotional disorders.

**clitoris**   A small organ containing erectile tissue that is covered by the labia minora. It contains sensitive tissue that is aroused during sexual stimulation and is similar to the penis in the male.

**closed fracture**   A simple fracture with no open skin or wound.

**coagulate**   When liquid is converted to a gel or solid, as in blood coagulation.

**coarctation of the aorta**   Severe congenital narrowing of the aorta.

**coccygeal**   Pertaining to the coccyx or tailbone.

**coccyx**   The tailbone, the four small fused vertebrae at the distal end of the vertebral column.

**cochlea**  A portion of the labyrinth associated with hearing. It is rolled in the shape of a snail shell. The organs of Corti line the cochlea.

**cochlear**  Pertaining to the cochlea.

**cochlear implant**  Mechanical device that is surgically placed under the skin behind the outer ear (pinna). It converts sound signals into magnetic impulses to stimulate the auditory nerve. Can be beneficial for those with profound sensorineural hearing loss.

**cochlear nerve**  The branch of the vestibulocochlear nerve that carries hearing information to the brain.

**cognitive disorders**  Deterioration of mental functions due to temporary brain or permanent brain dysfunction; includes dementia and Alzheimer's disease; also called organic mental disease.

**coitus**  Term for sexual intercourse.

**colectomy**  Surgical removal of the colon.

**collagen**  An insoluble fibrous protein present in connective tissue that forms a flexible mat to protect the skin and other parts of the body.

**collecting tubule**  A portion of the renal tubule.

**Colles' fracture**  A specific type of wrist fracture.

**colon**  Alos called the large intestines. Functions to reabsorb most of the fluid in the digested food. The material that remains after water reabsorption is the feces. The sections of the colon are the cecum, ascending colon, transverse colon, descending colon, and sigmoid colon.

**colonoscope**  Instrument to view inside the colon.

**colonoscopy**  A flexible fiberscope passed through the anus, rectum, and colon is used to examine the upper portion of the colon. Polyps and small growths can be removed during this procedure.

**color vision tests**  Use of polychromic (multicolored) charts to determine the ability of the patient to recognize color.

**colorectal**  Pertaining to the colon and rectum.

**colorectal carcinoma**  Cancerous tumor along the length of the colon and rectum.

**colostomy**  Surgical creation of an opening in some portion of the colon through the abdominal wall to the outside surface. The fecal material (stool) drains into a bag worn on the abdomen.

**colostrum**  A thin fluid first secreted by the breast after delivery; it does not contain much protein, but is rich in antibodies.

**colposcope**  Instrument to view inside the vagina.

**colposcopy**  Visual examination of the cervix and vagina using a colposcope or instrument with a magnifying lens.

**coma**  Abnormal deep sleep or stupor resulting from an illness or injury.

**combining form**  The word root plus the combining vowel. It is always written with a / between the word root and the combining vowel. For example, in the combining form *cardi/o*, *cardi* is the word root and /*o* is the combining vowel.

**combining vowel**  A vowel inserted between word parts that makes it possible to pronounce long medical terms. It is usually the vowel *o*.

**comedo**  Medical term for a blackhead. It is an accumulation of sebum in a sebaceous gland that has become blackened.

**comminuted fracture**  A fracture in which the bone is shattered, splintered, or crushed into many pieces or fragments. The fracture is completely through the bone.

**commissurotomy**  Surgical incision to change the size of an opening. For example, in mitral commissurotomy, a stenosis or narrowing is treated by cutting away at the adhesions around the mitral opening (orifice).

**common bile duct**  A duct that carries bile from the gallbladder to the duodenum.

**compact bone**  The hard exterior surface bone. Also called cortical bone.

**complete blood count (CBC)**  Blood test that consists of five tests; red blood cell count (RBC), white blood count (WBC), hemoglobin (Hg), hematocrit (Hct), and white blood cell differential.

**compound fracture**  An open fracture in which the skin has been broken through by the fracture.

**computed tomography scan (CT scan)**  An imaging technique that is able to produce a cross-sectional view of the body; X-ray pictures are taken at multiple angles through the body and a computer uses all these images to construct a composite cross-section.

**concussion**  Injury to the brain that results from a blow or impact from an object. Can result in unconsciousness, dizziness, vomiting, unequal pupil size, and shock.

**conductive hearing loss**  Loss of hearing as a result of the blocking of sound transmission in the middle ear and outer ear.

**condyle**  Refers to the rounded portion at the end of a bone.

**condyloma**  Wart-like growth on the external genitalia.

**cones**  The sensory receptors of the retina that are active in bright light and see in color.

**congenital anomaly**  Any abnormality present at birth. A birth defect.

**congenital septal defect (CSD)**  Defect, present at birth, in the wall separating two chambers of the heart. Results in a mixture of oxygenated and deoxygenated blood being carried to the surrounding tissues. There can be an atrial septal defect (ASD) and a ventricular septal defect (VSD).

**congestive heart failure (CHF)**  Pathological condition of the heart in which there is a reduced outflow of blood from the left side of the heart. Results in weakness, breathlessness, and edema.

**conization**  Surgical removal of a core of cervical tissue. Also refers to partial removal of the cervix.

**conjunctiva**  A protective mucous membrane lining on the underside of each eyelid and across the anterior surface of each eyeball.

**conjunctivitis**  Also referred to as pink eye or an inflammation of the conjunctiva.

**conjunctivoplasty**  Surgical repair of the conjunctiva.

**connective tissue**  The supporting and protecting tissue in body structures. Examples are fat or adipose tissue, cartilage, and bone.

**connective tissue membrane**  A membrane that contains only a single layer of connective tissue. It does not have an epithelial layer. The most common type of connective tissue membrane is the synovial membrane that lines synovial joints.

**conscious**  Condition of being awake and aware of surroundings.

**constipation**  Experiencing difficulty in defecation or infrequent defecation.

**consultation report**  Document in a patient's medical record. They are the reports given by specialists who the physician has requested to evaluate the patient.

**contracture**  An abnormal shortening of a muscle, making it difficult to stretch the muscle.

**contraindication**  Condition in which a particular drug should not be used.

**contrast studies**  A radiopaque substance is injected or swallowed; X-rays are then taken that outline the body structure containing the radiopaque substance.

**controlled substances**  Drugs that have a potential for being addictive (habit forming) or can be abused.

**contusion**  Injury caused by a blow to the body; causes swelling, pain, and bruising; the skin is not broken.

**convergence**  The moving inward of the eyes to see an object close to the face.

**conversion reaction**  A somatoform disorder in which the patient unconsciously substitutes physical signs or symptoms for anxiety. The most common physical signs or symptoms are blindness, deafness, and paralysis.

**convulsion**  Severe involuntary muscle contractions and relaxations. These have a variety of causes, such as epilepsy, fever, and toxic conditions.

**copulation**  Term for sexual intercourse.

**cor pulmonale**  Hypertrophy of the right ventricle of the heart as a result of lung disease.

**cordectomy**  Removal of part of the spinal cord.

**corium**  The living layer of skin located between the epidermis and the subcutaneous tissue. Also referred to as the dermis, it contains hair follicles, sweat glands, sebaceous glands, blood vessels, lymph vessels, nerve fibers, and muscle fibers.

**cornea**  A portion of the sclera that is clear and transparent and allows light to enter the interior of the eye. It also plays a role in bending light rays.

**corneal abrasion**  Scraping injury to the cornea; if it does not heal, it may develop into an ulcer.

**coronal plane**  A vertical plane that divides the body into front (anterior or ventral) and back (posterior or dorsal) sections. Also called the frontal plane.

**coronary**  Pertaining to the heart.

**coronary angiography**  Radiographic X-ray of the heart and large vessels after the injection of a radiopaque solution; X-rays are taken in rapid sequence as the material moves through the heart.

**coronary artery**  A group of three arteries that branch off the aorta and carry blood to the myocardium.

**coronary artery bypass graft (CABG)**  Open-heart surgery in which a blood vessel is grafted to route blood around the point of constriction in a diseased coronary artery.

**coronary artery disease**  Insufficient blood supply to the heart muscle due to an obstruction of one or more coronary arteries; may be caused by atherosclerosis and may cause angina pectoris and myocardial infarction.

**corpus**  The body or central portion of the uterus.

**cortex**  The outer layer of an organ. In the endocrine system, it refers to the outer layer of the adrenal glands.

**cortical**  Pertaining to the cortex.

**cortical bone**  The hard exterior surface bone. Also called compact bone.

**corticosteroids**  General term for the group of hormones secreted by the adrenal contex. They include mineralocorticoid hormones, glucocorticoid hormones, and steroid sex hormones.

**cortisol**  A steroid hormone secreted by the adrenal cortex. It regulates carbohydrate metabolism.

**costal**  Pertaining to the ribs.

**Cowper's gland**  Also called bulbourethral gland. These two small male reproductive system glands are located on either side of the urethra just distal to the prostate. The secretion from these glands neutralizes the acidity in the urethra and the vagina.

**cranial**  Pertaining to the skull.

**cranial cavity**  A dorsal body cavity. It is within the skull and contains the brain.

**cranial nerves**  Nerves that arise from the brain.

**craniotomy**  Incision into the skull.

**cranium**  The skull; bones that form a protective covering over the brain.

**creatine phosphokinase (CPK)**  A muscle enzyme found in skeletal muscle and cardiac muscle; blood test becomes elevated in disorders such as heart attack, muscular dystrophy, and other skeletal muscle pathologies.

**creatinine**  A waste product of muscle metabolism.

**crepitation**  Sound of broken bones rubbing together.

**cretinism**  Congenital condition due to a lack of thyroid that may result in arrested physical and mental development.

**Crohn's disease**  Form of chronic inflammatory bowel disease affecting the ileum and/or colon. Also called regional ileitis.

**cross-infection**  Occurs when a person, either a patient or health care worker, acquires a pathogen from another patient or health care worker.

**croup**  Acute viral respiratory infection common in infants and young children and characterized by a hoarse cough.

**crown**  Portion of a tooth that is covered by enamel. Also an artificial covering for the tooth created to replace the original enamel.

**crowning**  When the head of the baby is visible through the vaginal opening. A sign that birth is imminent.

**cryoextraction**  Procedure in which cataract is lifted from the lens with an extremely cold probe.

**cryoretinopexy**  Surgical fixation of the retina by using extreme cold.

**cryosurgery**  Exposing tissues to extreme cold in order to destroy them. Used in treating malignant tumors, and to control pain and bleeding.

**cryotherapy**  Using cold for therapeutic purposes.

**cryptorchidism**  Failure of the testes to descend into the scrotal sac before birth. Generally, the testes will descend before the boy is one year old. A surgical procedure called orchidopexy may be required to bring the testes down into the scrotum permanently. Failure of the testes to descend could result in sterility in the male.

**culdoscopy**   Examination of the female pelvic cavity by introducing an endoscope through the wall of the vagina.

**culture and sensitivity (C&S)**   A laboratory test in which a colony of pathogens that have been removed from an infected area are grown to identify the pathogen and then determine its sensitivity to a variety of antibiotics.

**cumulative action**   Action that occurs in the body when a drug is allowed to accumulate or stay in the body.

**curettage**   Removal of superficial skin lesions with a curette (surgical instrument shaped like a spoon) or scraper.

**curette**   A surgical instrument used to scrape and remove tissue.

**Cushing's syndrome**   Set of symptoms named after Harvey Cushing, an American neurosurgeon, that result from hypersecretion of the adrenal cortex. This may be the result of a tumor of the adrenal glands. The syndrome may present symptoms of weakness, edema, excess hair growth, skin discoloration, and osteoporosis.

**cuspids**   Permanent teeth located between the incisors and the bicuspids that assist in biting and cutting food. Humans have four cuspids. Also called canine teeth or eyeteeth.

**cusps**   The leaflets or flaps of a heart valve.

**cutaneous membrane**   This is another term for the skin.

**cuticle**   The thin skin-like layer overlapping the base of a nail.

**cyanosis**   Slightly bluish color of the skin due to a deficiency of oxygen and an excess of carbon dioxide in the blood. It is caused by a variety of disorder, ranging from chronic lung disease to congenital and chronic heart problems.

**cycloplegia**   Paralysis of the ciliary body.

**cycloplegic**   Drug that paralyzes the ciliary body; particularly useful during eye examinations and eye surgery.

**cyclotron**   Equipment consisting of a particle accelerator in which the particles are rotated between magnets.

**cyst**   Fluid-filled sac under the skin.

**cystalgia**   Bladder pain.

**cystectomy**   Excision of the bladder.

**cystic fibrosis**   Hereditary condition causing the exocrine glands to malfunction. The patient produces very thick mucous that causes severe congestion within the lungs and digestive system. Through more advanced treatment, many children are now living into adulthood with this disease.

**cystitis**   Inflammation of the bladder.

**cystocele**   Hernia or outpouching of the bladder that protrudes into the vagina. This may cause urinary frequency and urgency.

**cystography**   Process of instilling a contrast material or dye into the bladder by catheter to visualize the urinary bladder on X-ray.

**cystolith**   Bladder stone.

**cystoplasty**   Surgical repair of the bladder.

**cystorrhagia**   Rapid bleeding from the bladder.

**cystoscope**   Instrument used to visually examine the bladder.

**cystoscopy**   Visual examination of the urinary bladder using an instrument called a cystoscope.

**cystostomy**   Creation of an opening through the body wall and into the bladder.

**cystotomy**   Incision into the bladder.

**cytologic testing**   Examination of cells to determine their structure and origin. PAP smears are considered a form of cytologic testing.

**cytology**   The study of cells.

**cytotechnologist (CT)**   Laboratory professionals who use microscopes to analyze slides of cell specimens for abnormalities, especially cancer.

**cytotoxic**   Pertaining to poisoning cells.

**dacryocystitis**   Inflammation of tear sac.

**day surgery**   A type of outpatient surgery in which the patient is discharged on the same day he or she is admitted; also called ambulatory surgery.

**deafness**   The inability to hear or having some degree of hearing impairment.

**debridement**   Removal of foreign material and dead or damaged tissue from a wound.

**decibel (dB)**   Measures the intensity or loudness of a sound. Zero decibels is the quietest sound measured and 120 dB is the loudest sound commonly measured.

**deciduous teeth**   The 20 teeth that begin to erupt around the age of 6 months. Eventually pushed out by the permanent teeth.

**decongestant**   Reduces nasal congestion and swelling.

**decubitus ulcers**   Bedsores or pressure sores caused by pressure over bony prominences on the body. They are caused by a lack of blood flow.

**deep**   Directional term meaning away from the surface of the body.

**deep tendon reflex (DTR)**   Muscle contraction in response to a stretch caused by striking the muscle tendon with a reflex hammer; test used to determine if muscles are responding properly.

**defecation**   Evacuation of feces from the rectum.

**defibrillation**   A procedure that converts serious irregular heartbeats, such as fibrillation, by giving electric shocks to the heart.

**deglutination**   Swallowing.

**delirium**   State of mental confusion with a lack of orientation to time and place.

**delivery**   The emergence of the baby from the birth canal.

**delusions**   A false belief held with conviction even in the face of strong evidence to the contrary.

**dementia**   Progressive impairment of intellectual function that interferes with performing the activities of daily living. Patients have little awareness of their condition. Found in disorders such as Alzheimer's.

**dendrites**   Branched process off a neuron that receives impulses and carries them to the cell body.

**dental**   Pertaining to teeth

**dental assistant**   An assistant for a dentist.

**dental laboratory technician**   Specialist in fabricating dental prosthetics such as crowns, bridges, and dentures as prescribed by a dentist.

**dentalgia**   Tooth pain.

**dentin**   The main bulk of the tooth. It is covered by enamel.

**dentist**   Person who is authorized, based on education, training, and licensure, to practice dentistry.

**denture** Partial or complete set of artificial teeth that are set in plastic materials. Substitute for the natural teeth and related structures.

**deoxygenated** Blood in the veins that is low in oxygen content.

**depigmentation** Loss of normal skin color or pigment.

**dermabrasion** Abrasion or rubbing using wire brushes or sandpaper.

**dermatitis** Inflammation of the skin.

**dermatologist** A physician specialized in the diagnosis and treatment of diseases of the integumentary system.

**dermatology** The branch of medicine specializing in conditions of the integumentary system.

**dermatome** Instrument for cutting the skin or thin transplants of skin.

**dermatopathy** General term for skin disease.

**dermatoplasty** The surgical repair of the skin.

**dermis** The living layer of skin located between the epidermis and the subcutaneous tissue. It is also referred to as the corium or the *true skin*. It contains hair follicles, sweat glands, sebaceous glands, blood vessels, lymph vessels, nerve fibers, and muscle fibers.

**descending colon** The section of the colon that descends the left side of the abdomen.

**descending tracts** Nerve tracts carrying motor signals down the spinal cord to the muscles.

**diabetes insipidus (DI)** Disorder caused by the inadequate secretion of a hormone by the posterior lobe of the pituitary gland. There may be polyuria and polydipsia. This is more common in the young.

**diabetes mellitus** A serious disease in which the pancreas fails to produce insulin or the insulin does not work properly. Consequently, the patient has very high blood sugar. The kidney will attempt to lower the high blood sugar level by excreting excess sugar in the urine.

**diabetic nephropathy** Accumulation of damage to the glomerulus capillaries due to the chronic high blood sugars of diabetes mellitus.

**diabetic retinopathy** Secondary complication of diabetes that affects the blood vessels of the retina, resulting in visual changes and even blindness.

***Diagnostic and Statistical Manual of Mental Disorders* (DSM)** The guide for terminology and classifications relating to psychiatric disorders; published by the American Psychiatric Association.

**diagnostic medical sonographer** Performs ultrasound procedures as ordered by a physician.

**diagnostic reports** Found in a patient's medical record, it consists of the results of all diagnostic tests performed on the patient, principally from the lab and medical imaging (for example, X-ray and ultrasound).

**diaphoresis** Excessive or profuse sweating.

**diaphragm** The major muscle of inspiration. It separates the thoracic from the abdominal cavity.

**diaphragmatic** Pertaining to the diaphragm.

**diaphragmatocele** A protrusion of the stomach through the diaphragm into the chest cavity. Also called a hiatal hernia.

**diaphysis** The shaft portion of a long bone.

**diarrhea** Passing of frequent, watery bowel movements. Usually accompanies gastrointestinal (GI) disorders.

**diastole** The period of time during which a heart chamber is relaxed.

**diastolic pressure** The lower pressure within blood vessels during the relaxation phase of the heart beat.

**diencephalon** The portion of the brain that contains two of the most critical areas of the brain, the thalamus and the hypothalamus.

**dietetic assistant** Dietetic worker trained to assist a registered dietitian.

**dietetic technician** On-the-job trained worker who assists a registered dietitian.

**digestive enzymes** In addition to hormones, the pancreas also secretes digestive enzymes to digest food in the small intestines.

**digestive system** System that digests food and absorbs nutrients. Organs include the mouth, pharynx, esophagus, stomach, small and large intestines, liver, gallbladder, and anus. Also called the gastrointestinal system.

**digital rectal exam (DRE)** Manual examination for an enlarged prostate gland performed by palpating (feeling) the prostate gland through the wall of the rectum.

**dilation and curettage (D & C)** Surgical procedure in which the opening of the cervix is dilated and the uterus is scraped or suctioned of its lining or tissue. Often performed after a spontaneous abortion and to stop excessive bleeding from other causes.

**dilation stage** The first stage of labor. It begins with uterine contractions that press the fetus against the cervix causing it to dilate to 10 cm and become thin. The thinning of the cervix is called effacement.

**dilator** A surgical instrument used to enlarge an opening by stretching.

**dilute** To weaken the strength of a substance by adding something else.

**diphtheria** A bacterial infection of the respiratory system characterized by severe inflammation that can form a membrane coating in the upper respiratory tract that can cause marked difficulty breathing.

**diplopia** Double vision.

**discharge summary** Part of a patient's medical record. It is a comprehensive outline of the patient's entire hospital stay. It includes condition at time of admission, admitting diagnosis, test results, treatments and patient's response, final diagnosis, and follow-up plans.

**diskectomy** Removal of a herniated intervertebral disk.

**dislocation** Occurs when the bones in a joint are displaced from their normal alignment.

**disorders diagnosed in infancy and childhood** Mental disorders associated with childhood; includes mental retardation, attention deficit disorder, and autism.

**dissection** The surgical cutting of parts for separation and study.

**dissociative disorders** Disorders in which severe emotional conflict is so repressed that a split in the personality occurs; includes amnesia and multiple personality disorder.

**distal** Directional term meaning located farthest from the point of attachment to the body.

**distal convoluted tubule**   A portion of the renal tubule.

**diuresis**   Abnormal secretion of large amounts of urine.

**diuretic**   Increases the excretion of urine, which promotes the loss of water and salt from the body. Can assist in lowering blood pressure; therefore, these drugs are used to treat hypertension. Potassium in the body may by depleted with continued use of diuretics. Potassium-rich foods such as bananas, kiwi, and orange juice can help correct this deficiency.

**diverticulectomy**   Surgical removal of a diverticulum.

**diverticulitis**   Inflammation of a diverticulum or sac in the intestinal tract, especially in the colon.

**diverticulum**   An outpouching off the gut; may become inflamed if food becomes trapped within the pouch.

**doctor of medicine (MD)**   Physicians who examine patients, diagnose diseases, order treatments, perform surgery, and educate patients; also called allopathic physicians.

**doctor of osteopathy (DO)**   Emphasizes the role of the musculoskeletal system in the health of the body; examines patients, diagnoses diseases, orders treatments, performs surgery, and educates patients.

**dopaminergic drugs**   Group of medications to treat Parkinson's disease by either replacing the dopamine that is lacking or increasing the strength of the dopamine that is present.

**Doppler ultrasonography**   Measurement of sound-wave echos as they bounce off tissues and organs to produce an image. Can assist in determining heart and blood vessel damage.

**Doppler ultrasound**   Using an instrument placed externally over the uterus to examine the fetal heart.

**dorsal**   Directional term meaning near or on the back or spinal cord side of the body.

**dorsiflexion**   Backward bending, as of hand or foot.

**Down syndrome**   Disorder that produces moderate-to-severe mental retardation and multiple defects. The physical characteristics of a child with this disorder are a sloping forehead, flat nose or absent bridge to the nose, low-set eyes, and a general dwarfed physical growth. The disorder occurs more commonly when the mother is over 40.

**draping**   Process of covering the patient with sterile cloths that allow only the operative site to be exposed to the surgeon.

**Drug Enforcement Agency (DEA)**   The government agency that enforces regulation of controlled substances.

**drug interaction**   Occurs when the effect of one drug is altered because it was taken at the same time as another drug.

**drug tolerance**   Decrease in susceptibility to a drug after continued use of the drug.

**dry gangrene**   Late stages of gangrene characterized by the affected area becoming black and leathery.

**duodenostomy**   Create an opening into the duodenum.

**duodenum**   The first section of small intestines. Digestion is completed in the duodenum after the chyme mixes with digestive juices from the pancreas and gallbladder.

**dura mater**   The term means tough mother. It is the fibrous outermost meninges layer that forms a tough protective layer.

**dwarfism**   Condition of being abnormally small. It may be the result of a hereditary condition or an endocrine dysfunction.

**dyscrasia**   A general term indicating the presence of a disease affecting blood.

**dysentery**   Disease characterized by diarrhea, often with mucus and blood, severe abdominal pain, fever, and dehydration.

**dyskinesia**   Difficult or painful movement.

**dysmenorrhea**   Painful cramping that is associated with menstruation.

**dysorexia**   Abnormal appetite.

**dyspareunia**   Painful sexual intercourse.

**dyspepsia**   Indigestion.

**dysphagia**   Having difficulty eating.

**dysphasia**   Impairment of speech as a result of a brain lesion.

**dyshonia**   Abnormal voice.

**dyspnea**   Difficult, labored breathing.

**dystocia**   Abnormal or difficult labor and childbirth.

**dystrophy**   Abnormal or poor development.

**dysuria**   Painful or difficult urination. This is a symptom in many disorders, such as cystitis, urethritis, enlarged prostate in the male, and prolapsed uterus in the female.

**ear**   The sensory organ for hearing.

**eardrops**   Placed directly into the ear canal for the purpose of relieving pain or treating infection.

**eating disorders**   Abnormal behaviors related to eating; includes anorexia nervosa and bulimia.

**ecchymosis**   Skin discoloration or bruise caused by blood collecting under the skin.

**ecchocardiography**   Noninvasive diagnostic method using ultrasound to visualize internal cardiac structures; cardiac valve activity can be evaluated using this method.

**ecchoencephalography**   Recording of the ultrasonic echoes of the brain; useful in determining abnormal patterns of shifting in the brain.

**eclampsia**   Convulsive seizures and coma that can occur in a woman between the 20th week of pregnancy and the first week of postpartum. Often associated with hypertension.

**ectopic pregnancy**   Fetus that becomes abnormally implanted outside the uterine cavity. This is a condition requiring immediate surgery.

**ectropion**   Term referring to eversion (turning outward) of the eyelid.

**eczema**   Superficial dermatitis accompanied by papules, vesicles, and crusting.

**edema**   Condition in which the body tissues contain excessive amounts of fluid.

**effacement**   The thinning of the cervix during labor.

**efferent arteriole**   Arteriole that carries blood away from the glomerulus.

**efferent neurons**   Nerves that carry impulses away from the brain and spinal cord to the muscles and glands. Also called motor neurons.

**ejaculation**   The impulse of forcing seminal fluid from the male urethra.

**elective abortion**   The legal termination of a pregnancy for nonmedical reasons.

**electrocardiogram (ECG, EKG)**   Record of the electrical activity of the heart. Useful in the diagnosis of abnormal cardiac rhythm and heart muscle (myocardium) damage.

**electrocardiogram technician**   Conducts tests to record the electrical activity of the heart.

**electrocardiography**  Process of recording the electrical activity of the heart.

**electrocautery**  To destroy tissue with an electric current.

**electroconvulsive therapy (ECT)**  A procedure occasionally used for cases of prolonged major depression in which an electrode is placed on one or both sides of the patient's head and current is turned on briefly causing a convulsive seizure. A low level of voltage is used in modern ECT and the patient is administered a muscle relaxant and an anesthesia. Advocates of this treatment state that it is a more effective way to treat severe depression than with the use of drugs. It is not effective with disorders other than depression, such as schizophrenia and alcoholism.

**electroencephalogram**  A record of the brain's electrical activity.

**electroencephalography (EEG)**  Recording the electrical activity of the brain by placing electrodes at various positions on the scalp. Also used in sleep studies to determine if there is a normal pattern of activity during sleep.

**electrolyte**  Chemical compound that separates into charged particles, or ionizes, in a solution. Sodium chloride (NaCl) and potassium (K) are examples of electrolytes.

**electromyogram (EMG)**  Record of muscle electricity.

**electromyography**  Recording of the electrical patterns of a muscle in order to diagnose diseases.

**electron**  Minute particle with a negative electrical charge that is emitted from radioactive substances. These are called *rays*.

**electroneurodiagnostic technologist**  Performs diagnostic tests as ordered by a physician.

**elephantiasis**  Inflammation, obstruction, and destruction of the lymph vessels that results in enlarged tissues due to edema.

**elevation**  A muscle action that raises a body part, as in shrug the shoulders.

**ELISA (enzyme-linked immunosorbent assa)**  A blood test for an antibody to the AIDS virus. A positive test means that the person has been exposed to the virus. In the case of a false-positive reading, the Western blot test would be used to verify the results.

**embolectomy**  Surgical removal of an embolus or clot from a blood vessel.

**embolus**  Obstruction of a blood vessel by a blood clot that moves from another area.

**embryo**  The term to describe the developing infant from fertilization until the end of the eighth week.

**emergency medical technician–basic (EMT-B)**  Performs basic life support procedures such as establishing open airways, treating shock, assisting in childbirth, controlling bleeding, bandaging wounds, immobilizing fractures, and transporting patients.

**emergency medical technician–intermediate (EMT-I)**  Performs advanced life support procedures, completes patient assessments, administers intravenous fluids, and uses a defibrillator.

**emergency medical technician–paramedic (EMT-P)**  Performs advanced life support procedures, administers drugs, interprets electrocardiograms, intubates patients, and utilizes the most complex monitoring equipment.

**emesis**  Vomiting, usually with some force.

**emetic**  Induces vomiting.

**emmetropia (EM)**  State of normal vision.

**emphysema**  Pulmonary condition that can occur as a result of long-term heavy smoking. Air pollution also worsens this disease. The patient may not be able to breathe except in a sitting or standing position.

**empyema**  Pus within the pleural space, usually the result of infection.

**emulsification**  To make fats and lipids more soluble in water.

**enamel**  The hardest substance in the body. Covers the outer surface of teeth.

**encapsulated**  Growth enclosed in a sheath of tissue that prevents tumor cells from invading surrounding tissue.

**encephalitis**  Inflammation of the brain due to disease factors such as rabies, influenza, measles, or smallpox.

**encephalocele**  Protrusion of the brain through the cranial cavity.

**encephalomalacia**  Brain softening.

**encephalosclerosis**  Condition of hardening of the brain.

**endarterectomy**  Removal of the inside layer of an artery.

**endocarditis**  Inflammation of the inner lining layer of the heart. May be due to microorganisms or to an abnormal immunological response.

**endocardium**  The inner layer of the heart, which is very smooth and lines the chambers of the heart.

**endocervicitis**  Inflammation of the inner aspect of the cervix.

**endocrine glands**  A glandular system that secretes hormones directly into the bloodstream rather than into a duct. Endocrine glands are frequently referred to as ductless glands. The endocrine system includes the thyroid gland, adrenal glands, parathyroid glands, pituitary gland, pancreas (islets of Langerhans), testes, ovaries, and thymus gland.

**endocrine system**  The body system that consists of glands that secrete hormones directly into the blood stream. The endocrine glands include the adrenal glands, parathyroid glands, pancreas, pituitary gland, testes, ovaries, thymus gland, and thyroid gland.

**endocrinologist**  Physician who specializes in the treatment of endocrine glands, including diabetes.

**endocrinology**  The branch of medicine specializing in conditions of the endocrine system.

**endocrinopathy**  A disease of the endocrine system.

**endometrial biopsy**  Taking a sample of tissue from the lining of the uterus to test for abnormalities.

**endometrial cancer**  Cancer of the endometrial lining of the uterus.

**endometriosis**  Abnormal condition of endometrium tissue appearing throughout the pelvis or on the abdominal wall. This tissue is usually found within the uterus.

**endometritis**  Inflammation of the endometrial lining of the uterus.

**endometrium**  The inner lining of the uterus. It contains a rich blood supply and reacts to hormonal changes every month, which results in menstruation. During a pregnancy, the lining of the uterus does not leave the body but remains to nourish the unborn child.

**endoscopic retrograde cholanglopancreatography (ERCP)** Using an endoscope to X-ray the bile and pancreatic ducts.

**endoscopic surgery** Use of a lighted instrument to examine the interior of a cavity.

**endoscopy** A general term for a procedure to visually examine the inside of a body cavity or a hollow organ using an instrument called an endoscope. Specific examples of endoscopy relating to the digestive system include colonoscopy, gastrointestinal endoscopy, and gastroscopy.

**endotracheal** Pertaining to inside the trachea.

**endotracheal intubation** Placing a tube through the mouth to create an airway.

**enteralgia** Small intestine pain.

**enterectomy** Excision of the small intestines.

**enteritis** Inflammation of only the small intestine.

**enterorrhaphy** Suture small intestines.

**entropion** Term referring to inversion (turning inward) of the eyelid.

**enucleated** The loss of a cell's nucleus.

**enucleation** Surgical removal of an eyeball.

**enuresis** Involuntary discharge of urine after the age by which bladder control should have been established. This usually occurs by the age of five. Also called bedwetting at night.

**eosinophils** A granulocyte white blood cell that destroy parasites and increases during allergic reactions.

**epicardium** The outer layer of the heart. It forms part of the pericardium.

**epicondyle** A projection located above or on a condyle.

**epidermal** Pertaining to upon the skin.

**epidermis** The superficial layer of skin. It is composed of squamous epithelium cells. These are flat scale-like cells that are arranged in layers, called stratified squamous epithelium. The many layers of the epidermis create a barrier to infection. The epidermis does not have a blood supply, so it is dependent on the deeper layers of skin for nourishment. However, the deepest epidermis layer is called the basal layer. These cells are alive and constantly dividing. Older cells are pushed out toward the surface by new cells forming beneath. During this process, they shrink and die, becoming filled with a protein called keratin. The keratin-filled cells are sloughed off as dead cells.

**epididymectomy** Surgical excision of the epididymis.

**epididymis** The epididymis is a coiled tubule that lies on top of the tests within the scrotum. This tube stores sperm as they are produced and turns into the vas deferens.

**epididymitis** Inflammation of the epididymis that causes pain and swelling in the inguinal area.

**epidural hematoma** Mass of blood in the space outside the dura mater of the brain and spinal cord.

**epigastric** Pertaining to above the stomach. An anatomical division of the abdomen, the middle section of the upper row.

**epiglottis** A flap of cartilage that covers the larynx when a person swallows. This prevents food and drink from entering the larynx and trachea.

**epilepsy** Recurrent disorder of the brain in which convulsive seizures and loss of consciousness occur.

**epinephrine** A hormone produced by the adrenal medulla. Also known as adrenaline. Some of its actions include increased heart rate and force of contraction, bronchodilation, and relaxation of intestinal muscles.

**epiphysis** The wide ends of a long bone.

**episiorrhaphy** Suture the perineum.

**episiotomy** Surgical incision of the perineum to facilitate the delivery process. Can prevent an irregular tearing of tissue during birth.

**epispadias** Congenital opening of the urethra on the dorsal surface of the penis.

**epistaxis** Nosebleed.

**epithelial** Pertaining to the epithelium.

**epithelial membrane** Membranes that contain two layers of tissue: a superficial layer or epithelial tissue and an underlying connective tissue layer. The three common types of epithelial membranes are cutaneous, serous, and mucous membranes.

**epithelial tissue** Tissue found throughout the body as the skin, the outer covering of organs, and the inner lining for tubular or hollow structures.

**Epstein–Barr virus** Virus that is believed to be the cause of infectious mononucleosis, was discovered by Anthony Epstein, a British virologist, and Yvonne Barr, a French physician.

**equilibrium** The sense of balance.

**erectile dysfunction (ED)** Inability to copulate due to inability to maintain an erection; also called impotence.

**erectile dysfunction agents** Medication that temporarily produces an erection in patients with erectile dysfunction.

**erectile tissue** Tissue with numerous blood vessels and nerve endings. It becomes filled with blood and enlarges in size in response to sexual stimulation.

**ergonomics** The study of human work including how the requirements for performing work and the work environment affect the musculoskeletal and nervous system.

**eructation** Belching.

**erythema** Redness or flushing of the skin.

**erythroblastosis fetalis** Condition in which antibodies enter the fetus's blood and cause anemia, jaundice, edema, and enlargement of the liver and spleen. Also called hemolytic disease of the newborn.

**erythrocyte** Also called red blood cells or RBCs. Cells that contain hemoglobin, an iron-containing pigment that binds oxygen in order to transport it to the cells of the body.

**erythrocyte sedimentation rate (ESR)** Blood test to determine the rate at which mature red blood cells settle out of the blood after the addition of an anticoagulant. An indicator of the presence of an inflammatory disease.

**erythrocytosis** Too many red cells.

**erythroderma** Red skin.

**erythropenia** Too few red cells.

**erythropoiesis** The process of forming erythrocytes.

*Escherichia coli* **(E. coli)** Normal bacteria found in the intestinal track; the most common cause of lower urinary tract infections due to improper hygiene after bowel movements.

**esophageal stricture** Narrowing of the esophagus, which makes the flow of fluids and food difficult.

**esophageal varices** Enlarged and swollen varicose veins in the lower end of the esophagus; they can rupture and result in serious hemorrhage.

**esophagogastroduodenoscopy (EGD)**  Use of a flexible fiber-optic scope to visually examine the esophagus, stomach, and beginning of the duodenum.

**esophagoscopy and biopsy**  The esophagus is visualized by passing an instrument down the esophagus. A tissue sample for biopsy may be taken.

**esophagus**  The tube that carries food from the pharynx to the stomach.

**esotropia**  Inward turning of the eye. An example of a form of strabismus (muscle weakness of the eye).

**estimated date of confinement (EDC)**  Estimation date when the baby will be born based on a calculation from the last menstrual period of the mother.

**estrogen**  One of the hormones produced by the ovaries. It works with progesterone to control the menstrual cycle and it is responsible for producing the secondary sexual characteristics.

**ethmoid bone**  A cranial bone.

**eupnea**  Normal breathing.

**eustachian tube**  Tube or canal that connects the middle ear with the nasopharynx and allows for a balance of pressure between the outer and middle ear. Infection can travel via the mucous membranes of the eustachian tube, resulting in middle ear infections.

**euthyroid**  Normal thyroid.

**eversion**  Directional term meaning turning outward.

**Ewing's sarcoma**  Malignant growth found in the shaft of long bones that spreads through the periosteum. Removal is treatment of choice, as this tumor will metastasize or spread to other organs.

**excretory urography**  Injection of dye into the bloodstream followed by taking an X-ray to trace the action of the kidney as it excretes the dye.

**exfoliative cytology**  Scraping cells from tissue and then examining them under a microscope.

**exhalation**  To breathe air out of the lungs. Also called expiration.

**exocrine glands**  Glands that secrete substances into a duct. Tears and tear ducts are examples of an exocrine gland.

**exophthalmos**  Condition in which the eyeballs protrude, such as in Graves' disease. This is generally caused by an overproduction of thyroid hormone.

**exostosis**  A bone spur.

**exotropia**  Outward turning of the eye. Also an example of strabismus (muscle weakness of the eye).

**expectorant**  Assists in the removal of secretions from the bronchopulmonary membranes.

**expiration**  To breathe air out of the lungs. Also called exhalation.

**exploratory laparotomy**  Abdominal operation for the purpose of examining the abdominal organs and tissues for signs of disease or other abnormalities.

**exploratory surgery**  Surgery performed for the purpose of determining if there is cancer present or if a known cancer has spread. Biopsies are generally performed.

**explosive disorder**  An impulse control disorder in which the patient is unable to control violent rages.

**expulsion stage**  Stage of labor and delivery during which the baby is delivered.

**extension**  Movement that brings limb into or toward a straight condition.

**external ear**  The outermost portion of the ear. It consists of the auricle, auditory canal, and eardrum.

**external sphincter**  Ring of voluntary muscle that controls the emptying of urine from the bladder.

**extracorporeal circulation (ECC)**  During open heart surgery, the routing of blood to a heart-lung machine so it can be oxygenated and pumped to the rest of the body.

**extracorporeal shockwave lithotripsy (ESWL)**  Use of ultrasound waves to break up stones. Process does not require surgery.

**extraction**  Removing or "pulling" teeth.

**eye**  The sensory organs for vision.

**eye muscles**  There are six muscles that connect the eyeball to the orbit cavity. These muscles allow for rotation of the eyeball.

**eyeball**  The eye by itself, without any appendages such as the eye muscles or tear ducts.

**eyedrops**  Placed into the eye to control eye pressure in glaucoma. Also used during eye examinations to dilate the pupil of the eye for better examination of the interior of the eye.

**eyelashes**  Along the upper and lower edges of the eyelids; protect the eye from foreign particles; also called cilia.

**eyelids**  An upper and lower fold of skin that provides protection from foreign particles, injury from the sun and intense light, and trauma. Both the upper and lower edges of the eyelids have small hairs or cilia. In addition, sebaceous or oil glands are located in the eyelids. These secrete a lubricating oil.

**facial bones**  The skull bones that surround the mouth, nose, and eyes; muscles for chewing are attached to the facial bones.

**factitious disorders**  Intentionally feigning illness symptoms in order to gain attention such as malingering.

**falling test**  Test used to observe balance and equilibrium. The patient is observed balancing on one foot, then with one foot in front of the other, and then walking forward with eyes open. The same test is conducted with the patient's eyes closed. Swaying and falling with the eyes closed can indicate an ear and equilibrium malfunction.

**fallopian tubes**  Organ in the female reproductive system that transports eggs from the ovary to the uterus.

**fascia**  Connective tissue that wraps muscles. It tapers at each end of a skeletal muscle to form tendons.

**fasciitis**  Inflammation of fascia.

**fasciorrhaphy**  Suturing fascia.

**fasciotomy**  Incision into fascia.

**fasting blood sugar (FBS)**  Blood test to measure the amount of sugar circulating throughout the body after a 12-hour fast.

**fats**  Lipid molecules transported throughout the body dissolved in the blood.

**fecal occult blood test (FOBT)**  Laboratory test on the feces to determine if microscopic amounts of blood are present; also called hemoccult or stool guaiac.

**feces**  Food that cannot be digested becomes a waste product and is expelled or defecated as feces.

**female reproductive system**  System responsible for producing eggs for reproduction and provides place for growing baby. Organs include ovaries, fallopian tubes, uterus, vagina, and mammary glands.

**femoral**  Pertaining to the femur or thigh bone.

**femur**  Also called the thigh bone. It is a lower extremity bone.

**fertilization**  Also called impregnation. The fusion of an ova and sperm to produce an embryo.

**fetal monitoring**  Using electronic equipment placed on the mother's abdomen to check the baby's heart rate and strength during labor.

**fetus**  The term to describe the developing newborn from the end of the eighth week until birth.

**fibrillation**  Abnormal quivering or contractions of heart fibers. When this occurs within the fibers of the ventricle of the heart, arrest and death can occur. Emergency equipment to defibrillate, or convert the heart to a normal beat, is necessary.

**fibrin**  Whitish protein formed by the action of thrombin and fibrinogen, which is the basis for the clotting of blood.

**fibrinogen**  Blood protein that is essential for clotting to take place.

**fibrinolysis**  Destruction of fibers.

**fibrocystic breast disease**  Benign cysts forming in the breast.

**fibroid tumor**  Benign tumor or growth that contains fiber-like tissue. Uterine fibroid tumors are the most common tumors in women.

**fibromyalgia**  A condition with widespread aching and pain in the muscles and soft tissue.

**fibrous joint**  A joint that has almost no movement because the ends of the bones are joined together by thick fibrous tissue. The sutures of the skull are an example of a fibrous joint.

**fibula**  One of the lower leg bones in the lower extremity.

**fibular**  Pertaining to the fibula, a lower leg bone.

**film**  Thin sheet of cellulose material coated with a light-sensitive substance that is used in taking photographs. There is a special photographic film that is sensitive to X-rays.

**film badge**  Badge containing film that is sensitive to X-rays. This is worn by all personnel in radiology to measure the amount of X-rays to which they are exposed.

**filtration**  First stage of urine production during which waste products are filtered from the blood.

**fimbriae**  The fingerlike extensions on the end of the fallopian tubes. The fimbriae drape over each ovary in order to direct the ovum into the fallopian tube after it is expelled by the ovary.

**fine motor skills**  The use of precise and coordinated movements in such activities as writing, buttoning, and cutting.

**fingerspelling**  Using various hand and finger shapes and positions to represent the written alphabet. These positions can be strung together to form words.

**fissure**  A deep groove or slit-type opening.

**fistulectomy**  Excision of a fistula.

**flat bone**  A type of bone with a thin flattened shape. Examples include the scapula, ribs, and pelvic bones.

**flatus**  Passing gas.

**flexion**  Act of bending or being bent.

**fluorescein angiography**  Process of injecting a dye (fluorescein) to observe the movement of blood for detecting lesions in the macular area of the retina. Used to determine if there is a detachment of the retina.

**fluorescein staining**  Applying dye eyedrops that are a bright green fluorescent color; used to look for corneal abrasions or ulcers.

**fluoroscopy**  Use of a fluoroscope to picture the shadows of objects. Also referred to as X-rays.

**flutter**  An arrhythmia in which the atria beat too rapidly, but in a regular pattern.

**focal seizure**  A localized epileptic seizure often affecting one limb.

**follicle-stimulating hormone (FSH)**  A hormone secreted by the anterior pituitary gland. It stimulates growth of eggs in females and sperm in males.

**foramen**  A passage or opening through a bone for nerves and blood vessels.

**forceps**  A surgical instrument used to grasp tissues.

**foreskin**  Also called the prepuce. A protective covering over the glans penis. It is this covering of skin that is removed during circumcision.

**formed elements**  The solid, cellular portion of blood. It consists of erythrocytes, leukocytes, and platelets.

**fossa**  A shallow cavity or depression within or on the surface of a bone.

**fovea centralis**  The area of the retina that has the sharpest vision.

**Fowler position**  Surgical position in which the patient is sitting with back positioned at a 45° angle.

**fracture**  An injury to a bone that causes it to break. Fractures are named to describe the type of damage to the bone.

**fraternal twins**  Twins that develop from two different ova fertilized by two different sperm; although twins, these siblings do not have identical DNA.

**free edge**  The exposed edge of a nail that is trimmed when nails become too long.

**frequency**  A greater than normal occurrence in the urge to urinate, without an increase in the total daily volume of urine. Frequency is an indication of inflammation of the bladder or urethra.

**frontal bone**  The forehead bone of the skull.

**frontal lobe**  One of the four cerebral hemisphere lobes. It controls motor functions.

**frontal plane**  A vertical plane that divides the body into front (anterior or ventral) and back (posterior or dorsal) sections. Also called the coronal plane.

**frostbite**  Freezing or the effect of freezing a part of the body. Exposed areas such as ears, nose, cheeks, fingers, and toes are generally affected.

**frozen section (FS)**  A thin piece of tissue is cut from a frozen specimen for rapid examination under a microscope.

**fundus**  The domed upper portion of an organ such as the stomach or uterus.

**fungal scrapings**  Scrapings, taken with a curette or scraper, of tissue from lesions are placed on a growth medium and examined under a microscope to identify fungal growth.

**fungi**   Organisms found in the Kingdom Fungi. Some are capable of causing disease in humans, such as yeast infections or histoplasmosis.

**furuncle**   Staphylococcal skin abscess with redness, pain, and swelling. Also called a boil.

**gait**   Manner of walking.

**gallbladder**   This small organ is located just under the liver. It functions to store the bile produced by the liver. The gallbladder releases bile into the duodenum through the common bile duct.

**gallstones**   Stones that form in the gallbladder, usually from excess cholesterol.

**gametes**   The reproductive sex cells—ova and sperm.

**gamma globulin**   Protein component of blood containing antibodies that help to resist infection.

**ganglion**   Knot-like mass of nerve tissue located outside the brain and spinal cord.

**gangrene**   Necrosis of the skin usually due to deficient blood supply.

**gastrectomy**   Surgical removal of the stomach.

**gastric carcinoma**   Cancerous tumor of the stomach.

**gastritis**   Inflammation of the stomach that can result in pain, tenderness, nausea, and vomiting.

**gastrodynia**   Stomach pain.

**gastroenteritis**   Inflammation of the stomach and small intestines.

**gastroenterologist**   A physician specialized in treating diseases and conditions of the gastrointestinal tract.

**gastroenterology**   Branch of medicine specializing in conditions of the gastrointestinal system.

**gastroesophageal reflux disease (GERD)**   Acid from the stomach backs up into the esophagus causing inflammation and pain.

**gastrointestinal system (GI)**   System that digests food and absorbs nutrients. Organs include the mouth, pharynx, esophagus, stomach, small and large intestines, liver, gallbladder, and anus. Also called the digestive system.

**gastromalacia**   Softening of the stomach.

**gastroscope**   Instrument to view inside the stomach.

**gastroscopy**   A flexible gastroscope is passed through the mouth and down the esophagus in order to visualize inside the stomach; used to diagnose peptic ulcers and gastric carcinoma.

**gastrostomy**   Surgical creation of a gastric fistula or opening through the abdominal wall. The opening is used to place food into the stomach when the esophagus is not entirely open (esophageal stricture).

**gavage**   Using a nasogastric tube to place liquid nourishment directly into the stomach.

**Geiger counter**   Instrument used for detecting radiation.

**general anesthesia**   General anesthesia produces a loss of consciousness including an absence of pain sensation. It is administered to a patient by either an intravenous or inhalation method. The patient's vital signs are carefully monitored when using a general anesthetic.

**general hospital**   Hospitals that typically provide services to diagnose (laboratory, diagnostic imaging) and treat (surgery, medications, therapy) diseases for a short period of time. In addition, they usually provide emergency and obstetrical care. Also called an acute care hospital.

**generic name**   The recognized and accepted official name for a drug. Each drug has only one generic name. This name is not subject to trademark, so any pharmaceutical manufacturer may use it. Also called nonproprietary name.

**genetic counseling**   Evaluation of parents' potential for producing a child with a genetic disease; especially important for families with a history of genetic diseases.

**genital herpes**   Creeping skin disease that can appear like a blister or vesicle, caused by a sexually transmitted virus.

**genital warts**   Growths and elevations of warts on the genitalia of both males and females that can lead to cancer of the cervix in females.

**genitalia**   The male and female reproductive organs.

**genitourinary**   Referring to the organs of the urinary system and the female or male sexual organs.

**gestation**   Length of time from conception to birth, generally nine months. Calculated from the first day of the last menstrual period, with a range of from 259 days to 280 days.

**gigantism**   Excessive development of the body due to the overproduction of the growth hormone by the pituitary gland. The opposite of dwarfism.

**gingivectomy**   Excision of the gums.

**gingivitis**   Inflammation of the gums characterized by swelling, redness, and a tendency to bleed.

**glands**   The organs of the body that release secretions. Exocrine glands, like sweat glands, release their secretions into ducts. Endocrine glands, such as the thyroid gland, release their hormones directly into the blood stream.

**glans penis**   The larger and softer tip of the penis. It is protected by a covering called the prepuce or foreskin.

**glaucoma**   Increase in intraocular pressure, which, if untreated, may result in atrophy (wasting away) of the optic nerve and blindness. Glaucoma is treated with medication and surgery. There is an increased risk of developing glaucoma in persons over 60 years of age, people of African ancestry, persons who have sustained a serious eye injury, and anyone with a family history of diabetes or glaucoma.

**globulins**   One type of protein found dissolved in the plasma.

**glomerular capsule**   Also called Bowman's capsule. Part of the renal corpuscle. It is a double-walled cup-like structure that encircles the glomerulus. In the filtration stage of urine production, waste products filtered from the blood enter Bowman's capsule as the glomerular filtrate.

**glomerular filtrate**   The product of the filtration stage of urine production. Water, electrolytes, nutrients, wastes, and toxins that are filtered from blood passing through the glomerulus. The filtrate enters Bowman's capsule.

**glomerulonephritis**   Inflammation of the kidney (primarily of the glomerulus). Since the glomerular membrane is inflamed, it becomes more permeable and will allow protein and blood cells to enter the filtrate. Results in protein in the urine (proteinuria) and hematuria.

**glomerulus**   Ball of capillaries encased by Bowman's capsule. In the filtration stage of urine production, wastes filtered from the blood leave the glomerulus capillaries and enter Bowman's capsule.

**glossectomy**   Complete or partial removal of the tongue.

**glottis**   The opening between the vocal cords. Air passes through the glottis as it moves through the larynx. Changing the tension of the vocal cords changes the size of the opening.

**glucagon**   A hormone secreted by the pancreas. It stimulates the liver to release glucose into the blood.

**glucocorticoid**   A group of hormones secreted by the adrenal cortex. They regulate carbohydrate levels in the body. Cortisol is an example of a glucocorticoid.

**glucose**   The form of sugar used by the cells of the body to make energy. It is transported to the cells in the blood.

**glucose tolerance test (GTT)**   Test to determine the blood sugar level. A measured dose of glucose is given to a patient either orally or intravenously. Blood samples are then drawn at certain intervals to determine the ability of the patient to utilize glucose. Used for diabetic patients to determine their insulin reponse to glucose.

**gluteus maximus**   A muscle named for its size and location: gluteus means *rump area* and maximus means *large.*

**glycosuria**   Presence of an excess of sugar in the urine.

**goiter**   Enlargement of the thyroid gland.

**gonads**   The organs responsible for producing sex cells. The female gonads are the ovaries and they produce ova. The male gonads are the testes and they produce sperm.

**gonioscopy**   Use of an instrument called a gonioscope to examine the anterior chamber of the eye to determine ocular motility and rotation.

**gonorrhea**   Sexually transmitted inflammation of the mucous membranes of either sex. Can be passed on to an infant during the birth process.

**gout**   Inflammation of the joints caused by excessive uric acid.

**grade**   A tumor can be graded from grade I through grade IV. The grade is based on the microscopic appearance of the tumor cells. A grade I tumor is well differentiated and is easier to treat than the more advanced grades.

**graft vs. host disease (GVHD)**   Serious complication of bone marrow transplant; immune cells from the donor bone marrow (graft) attack the recipient's (host's) tissues.

**grand mal**   A type of severe epilepsy seizure characterized by a loss of consciousness and convulsions. It is also called a tonic-clonic seizure, indicating that the seizure alternates between strong continuous muscle spasms (tonic) and rhythmic muscle contraction and relaxation (clonic).

**granulocytes**   Granular polymorphonuclear leukocyte. There are three types: neutrophil, eosinophil, and basophil.

**Graves' disease**   Condition, named for Robert Graves, an Irish physician, that results in overactivity of the thyroid gland and can result in a crisis situation. Also called hyperthyroidism.

**gray matter**   Tissue within the central nervous system. It consists of unsheathed or uncovered nerve cell bodies and dendrites.

**greenstick fracture**   Fracture in which there is an incomplete break; one side of the bone is broken and the other side is bent. This type of fracture is commonly found in children due to their softer and more pliable bone structure.

**gross motor skills**   The use of large muscle groups that coordinate body movements such as walking, running, jumping, and balance.

**growth hormone**   A hormone secreted by the anterior pituitary that stimulates growth of the body.

**Guillan-Barré syndrome**   Disease of the nervous system in which nerves lose their myelin covering; may be caused by an autoimmune reaction; characterized by loss of sensation and/or muscle control in the arms and legs; symptoms then move toward the trunk and may even result in paralysis of the diaphragm.

**gut**   Name for the continuous muscular tube that stretches between the mouth and anus; also called the alimentary canal.

**gynecologist**   A physician specialized in treating conditions and diseases of the female reproductive system.

**gynecology**   Branch of medicine specializing in conditions of the female reproductive system.

**gynecomastia**   The development of breast tissue in males; may be a symptom of adrenal feminization.

**gyri**   The convoluted, elevated portions of the cerebral cortex. They are separated by fissures or sulci.

**H$_2$-receptor antagonist**   Blocks the production of stomach acids.

**habituation**   Development of an emotional dependence on a drug due to repeated use.

**hair**   A structure in the integumentary system.

**hair follicle**   Cavities in the dermis that contain the hair root. Hair grows longer from the root.

**hair root**   Deeper cells that divide to grow a hair longer.

**hair shaft**   Older keratinized cells that form most of the length of a hair.

**halitosis**   Bad or offensive breath, which can often be a sign of disease.

**hallucinations**   The perception of an object that is not there or event that has not happened. Hallucinations may be visual, auditory, olfactory, gustatory, or tactile.

**Hashimoto's disease**   Chronic form of thyroiditis, named for a Japanese surgeon.

**head**   The large ball-shaped end of a bone. It may be separated from the shaft of the bone by an area called the neck.

**health maintenance organization (HMO)**   An organization that contracts with a group of physicians and other health care workers to provide care exclusively for its members. The HMO pays the health care workers a prepaid fixed amount per member whether that member requires medical attention or not.

**hearing**   One of the special senses; sound waves detected by the ear.

**hearing aid**   Apparatus or mechanical device used by persons with impaired hearing to amplify sound. Same as amplification device.

**hearing impairment**   Loss of hearing sufficient to interfere with a person's ability to communicate.

**hearing level**   Audiometer reading in decibels (dB) that corresponds to the listener's hearing threshold ratio, which is the softest sound the listener can hear, expressed in decibels (dB).

**heart**   Organ of the cardiovascular system that contracts to pump blood through the blood vessels.

**heart block**   Occurs when the electrical impulse is blocked from traveling down the bundle of His or bundle branches; results in the ventricles beating at a different rate than the atria; also called a bundle branch block.

**heart transplantation**   Replacement of a diseased or malfunctioning heart with a donor's heart.

**heart valve prolapse**   The cusps or flaps of the heart valve are too loose and fail to shut tightly, allowing blood to flow backwards through the valve when the heart chamber contracts. Most commonly occurs in the mitral valve, but may affect any of the heart valves.

**heart valve stenosis**   The cusps or flaps of the heart valve are too stiff. Therefore, they are unable to open fully, making it difficult for blood to flow through, or to shut tightly, allowing blood to flow backwards. This condition may affect any of the heart valves.

**Heimlich maneuver**   Technique for removing a foreign body or food from the trachea or pharynx when it is choking a person. The maneuver consists of applying pressure just under the diaphragm to pop the obstruction out.

*Helicobacter pylori* **(H. pylori)**   A bacteria that may cause inflammation of the stomach lining and peptic ulcers in some people.

**hemangioma**   Common benign, vascular tumor usually located on the skull or vertebral body.

**hematemesis**   To vomit blood from the gastrointestinal tract, often looks like coffee grounds.

**hematic system**   The system that consists of plasma and blood cells—erythrocytes, leukocytes, and platelets; responsible for transporting oxygen, protecting against pathogens, and controlling bleeding.

**hematinic**   Substance that increases the number of erythrocytes or the amount of hemoglobin in the blood.

**hematochezia**   Passing bright red blood in the stools.

**hematocrit (HCT, Hct, crit)**   Blood test to measure the volume of red blood cells (erythrocytes) within the total volume of blood.

**hematocytopenia**   Condition of too few blood cells in the circulation.

**hematologist**   A physician who specializes in treating diseases and conditions of the blood.

**hematology**   Branch of medicine specializing in conditions of the hematic system.

**hematoma**   Swelling or mass of blood caused by a break in a vessel in an organ or tissue, or beneath the skin.

**hematopoiesis**   The process of forming blood.

**hematosalpinx**   Condition of having blood in the fallopian tubes.

**hematuria**   Condition of blood in the urine.

**hemianopia**   Loss of vision in half of the visual field. A stroke patient may suffer from this disorder.

**hemiparesis**   Weakness or loss of motion on one side of the body.

**hemiplegia**   Paralysis on only one side of the body.

**hemodialysis (HD)**   Use of an artificial kidney machine that filters the blood of a person to remove waste products. Use of this technique in patients who have defective kidneys is lifesaving.

**hemoglobin (Hg)**   Iron-containing pigment of red blood cells that carries oxygen from the lungs to the tissue.

**hemolysis**   The destruction of blood cells.

**hemolytic anemia**   An anemia that develops as the result of the excessive loss of erythrocytes.

**hemolytic disease of the newborn**   Condition in which antibodies in the mother's blood enter the fetus's blood and cause anemia, jaundice, edema, and enlargement of the liver and spleen. Also called erythroblastosis fetalis.

**hemophilia**   Hereditary blood disease in which there is a prolonged blood clotting time. It is transmitted by a sex-linked trait from females to males. It appears almost exclusively in males.

**hemoptysis**   Coughing up blood or blood-stained sputum.

**hemorrhage**   Blood flow, the escape of blood from a blood vessel.

**hemorrhoidectomy**   Surgical excision of hemorrhoids from the anorectal area.

**hemorrhoids**   Varicose veins in the rectum.

**hemostasis**   To stop bleeding or the stagnation of the circulating blood.

**hemostat**   A surgical instrument used to grasp blood vessels to control bleeding.

**hemostatic**   Any drug, medicine, or clotting protein from blood that stops bleeding, such as vitamin K or factor VIII (the clotting factor missing in hemophiliacs).

**hemothorax**   Condition of having blood in the chest cavity.

**hepatic lobectomy**   Surgical removal of a lobe of the liver.

**hepatitis**   Infectious, inflammatory disease of the liver. Hepatitis B and C types are spread by contact with blood and bodily fluids of an infected person.

**hepatoma**   Liver tumor.

**herniated nucleus pulposus (HNP)**   A rupture of the fibro-cartilage disk between two vertebrae. This results in pressure on a spinal nerve and causes pain, weakness, and nerve damage. Also called a slipped disk.

**hernioplasty**   Surgical repair of a hernia; also called herniorrhaphy.

**hertz (HZ)**   Measurement of the frequency or pitch of sound. The lowest pitch on an audiogram is 250 Hz. The measurement can go as high as 8000 Hz, which is the highest pitch measured.

**hesitancy**   A decrease in the force of the urine stream, often with difficulty initiating the flow. It is often a symptom of a blockage along the urethra, such as an enlarged prostate gland.

**heterograft**   Skin graft from an animal of another species (usually a pig) to a human; also called a xenograft.

**hiatal hernia**   Protrusion of the stomach through the diaphragm and extending into the thoracic cavity; gastroesophageal reflux disease is a common symptom.

**hilum**   Center of the concave side of the kidney which is an important landmark on the kidney. It is the site where the renal artery enters, the renal vien leaves, the ureter leaves, and nerves enter and leave the kidney.

**hirsutism**   Excessive hair growth over the body.

**histology**   The study of tissues.

**histoplasmosis**   Pulmonary disease caused by a fungus found in dust in the droppings of pigeons and chickens.

**history and physical**   Medical record document written by the admitting physician. It details the patient's history, results of the physician's examination, initial diagnoses, and physician's plan of treatment.

**hives**  Appearance of wheals as part of an allergic reaction.

**Hodgkin's disease**  Also called Hodgkin's lymphoma. Cancer of the lymphatic cells found in concentration in the lymph nodes.

**Holter monitor**  Portable ECG monitor worn by the patient for a period of a few hours to a few days to assess the heart and pulse activity as the person goes through the activities of daily living.

**home health care**  Agencies that provide nursing, therapy, personal care, or housekeeping services in the patient's own home.

**homeostasis**  Steady state or state of balance within the body. The kidneys assist in maintaining this regulatory, steady state.

**homologous transfusion**  Replacement of blood by transfusion of blood received from another person.

**hordeolum**  Refers to a stye (or *sty*), a small purulent inflammatory infection of a sebaceous gland of the eye, treated with hot compresses and surgical incision.

**horizontal plane**  A horizontal plane that divides the body into upper (superior) and lower (inferior) sections. Also called the transverse plane.

**hormone**  A chemical substance secreted by an endocrine gland. It enters the blood stream and is carried to target tissue. Hormones work to control the functioning of the target tissue. Given to replace the loss of natural hormones or to treat disease by stimulating hormonal effects.

**hormone replacement therapy (HRT)**  Menopause or the surgical loss of the ovaries results in the lack of estrogen production; replacing this estrogen with an oral medication prevents some of the consequences of menopause, especially in younger women who have surgically lost their ovaries.

**hormone therapy**  Treatment of cancer with natural hormones or with chemicals that produce hormone-like effects.

**hospices**  An organized group of health care workers that provide supportive treatment to dying patients and their families.

**human growth hormone therapy**  Therapy with human growth hormone in order to stimulate skeletal growth; used to treat children with abnormally short stature.

**human immunodeficiency virus (HIV)**  Virus that causes AIDS; also known as a retrovirus.

**humeral**  Pertaining to the humerus or upper arm bone.

**humerus**  The upper arm bone in the upper extremity.

**humoral immunity**  Immunity that responds to antigens, such as bacteria and foreign agents, by producing antibodies. Also called antibody-mediated immunity.

**Huntington's chorea**  Rare condition characterized by bizarre involuntary movements called chorea. The patient may have progressive mental and physical disturbances that generally begin around 40.

**hydrocele**  Accumulation of fluid within the testes.

**hydrocephalus**  Accumulation of cerebrospinal fluid within the ventricles of the brain, causing the head to be enlarged. It is treated by creating an artificial shunt for the fluid to leave the brain.

**hydrochloric acid**  Acid secreted by the stomach lining. Aids in digestion.

**hydronephrosis**  Distention of the pelvis due to urine collecting in the kidney resulting from an obstruction.

**hydrotherapy**  Using water for treatment purposes.

**hymen**  A thin membranous tissue that covers the external vaginal opening or orifice. The membrane is broken during the first sexual encounter of the female. It can also be broken prematurely by the use of tampons or during some sports activities.

**hymenectomy**  Surgical removal of the hymen. Performed when the hymen tissue is particularly tough.

**hyoid bone**  A single, U-shaped bone suspended in the neck between the mandible and larynx. It is a point of attachment for swallowing and speech muscles.

**hyperbaric oxygen therapy**  Use of oxygen under greater than normal pressure to treat cases of smoke inhalation, carbon monoxide poisoning, and other conditions. In some cases the patient is placed in a hyperbaric oxygen chamber for this treatment.

**hypercalcemia**  Condition of having an excessive amount of calcium in the blood.

**hypercapnia**  Excessive carbon dioxide.

**hyperemia**  Redness of the skin caused by increased blood flow to the skin.

**hyperesthesia**  Having excessive sensation.

**hyperglycemia**  Having an excessive amount of glucose (sugar) in the blood.

**hyperhidrosis**  Abnormal condition of excessive sweat.

**hyperkalemia**  Condition of having an excessive amount of potassium in the blood.

**hyperkinesia**  An excessive amount of movement.

**hyperlipidemia**  Condition of having too high a level of lipids such as cholesterol in the bloodstream; a risk factor for developing atherosclerosis and coronary artery disease.

**hyperopia**  With this condition a person can see things in the distance but has trouble reading material at close vision. Also known as farsightedness.

**hyperpigmentation**  Abnormal amount of pigmentation in the skin, which is seen in diseases such as acromegaly and adrenal insufficiency.

**hyperplasia**  Excessive development of normal cells within an organ.

**hyperpnea**  Excessive deep breathing.

**hypersecretion**  Excessive hormone production by an endocrine gland.

**hypertension**  High blood pressure.

**hypertensive heart disease**  Heart disease as a result of persistently high blood pressure, which damages the blood vessels and ultimately the heart.

**hyperthyroidism**  Condition resulting from overactivity of the thyroid gland that can result in a crisis situation. Also called Graves' disease.

**hypertrophy**  An increase in the bulk or size of a tissue or structure.

**hyperventilation**  To breathe both fast (tachypnea) and deep (hyperpnea).

**hypnotic**  Used to produce sleep or hypnosis.

**hypocalcemia**  Condition of having a low calcium level in the blood.

**hypochondria**   A somatoform disorder involving a preoccupation with health concerns.

**hypochromic anemia**   Anemia resulting from having insufficient hemoglobin in the erythrocytes; named because the hemoglobin molecule is responsible for the dark red color of the erythrocytes.

**hypodermic**   Pertaining to under the skin.

**hypogastric**   Pertaining to below the stomach. An anatomical division of the abdomen, the middle section of the bottom row.

**hypoglossal**   Pertaining to under the tongue.

**hypoglycemia**   Condition of having a low sugar level in the blood.

**hyponatremia**   Condition of having a low sodium level in the blood.

**hypopnea**   Insufficient or shallow breathing.

**hyposecretion**   Deficient hormone production by an endocrine gland.

**hypospadias**   Congenital opening of the male urethra on the underside of the penis.

**hypotension**   Low blood pressure.

**hypothalamus**   The hypothalamus is a portion of the diencephalon that lies just below the thalamus. It controls body temperature, appetite, sleep, sexual desire, and emotions such as fear. It also regulates the release of hormones from the pituitary gland and regulates the parasympathetic and sympathetic nervous systems.

**hypothyroidism**   Result of a deficiency in secretion by the thyroid gland. This results in a lowered basal metabolism rate with obesity, dry skin, slow pulse, low blood pressure, sluggishness, and goiter. Treatment is replacement with synthetic thyroid hormone.

**hypoventilation**   To breathe both slow (bradypnea) and shallow (hypopnea).

**hypoxemia**   Deficiency of oxygen in the blood.

**hypoxia**   Absence of oxygen in the tissues.

**hysterectomy**   Removal of the uterus.

**hysteropexy**   Surgical fixation of the uterus.

**hysterorrhexis**   Rupture of the uterus.

**hysterosalpingography**   Process of taking an X-ray of the uterus and oviducts after a radiopaque material is injected into the organs.

**iatrogenic**   Usually an unfavorable response that results from taking a medication.

**ice packs**   Using ice in a bag or container to treat localized conditions.

**ichthyoderma**   Dry and scaly skin condition.

**ichthyosis**   Condition in which the skin becomes dry, scaly, and keratinized.

**identical twins**   Twins that develop from the splitting of one fertilized ovum; these siblings have identical DNA.

**idiosyncrasy**   Unusual or abnormal response to a drug or food.

**ileocecal valve**   Sphincter between the ileum and the cecum.

**ileostomy**   Surgical creation of a passage through the abdominal wall into the ileum.

**ileum**   The third portion of the small intestines. Joins the colon at the cecum. The ileum and cecum are separated by the ileocecal valve.

**ileus**   Severe abdominal pain, inability to pass stools, vomiting, and abdominal distention as a result of an intestinal blockage; may require surgery to reverse the blockage.

**iliac**   Pertaining to the ilium; one of the pelvic bones.

**ilium**   One of three bones that form the os coxae or innominate bone of the pelvis.

**immune response**   Ability of lymphocytes to respond to specific antigens.

**immunity**   The body's ability to defend itself against pathogens.

**immunization**   Providing protection against communicable diseases by stimulating the immune system to produce antibodies against that disease. Children can now be immunized for the following diseases; hepatitis B, diphtheria, tetanus, pertussis, tetanus, *Haemophilus influenzae* type b, polio, measles, mumps, rubella, and chickenpox. Also called vaccination.

**immunocompromised**   Having an immune system that is unable to respond properly to pathogens.

**immunoglobulins**   Antibodies secreted by the B cells. All antibodies are immunoglobulins. They assist in protecting the body and its surfaces from the invasion of bacteria. For example, the immunoglobulin IgA in colostrum, the first milk from the mother, helps to protect the newborn from infection.

**immunologist**   A physician who specializes in treating infectious diseases and other disorders of the immune system.

**immunology**   Branch of medicine specializing in conditions of the lymphatic and immune systems.

**immunosuppressants**   Blocks certain actions of the immune system; required to prevent rejection of a transplanted organ.

**immunotherapy**   The production or strengthening of a patient's immune system in order to treat a disease.

**impacted fracture**   Fracture in which bone fragments are pushed into each other.

**impacted wisdom tooth**   Wisdom tooth that is tightly wedged into the jawbone so that it is unable to erupt.

**impetigo**   A highly contagious staphylococcal skin infection, most commonly occurring on the faces of children. It begins as blisters that then rupture and dry into a thick, yellow crust.

**implant**   Prosthetic device placed in the jaw to which a tooth or denture may be anchored.

**impotence**   Inability to copulate due to inability to maintain an erection; also called erectile dysfunction.

**impregnation**   Also called fertilization. The fusion of an ova and sperm to produce an embryo.

**impulse control disorders**   Inability to resist an impulse to perform some act that is harmful to the individual or others; includes kleptomania, pyromania, explosive disorder, and pathological gambling.

**incision and drainage (I&D)**   Making an incision to create an opening for the drainage of material such as pus.

**incisors**   Biting teeth in the very front of the mouth that function to cut food into smaller pieces. Humans have eight incisors.

**incus**   One of the three ossicles of the middle ear. Also called the anvil.

**infarct**   Area of tissue within an organ that undergoes necrosis (death) following the loss of blood supply.

**inferior**   Directional term meaning toward the feet or tail, or below.

**inferior venae cavae**   The branch of the venae cavae that drains blood from the abdomen and lower body.

**infertility**   Inability to produce children; generally defined as no pregnancy after properly timed intercourse for 1 year.

**inflammation**   The tissue response to injury from pathogens or physical agents; characterized by redness, pain, swelling, and feeling hot to touch.

**inflammatory bowel disease (IBD)**   Ulceration of the mucous membranes of the colon of unknown origin. Also known as ulcerative colitis.

**influenza**   Viral infection of the respiratory system characterized by chills, fever, body aches, and fatigue. Commonly called the flu.

**informed consent**   A medical record document, voluntarily signed by the patient or a responsible party, that clearly describes the purpose, methods, procedures, benefits, and risks of a diagnostic or treatment procedure.

**inguinal**   Commonly referred to as the groin. There is a collection of lymph nodes in this region that drain each leg.

**inguinal hernia**   Hernia or outpouching of intestines into the inguinal region of the body.

**inhalation**   To breathe air into the lungs. Also called inspiration.

**innate immunity**   Immunity that is not specific to a particular disease and does not require prior exposure to the pathogen. Also called natural immunity.

**inner ear**   The innermost section of the ear. It contains the cochlea, semicircular canals, saccule, and utricle.

**innominate bone**   Also called the os coxae or hip bone. It is the pelvis portion of the lower extremity. It consists of the ilium, ischium, and pubis and unites with the sacrum and coccyx to form the pelvis.

**insertion**   The attachment of a skeletal muscle to the more movable bone in the joint.

**insomnia**   A sleeping disorder characterized by a marked inability to fall asleep.

**inspiration**   To breathe air into the lungs. Also called inhalation.

**insulin**   The hormone secreted by the pancreas. It regulates the level of sugar in the blood stream. The more insulin present in the blood, the lower the blood sugar will be.

**insulin-dependent diabetes mellitus (IDDM)**   Also called type 1 diabetes mellitus; it develops early in life when the pancreas stops insulin production. Persons with IDDM must take daily insulin injections.

**insulinoma**   Tumor of the islets of Langerhans cells of the pancreas that secretes an excessive amount of insulin.

**integument**   Another term for skin.

**integumentary system**   The skin and its appendages including sweat glands, oil glands, hair, and nails. Sense organs that allow us to respond to changes in temperature, pain, touch, and pressure are located in the skin. It is the largest organ in the body.

**interatrial**   Pertaining to between the atria.

**interatrial septum**   The wall or septum that divides the left and right atria.

**intercostal muscles**   Muscles between the ribs. When they contract they raise the ribs, which helps to enlarge the thoracic cavity.

**intermittent positive pressure breathing (IPPB)**   Method for assisting patients to breathe using a mask connected to a machine that produces an increased pressure.

**internal sphincter**   Ring of involuntary muscle that keeps urine within the bladder.

**internist**   A physician specialized in treating diseases and conditions of internal organs such as the respiratory system.

**interpreter**   Person with training in areas such as sign language, fingerspelling, and speech, who can transmit verbal or written messages to the person with a hearing impairment.

**interstitial cystitis**   Disease of unknown cause in which there is inflammation and irritation of the bladder. Most commonly seen in middle-aged women.

**interventricular**   Pertaining to between the ventricles.

**interventricular septum**   The wall or septum that divides the left and right ventricles.

**intervertebral**   Pertaining to between vertebrae.

**intracavitary**   Injection into a body cavity such as the peritoneal and chest cavity.

**intracoronary artery stent**   Placing a stent within a coronary artery to treat coronary ischemia due to atherosclerosis.

**intracranial**   Pertaining to inside the skull.

**intradermal**   Pertaining to within the skin.

**intramuscular**   Pertaining to within the muscle.

**intraocular**   Pertaining to within the eye.

**intrathecal**   Injection into the meninges space surrounding the brain and spinal cord.

**intrauterine device (IUD)**   Device that is inserted into the uterus by a physician for the purpose of contraception.

**intravenous (IV)**   Injection into the veins. This route can be set up so that there is a continuous administration of medication.

**intravenous cholangiography (IVC)**   A dye is administered intravenously to the patient that allows for X-ray visualization of the bile ducts.

**intravenous cholecystography**   A dye is administered intravenously to the patient that allows for X-ray visualization of the gallbladder.

**intravenous pyelogram (IVP)**   Injecting a contrast medium into a vein and then taking an X-ray to visualize the renal pelvis.

**intussusception**   An intestinal condition in which one portion of the intestine telescopes into an adjacent portion causing an obstruction, and gangrene if untreated.

**invasive disease**   Tendency of a malignant tumor to spread to immediately surrounding tissue and organs.

**inversion**   Directional term meaning turning inward or inside out.

**iodine**   A mineral required by the thyroid to produce its hormones.

**iridectomy**   Excision of the iris.

**iridoplegia**   Paralysis of the iris.

**iridosclerotomy**   Incision into the iris and sclera.

**iris**   The colored portion of the eye. It can dilate or constrict to change the size of the pupil and control the amount of light entering the interior of the eye.

**iritis**   Inflammation of the iris.

**iron-deficiency anemia**   Anemia that results from having insufficient iron to manufacture hemoglobin.

**irregular bones** A type of bone having an irregular shape. Vertebrae are irregular bones.

**irritable bowel syndrome (IBS)** Disturbance in the functions of the intestine from unknown causes. Symptoms generally include abdominal discomfort and an alteration in bowel activity.

**ischemia** Localized and temporary deficiency of blood supply due to an obstruction of the circulation.

**ischial** Pertaining to the ischium, one of the pelvic bones.

**ischium** One of the three bones that form the os coxae or innominate bone of the pelvis.

**islets of Langerhans** The regions within the pancreas that secrete insulin and glucagon.

**jaundice** Yellow cast to the skin, mucous membranes, and the whites of the eyes caused by the deposit of bile pigment from too much bilirubin in the blood. Bilirubin is a waste product produced when worn out red blood cells are broken down. May be symptom of disorders such as gallstones blocking the common bile duct or carcinoma of the liver.

**jejunostomy** Surgical creation of a permanent opening into the jejunum.

**jejunum** The middle portion of the small intestines. Site of nutrient absorption.

**joint capsule** Elastic capsule that encloses synovial joints.

**joints** The point at which two bones meet. It provides flexibility.

**Kaposi's sarcoma** Form of skin cancer frequently seen in acquired immunodeficiency syndrome (AIDS) patients. Consists of brownish-purple papules that spread from the skin and metastasize to internal organs.

**kegel exercises** Exercises to strengthen female pubic muscles. The exercises are useful in treating incontinence and as an aid in the childbirth process.

**keloid** Formation of a scar after an injury or surgery that results in a raised, thickened red area.

**keratin** A hard protein substance produced by the body. It is found in hair and nails, and filling the inside of epidermal cells.

**keratitis** Inflammation of the cornea.

**keratometry** Measurement of the curvature of the cornea using an instrument called a keratometer.

**keratoplasty** Surgical repair of the cornea (corneal transplant).

**keratosis** Overgrowth and thickening of the epithelium.

**keratotomy** Incision into the cornea.

**ketoacidosis** Acidosis due to an excess of ketone bodies (waste products). A serious condition that requires immediate treatment and can result in death for the diabetic patient if not reversed.

**ketonuria** Ketones in the urine.

**kidney** The two kidneys are located in the lumbar region of the back behind the parietal peritoneum. They are under the muscles of the back, just a little above the waist. The kidneys have a concave or depressed area that gives them a bean-shaped appearance. The center of this concavity is called the hilum.

**kidneys, ureters, bladder** X-ray taken of the abdomen demonstrating the kidneys, ureters, and bladder without using any contrast dye; also called a flat-plate abdomen.

**kleptomania** An impulse control disorder in which the patient is unable to refrain from stealing. The items are often trivial and unneeded.

**kyphosis** Abnormal increase in the outward curvature of the thoracic spine. Also known as hunchback or humpback.

**labia majora** The outer folds of skin that serves as protection for the female external genitalia and urethral meatus.

**labia minora** The inner folds of skin that serves as protection for the female external genitalia and urethral meatus.

**labor** The period of time beginning with uterine contractions and ending with the birth of the baby. There are three stages: the dilation stage, the expulsion stage, and the placental stage.

**labyrinth** The term that refers to the inner ear. It is several fluid-filled cavities within the temporal bone. The labyrinth consists of the cochlea, vestibule, and three semicircular canals. Hair cells called the organs of Corti line the inner ear. These hair cells change the sound vibrations to electrical impulses and send the impulses to the brain via the vestibulocochlear nerve.

**labyrinthectomy** Excision of the labyrinth.

**labyrinthitis** Labyrinth inflammation.

**lacrimal** Pertaining to tears.

**lacrimal bone** A facial bone.

**lacrimal ducts** Tear ducts located in the inner corner of the eye socket. They collect the tears and drain them into the lacrimal sac.

**lacrimal gland** A gland located in the outer corner of each eyelid. It washes the anterior surface of the eye with fluid called tears.

**lactation** The function of secreting milk after childbirth from the breasts or mammary glands.

**lactic** Pertaining to milk.

**lactiferous ducts** Carries milk from the milk-producing glands to the nipple.

**lactiferous glands** Milk-producing glands in the breast.

**lactorrhea** Discharge of milk.

**laminectomy** Removal of a portion of a vertebra in order to relieve pressure on the spinal nerve.

**laparoscope** Instrument to view inside the abdomen.

**laparoscopic adrenalectomy** Excision of the adrenal gland through a small incision in the abdomen and using endoscopic instruments.

**laparoscopy** An instrument or scope is passed into the abdominal wall through a small incision. The abdominal cavity is then examined for tumors and other conditions with this lighted instrument. Also called peritoneoscopy.

**laparotomy** Incision into the abdomen.

**laryngectomy** Surgical removal of the larynx. This procedure is most frequently performed for excision of cancer.

**laryngitis** Inflammation of the larynx causing difficulty in speaking.

**laryngopharynx** The inferior section of the pharynx. It lies at the same level in the neck as the larynx. Air has already entered the larynx, therefore the laryngopharynx carries food and drink to the esophagus.

**laryngoplasty** Surgical repair of the larynx.

**laryngoplegia**  Paralysis of the voice box.

**laryngoscopy**  Examination of the interior of the larynx with a lighted instrument.

**laryngospasm**  Muscle spasms in the voice box.

**larynx**  Also called the voice box. Respiratory system organ responsible for producing speech. It is located just below the pharynx.

**laser-assisted in-situ keratomileusis (LASIK)**  Correction of myopia using laser surgery to remove corneal tissue.

**laser photocoagulation**  The use of a laser beam to destroy very small precise areas of the retina; may be used to treat retinal detachment or macular degeneration.

**laser surgery**  Use of a controlled beam of light for cutting, hemostasis, or tissue destruction.

**laser therapy**  Removal of skin lesions and birthmarks using a laser beam that emits intense heat and power at a close range. The laser converts frequencies of light into one small, powerful beam.

**last mentrual period (LMP)**  Date when the last menstrual period started.

**lateral (lat)**  Directional term meaning to the side.

**lateral epicondylitis**  Inflammation of the muscle attachment to the lateral epicondyle of the elbow; often caused by strongly gripping. Commonly called tennis elbow.

**lateral recumbent**  Lying on either the left or right side.

**lateral view**  Positioning the patient so that the side of the body faces the X-ray machine.

**lavage**  Using an NG tube to wash out the stomach.

**laxative**  A mild cathartic.

**left hypochondriac**  An anatomical division of the abdomen, the left side of the upper row.

**left iliac**  An anatomical division of the abdomen, the left side of the upper row.

**left lower quadrant (LLQ)**  A clinical division of the abdomen. It contains portions of small and large intestines, left ovary and fallopian tube, and left ureter.

**left lumbar**  An anatomical division of the abdomen, the left side of the middle row.

**left upper quadrant (LUQ)**  A clinical division of the abdomen. It contains the left lobe of the liver, spleen, stomach, portion of the pancreas, and portion of small and large intestines.

**Legionnaire's disease**  Severe, often fatal disease characterized by pneumonia and gastrointestinal symptoms. Caused by a gram-negative bacillus and named after people who came down with it at an American Legion convention in 1976.

**leiomyofibroma**  Fibrous smooth muscle tumor.

**leiomyoma**  Smooth muscle tumor.

**lens**  The transparent structure behind the pupil and iris. It functions to bend light rays so they land on the retina.

**lethargy**  Condition of sluggishness or stupor.

**leukemia**  Cancer of the WBC-forming bone marrow; results in a large number of abnormal WBCs circulating in the blood.

**leukocytes**  Also called white blood cells or WBCs. A group of several different types of cells that provide protection against the invasion of bacteria and other foreign material. They are able to leave the bloodstream and search out the foreign invaders (bacteria, virus, and toxins), where they perform phagocytosis.

**leukocytopenia**  Too few white cells.

**leukocytosis**  Too many white cells.

**leukoderma**  Disappearance of pigment from the skin in patches, causing a milk-white appearance. Also called vitiligo.

**leukoplakia**  Formation of white patches or spots on the mucous membranes of the cheek or tongue. These lesions may become malignant.

**licensed practical nurse (LPN)**  Trained in basic nursing techniques such as administering medications, dressing wounds, and collecting specimens for laboratory tests.

**licensed vocational nurse (LVN)**  Trained in basic nursing techniques such as administering medications, dressing wounds, and collecting specimens for laboratory tests.

**ligaments**  Very strong bands of connective tissue that bind bones together at a joint.

**ligation and stripping**  Surgical treatment for varicose veins; the damaged vein is tied off (ligation) and removed (stripping).

**lingual tonsils**  Tonsils located on the very posterior section of the tongue as it joins with the pharynx.

**lipectomy**  Surgical removal of fat.

**lipocytes**  Medical term for cells that contain fat molecules.

**lipoma**  Fatty tumor that generally does not metastasize.

**liposuction**  Removal of fat beneath the skin by means of suction.

**lips**  The anterior opening of the oral cavity.

**lithotomy**  Surgical incision to remove kidney stones.

**lithotomy position**  Lying face up with hips and knees bent at 90° angles.

**lithotripsy**  Destroying or crushing kidney stones in the bladder or urethra with a device called a lithotriptor.

**liver**  A large organ located in the right upper quadrant of the abdomen. It serves many functions in the body. Its digestive system role includes producing bile, processing the absorbed nutrients, and detoxifying harmful substances.

**liver biopsy**  Excision of a small piece of liver tissue for microscopic examination. Generally used to determine if cancer is present.

**liver scan**  A radioactive substance is administered to the patient by an intravenous (IV) route. When the substance enters the liver cells, the organ can be visualized. This is used to detect tumors, abscesses, and other pathologies that result in hepatomegaly (an enlarged liver).

**liver transplant**  Transplant of a liver from a donor.

**lobectomy**  Surgical removal of a lobe of the lung. Often the treatment of choice for lung cancer.

**local anesthesia**  Local anesthesia produces a loss of sensation in one localized part of the body. The patient remains conscious when this type of anesthetic is used. It is administered either topically or via a subcutaneous route.

**long bone**  A type of bone that is longer than it is wide. Examples include the femur, humerus, and phalanges.

**long-term care facility**  A facility that provides long-term care for patients who need extra time to recover from an illness or accident before they return home or for persons who can no longer care for themselves. Also called a nursing home.

**loop of Henle**  A portion of the renal tubule.

**lordosis**   Abnormal increase in the forward curvature of the lumbar spine. Also known as swayback.

**low birth weight (LBW)**   Abnormally low weight in a newborn. It is usually considered to be less than 5.5 pounds.

**low sex drive**   A sexual disorder characterized by having a decreased interest in sexual intimacy.

**lower esophageal sphincter**   Also called the cardiac sphincter. Prevents food and gastric juices from backing up into the esophagus.

**lower extremity (LE)**   The leg.

**lower gastrointestinal series (lower GI series)**   X-ray image of the colon and rectum is taken after the administration of barium by enema; also called a barium enema.

**lumbar**   Pertaining to the five low back vertebrae.

**lumbar puncture (LP)**   Puncture with a needle into the lumbar area (usually the fourth intervertebral space) to withdraw fluid for examination and for the injection of anesthesia. Also called spinal puncture or spinal tap.

**lumbar vertebrae**   The five vertebrae in the low back region.

**lumen**   The space, cavity, or channel within a tube or tubular organ or structure in the body.

**lumpectomy**   Excision of only a breast tumor and the tissue immediately surrounding it.

**lungs**   The major organs of respiration. The lungs consist of air passageways, the bronchi and bronchioles, and the air sacs, alveoli. Gas exchange takes place within the alveoli.

**lunula**   The lighter colored, half-moon region at the base of a nail.

**luteinizing hormone**   A hormone secreted by the anterior pituitary. It regulates function of male and female gonads and plays a role in releasing ova in females.

**lymph**   Clear, transparent, colorless fluid found in the lymphatic vessels and the cisterna chyli.

**lymph capillaries**   The smallest lymph vessels; they collect excessive tissue fluid.

**lymph ducts**   The two largest vessels in the lymphatic system, the lymphatic duct and the thoracic duct.

**lymph glands**   Another name for lymph nodes; small organs composed of lymphatic tissue located along the route of the lymphatic vessels; remove impurities from the lymph and manufacture lymphocytes and antibodies.

**lymph nodes**   Small organs in the lymphatic system that filter bacteria and other foreign organisms from the body fluids.

**lymph vessels**   Vessels in the lymphatic system that carry lymph fluid throughout the body.

**lymphadenectomy**   Excision of the lymph node. This is usually done to test for malignancy.

**lymphadenitis**   Inflammation of the lympth glands. Referred to as swollen glands.

**lymphadenopathy**   Disease of the lymph nodes.

**lymphangiogram**   X-ray taken of the lymph vessels after the injection of dye. The lymph flow through the chest is traced.

**lymphangiography**   Process of taking an X-ray of the lymph vessels after the injection of a radiopaque material.

**lymphatic**   Pertaining to lymph.

**lymphatic system**   System that helps the body fight infection. Organs include the spleen, lymph vessels, and lymph nodes.

**lymphatic vessels**   Extensive network of vessels throughout the entire body; conduct lymph from the tissue toward the thoracic cavity.

**lymphedema**   Edema appearing in the extremities due to an obstruction of the lymph flow through the lymphatic vessels.

**lymphocytes**   An agranulocyte white blood cell that provides protection through the immune response.

**lymphoma**   A tumor of lymphatic tissue.

**macrophage**   Phagocytic cells that are found in large quantities in the lymph nodes. They engulf foreign particles.

**macrotia**   Abnormally large ears.

**macula lutea**   Images are projected onto the area of the retina.

**macular degeneration**   Deterioration of the macular area of the retina of the eye. May be treated with laser surgery to destroy the blood vessels beneath the macula.

**macule**   Flat, discolored area that is flush with the skin surface. An example would be a freckle or a birthmark.

**magnetic resonance imaging (MRI)**   Medical imaging that uses radio-frequency radiation as its source of energy. It does not require the injection of contrast medium or exposure to ionizing radiation. The technique is useful for visualizing large blood vessels, the heart, the brain, and soft tissues.

**major depression**   A mood disorder characterized by a marked loss of interest in usually enjoyable activities, disturbances in sleep and eating patterns, fatigue, suicidal thoughts, and feelings of hopelessness, worthlessness, and guilt.

**malabsorption syndrome**   Inadequate absorption of nutrients from the intestinal tract. May be caused by a variety of diseases and disorders, such as infections and pancreatic deficiency.

**male pattern baldness**   Genetically determined pattern of progressive hair loss. It begins with a receding hairline at the forehead and eventually leads to loss of hair on the top of the head.

**male reproductive system**   System responsible for producing sperm for reproduction; organs include testes, vas deferens, urethra, prostate gland, and penis.

**malignant**   A tumor that is cancerous. Malignant tumors are generally progressive and recurring.

**malignant lymphoma**   Cancerous tumor of lymphatic tissue; most commonly occurs in lymph nodes, the spleen, or other body sites containing large amounts of lymphatic cells.

**malignant melanoma**   Malignant, darkly pigmented tumor or mole of the skin.

**malingering**   A type of factitious disorder in which the patient intentionally feigns illness for attention or secondary gain.

**malleus**   One of the three ossicles of the middle ear. Also called the hammer.

**mammary glands**   The breasts; milk-producing glands to provide nutrition for newborn.

**mammogram**   X-ray record of the breast.

**mammography**   Process of X-raying the breast.

**mammoplasty**   Surgical repair of the breast.

**mandible**   The lower jawbone.

**mandibular**   Pertaining to the mandible or lower jaw.

**mania**   A mood disorder characterized by extreme elation and euphoria. The patient displays rapid speech, flight of ideas, decreased sleep, distractibility, grandiosity, and poor judgment.

**masochism**   A sexual disorder characterized by receiving sexual gratification from being hurt or abused.

**massage**   Kneading or applying pressure by hands to a part of the patient's body to promote muscle relaxation and reduce tension.

**mastalgia**   Breast pain.

**mastectomy**   Excision of the breast.

**mastication**   Chewing.

**mastitis**   Inflammation of the breast, which is common during lactation but can occur at any age.

**maxilla**   The upper jawbone.

**maxillary**   Pertaining to the maxilla or upper jaw.

**meatotomy**   Surgical enlargement of the urinary opening (meatus).

**meconium**   A substance that collects in the intestines of a fetus and becomes the first stool of a newborn.

**medial**   Directional term meaning to the middle or near the middle of the body or the structure.

**median plane**   Plane that runs lengthwise from front to back and divides the body or any of its parts into right and left portions; also called the sagittal plane.

**mediastinal**   There is a collection of lymph nodes located in the mediastinum (central chest area) that drain the chest.

**mediastinum**   The central region of the chest cavity. It contains the organs between the lungs, including the heart, aorta, esophagus, and trachea.

**medical laboratory technician (MLT)**   Performs laboratory tests under the supervision of the medical technologist.

**medical record**   Documents the details of a patient's hospital stay. Each health care professional that has contact with the patient in any capacity completes the appropriate report of that contact and adds it to the medical chart. This results in a permanent physical record of the patient's day-to-day condition, when and what services he or she receives, and the response to treatment. Also called a chart.

**medical technologist (MT)**   Performs laboratory tests as ordered by a physician.

**medical transcriptionist**   Transcribes dictated medical notes.

**medulla**   The central area of an organ. In the endocrine system it refers to the adrenal medulla.

**medulla oblongata**   A portion of the brain stem that connects the spinal cord with the brain. It contains the respiratory, cardiac, and blood pressure control centers.

**medullary cavity**   The large open cavity that extends the length of the shaft of a long bone; contains yellow bone marrow.

**melanin**   The black color pigment in the skin. It helps to prevent the sun's ultraviolet rays from entering the body.

**melanocytes**   Special cells in the basal layer of the epidermis. They contain the black pigment melanin that gives skin its color and protects against the ultraviolet rays of the sun.

**melanocyte-stimulating hormone**   A hormone secreted by the anterior pituitary. It stimulates pigment production in the skin.

**melanoma**   Also called malignant melanoma. A dangerous form of skin cancer caused by an overgrowth of melanin in a melanocyte. It may metastasize or spread. Exposure to ultraviolet light is a risk factor for developing melanoma.

**melatonin**   Hormone secreted by the pineal gland; plays a role in regulating the body's circadian rhythm.

**melena**   Passage of dark tarry stools; color is the result of digestive enzymes working on blood in the stool.

**membrane**   Thin structures that cover and protect the body surface, line body cavities, and line some of the internal organs, such as the digestive and respiratory passages. Membranes also secrete lubricating fluids to reduce friction during some processes, such as respiration, and serve to anchor organs and bones. There are two major types of membranes, epithelial and connective tissue.

**menarche**   The first menstrual period.

**Ménière's disease**   Abnormal condition within the labyrinth of the inner ear that can lead to a progressive loss of hearing. The symptoms are dizziness or vertigo, hearing loss, and tinnitus (ringing in the ears).

**meninges**   Three connective tissue membrane layers that surround the brain and spinal cord. The three layers are dura mater, arachnoid layer, and pia mater. The dura mater and arachnoid layer are separated by the subdural space. The arachnoid layer and pia mater are separated by the subarachnoid space.

**meningioma**   Slow-growing tumor in the meninges of the brain.

**meningitis**   Inflammation of the membranes of the spinal cord and brain that is caused by a microorganism.

**meningocele**   Congenital hernia in which the meninges, or membranes, protrude through an opening in the spinal column or brain.

**menopause**   Cessation or ending of menstrual activity. This is generally between the ages of 40 and 55.

**menorrhagia**   Excessive bleeding during the menstrual period. Can be either in the total number of days or the amount of blood or both.

**menstrual cycle**   The 28-day fertility cycle in women; includes ovulation and sloughing off the endometrium if a pregnancy does not occur.

**menstrual period**   Another name for the menstrual cycle.

**menstruation**   The loss of blood and tissue as the endometrium in shed by the uterus. The flow exits the body through the cervix and vagina. The flow occurs approximately every 28 days.

**mental retardation**   A disorder characterized by a diminished ability to process intellectual functions.

**metabolism**   The sum of all the chemical processes taking place in the body.

**metacarpals**   The hand bones in the upper extremity.

**metastases**   The spreading of a cancerous tumor from its original site to different locations of the body. Singular is metastasis.

**metastasis (mets)**   Movement and spread of cancer cells from one part of the body to another. Metastases is plural.

**metastasized**   When cancerous cells migrate away from a tumor site. They commonly move through the lymphatic system and become trapped in lymph nodes.

**metatarsals**   The ankle bones in the lower extremity.

**metrorrhagia**  Rapid (menstrual) blood flow from the uterus.

**metrorrhea**  Discharge from the uterus.

**microtia**  Abnormally small ears.

**micturition**  Another term for urination.

**midbrain**  A portion of the brain stem.

**middle ear**  The middle section of the ear. It contains the ossicles.

**migraine**  A specific type of headache characterized by severe head pain, photophobia, vertigo, and nausea.

**mineralocorticoid**  A group of hormones secreted by the adrenal cortex. They regulate electrolytes and fluid volume in the body. Aldosterone is an example of a mineralocorticoid.

**miotic**  Any substance that causes the pupil to constrict.

**miscarriage**  The unplanned loss of a fetus. Also called a spontaneous abortion.

**mitral valve**  A valve between the left atrium and ventricle in the heart. It prevents blood from flowing backwards into the atrium. It is also called the bicuspid valve because it has two cusps or flaps.

**mobility**  State of having normal movement of all body parts.

**moist hot packs**  Applying moist warmth to a body part to produce the slight dilation of blood vessels in the skin; causes muscle relaxation in the deeper regions of the body and increases circulation, which aids healing.

**molars**  Large somewhat flat-topped back teeth. Function to grind food. Humans have up to 12 molars.

**monoaural**  Referring to one ear.

**monochromatism**  Unable to perceive one color.

**monocytes**  An agranulocyte white blood cell that is important for phagocytosis.

**mononucleosis**  Acute infectious disease with a large number of atypical lymphocytes. Caused by the Epstein–Barr virus. There may be abnormal liver function.

**monoparesis**  Weakness of one extremity.

**monoplegia**  Paralysis of one extremity.

**monospot**  Test of infectious mononucleosis in which there is a nonspecific antibody called heterophile antibody.

**mood disorders**  Characterized by instability in mood; includes major depression, mania, and bipolar disorder.

**morbidity**  Number that represents the number of sick persons in a particular population.

**mortality**  Number that represents the number of deaths in a particular population.

**motor neurons**  Nerves that carry activity instruction from the CNS to muscles or glands out in the body; also called efferent neurons.

**mouth**  The external opening of the alimentary canal. It contains the teeth and tongue for biting and chewing food.

**mucolytic**  Liquefies mucus so it is easier to cough and clear it from the respiratory tract.

**mucous membrane**  These membranes line body passages that open directly to the exterior of the body, such as the mouth and reproductive tract, and secrete a thick substance, or mucus.

**mucus**  Sticky fluid secreted by mucous membrane lining of the respiratory tract. Assists in cleansing air by trapping dust and bacteria.

**multigravida**  Woman who has had more than one pregnancy.

**multipara**  Woman who has given birth to more than one child.

**multiple personality disorder**  A type of dissociative disorder in which the person displays two or more distinct conscious personalities that alternate in controlling the body. The alternate personalities may or may not be aware of each other.

**multiple sclerosis (MS)**  Inflammatory disease of the central nervous system. Rare in children. Generally strikes adults between the ages of 20 and 40. There is progressive weakness and numbness.

**murmur**  An abnormal heart sound as a soft blowing sound or a harsh click. They may be soft and heard only with a stethoscope, or so loud they can be heard several feet away.

**muscle biopsy**  Removal of muscle tissue for pathological examination.

**muscle relaxant**  Produces the relaxation of skeletal muscle.

**muscle tissue**  Tissue that is able to contract and shorten its length, thereby producing movement. Muscle tissue may be under voluntary control (attached to the bones) or involuntary control (heart and digestive organs).

**muscle tissue fibers**  The bundles of muscle tissue that form a muscle.

**muscles**  Muscles are bundles of parallel muscle tissue fibers. As the fibers contract (shorten in length) they pull whatever they are attached to closer together. This may move two bones closer together or make an opening more narrow. A muscle contraction occurs when a message is transmitted from the brain through the nervous system to the muscles.

**muscular**  Pertaining to muscles.

**muscular dystrophy**  Inherited disease causing a progressive muscle weakness and atrophy.

**musculoskeletal system (MS)**  System that provides support for the body and produces movement. Organs of the musculoskeletal system includes muscles, tendons, bones, joints, and cartilage.

**mutation**  Change or transformation from the original.

**myasthenia**  Lack of muscle strength.

**myasthenia gravis**  Disorder causing loss of muscle strength and paralysis. This is an autoimmune disease.

**mydriatic**  Any substance that causes the pupil to dilate.

**myelin**  Tissue that wraps around many of the nerve fibers. It is composed of fatty material and functions as an insulator.

**myelinated**  Nerve fibers covered with a layer of myelin.

**myelitis**  Inflammation of the spinal cord.

**myelogram**  X-ray record of the spinal cord following injection of meninges with radiopaque dye.

**myelography**  Injection of a radiopaque dye into the spinal canal. An X-ray is then taken to examine the normal and abnormal outlines made by the dye.

**myeloma**  Malignant neoplasm originating in plasma cells in the bone.

**myelomalacia**  Spinal cord softening.

**myelomeningocele**  A hernia composed of meninges and spinal cord.

**myocardial**  Pertaining to heart muscle.

**myocardial infarction (MI)**  Condition caused by the partial or complete occlusion or closing of one or more of the coronary arteries. Symptoms include severe chest pain or heavy pressure in the middle of the chest. A delay in treatment could result in death. Also referred to as MI or heart attack.

**myocarditis**   Inflammation of heart muscle.

**myocardium**   The middle layer of the muscle. It is thick and composed of cardiac muscle. This layer produces the heart contraction.

**myometrium**   The middle muscle layer of the uterus.

**myoneural junction**   The point at which a nerve contacts a muscle fiber.

**myopathy**   Any disease of muscles.

**myopia (MY)**   With this condition a person can see things that are close up but distance vision is blurred. Also known as nearsightedness.

**myoplasty**   Surgical repair of muscle.

**myorrhaphy**   Suture a muscle.

**myringectomy**   Excision of the eardrum.

**myringitis**   Eardrum inflammation.

**myringoplasty**   Surgical reconstruction of the eardrum. Also called tympanoplasty.

**myringotomy**   Surgical puncture of the eardrum with removal of fluid and pus from the middle ear, to eliminate a persistent ear infection and excessive pressure on the tympanic membrane. A polyethylene tube is placed in the tympanic membrane to allow for drainage of the middle ear cavity.

**myxedema**   Condition resulting from a hypofunction of the thyroid gland. Symptoms can include anemia, slow speech, enlarged tongue and facial features, edematous skin, drowsiness, and mental apathy.

**nail body**   Flat plate of keratin that forms most of the nails.

**nail root**   Base of a nail; nails grow longer from the root.

**nailbed**   Connects nail body to connective tissue underneath.

**nails**   A structure in the integumentary system.

**narcissistic personality**   A personality disorder characterized by an abnormal sense of self-importance.

**narcolepsy**   Chronic disorder in which there is an extreme uncontrollable desire to sleep.

**narcotic**   Produces sleep or stupor. In moderate doses this drug will depress the central nervous system and relieve pain. In excessive doses it will cause stupor, coma, and even death. Can become habit forming (addictive).

**nares**   External openings of the nose that open into the nasal cavity.

**nasal bone**   A facial bone.

**nasal canula**   Two-pronged plastic device for delivering oxygen into the nose; one prong is inserted into each nare.

**nasal cavity**   Large cavity just behind the external nose that receives the outside air. It is covered with mucous membrane to cleanse the air. The nasal septum divides the nasal cavity into left and right halves.

**nasal septum**   A flexible cartilage wall that divides the nasal cavity into left and right halves. It is covered by mucous membrane.

**nasogastric**   Pertaining to the nose and stomach.

**nasogastric intubation (NG tube)**   A flexible catheter is inserted into the nose and down the esophagus to the stomach; may be used for feeding or to suction out stomach fluids.

**nasolacrimal duct**   Duct that collects tears from the inner corner of the eye socket and drains them into the nasal cavity.

**nasopharynx**   The superior section of the pharynx that receives air from the nose.

**natural immunity**   Immunity that is not specific to a particular disease and does not require prior exposure to the pathogen. Also called innate immunity.

**natural killer (NK) cells**   T cells that can kill by entrapping foreign cells, tumor cells, and bacteria. Also called T8 cells.

**nausea**   A feeling of needing to vomit.

**neck**   A narrow length of bone that connects the ball of a ball-and-socket joint to the diaphysis of a long bone.

**necrosis**   Dead tissue.

**needle biopsy**   Using a sterile needle to remove tissue for examination under a microscope.

**neonate**   Term used to describe the newborn infant during the first 4 weeks of life.

**neonatology**   Study of the newborn.

**neoplasm**   An abnormal growth of tissue that may be benign or malignant. Also called a tumor.

**nephrectomy**   Excision of a kidney.

**nephritis**   Inflammation of the kidney.

**nephrogram**   X-ray of the kidney.

**nephrolithiasis**   The presence of calculi in the kidney.

**nephrology**   Branch of medicine specializing in conditions of the urinary system.

**nephroma**   Kidney tumor.

**nephromalacia**   Softening of the kidney.

**nephromegaly**   Enlarged kidney.

**nephron**   The functional or working unit of the kidney that filters the blood and produces the urine. There are more than 1 million nephrons in an adult kidney. Each nephron consists of a renal corpuscle and the renal tubules.

**nephropathy**   Kidney disease.

**nephropexy**   Surgical fixation of a kidney.

**nephroptosis**   Drooping kidney.

**nephrosclerosis**   Hardening of the kidney.

**nephrosis**   Abnormal condition (degeneration) of the kidney.

**nephrostomy**   Create a new opening across the body wall into the kidney.

**nephrotomy**   Incision into a kidney.

**nerve block**   Also referred to as regional anesthesia. This anesthetic interrupts a patient's pain sensation in a particular region of the body. The anesthetic is injected near the nerve that will be blocked from sensation. The patient usually remains conscious.

**nerve cell body**   The portion of the nerve cell that includes the nucleus.

**nerve conduction velocity**   A test to determine if nerves have been damaged by recording the rate at which an electrical impulse travels along a nerve. If the nerve is damaged, the velocity will be decreased.

**nerve root**   The point where a spinal or cranial nerve is attached to the CNS.

**nerves**   Structures in the nervous system that conduct electrical impulses from the brain and spinal cord to muscles and other organs.

**nervous system**   System that coordinates all the conscious and subconscious activities of the body. Organs include the brain, spinal cord, and nerves.

**nervous tissue** Nervous tissue conducts electrical impulses to and from the brain and the rest of the body.

**neural** Pertaining to nerves.

**neuralgia** Nerve pain.

**neurectomy** Excision of a nerve.

**neuroglial cells** Cells that perform support functions for neurons.

**neurologist** Physician who specializes in disorders of the nervous system.

**neurology** Branch of medicine specializing in conditions of the nervous system.

**neurolysis** Nerve destruction.

**neuroma** Nerve tumor.

**neuron** The name for an individual nerve cell. Neurons group together to form nerves and other nervous tissue.

**neuroplasty** Surgical repair of nerves.

**neurorrhaphy** Suture a nerve.

**neurosis** Mental disorder in which there are symptoms such as depression and anxiety.

**neurosurgeon** A physician specializing in treating conditions and diseases of the nervous systems by surgical means.

**neurosurgery** Branch of medicine specializing in surgery on the nervous system.

**neurotomy** Incision into a nerve.

**neurotransmitter** Chemical messenger that carries an electrical impulse across the gap between two neurons.

**neutrophils** A granulocyte white blood cell that is important for phagocytosis. It is also the most numerous of the leukocytes.

**nevus** Pigmented (colored) congenital skin blemish, birthmark, or mole. Usually benign but may become cancerous.

**nipple** Point at which milk is released from the breast.

**nitrogenous wastes** Waste products that contain nitrogen. These products, such as ammonia and urea, are produced during protein metabolism.

**nocturia** Excessive urination during the night. May or may not be abnormal.

**nodule** Solid, raised group of cells.

**non-Hodgkin's lymphoma (NHL)** Cancer of the lymphatic tissues other than Hodgkin's lymphoma.

**noninsulin–dependent diabetes mellitus** Also called type 2 diabetes mellitus. It develops later in life when the pancreas produces insufficient insulin; persons may take oral hypoglycemics to stimulate insulin secretion, or may eventually have to take insulin.

**nonprescription drug** Drugs that are accessible in drugstores without a prescription. Also called over-the-counter (OTC) drugs.

**nonproprietary name** The recognized and accepted official name for a drug. Each drug has only one generic name, which is not subject to trademark, so any pharmaceutical manufacturer may use it. Also called generic name.

**nonsteroidal anti-inflammatory drugs (NSAID)** A large group of drugs including aspirin and ibuprofen that provide mild pain relief and anti-inflammatory benefits for conditions such as arthritis.

**norepinephrine** A hormone secreted by the adrenal medulla. It is a strong vasoconstrictor.

**normal psychology** Behaviors that include how the personality develops, how people handle stress, and the stages of mental development.

**nose** Outside air enters the respiratory system through the nose. The nose includes the external nasal opening and the nasal cavity.

**nosocomial infection** An infection acquired as a result of hospital exposure.

**nuclear medicine** Use of radioactive substances to diagnose diseases. A radioactive substance known to accumulate in certain body tissues is injected or inhaled. After waiting for the substance to travel to the body area of interest the radioactivity level is recorded. Commonly referred to as a scan.

**nuclear medicine technologist** Performs nuclear medicine scans as ordered by a physician.

**nulligravida** Woman who has never been pregnant.

**nullipara** Woman who has never produced a viable baby.

**nurse** To breastfeed a baby.

**nurse anesthetist** A registered nurse who has received additional training and education in the administration of anesthetic medications.

**nurse practitioner (NP)** A registered nurse who receives advanced training in a specialized area of nursing such as family health, women's health, pediatric health, gerontological health, or acute care.

**nurse's notes** Medical record document that records the patient's care throughout the day. It includes vital signs, treatment specifics, patient's response to treatment, and patient's condition.

**nursing home** A facility that provides long-term care for patients who need extra time to recover from all illness or accident before they return home or for persons who can no longer care for themselves. Also called a long-term care facility.

**nutrients** Substances necessary for the functioning of the body, such as glucose and amino acids.

**nyctalopia** Difficulty seeing in dim light; usually due to damaged rods.

**nystagmus** Jerky-appearing involuntary eye movement.

**obesity** Having an abnormal amount of fat in the body.

**oblique fracture** Fracture at an angle to the bone.

**oblique muscle** Oblique means slanted. Two of the eye muscles are oblique muscles.

**oblique view** Positioning the patient so that the X-rays pass through the body on an angle.

**obsessive-compulsive behavior** A type of anxiety disorder in which the person performs repetitive rituals in order to reduce anxiety.

**obstetrician** A physician specialized in providing care for pregnant women and delivering infants.

**obstetrics (OB)** Branch of medicine that treats women during pregnancy and childbirth, and immediately after childbirth.

**occipital bone** A cranial bone.

**occipital lobe** One of the four cerebral hemisphere lobes. It controls eyesight.

**Occupational Safety and Health Administration (OSHA)** Federal agency that issued mandatory guidelines to ensure that all employees at risk of exposure to body fluids are provided with personal protective equipment.

**occupational therapist (OTR)**   Specializes in rehabilitating patients to perform activities that are essential for daily living.

**occupational therapy (OT)**   Assists patients to regain, develop, and improve skills that are important for independent functioning. Occupational therapy personnel work with people who, because of illness, injury, developmental, or psychological impairments, require specialized training in skills that will enable them to lead independent, productive, and satisfying lives. Occupational therapists instruct patients in the use of adaptive equipment and techniques, body mechanics, and energy conservation. They also employ modalities such as heat, cold, and therapeutic exercise.

**occupational therapy assistant (OTA)**   Performs occupational therapy procedures under the supervision of an occupational therapist.

**oculomycosis**   Condition of eye fungus.

**oligomenorrhea**   Scanty menstrual flow.

**oligospermia**   Condition of having few sperm.

**oliguria**   Condition of scanty amount of urine.

**oncogenic**   Cancer causing.

**oncology**   The branch of medicine dealing with tumors.

**onychectomy**   Excision of a nail.

**onychia**   Infected nailbed.

**onychomalacia**   Softening of nails.

**onychomycosis**   Abnormal condition of nail fungus.

**onychophagia**   Nail biting.

**oophorectomy**   Removal of an ovary.

**oophoritis**   Inflammation of an ovary.

**open fracture**   Fracture in which the skin has been broken through to the fracture.

**open-heart surgery**   Surgery that involves incision of the heart, coronary arteries, or the heart valves.

**operative report**   A medical record report from the surgeon detailing an operation. It includes a pre- and postprocedure itself, and how the patient tolerated the procedure.

**ophthalmalgia**   Eye pain.

**ophthalmic**   Pertaining to the eyes.

**ophthalmologist**   A physician specialized in treating conditions and diseases of the eye.

**ophthalmology**   Branch of medicine specializing in condition of the eye.

**ophthalmoplegia**   Paralysis of the eye.

**ophthalmorrhagia**   Rapid bleeding from the eye.

**ophthalmoscope**   Instrument to view inside the eye.

**ophthalmoscopy**   Examination of the interior of the eyes using an instrument called an ophthalmoscope. The physician will dilate the pupil in order to see the cornea, lens, and retina. Identifies abnormalities in the blood vessels of the eye and some systemic diseases.

**opportunistic infections**   Infectious diseases that are associated with AIDS since they occur as a result of the lowered immune system and resistance of the body to infections and parasites.

**opposition**   Moves thumb away from palm; the ability to move the thumb into contact with the other fingers.

**optic**   Pertaining to the eye.

**optic disk**   The area of the retina associated with the optic nerve. Also called the blind spot.

**optic nerve**   The second cranial nerve that carries impulses from the retinas to the brain.

**optician**   Grinds and fits prescription lenses and contacts as prescribed by a physician or optometrist.

**optometer**   Instrument to measure vision.

**optometrist (OD)**   Doctor of optometry; provides care for the eyes including examining the eyes for diseases, assessing visual acuity, prescribing corrective lenses and eye treatments, and educating patients.

**optometry**   Process of measuring vision.

**oral**   Pertaining to the mouth.

**oral antibiotics**   Oral antibiotics are required to treat otitis media and labyrinthitis because the tympanic membrane prevents eardrops from reaching the middle ear cavity.

**oral cavity**   The mouth.

**oral contraceptive pills (OCPs)**   Birth control medication that uses low doses of female hormones to prevent conception by blocking ovulation.

**oral hypoglycemic agent**   Medication taken by mouth that causes a decrease in blood sugar. This is not used for insulin-dependent patients. There is no proof that this medication will prevent the long-term complications of diabetes mellitus.

**oral leukoplakia**   Development of white patches on the mucous membrane inside the mouth; may develop into cancer.

**orchidectomy**   Excision of the testes.

**orchidopexy**   Surgical fixation to move undescended testes into the scrotum and attaching to prevent retraction.

**orchiectomy**   Surgical removal of the testes.

**orchioplasty**   Surgical repair of the testes.

**orchiotomy**   Incision into the testes.

**organic mental disease**   Deterioration of mental functions due to temporary brain or permanent brain dysfunction; includes dementia and Alzheimer's disease; also called cognitive disorders.

**organism**   A whole, living individual. The sum of all the cells, tissues, organs, and systems working together to sustain life.

**organs**   Groups of different types of tissue coming together to perform special functions. For example, the heart contains muscular fibers, nerve tissue, and blood vessels.

**organs of Corti**   The sensory receptor hair cells lining the cochlea. These cells change the sound vibrations to electrical impulses and send the impulses to the brain via the vestibulocochlear nerve.

**origin**   The attachment of a skeletal muscle to the less movable bone in the joint.

**oropharynx**   The middle section of the pharynx that receives food and drink from the mouth.

**orthodontics**   The dental specialty concerned with straightening teeth.

**orthodontist**   Dentist who is an expert in orthodontia, which is straightening teeth.

**orthopedic surgery**   The branch of medicine specializing in surgical treatments of the musculoskeletal system.

**orthopedics**   Branch of medicine specializing in the diagnosis and treatment of conditions of the musculoskeletal system.

**orthopedist**   Physician who specializes in treatment of conditions of the musculoskeletal system.

**orthopnea**   Term to describe a patient who needs to sit up straight in order to breathe comfortably.

**orthotics**   The use of equipment, such as splints and braces, to support a paralyzed muscle, promote a specific motion, or correct musculoskeletal deformities.

**orthotist**   Person skilled in orthotics.

**os coxae**   Also called the innominate bone or hip bone. It is the pelvis portion of the lower extremity. It consists of the ilium, ischium, and pubis and unites with the sacrum and coccyx to form the pelvis.

**osseous tissue**   Bony tissue. One of the hardest tissues in the body.

**ossicles**   The three small bones in the middle ear. The bones are the incus, malleus, and stapes. The ossicles amplify and conduct the sound waves to the inner ear.

**ossification**   The process of bone formation.

**osteoarthritis**   Noninflammatory type of arthritis resulting in degeneration of the bones and joints, especially those bearing weight.

**osteoblast**   An embryonic bone cell.

**osteocarcinoma**   Cancer of the bone.

**osteochondroma**   Tumor composed of both cartilage and bony substance.

**osteoclasia**   Intentional breaking of a bone in order to correct a deformity.

**osteocyte**   Mature bone cells.

**osteogenic sarcoma**   The most common type of bone cancer; usually begins in osteocytes found at the ends of long bones.

**osteomalacia**   Softening of the bones caused by a deficiency of phosphorus or calcium. It is thought that in children the cause is insufficient sunlight and vitamin D.

**osteomyelitis**   Inflammation of the bone and bone marrow due to infection; can be difficult to treat.

**osteopathy**   Form of medicine that places great emphasis on the musculoskeletal system and the body system as a whole. Manipulation is also used as part of the treatment.

**osteoporosis**   Decrease in bone mass that results in a thinning and weakening of the bone with resulting fractures. The bone becomes more porous, especially in the spine and pelvis.

**osteotome**   An instrument to cut bone.

**osteotomy**   Incision into a bone.

**otalgia**   Ear pain.

**otic**   Pertaining to the ear.

**otitis**   Ear inflammation.

**otitis externa (OE)**   External ear infection; most commonly caused by fungus. Also called otomycosis and commonly referred to as swimmer's ear.

**otitis media (OM)**   Commonly referred to as middle ear infection; seen frequently in children. Often preceded by an upper respiratory infection.

**otologist**   A physician specialized in the diagnosis and treatment of diseases of the ear.

**otology**   Study of ear.

**otomycosis**   Fungal infection of the ear, usually in the auditory canal.

**otoplasty**   Corrective surgery to change the size of the external ear or pinna. The surgery can either enlarge or lessen the size of the pinna.

**otopyorrhea**   Pus discharge from the ear.

**otorhinolaryngologist**   A physician who specializes in the treatment of diseases of the ear, nose, and throat.

**otorhinolaryngology**   Branch of medicine that treats diseases of the ears, nose, and throat. Also referred to as ENT.

**otosclerosis**   Progressive hearing loss caused by immobility of the stapes bone.

**otoscope**   Instrument to view inside the ear.

**otoscopy**   Examination of the ear canal, eardrum, and outer ear using the otoscope. Foreign material can be removed from the ear canal with this procedure.

**outpatient clinic**   A facility that provides services that do not require overnight hospitalization. The services range from simple surgeries to diagnostic testing to therapy. Also called an ambulatory care center or a surgical center.

**ova**   The female sex cell or gamete produced in the ovary. An ovum fuses with a sperm to produce an embryo. Singular is ovum.

**ova and parasites**   Laboratory examination of feces with a microscope for the presence of parasites or their eggs.

**oval window**   The division between the middle and inner ear.

**ovarian carcinoma**   Cancer of the ovary.

**ovarian cyst**   Sac that develops within the ovary.

**ovaries**   The female gonads. These two glands are located on either side of the lower abdominopelvic region of the female. They are responsible for the production of the sex cells, ova, and the hormones estrogen and progesterone.

**over-the-counter**   Drugs that are accessible in drugstores without a prescription. Also called nonprescription drugs.

**oviducts**   Tubes that carry the ovum from the ovary to the uterus; also called fallopian tubes or uterine tubes.

**ovulation**   The release of an ovum from the ovary.

**ovum**   The female sex cell or gamete. It is produced in the ovary. An ovum fuses with a sperm to produce an embryo. Plural is ova.

**oxygen**   Gaseous element absorbed by the blood from the air sacs in the lungs. It is necessary for cells to make energy.

**oxygenated**   Term for blood with a high oxygen level.

**oxytocin**   A hormone secreted by the posterior pituitary. It stimulates uterine contractions during labor and delivery.

**pacemaker**   Another name for the sinoatrial node of the heart.

**pacemaker implantation**   Electrical device that substitutes for the natural pacemaker of the heart. It controls the beating of the heart by a series of rhythmic electrical impulses. An external pacemaker has the electrodes on the outside of the body; an internal pacemaker has the electrodes surgically implanted within the chest wall.

**pachyderma**   Thickening of the skin.

**packed cells**   A transfusion of only the formed elements and without plasma.

**Paget's disease**   A fairly common metabolic disease of the bone from unknown causes. It usually attacks middle-aged and elderly people and is characterized by bone destruction and deformity.

**pain control**   Managing pain through the use of a variety of means, including medications, biofeedback, and mechanical devices.

**palate**   The roof of the mouth. The anterior portion is hard or bony, and the posterior portion is soft or flexible.

**palatine bone**   A facial bone.

**palatine tonsils**   Tonsils located in the lateral wall of the pharynx close to the mouth.

**palliative therapy**   Treatment designed to reduce the intensity of painful symptoms, but not to produce a cure.

**palpitations**   Pounding, racing heartbeat.

**palsy**   Temporary or permanent loss of the ability to control movement.

**pancreas**   Organ in the digestive system that produces digestive enzymes. Also a gland in the endocrine system that produces two hormones, insulin and glucagon.

**pancreatic enzymes**   Digestive enzymes produced by the pancreas and added to the chyme in the duodenum.

**pancreatitis**   Inflammation of the pancreas.

**pancytopenia**   Too few of all types of blood cells.

**panhypopituitarianism**   Deficiency in all the hormones secreted by the pituitary gland; often recognized because of problems with the glands regulated by the pituitary—adrenal cortex, thyroid, ovaries, and testes.

**panic attacks**   A type of anxiety disorder characterized by a sudden onset of intense apprehension, fear, terror, or impending doom often accompanied by a racing heart rate.

**pansinusitis**   Inflammation of all the sinuses.

**PAP (Papanicolaou) smear**   Test for the early detection of cancer of the cervix named after the developer of the test, George Papanicolaou, a Greek physician. A scraping of cells is removed from the cervix for examination under a microscope.

**papilledema**   Swelling of the optic disk, often as a result of increased intraocular pressure. Also called choked disk.

**papule**   Small, solid, circular raised spot on the surface of the skin, often as a result of an inflammation in an oil gland.

**paracentesis**   Insertion of a needle into the abdominal cavity to withdraw fluid; tests to diagnose disease may be conducted on the fluid.

**paralysis**   Temporary or permanent loss of function or voluntary movement.

**paranasal sinuses**   Air-filled cavities within the facial bones that open into the nasal cavity; act as an echo chamber during sound production.

**paranoid personality**   A personality disorder characterized by exaggerated feelings of persecution.

**paraplegia**   Paralysis of the lower portion of the body and both legs.

**parasympathetic**   A branch of the autonomic nervous system. This system serves as a counterbalance for the sympathetic nerves. Therefore, it causes the heart rate to slow down, lower the blood pressure, constrict eye pupils, and increase digestion.

**parathyroid glands**   Four small glands located on the back surface of the thyroid gland. The parathyroid hormone secreted by these glands regulates the amount of calcium in the blood.

**parathyroid hormone**   The hormone secreted by the parathyroid glands. The more hormone, the higher the calcium level in the blood and the lower the level stored in bone. A low hormone level will cause tetany.

**parathyroidectomy**   Excision of one or more of the parathyroid glands. This is performed to halt the progress of hyperparathyroidism.

**parathyroidoma**   A parathyroid gland tumor.

**parenteral**   A route for introducing medication other than through the gastrointestinal tract; most commonly involves injection into the body through a needle and syringe.

**paresthesia**   An abnormal sensation such as burning or tingling.

**parietal**   Term meaning the outermost layer.

**parietal bone**   A cranial bone.

**parietal layer**   The outer pleural layer around the lungs. It lines the inside of the chest cavity.

**parietal lobe**   One of the four cerebral hemisphere lobes. It receives and interprets nerve impulses from sensory receptors.

**parietal pericardium**   The outer layer of the pericardium surrounding the heart.

**parietal peritoneum**   The outer layer of the serous membrane sac lining the abdominopelvic cavity.

**parietal pleura**   The outer layer of the serous membrane sac lining the thoracic cavity.

**Parkinson's disease**   Chronic disorder of the nervous system with fine tremors, muscular weakness, rigidity, and a shuffling gait.

**paronychia**   Infection around a nail.

**parotid glands**   A pair of salivary glands located in front of the ears.

**paroxysmal nocturnal dyspnea (PND)**   Attacks of shortness of breath (SOB) that occur only at night and awaken the patient.

**parturition**   Childbirth.

**passive acquired immunity**   Immunity that results when a person receives protective substances produced by another human or animal. This may take the form of maternal antibodies crossing the placenta to a baby or an antitoxin injection.

**passive aggressive personality**   A personality disorder in which the person expresses feelings or anger or hostility through indirect or covert actions.

**passive range of motion (PROM)**   Therapist putting a patient's joints through a full range of motion without assistance from the patient.

**patella**   Also called the kneecap. It is a lower extremity bone.

**patellar**   Pertaining to the patella or kneecap.

**patent**   Open or unblocked, such as a patent airway.

**patent ductus arteriosus**   Congenital heart anomaly in which the opening between the pulmonary artery and the aorta fails to close at birth. This condition requires surgery.

**pathogenic**   Microscopic organisms, such as bacteria, that are capable of causing disease.

**pathogens**   Disease-bearing organisms.

**pathologic fracture** Fracture caused by diseased or weakened bone.

**pathological gambling** An impulse control disorder in which the patient is unable to control the urge to gamble.

**pathologist** A physician who specializes in evaluating specimens removed from living or dead patients.

**Pathologist's Report** A medical record report given by a pathologist who studies tissue removed from the patient (for example: bone marrow, blood, or tissue biopsy).

**pathology** The branch of medicine specializing in studying how disease affects the body.

**pectoral girdle** Consists of the clavicle and scapula; functions to attach the upper extremity to the axial skeleton.

**pediculosis** Infestation with lice.

**pedophilia** A sexual disorder characterized by having sexual interest in children.

**pelvic** Pertaining to the pelvis.

**pelvic cavity** The inferior portion of the abdominopelvic cavity.

**pelvic examination** Physical examination of the vagina and adjacent organs performed by a physician placing the fingers of one hand into the vagina. A visual examination is performed using a speculum.

**pelvic girdle** Consists of the ilium, ischium, and pubis; functions to attach the lower extremity to the axial skeleton.

**pelvic inflammatory disease (PID)** Any inflammation of the female reproductive organs, generally bacterial in nature.

**pelvic ultrasonography** Use of ultrasound waves to produce an image or photograph of an organ, such as the uterus, ovaries, or fetus.

**pelvimetry** Measurement of the pelvic area, which helps in determining if the fetus can be delivered vaginally.

**pemphigus vulgaris** Blisters forming in the skin and mucous membranes.

**penis** The penis is the male sex organ. It is composed of erectile tissue that becomes erect during sexual stimulation, allowing it to be placed within the female vagina for ejaculation of semen. The larger, soft tip is referred to as the glans penis.

**peptic ulcer** Ulcer occurring in the lower portion of the esophagus, stomach, and duodenum and thought to be caused by the acid of gastric juices.

**percussion** Use of the fingertips to tap the body lightly and sharply. Aids in determining the size, position, and consistency of the underlying body part.

**percutaneous transhepatic cholangiography (PTC)** A contrast medium is injected directly into the liver to visualize the bile ducts. Used to detect obstructions.

**percutaneous transluminal coronary angioplasty (PTCA)** Method for treating localized coronary artery narrowing. A balloon catheter is inserted through the skin into the coronary artery and inflated to dilate the narrow blood vessel.

**pericardial cavity** Cavity formed by the serous membrane sac surrounding the heart.

**pericardiocentesis** Insertion of a needle into the pericardial sac for the purpose of aspirating excess fluid around the heart.

**pericarditis** Inflammatory process or disease of the pericardium.

**pericardium** The double-walled outer sac around the heart. The inner layer of the pericardium is called the epicardium, the outer layer is the heart itself. This sac contains pericardial fluid that reduces friction caused by the heart beating.

**peridontal disease** Disease of the supporting structures of the teeth, including the gums and bones.

**perimetritis** Inflammation around the uterus.

**perimetrium** The outer layer of the uterus.

**perineum** In the male, the external region between the scrotum and anus. In the female, the external region between the vagina and anus.

**perioperative** The period of time that includes before, during, and after a surgical procedure.

**periosteum** The membrane that covers most bones. It contains numerous nerves and lymphatic vessels.

**peripheral nervous system** The portion of the nervous system that contains the cranial nerves and spinal nerves. These nerves are mainly responsible for voluntary muscle movement, smell, taste, sight, and hearing.

**peripheral neuropathy** Damage to the nerves in the lower legs and hands as a result of diabetes mellitus; symptoms include either extreme sensitivity or numbness and tingling.

**peripheral vascular disease** Any abnormal condition affecting blood vessels outside the heart; symptoms may include pain, pallor, numbness, and loss of circulation and pulses.

**peristalsis** The wave-like muscular movements in the wall of the digestive system tube—esophagus, stomach, small intestines, and colon—that function to move food along the tube.

**peristaltic waves** The wave-like contractions of the muscles in a tubular organ, such as the ureters, that propel forward any substance inside the tube.

**peritoneal dialysis** Removal of toxic waste substances from the body by placing warm chemically balanced solutions into the peritoneal cavity. Used in treating renal failure and certain poisonings.

**peritoneum** Membranous sac that lines the abdominal cavity and encases the abdominopelvic organs. The kidneys are an exception since they lay outside the peritoneum and alongside the vertebral column.

**peritonsillar abscess** Infection of the tissues between the tonsils and the pharynx. Also called a quinsy sore throat.

**peritubular capillaries** Capillary bed surrounding the renal tubules.

**permanent teeth** The 32 permanent teeth begin to erupt at about the age of 6. Generally complete by the age of 16.

**pernicious anemia** Anemia associated with insufficient absorption of vitamin $B_{12}$ by the digestive system.

**personality disorders** Inflexible or maladaptive behavior patterns that affect a person's ability to function in society. Includes paranoid personality disorder, narcissistic personality disorder, antisocial personality disorder, and passive aggressive personality.

**perspiration** Another term for sweating.

**pertussis** A contagious bacterial infection of the larynx, trachea, and bronchi characterized by coughing attacks that end with a whooping sound. Also called whooping cough.

**petechiae** Flat, pinpoint, purplish spots from bleeding under the skin.

**petit mal**  A type of epilepsy seizure that lasts only a few seconds to half a minute, characterized by a loss of awareness and an absence of activity. It is also called an absence seizure.

**pH**  A number between 1 and 14 that indicates how acidic or basic a substance is. A solution with a pH of 1 is very acidic, 7 is neutral, and 14 is very basic.

**phacoemulsification**  Use of high-frequency sound waves to emulsify (liquefy) a lens with a cataract, which is then aspirated (removed by suction) with a needle.

**phagocyte**  Neutrophil component of the blood; has the ability to ingest and destroy bacteria.

**phagocytosis**  The process of engulfing or ingesting material. Several types of white blood cells function by engulfing bacteria.

**phalangeal**  Pertaining to the phalanges or finger and toe bones.

**phalanges**  The finger bones in the upper extremities and the toe bones in the lower extremities.

**pharmaceutical**  Related to medications or pharmacies.

**pharmacist (RPh or PharmD)**  Receives drug requests made by physicians, and gathers pertinent information that would affect the dispensing of certain drugs, reviews patients' medications for drug interactions, provides health care workers with information regarding drugs, and educates the public.

**pharmacology**  Study of the origins, nature, properties, and effects of drugs on the living organism.

**pharmacy technician**  Works under the supervision of a pharmacist. Duties include computer order entry, generating prescription labels, and keeping electronic patient profiles.

**pharyngeal tonsils**  Another term for adenoids. The tonsils are a collection of lymphatic tissue found in the nasopharynx to combat microorganisms entering the body through the nose.

**pharyngitis**  Inflammation of the mucous membrane of the pharynx, usually caused by a viral or bacterial infection. Commonly called a sore throat.

**pharynx**  Medical term for the throat. The passageway that conducts air from the nasal cavity to the trachea, and also carries food and drink from the mouth to the esophagus. The pharynx is divided into three sections: the nasopharynx, oropharynx, and laryngopharynx.

**pheochromocytoma**  Usually benign tumor of the adrenal medulla that secretes epinephrine; symptoms include anxiety, heart palpitations, dyspnea, profuse sweating, headache, and nausea.

**phimosis**  Narrowing of the foreskin over the glans penis that results in difficulty with hygiene. This condition can lead to infection or difficulty with urination. It is treated with circumcision, the surgical removal of the foreskin.

**phlebitis**  Inflammation of a vein.

**phleborrhaphy**  Suturing a vein.

**phlebotomist**  A specialist in drawing venous blood samples.

**phlebotomy**  Creating an opening into a vein to withdraw blood.

**phlegm**  Thick mucus secreted by the membranes that line the respiratory tract. When phlegm is coughed through the mouth, it is called *sputum*. Phlegm is examined for color, odor, and consistency.

**phobias**  A type of anxiety disorder in which a person has irrational fears. An example is photophobia, the fear of light.

**phonophoresis**  The use of ultrasound waves to introduce medication across the skin into the subcutaneous tissues.

**photon absorptiometry**  Measurement of bone density using an instrument for the purpose of detecting osteoporosis.

**photophobia**  Fear of light.

**photorefractive keratectomy (PRK)**  Use of a laser to reshape the cornea to correct errors of refraction.

**photosensitivity**  Condition in which the skin reacts abnormally when exposed to light such as the ultraviolet rays of the sun.

**physiatrist**  Physician specializing in rehabilitation or physical medicine.

**physical medicine**  Use of natural methods, including physical therapy, to cure diseases and disorders.

**physical therapist (PT or DPT)**  Specializes in programs for movement dysfunction and physical disabilities resulting from muscle, bone, joint, and nerve injuries or disease.

**physical therapy (PT)**  Treating disorders using physical means and methods. Physical therapy personnel assess joint motion, muscle strength and endurance, function of heart and lungs, and performance of activities required in daily living, along with other responsibilities. Physical therapy treatment includes gait training, therapeutic exercise, massage, joint and soft tissue mobilization, thermal and cryotherapy, electrical stimulation, ultrasound, and hydrotherapy. These methods strengthen muscles, improve motion and circulation, reduce pain, and increase function.

**physical therapy assistant (PTA)**  Performs physical therapy procedures under the supervision of a physical therapist.

**physician assistant (PA)**  Performs many of the tasks traditionally performed by physicians, such as conducting physical examinations, ordering tests and treatments, making diagnoses, counseling patients, assisting in surgery, and writing prescriptions.

***Physician's Desk Reference***  A resource for drug information. It is an easy-to-use resource and should be in every physician's office or medical facility.

**physician's offices**  Individual or groups of physicians providing diagnostic and treatment services in a private office setting rather than a hospital.

**physician's orders**  Medical record document that contains a complete list of the care, medications, tests, and treatments the physician orders for the patient.

**physician's progress notes**  Part of a patient's medical record. It is the physician's daily record of the patient's condition, results of the physician's examinations, summary of test results, updated assessment and diagnoses, and further plans for the patient's care.

**pia mater**  The term means soft mother. This thin innermost meninges layer is applied directly to the surface of the brain.

**pineal gland**  A gland in the endocrine system that produces a hormone called melatonin.

**pink eye**  A common term for conjunctivitis.

**pinna**  Also called the auricle. The external ear, which functions to capture sound waves as they go past the outer ear.

**pituitary gland**   An endocrine gland located behind the optic nerve in the brain. It is also called the master gland since it controls the functions of many other endocrine glands. It is divided into two lobes: anterior and posterior. The anterior pituitary gland secretes hormones that aid in controlling growth and stimulating the thyroid gland, sexual glands, and adrenal cortex. The posterior pituitary is responsible for the antidiuretic hormone and oxytocin.

**placebo**   Inactive, harmless substance used to satisfy a patient's desire for medication. It is also given to control groups of patients in research studies in which another group receives a drug. The effect of the placebo versus the drug is then observed.

**placenta**   Also called afterbirth. An organ attached to the uterine wall that is composed of maternal and fetal tissues. Oxygen, nutrients, carbon dioxide, and wastes are exchanged between the mother and baby through the placenta. The baby is attached to the placenta by way of the umbilical cord.

**placenta previa**   Occurs when the placenta is in the lower portion of the uterus and thus blocks the birth canal.

**placental stage**   The third stage of labor, which takes place after delivery of the infant. The uterus resumes strong contractions and the placenta detaches from the uterine wall and is delivered through the vagina.

**plantar flexion**   Bend sole of foot; point toes downward.

**plaque**   Gummy mass of microorganisms that grows on the crowns of teeth and spreads along the roots. It is colorless and transparent.

**plasma**   The liquid portion of blood containing 90% water. The remaining 10% consists of plasma proteins (serum albumin, serum globulin, fibrinogen, and prothrombin), inorganic substances (calcium, potassium, and sodium), organic components (glucose, amino acids, cholesterol), and waste products (urea, uric acid, ammonia, and creatinine).

**plasma proteins**   Proteins that are found in plasma. Includes serum albumin, serum globulin, fibrinogen, and prothrombin.

**plasmapheresis**   Method of removing plasma from the body without depleting the formed elements; whole blood is removed and the cells and plasma are separated; the cells are returned to the patient along with a donor plasma transfusion.

**platelet count**   Blood test to determine the number of platelets in a given volume of blood.

**platelets**   Cells responsible for the coagulation of blood. These are also called thrombocytes and contain no hemoglobin.

**pleura**   A protective double layer of serous membrane around the lungs. The parietal membrane is the outer layer and the visceral layer is the inner membrane. It secretes a thin, watery fluid to reduce friction associated with lung movement.

**pleural cavity**   Cavity formed by the serous membrane sac surrounding the lungs.

**pleural effusion**   Abnormal presence of fluid or gas in the pleural cavity. Physicians can detect the presence of fluid by tapping the chest (percussion) or listening with a stethoscope (auscultation).

**pleural rub**   Grating sound made when two surfaces, such as the pleura surfaces, rub together during respiration. It is caused when one of the surfaces becomes thicker as a result of inflammation or other disease conditions. This rub can be felt through the fingertips when they are placed on the chest wall or heard through the stethoscope.

**pleurisy**   Inflammation of the pleura.

**pleurocentesis**   A puncture of the pleura to withdraw fluid from the thoracic cavity in order to diagnose disease.

**pleuropexy**   Surgical fixation of the pleura.

**plication**   Taking tucks surgically in a structure to shorten it.

**pneumoconiosis**   Condition resulting from inhaling environmental particles that become toxic, such as coal dust (anthracosis) or asbestos (asbestosis).

*Pneumocystis carinii* **pneumonia (PCP)**   Pneumonia with a nonproductive cough, very little fever, and dyspnea. Seen in persons with weakened immune systems, such as patients with AIDS.

**pneumoencephalography (PEG)**   X-ray examination of the brain following withdrawal of cerebrospinal fluid and injection of air or gas via spinal puncture.

**pneumonectomy**   Surgical removal of lung tissue.

**pneumonia**   Inflammatory condition of the lung, which can be caused by bacterial and viral infections, diseases, and chemicals.

**pneumonomycosis**   Disease of the lungs caused by a fungus.

**pneumothorax**   Collection of air or gas in the pleural cavity, which can result in the collapse of a lung.

**podiatrist**   Specialist in treating disorders of the feet.

**poliomyelitis**   Acute viral disease that causes an inflammation of the gray matter of the spinal cord, resulting in paralysis in some cases. Has been brought under almost total control through vaccinations.

**polyarteritis**   Inflammation of many arteries.

**polycystic kidneys**   Formation of multiple cysts within the kidney tissue; results in the destruction of normal kidney tissue and uremia.

**polycythemia vera**   Production of too many red blood cells in the bone marrow.

**ploydipsia**   Condition of having an excessive amount of thirst, such as in diabetes.

**polyethylene tube (PE tube)**   Small tube surgically placed in a child's ear to assist in drainage of infection.

**polymyositis**   Disease involving muscle inflammation and weakness from an unknown cause.

**polyneuritis**   Inflammation of many nerves.

**polyp**   Small tumor with a pedicle or stem attachment. They are commonly found in vascular organs such as the nose, uterus, and rectum.

**polyphagia**   To eat excessively.

**polyposis**   Small tumors that contain a pedicle or foot-like attachment in the mucous membranes of the large intestine (colon).

**polyuria**   Condition of having excessive urine production. This can be a symptom of disease conditions such as diabetes.

**pons**   This portion of the brain stem forms a bridge between the cerebellum and cerebrum. It is also where nerve fibers cross from one side of the brain to control functions and movement on the other side of the brain.

**positron emission tomography (PET)**   Use of positive radionuclides to reconstruct brain sections. Measurements can be taken of oxygen and glucose uptake, cerebral blood flow, and blood volume.

**posterior**  Directional term meaning near or on the back or spinal cord side of the body.

**posterior lobe**  The posterior portion of the pituitary gland. It secretes antidiuretic hormone and oxytocin.

**posteroanterior (PA) and lateral of the chest**  Routine X-ray of the heart and lungs.

**postoperative**  The period of time immediately following the surgery.

**postpartum**  Period immediately after delivery or childbirth.

**postprandial**  Pertaining to after a meal.

**postural drainage**  Draining secretions from the bronchi by placing the patient in a position that uses gravity to promote drainage. Used for the treatment of cystic fibrosis and bronchiectasis, and before lobectomy surgery.

**postural drainage with clapping**  Drainage of secretions from the bronchi or a lung cavity by having the patient lie so that gravity allows drainage to occur. Clapping is using the hand in a cupped position to perform percussion on the chest. Assists in loosening secretions and mucus.

**potassium**  An inorganic substance found in plasma. It is important for bones and muscles.

**potentiation**  Giving a patient a second drug to boost (potentiate) the effect of another drug; the total strength of the drugs is greater than the sum of the strength of the individual drugs.

**preeclampsia**  Toxemia of pregnancy that, if untreated, can result in true eclampsia. Symptoms include hypertension, headaches, albumin in the urine, and edema.

**prefix**  A word part added in front of the word root. It frequently gives information abou the location of the organ, the number of parts or the time (frequency). Not all medical terms have a prefix.

**pregnancy**  The time from fertilization of an ovum to the birth of the newborn.

**pregnancy test**  Chemical test that can determine a pregnancy during the first few weeks. Can be performed in a physician's office or with a home-testing kit.

**premature**  Early.

**premature ejaculation**  A sexual disorder characterized by rapid sexual climax and ejaculation.

**premenstrual syndrome (PMS)**  Symptoms that develop just prior to the onset of a menstrual period, which can include irritability, headache, tender breasts, and anxiety.

**premolar**  Another term for the bicuspid teeth.

**prenatal visits**  Appointments with a physician or nurse practitioner for the purpose of monitoring the mother's pregnancy.

**preoperative (preop, pre-op)**  The period of time preceding surgery.

**prepuce**  Also called the foreskin. A protective covering over the glans penis. It is this covering of the skin that is removed during circumcision.

**presbycusis**  Loss of hearing that can accompany the aging process.

**presbyopia**  Visual loss due to old age, resulting in difficulty in focusing for near vision (such as reading).

**prescription**  A written explanation to the pharmacist regarding the name of the medication, the dosage, and the times of administration.

**prescription drug**  A drug that can only be ordered by a licensed physician, dentist, or veterinarian.

**primary site**  Designates where a malignant tumor first appeared.

**primigravida**  Woman who has been pregnant once.

**primipara**  Woman who has given birth once.

**probe**  A surgical instrument used to explore tissue.

**process**  A projection from the surface of a bone.

**proctology**  Branch of medicine specializing in conditions of the lower gastrointestinal system.

**proctoplasty**  Plastic surgery of the anus and rectum.

**proctoptosis**  Drooping rectum.

**proctoscopy**  Examination of the anus and rectum with an endoscope inserted through the rectum.

**progesterone**  One of the hormones produced by the ovaries. It works with estrogen to control the menstrual cycle.

**prolactin**  A hormone secreted by the anterior pituitary. It stimulates milk production.

**prolapsed umbilical cord**  When the umbilical cord of the baby is expelled first during delivery and is squeezed between the baby's head and the vaginal wall. This presents an emergency situation since the baby's circulation is compromised.

**prolapsed uterus**  Fallen uterus that can cause the cervix to protrude through the vaginal opening. Generally caused by weakened muscles from vaginal delivery or as the result of pelvic tumors pressing down.

**pronation**  To turn downward or backward, as with the hand or foot.

**prone**  Directional term meaning lying horizontally facing downward.

**prophylaxis**  Prevention of disease. For example, an antibiotic can be used to prevent the occurrence of a disease.

**proprietary name**  The name a pharmaceutical company chooses as the trademark or market name for its drug. Also called brand or trade name.

**prostate cancer**  Slow-growing cancer that affects a large number of males after age 50. The PSA (prostate-specific antigen) test is used to assist in early detection of this disease.

**prostate gland**  A gland in the male reproductive system that produces fluids that nourish the sperm.

**prostate-specific antigen (PSA)**  A blood test to screen for prostate cancer. Elevated blood levels of PSA are associated with prostate cancer.

**prostatectomy**  Surgical removal of the prostate gland.

**prostatitis**  Inflamed condition of the prostate gland that may be a result of an infection.

**prostatolith**  Prostate stone.

**prostatolithotomy**  Incision into the prostate in order to remove a stone.

**prostatorrhea**  Discharge from the prostate gland.

**prosthesis**  Artificial device used as a substitute for a body part that is either congenitally missing or absent as a result of accident or disease; for instance, an artificial leg or hip prosthesis.

**prosthetics**  Artificial devices, such as limbs and joints, that replace a missing body part.

**prosthetist**  Person who fabricates and fits prostheses.

**protein-bound iodine test (PBI)**  Blood test to measure the concentration of thyroxine ($T_4$) circulating in the blood stream. The iodine becomes bound to the protein in the blood and can be measured. Useful in establishing thyroid function.

**prothrombin**  Protein element within the blood that interacts with calcium salts to form thrombin.

**prothrombin time (Pro time)**  Measurement of the time it takes for a sample of blood to coagulate.

**protocol**  The actual plan of care, including the medications, surgeries, and treatments for the care of a patient. Often, the entire health care team, including the physician, oncologist, radiologist, nurse, and patient, will assist in designing the treatment plan.

**proton pump inhibitor**  Blocks the stomach's ability to secrete acid. Used to treat peptic ulcers and gastroesophageal reflux disease.

**protozoans**  Single-celled organisms that can infect the body.

**proximal**  Directional term meaning located closest to the point of attachment to the body.

**proximal convoluted tubule**  A portion of the renal tubule.

**pruritus**  Severe itching.

**pseudocyesis**  False pregnancy.

**pseudohypertrophic muscular dystrophy**  One type of inherited muscular dystrophy in which the muscle tissue is gradually replaced by fatty tissue, making the muscle look strong.

**psoriasis**  Chronic inflammatory condition consisting of crusty papules forming patches with circular borders.

**psychiatric mental health technician**  Works under the supervision of physicians, psychologists, and nurses; also known as psychiatric aides.

**psychiatric nurse**  A nurse with additional training in the care of patients with mental, emotional, and behavioral disorders.

**psychiatric social worker**  A social worker with additional training in the care of patients with mental, emotional, or behavioral disorders.

**psychiatrist (MD or DO)**  A physician with specialized training in diagnosing and treating mental disorders; prescribes medication and conducts counseling.

**psychiatry**  The branch of medicine that deals with the diagnosis, treatment, and prevention of mental disorders.

**psychologist**  Specialist trained in the study of psychological analysis, therapy, and research.

**psychology**  The study of human behavior and thought process. This behavioral science is primarily concerned with understanding how human beings interact with their physical environment and with each other.

**psychopathy**  Disease of the mind.

**psychopharmacology**  The study of the effects of drugs on the mind and particularly the use of drugs in treating mental disorders. The main classes of drugs for the treatment of mental disorders are antipsychotic drugs, antidepressant drugs, minor tranquilizers, and lithium.

**psychosis**  Severe mental disorder with symptoms such as depression and anxiety. The patient is not in touch with reality and may withdraw into an inner world, as in schizophrenia, or become severely emotionally impaired, as in mania.

**psychotherapy**  A method of treating mental disorders by mental rather than chemical or physical means. It includes psychoanalysis, humanistic therapies, and family and group therapy.

**puberty**  Beginning of menstruation and the ability to reproduce. Usually occurs around 16 years of age.

**pubic**  Pertaining to the pubis; one of the pelvic bones.

**pubic symphysis**  The point where the left and right pubic bones meet and are held together by a thick piece of cartilage, making it a cartilaginous joint.

**pubis**  One of the three bones that form the os coxae or innominate bone.

**puerperium**  Term used when discussing the mother's first 3 to 6 weeks after childbirth.

**pulmonary**  Pertaining to the lung.

**pulmonary angiography**  Injecting dye into a blood vessel for the purpose of taking an X-ray of the arteries and veins of the lungs.

**pulmonary artery**  The large artery that carries deoxygenated blood from the right ventricle to the lung.

**pulmonary capillaries**  Network of capillaries in the lungs that tightly encase each alveolus; sight of gas exchange.

**pulmonary circulation**  The pulmonary circulation transports deoxygenated blood from the right side of the heart to the lungs where oxygen and carbon dioxide are exchanged. Then it carries oxygenated blood back to the left side of the heart.

**pulmonary edema**  Condition in which lung tissue retains an excessive amount of fluid. Results in labored breathing.

**pulmonary embolism**  Blood clot or air bubble in the pulmonary artery or one of its branches.

**pulmonary function test (PFT)**  Breathing equipment used to determine respiratory function and measure lung volumes and gas exchange.

**pulmonary medicine**  The study of diseases of the respiratory system. Also called thoracic medicine.

**pulmonary valve**  The semilunar valve between the right ventricle and pulmonary artery in the heart. It prevents blood from flowing backwards into the ventricle.

**pulmonary vein**  Large vein that returns oxygenated blood from the lungs to the left atrium.

**pulmonologist**  A physician specialized in treating diseases and disorders of the respiratory system.

**pulmonology**  Branch of medicine specializing in conditions of the respiratory system.

**pulp cavity**  The hollow interior of a tooth; contains soft tissue made up of blood vessels, nerves, and lymph vessels.

**pulse**  Expansion and contraction produced by blood as it moves through an artery. The pulse can be taken at several pulse points throughout the body where an artery is close to the surface.

**pupil**  The hole in the center of the iris. The size of the pupil is changed by the iris dilating or constricting.

**Purkinje fibers**   Part of the conduction system of the heart; found in the ventricular myocardium.

**purpura**   Hemorrhages into the skin and mucous membranes.

**purulent**   Pus-filled sputum, which can be the result of infection.

**pustule**   Raised spot on the skin containing pus.

**pyelitis**   Inflammation of the renal pelvis.

**pyelogram**   X-ray record of the renal pelvis after injection of a radiopaque dye.

**pyelonephritis**   Inflammation of the renal pelvis and the kidney. One of the most common types of kidney disease. It may be the result of a lower urinary tract infection that moved up to the kidney by way of the ureters. There may be large quantities of white blood cells and bacteria in the urine, and blood (hematuria) may even be present in the urine in this condition. Can occur with any untreated or persistent case of cystitis.

**pyeloplasty**   Surgical repair of the renal pelvis.

**pyloric sphincter**   Sphincter at the distal end of the stomach. Controls the passage of food into the duodenum.

**pyloric stenosis**   Condition in which the pyloric sphincter becomes abnormally narrow. Food is not able to pass from the stomach into the small intestines. The main symptom is emesis or vomiting.

**pyogenic**   Pus-forming.

**pyorrhea**   Discharge of purulent material from dental tissue.

**pyosalpinx**   Condition of having pus in the fallopian tubes.

**pyothorax**   Condition of having pus in the chest cavity.

**pyromania**   An impulse control disorder in which the patient is unable to control the impulse to start fires.

**pyuria**   Presence of pus in the urine.

**quadriplegia**   Paralysis of all four extremities. Same as tetraplegia.

**radial**   Pertaining to the radius; a lower arm bone.

**radial keratotomy**   Spoke-like incisions around the cornea that result in it becoming flatter; a surgical treatment for myopia.

**radiation therapy**   Use of X-rays to treat disease, especially cancer.

**radical mastectomy**   Surgical removal of the breast tissue plus chest muscles and axillary lymph nodes.

**radical surgery**   Extensive surgery to remove as much tissue associated with a tumor as possible.

**radiculitis**   Nerve root inflammation.

**radioactive**   Substance capable of emitting or sending out radiant energy.

**radioactive implant**   Embedding a radioactive source directly into tissue to provide a highly localized radiation dosage to damage nearby cancerous cells. Also called brachytherapy.

**radioactive iodine uptake test (RAIU)**   Test in which radioactive iodine is taken orally (PO) or intravenously (IV) and the amount that is eventually taken into the thyroid gland (the uptake) is measured to assist in determining thyroid function.

**radiography**   Making of X-ray pictures.

**radioimmunoassay (RIA)**   Test used to measure the levels of hormones in the plasma of the blood.

**radioisotope**   Radioactive form of an element.

**radiologist**   Physician who practices diagnosis and treatment by the use of radiant energy. He or she is responsible for interpreting X-ray films.

**radiology**   The branch of medicine that uses radioactive substances such as X-rays, isotopes, and radiation to prevent, diagnose, and treat diseases.

**radiolucent**   Structures that allow X-rays to pass through and expose the photographic plate, making it appear as a black area on the X-ray, are termed radiolucent.

**radiopaque**   Structures that are impenetrable to X-rays, appearing as a light area on the radiograph (X-ray).

**radius**   One of the forearm bones in the upper extermity.

**rales**   Abnormal crackling sound made during inspiration. Usually indicates the presence of moisture and can indicate a pneumonia condition.

**range of motion**   The range of movement of a joint, from maximum flexion through maximum extension. It is measured as degrees of a circle.

**Raynaud's phenomenon**   Periodic ischemic attacks affecting the extremities of the body, especially the fingers, toes, ears, and nose. The affected extremities become cyanotic and very painful. These attacks are brought on by arterial constriction due to extreme cold or emotional stress.

**reabsorption**   Second phase of urine production; substances needed by the body are reabsorbed as the filtrate passes through the kidney tubules.

**rectal**   Introduced directly into the rectal cavity in the form of suppositories or solution. Drugs may have to be administered by this route if the patient is unable to take them by mouth due to nausea, vomiting, and surgery.

**rectocele**   Protrusion or herniation of the rectum into the vagina.

**rectum**   An area at the end of the digestive tube for storage of feces that leads to the anus.

**rectus abdominis**   A muscle named for its location and the direction of its fibers: rectus means straight and abdominis means abdominal.

**rectus muscle**   Rectus means straight. Four of the eye muscles are rectus muscles.

**red blood cell count (RBC)**   Blood test to determine the number of erythrocytes in a volume of blood; a decrease in red blood cells may indicate anemia; an increase may indicate polycythemia.

**red blood cell morphology**   Examination of blood for abnormalities in the shape (morphology) of the erythrocytes. Used to determine diseases like sickle-cell anemia.

**red blood cells**   Also called erythrocytes or RBCs. Cells that contain hemoglobin, and iron-containing pigment that binds oxygen in order to transport it to the cells of the body.

**red bone marrow**   Tissue that manufactures most of the blood cells. It is found in cancellous bone cavities.

**reduction**   Correcting a fracture by realigning the bone fragments. Closed reduction is doing this without entering the body. Open reduction is making a surgical incision at the site of the fracture to do the reduction, often necessary where there are bony fragments to be removed.

**refraction**   Eye examination performed by a physician to determine and correct refractive errors in the eye.

**refractive error**   Defect in the ability of the eye to focus accurately on the image hitting it. Occurs in farsightedness and nearsightedness.

**regional anesthesia**   Regional anesthesia is also referred to as a nerve block. This anesthetic interrupts a patient's pain sensation in a particular region of the body. The anesthetic is injected near the nerve that will be blocked from sensation. The patient usually remains conscious.

**registered dental hygienist (RDH)**   Specializes in cleaning teeth and taking X-rays.

**registered dietitian (RD)**   Promotes health and prevents or treats illnesses through diet modification and nutritional education.

**registered health information administrator (RHIA)**   Directs the functioning of a health information department.

**registered health information technician (RHIT)**   Makes certain that medical records are complete and accurate.

**registered nurse (RN)**   Assesses patient status and progress, provides patient care, administers medications, and provides patient education.

**registered radiologic technologist (RRT)**   Performs imaging procedures as ordered by a physician including X-rays, computed tomography, MRI, and fluoroscopy.

**registered respiratory therapist (RRT)**   Develops and implements respiratory care plans, performs diagnostic tests, provides respiratory treatments, and participates in patient education.

**regurgitation**   Return of fluids and solids from the stomach into the mouth. Similar to *emesis* but without the force.

**rehabilitation**   Process of treatment and exercise that can help a person with a disability attain maximum function and well-being.

**rehabilitation centers**   Facilities that provide intensive physical and occupational therapy. They include inpatient and outpatient treatment.

**reinfection**   An infection that occurs when a person becomes infected again with the same pathogen that originally brought him or her to the hospital.

**remission**   Period during which the symptoms of a disease or disorder leave. Can be temporary.

**renal artery**   Artery that originates from the abdominal aorta and carries blood to the nephrons of the kidney.

**renal colic**   Pain caused by a kidney stone, which can be excruciating and generally requires medical treatment.

**renal corpuscle**   Part of a nephron. It is a double-walled cup-like structure called the glomerular capsule or Bowman's capsule and contains a capillary network called the glomerulus. An afferent arteriole carries blood to the glomerulus and an efferent arteriole carries blood away from the glomerulus. The filtration stage of urine production occurs in the renal corpuscle as wastes are filtered from the blood in the glomerulus and enter Bowman's capsule.

**renal failure**   Inability of the kidneys to filter wastes from the blood resulting in uremia; may be acute or chronic; major reason for a patient being placed on dialysis.

**renal papilla**   Tip of a renal pyramid.

**renal pelvis**   Large collecting site for urine within the kidney. Collects urine from each calyx. Urine leaves the renal pelvis via the ureter.

**renal pyramids**   Triangular-shaped region of the renal medulla.

**renal transplant**   Surgical replacement of a donor kidney.

**renal tubule**   Network to tubes found in a nephron. It consists of the proximal convoluted tubule, the loop of Henle, the distal tubule, and the collecting tubule. The reabsorption and secretion stages of urine production occur within the renal tubule. As the glomerular filtrate passes through the renal tubule, most of the water and some of the dissolved substances, such as amino acids and electrolytes, are reabsorbed. At the same time, substances that are too large to filter into Bowman's capsule, such as urea, are secreted directly from the bloodstream into the renal tubule. The filtrate that reaches the collecting tubule becomes urine.

**renal vein**   Vein that carries blood away from the kidneys.

**resection**   To surgically cut out; excision.

**residual hearing**   Amount of hearing that is still present after damage has occurred to the auditory mechanism.

**respiratory membrane**   Formed by the tight association of the walls of alveoli and capillaries; gas exchange between lungs and blood occurs across this membrane.

**respiratory system**   System that brings oxygen into the lungs and expels carbon dioxide. Organs include the nose, pharynx, larynx, trachea, bronchial tubes, and lungs.

**retina**   The innermost layer of the eye. It contains the visual receptors called rods and cones. The rods and cones receive the light impulses and transmit them to the brain via the optic nerve.

**retinal**   Pertaining to the retina.

**retinal blood vessels**   The blood vessels that supply oxygen to the rods and cones of the retina.

**retinal detachment**   Occurs when the retina becomes separated from the choroids layer. This separation seriously damages blood vessels and nerves resulting in blindness.

**retinitis pigmentosa**   Progressive disease of the eye that results in the retina becoming hard (sclerosed), pigmented (colored), and atrophied (wasting away). There is no known cure for this condition.

**retinoblastoma**   Malignant glioma of the retina.

**retinopathy**   Retinal disease.

**retinopexy**   Surgical fixation of the retina.

**retrograde pyelogram**   A diagnostic X-ray in which dye is inserted through the urethra to outline the bladder, ureters, and renal pelvis.

**retroperitoneal**   Pertaining to behind the peritoneum. Used to describe the position of the kidneys, which is outside of the peritoneal sac alongside the spine.

**retrovirus**   Virus, such as HIV, in which the virus copies itself using the host's DNA.

**Reye's syndrome**   A brain inflammation that occurs in children following a viral infection, usually the flu or chickenpox. It is characterized by vomiting and lethargy and may lead to coma and death.

**Rh factor**   An antigen marker found on erythrocytes of persons with Rh+ blood.

**rhabdomyolysis**  Skeletal muscle destruction.

**rhabdomyoma**  Skeletal muscle tumor.

**rheumatic heart disease**  Valvular heart disease as a result of having had rheumatic fever.

**rheumatoid arthritis (RA)**  Chronic form of arthritis with inflammation of the joints, swelling, stiffness, pain, and changes in the cartilage that can result in crippling deformities.

**rhinitis**  Inflammation of the nose.

**rhinomycosis**  Condition of having a fungal infection in the nose.

**rhinoplasty**  Plastic surgery of the nose.

**rhinorrhagia**  Rapid and excessive flow of blood from the nose.

**rhinorrhea**  Watery discharge from the nose, especially with allergies or a cold, runny nose.

**Rh-negative**  A person with Rh- blood type. The person's RBCs do not have the Rh marker and will make antibodies against Rh+ blood.

**rhonchi**  Somewhat musical sound during expiration, often found in asthma or infection, and caused by spasms of the bronchial tubes. Also called wheezing.

**Rh-positive**  A person with Rh+ blood type. The person's RBCs have the Rh marker.

**rhytidectomy**  Surgical removal of excess skin to eliminate wrinkles. Commonly referred to as a facelift.

**rhytidoplasty**  Excision of wrinkles.

**rib cage**  Also called the chest cavity. It is the cavity formed by the curved ribs extending from the vertebral column around the sides and attaching to the sternum. The ribs are part of the axial skeleton.

**rickets**  Deficiency in calcium and vitamin D found in early childhood that results in bone deformities, especially bowed legs.

**right hypochondriac**  An anatomical division of the abdomen; the right upper row.

**right iliac**  An anatomical division of the abdomen; the right lower row. Also called the right inguinal.

**right lower quadrant (RLQ)**  A clinical division of the abdomen. It contains portions of small and large intestines, right ovary and fallopian tube, appendix, right ureter.

**right lumbar**  An anatomical division of the abdomen, the right middle row.

**right lymphatic duct**  One of two large lymphatic ducts. It drains right arm and the right side of the neck and chest; empties lymph into the right subclavian vein.

**right upper quadrant (RUQ)**  A clinical division of the abdomen. It contains the right lobe of the liver, the gallbladder, a portion of the pancreas, and portions of small and large intestine.

**Rinne and Weber tuning-fork tests**  The physician holds a tuning fork, an instrument that produces a constant pitch when it is struck against or near the bones on the side of the head. These tests assess both nerve and bone conduction of sound.

**rods**  The sensory receptors of the retina that are active in dim light and do not perceive color.

**roentgen**  Unit for describing an exposure dose of radiation.

**roentgenology**  X-rays.

**Romberg's test**  Test used to establish neurological function in which the person is asked to close his or her eyes and place their feet together. This test for body balance is positive if the patient sways when the eyes are closed.

**root**  The portion of a tooth below the gum line.

**root canal**  Dental treatment involving the pulp cavity of the root of a tooth. Procedure is used to save a tooth that is badly infected or abscessed.

**rotation**  Moving around a central axis.

**rubella**  Contagious viral skin infection; commonly called German measles.

**rugae**  The prominent folds in the mucosa of the stomach. They smooth out and almost disappear allowing the stomach to expand when it is full of food.

**saccule**  Found in the inner ear. It plays a role in equilibrium.

**sacral**  Pertaining to the sacrum.

**sacrum**  The five fused vertebrae that form a large flat bone in the upper buttock region.

**sagittal plane**  A vertical plane that divides the body into left and right sections.

**saliva**  Watery fluid secreted into the mouth from the salivary glands; contains digestive enzymes that break down carbohydrates and lubricants that make it easier to swallow food.

**salivary glands**  Exocrine glands with ducts that open into the mouth. They produce saliva, which makes the bolus of food easier to swallow and begins the digestive process. There are three pairs of salivary glands: parotid, submandibular, and sublingual.

**salpingitis**  Inflammation of the fallopian tube or tubes.

**salpingocyesis**  Tubal pregnancy.

**salpingostomy**  The creation of an artificial opening in a fallopian tube.

**salpingotomy**  Incision into the fallopian tubes.

**sanguinous**  Pertaining to blood.

**sarcoidosis**  Inflammatory disease of the lymph system in which lesions may appear in the liver, skin, lungs, lymph nodes, spleen, eyes, and small bones of the hands and feet.

**scabies**  Contagious skin disease caused by an egg-laying mite that causes intense itching; often seen in children.

**scalpel**  A surgical instrument used to cut and separate tissue.

**scan**  Recording the emission of radioactive waves on a photographic plate after a substance has been injected into the body.

**scapula**  Also called the shoulder blade. An upper extremity bone.

**scapular**  Pertaining to the scapula or shoulder blade.

**schizophrenia**  Mental disorders characterized by distortions of reality such as delusions and hallucinations.

**sciatica**  Pain in the low back that radiates down the back of a leg caused by pressure on the sciatic nerve from a herniated nucleus pulposus.

**sclera**  The tough protective outer layer of the eyeball. It is commonly referred to as the white of the eye.

**scleral buckling**  Placing a band of silicone around the outside of the sclera to stabilize a detaching retina.

**scleritis**   Inflammation of the sclera.

**scleroderma**   Disorder in which the skin becomes taut, thick, and leather-like.

**scleromalacia**   Softening of the sclera.

**sclerotomy**   Incision into the sclera.

**scoliosis**   Abnormal lateral curvature of the spine.

**scratch test**   Form of allergy testing in which the body is exposed to an allergen through a light scratch in the skin.

**scrotum**   A sac that serves as a container for the testes. This sac, which is divided by a septum, supports the testicles and lies between the legs and behind the penis.

**scrub nurse**   Surgical assistant who hands instruments to the surgeon. This person wears sterile clothing and maintains the sterile operative field.

**sebaceous cyst**   Sac under the skin filled with sebum or oil from a sebaceous gland. This can grow to a large size and may need to be excised.

**sebaceous gland**   Also called oil glands. They produce a substance called sebum that lubricates the skin surface.

**seborrhea**   Excessive discharge of sebum.

**sebum**   Thick, oily substance secreted by sebaceous glands that lubricates the skin to prevent drying out. When sebum accumulates, it can cause congestion in the sebaceous glands and whiteheads or pimples may form. When the sebum becomes dark it is referred to as a comedo or blackhead.

**secretion**   Third phase of urine production; additional waste products are added to the filtrate as it passes through the kidney tubules.

**sedative**   Produces relaxation without causing sleep.

**seizure**   Sudden attack of severe muscular contractions associated with a loss of consciousness. This is seen in grand mal epilepsy.

**self-innoculation**   Infection that occurs when a person becomes infected in a different part of the body by a pathogen from another part of his or her own body, such as intestinal bacteria spreading to the urethra.

**semen**   Semen contains sperm and fluids secreted by male reproductive system glands. It leaves the body through the urethra.

**semen analysis**   This procedure is used when performing a fertility workup to determine if the male is able to produce sperm. Semen is collected by the patient afer abstaining from sexual intercourse for a period of three to five days. The sperm in the semen are analyzed for number, swimming strength, and shape. This is also used to determine if a vasectomy has been successful. After a period of six weeks, no sperm should be present in a sample from the patient.

**semicircular canals**   A portion of the labyrinth associated with balance and equilibrium.

**semilunar valve**   The heart valves located between the ventricles and the great arteries leaving the heart. The pulmonary valve is located between the right ventricle, and the pulmonary artery and the aortic valve are located between the left ventricle and the aorta.

**seminal vesicles**   Two male reproductive system glands located at the base of the bladder. They secrete a fluid that nourishes

the sperm into the vas deferens. This fluid plus the sperm constitutes much of the semen.

**seminiferous tubules**   Network of coiled tubes that make up the bulk of the testes. Sperm development takes place in the walls of the tubules and the mature sperm are released into the tubule in order to leave the testes.

**sensorineural hearing loss**   Type of hearing loss in which the sound is conducted normally through the external and middle ear but there is a defect in the inner ear or with the cochlear nerve, resulting in the inability to hear. A hearing aid may help.

**sensory neurons**   Nerves that carry sensory information from sensory receptors to the brain; also called afferent neurons.

**sensory receptors**   Nerve fibers that are located directly under the surface of the skin. These receptors detect temperature, pain, touch, and pressure. The messages for these sensations are conveyed to the brain and spinal cord from the nerve endings in the skin.

**septicemia**   Having bacteria in the blood stream; commonly referred to as blood poisoning.

**septoplasty**   Surgical repair of the septum.

**sequential multiple analyzer computer (SMAC)**   Machine for doing multiple blood chemistry tests automatically.

**serous**   Watery secretion of serous membranes.

**serous membrane**   These membranes are found lining body cavities and secrete a thin, watery fluid that acts as a lubricant as organs rub against one another.

**serum**   Clear, sticky fluid that remains after the blood has clotted.

**serum bilirubin**   Blood test to determine the amount of the waste product bilirubin in the bloodstream; elevated levels indicate liver disease.

**serum electrolyte level**   A laboratory test to measure the amount of sodium, potassium, and chloride ions in the blood.

**serum glucose tests**   Blood test performed to assist in determining insulin levels and useful for adjusting medication dosage.

**serum lipoprotein level**   A laboratory test to measure the amount of cholesterol and triglycerides in the blood.

**severe combined immunodeficiency syndrome (SCIDS)**   Disease seen in children born with a nonfunctioning immune system; often forced to live in sealed sterile rooms.

**sexual disorders**   Disorders include aberrant sexual activity and sexual dysfunction; includes pedophilia, masochism, voyeurism, low sex drive, and premature ejaculation.

**sexually transmitted disease (STD)**   Disease usually acquired as the result of sexual intercourse; formerly more commonly referred to as venereal disease.

**shield**   Protective device used to protect against radiation.

**shingles**   Eruption of vesicles along a nerve, causing a rash and pain. Caused by the same virus as chickenpox.

**short bone**   A type of bone that is roughly cube shaped. The carpals are short bones.

**shortness of breath (SOB)**   Term used to indicate that a patient is having some difficulty breathing. The cause can range from mild SOB after exercise to SOB associated with heart disease.

**sialadenitis**   Inflammation of a salivary gland.

**sialolith**   A salivary gland stone.

**sickle cell anemia**   Severe, chronic, incurable disorder that results in anemia and causes joint pain, chronic weakness, and infections. It is more common in people of Mediterranean and African heritage. The actual blood cell is crescent shaped.

**side effect**   Response to a drug other than the effect desired.

**sigmoid colon**   The final section of colon. It follows an S-shaped path and terminates in the rectum.

**sigmoidoscope**   Instrument to view inside the sigmoid colon.

**sigmoidoscopy**   Using a flexible sigmoidoscope to visually examine the sigmoid colon; commonly done to diagnose cancer and polyps.

**Signing Exact English (SEE-2)**   Translation of English into signs. American Sign Language (ASL) is used in combination with other sign languages and fingerspelling to correspond exactly to the spoken English.

**silicosis**   Form of respiratory disease resulting from the inhalation of silica (quartz) dust. Considered an occupational disease.

**simple fracture**   Fracture with no open skin or wound.

**simple mastectomy**   Surgical removal of the breast tissue.

**sinoatrial node (SA)**   Also called the pacemaker of the heart. It is an area of the right atria that initiates the electrical pulse that causes the heart to contract.

**sinus**   A hollow cavity within a bone.

**skeletal muscle**   A voluntary muscle that is attached to bones by a tendon.

**skin**   The major organ of the integumentary system. It forms a barrier between the external and internal environments.

**skin graft**   The transfer of skin from a normal area to cover another site. Used to treat burn victims and after some surgical procedures.

**skin test (ST)**   Test to determine the patient's reaction to a suspected allergen by injecting a small amount under the skin (interdermal) with a needle. The reaction of the patient to this material is then read to indicate any allergy. Examples of such tests are the tuberculin (TB) test, Mantoux (PPD) test, patch test, and Schick test.

**sleep disorder**   Any condition that interferes with sleep other than environmental noises. Can include difficulty sleeping (insomnia), nightmares, night terrors, sleepwalking, and apnea.

**sleepwalking**   A sleeping disorder in which the patient performs complex activities while asleep.

**slit lamp microscope**   Instrument used in ophthalmology for examining the posterior surface of the cornea.

**small intestine**   The portion of the digestive tube between the stomach and colon, and the major site of nutrient absorption. There are three sections: duodenum, jejunum, and ileum.

**smooth muscle**   An involuntary muscle found in internal organs such as the digestive organs or blood vessels.

**Snellen's chart**   Chart used for testing distance vision. It contains letters of varying size and is administered from a distance of 20 feet. A person who can read at 20 feet what the average person can read at that distance is said to have 20/20 vision.

**sodium**   An inorganic substance found in plasma.

**somatic**   Pertaining to the body.

**somatic nerves**   Nerves that serve the skin and skeletal muscles and are mainly involved with the conscious and voluntary activities of the body.

**somatoform disorders**   Patient has physical symptoms for which no physical disease can be determined; includes hypochondria and conversion reaction.

**somatotropin**   Another name for growth hormone; a hormone that promotes growth of the body by stimulating cells to rapidly increase in size and divide.

**spasm**   A sudden, involuntary, strong muscle contraction.

**special sense organs**   The special sense organs perceive environmental conditions. The eyes, ears, nose, and tongue contain special sense organs.

**specialty care hospitals**   Hospitals that provide care for very specific types of disease. A good example is a psychiatric hospital.

**speculum**   A surgical instrument used to spread apart walls of a cavity.

**speech-language pathologist (CCC)**   Evaluates and treats communication disorders.

**speechreading**   Ability to watch a person's mouth and word formation during speaking to interpret what they are saying. Also referred to as lipreading.

**sperm**   Also called spermatozoon (plural is spermatozoa). The male sex cell. One sperm fuses with the ova to produce a new being.

**spermatic cord**   The term for the cord-like collection of structures that include the vas deferens, arteries, veins, nerves, and lymph vessels. The spermatic cord suspends the testes within the scrotum.

**spermatogenesis**   Formation of mature sperm.

**spermatolysis**   Destruction of sperm.

**spermatolytic**   Destruction of spermatozoa.

**spermatozoa**   Also called sperm, the singular is spermatozoon. The male sex cell. One sperm fuses with the ova to produce a new being.

**spermatozoon**   Also called sperm, the plural is spermatozoa. The male sex cell. One sperm fuses with the ova to produce a new being.

**sphenoid bone**   A cranial bone.

**sphincter**   A ring of muscle around a tubular organ. It can contract to control the opening of the tube.

**sphygmomanometer**   Instrument for measuring blood pressure. Also referred to as a blood pressure cuff.

**spina bifida**   Congenital defect in the walls of the spinal canal in which the laminae of the vertebra do not meet or close. Results in membranes of the spinal cord being pushed through the opening. Can also result in other defects, such as hydrocephalus.

**spinal**   Pertaining to the spine.

**spinal cavity**   A dorsal body cavity within the spinal column that contains the spinal cord.

**spinal cord**   The spinal cord provides a pathway for impulses traveling to and from the brain. It is a column of nerve fibers that extends from the medulla oblongata of the brain down to the level of the second lumbar vertebra.

**spinal cord injury (SCI)**   Bruising or severing of the spinal cord from a blow to the vertebral column resulting in muscle paralysis and sensory impairment below the injury level.

**spinal fusion**   Surgical immobilization of adjacent vertebrae. This may be done for several reasons, including correction for a herniated disk.

**spinal nerves**   The nerves that arise from the spinal cord.

**spinal stenosis**   Narrowing of the spinal canal causing pressure on the cord and nerves.

**spiral fracture**   Fracture in an "S"-shaped spiral. It can be caused by a twisting injury.

**spirometer**   Instrument consisting of a container into which a patient can exhale for the purpose of measuring the air capacity of the lungs.

**spirometry**   Using a device to measure the breathing capacity of the lungs.

**spleen**   Organ in the lymphatic system that filters microorganisms and old red blood cells from the blood.

**splenectomy**   Excision of the spleen.

**splenomegaly**   Enlargement of the spleen.

**splenopexy**   Artificial fixation of a movable spleen.

**spondylolisthesis**   The forward sliding of a lumbar vertebra over the vertebra below it.

**spondylosis**   A degenerative condition of the vertebral column.

**spongy bone**   The bony tissue found inside a bone. It contains cavities that hold red bone marrow. Also called cancellous bone.

**spontaneous abortion**   Loss of a fetus without any artificial aid. Also called a miscarriage.

**sprain**   Pain and disability caused by trauma to a joint. A ligament may be torn in severe sprains.

**sputum**   Mucus or phlegm that is coughed up from the lining of the respiratory tract. Tested to determine what type of bacteria of virus is present as an aid in selecting the proper antibiotic treatment.

**sputum culture and sensitivity (C&S)**   Testing sputum by placing it on a culture medium and observing any bacterial growth. The specimen is then tested to determine antibiotic effectiveness.

**sputum cytology**   Testing for malignant cells in sputum.

**squamous cell carcinoma**   Epidermal cancer that may go into deeper tissue but does not generally metastasize.

**staging**   The process of classifying tumors based on their degree of tissue invasion and the potential response to therapy. The TNM staging system is frequently used. The T refers to the tumor's size and invasion, the N refers to lymph node involvement, and the M refers to the presence of metastases of the tumor cells.

**staging laparotomy**   Surgical procedure in which the abdomen is entered to determine the extent and staging of a tumor.

**stapedectomy**   Removal of the stapes bone to treat otosclerosis (hardening of the bone). A prosthesis or artificial stapes may be implanted.

**stapes**   One of the three ossicles of the middle ear. It is attached to the oval window leading to the inner ear. Also called the stirrup.

**steatorrhea**   Passage of a large amount of fat in the stool; caused by an inability to digest fats usually due to a problem with the pancreatic enzymes.

**stent**   A stainless steel tube placed within a blood vessel or a duct to widen the lumen.

**sterility**   Inability to father children due to a problem with spermatogenesis.

**sterilization**   Process of rendering a male or female sterile or unable to conceive children.

**sternal**   Pertaining to the sternum or breast bone.

**sternum**   Also called the breast bone. It is part of the axial skeleton and the anterior attachment for ribs.

**steroid sex hormones**   A class of hormones secreted by the adrenal cortex. It includes aldosterone, cortisol, androgens, estrogens, and progestins.

**stethoscope**   Instrument for listening to body sounds, such as the chest, heart, or intestines.

**stillbirth**   Birth in which a viable-aged fetus dies before or at the time of delivery.

**stomach**   A J-shaped muscular organ that acts as a sac to collect, churn, digest, and store food. It is composed of three parts: the fundus, body, and antrum. Hydrochloric acid is secreted by glands in the mucous membrane lining of the stomach. Food mixes with other gastric juices and the hydrochloric acid to form a semisoft mixture called chyme, which then passes into the duodenum.

**stool culture**   A laboratory test of feces to determine if there are any pathogenic bacteria present.

**strabismus**   An eye muscle weakness resulting in each eye looking in a different direction at the same time. May be corrected with glasses, eye exercises, and/or surgery. Also called lazy eye or crossed eyes.

**strabotomy**   Incision into the eye muscles in order to correct strabismus.

**strain**   Trauma to muscle from excessive stretching or pulling.

**stratified squamous epithelial**   Describes the layers of flat or scale-like cells found in the epidermis. Stratified means multiple layers and squamous means flat.

**stress/exercise testing**   Method for evaluating cardiovascular fitness. The patient is placed on a treadmill or a bicycle and then subjected to steadily increasing levels of work. An EKG and oxygen levels are taken while the patient exercises.

**stricture**   Narrowing of a passageway in the urinary system.

**stridor**   Harsh, high-pitched, noisy breathing sound that is made when there is an obstruction of the bronchus or larynx. Found in conditions such as croup in children.

**subarachnoid space**   The space located between the arachnoid layer and pia mater. It contains cerebrospinal fluid.

**subcutaneous**   Pertaining to under the skin.

**subcutaneous layer**   This is the deepest layer of the skin where fat is formed. This layer of fatty tissue protects the deeper tissues of the body and acts as an insulation for heat and cold.

**subdural hematoma**   Mass of blood forming beneath the dura mater of the brain.

**subdural space**   The space located between the dura mater and the arachnoid layer.

**sublingual**   Pertaining to under the tongue.

**sublingual glands**   A pair of salivary glands in the floor of the mouth.

**submandibular glands**   A pair of salivary glands in the floor of the mouth.

**substance-related disorders**   Overindulgence or dependence on chemical substances including alcohol, illegal drugs, and prescription drugs.

**sudden infant death syndrome (SIDS)**   The sudden, unexplained death of an infant in which a postmortem examination fails to determine the cause of death.

**suffix**   A word part attached to the end of a word. It frequently indicates a condition, disease, or procedure. Almost all medical terms have a suffix.

**sulci**   Also called fissures. The grooves that separate the gyri of the cerebral cortex.

**superficial**   Directional term meaning toward the surface of the body.

**superior**   Directional term meaning toward the head, or above.

**superior venae cavae**   The branch of the vena cavae that drains blood from the chest and upper body.

**supination**   Turn the palm or foot upward.

**supine**   Directional term meaning lying horizontally and facing upward.

**suppositories**   A method for administering medication by placing it in a substance that will melt after being placed in a body cavity, usually rectally, and release the medication.

**suppurative**   Containing or producing pus.

**surgeon**   A physician who has completed additional training of 5 years or more in a surgical specialty area. The specialty areas include orthopedics, neurosurgery, gynecology, ophthalmology, urology, and thoracic, vascular, cardiac, plastic, and general surgery.

**surgery**   The branch of medicine dealing with operative procedures to correct deformities and defects, repair injuries, and diagnose and cure diseases.

**surgical center**   A facility that provides services that range from simple surgeries to diagnostic testing to therapy and do not require overnight hospitalization. Also called an ambulatory care center or an outpatient clinic.

**surgical technologist**   Assists physicians and other health care workers before, during, and after surgery.

**suture material**   Used to close a wound or incision. Examples are catgut, silk thread, or staples. They may or may not be removed when the wound heals, depending on the type of material that is used.

**sutures**   The fibrous joints formed between the cranial bones.

**sweat duct**   Duct leading from a sweat gland to the surface of the skin; carries sweat.

**sweat glands**   Glands that produce sweat, which assists the body in maintaining its internal temperature by creating a cooling effect when it evaporates.

**sweat pore**   The surface opening of a sweat duct.

**sweat test**   Test performed on sweat to determine the level of chloride. There is an increase in skin chloride in the disease cystic fibrosis.

**sympathectomy**   Excision of a portion of the sympathetic nervous system. Could include a nerve or a ganglion.

**sympathetic**   A branch of the autonomic nervous system. This system stimulates the body in times of stress and crisis by increasing heart rate, dilating airways to allow for more oxygen, increasing blood pressure, inhibiting digestion, and stimulating the production of adrenaline during a crisis.

**synapse**   The point at which the axon of one neuron meets the dendrite of the next neuron.

**syncope**   Fainting

**syndrome**   Group of symptoms and signs that when combined present a clinical picture of a disease or condition.

**synovial fluid**   The fluid secreted by a synovial membrane in a synovial joint. It lubricates the joint and reduces friction.

**synovial joint**   A freely moving joint that is lubricated by synovial fluid.

**synovial membrane**   The membrane that lines a synovial joint. It secretes a lubricating fluid called synovial fluid.

**syphilis**   Infectious, chronic, venereal disease that can involve any organ. May exist for years without symptoms. Treated with the antibiotic pencillin.

**systemic**   Pertaining to a system.

**systemic circulation**   The systematic circulation transports oxygenated blood from the left side of the heart to the cells of the body and then back to the right side of the heart.

**systemic lupus erythematosus (SLE)**   Chronic disease of the connective tissue that injures the skin, joints, kidneys, nervous system, and mucous membranes. May produce a characteristic butterfly rash across the cheeks and nose.

**systems**   A system is composed of several organs working in a compatible manner to perform a complex function or functions. Examples include the digestive system, the cardiovascular system, and the respiratory system.

**systole**   The period of time during which a heart chamber is contracting.

**systolic pressure**   The maximum pressure within blood vessels during a heart contraction.

$T_3$   Abbreviation for triiodothyronine, a thyroid hormone.

$T_4$   Abbreviation for thyroxine, a thyroid hormone.

**T cells**   A lymphocyte active in cellular immunity.

**T lymphocytes**   A type of lymphocyte involved with producing cells that physically attack and destroy pathogens.

**tachycardia**   Abnormally fast heart rate, over 100 bpm.

**tachypnea**   Rapid breathing rate.

**tagging**   Attachment of a radioactive material to a chemical and tracing it as it moves through the body.

**talipes**   Congenital deformity of the foot. Also referred to as a clubfoot.

**target organs**   The organs that hormones act on to either increase or decrease the organ's activity level.

**tarsals**   The ankle bones in the lower extremity.

**taste buds**   Found on the surface of the tongue; designed to detect bitter, sweet, sour, and salty flavors in our food.

**tears**   Fluid that washes and lubricates the anterior surface of the eyeball.

**teeth**   Structures in mouth that mechanically break up food into smaller pieces during chewing.

**temporal bone**   A cranial bone.

**temporal lobe** One of the four cerebral hemisphere lobes. It controls hearing and smell.

**temporomandibular joint (TMJ) disease** Inflammation of the jaw joint resulting in pain and poor bite.

**tenaculum** A long-handled clamp surgical instrument.

**tendinous** Pertaining to a tendon.

**tendon** The strong connective tissue cords that attach skeletal muscles to bones.

**tendonitis** Inflammation of tendon.

**tendoplasty** Surgical repair of a tendon.

**tendotomy** Incision into a tendon.

**tenodynia** Pain in a tendon.

**tenomyopathy** Disease of tendons and muscles.

**tenorrhaphy** Suture a tendon.

**testes** The male gonads. The testes are oval glands located in the scrotum that produce sperm and the male hormone, testosterone.

**testicles** Also called testes (singular is testis). These oval-shaped organs are responsible for the development of sperm within the seminiferous tubules. The testes must be maintained at the proper temperature for the sperm to survive. This lower temperature level is controlled by the placement of the scrotum outside the body. The hormone testosterone, which is responsible for the growth and development of the male reproductive organs, is also produced by the testes.

**testicular carcinoma** Cancer of one or both testicles.

**testicular torsion** A twisting of the spermatic cord.

**testosterone** Male hormone produced in the testes. It is responsible for the growth and development of the male reproductive organs.

**tetany** A condition the results from a calcium deficiency in the blood. It is characterized by muscle twitches, cramps, and spasms.

**tetralogy of Fallot** Combination of four congenital anomalies: pulmonary stenosis, an interventricular septal defect, abnormal blood supply to the aorta, and hypertrophy of the right ventricle. Needs immediate surgery to correct.

**tetraplegia** Paralysis of all four limbs. Same as quadriplegia.

**thalamus** The thalamus is a portion of the diencephalon. It is composed of gray matter and acts as a center for relaying impulses from the eyes, ears, and skin to the cerebrum. Pain perception is also controlled by the thalamus.

**thalassemia** A genetic disorder in which the person is unable to make functioning hemoglobin; results in anemia.

**therapeutic abortion** The termination of a pregnancy for the health of the mother.

**therapeutic exercise** Exercise planned and carried out to achieve a specific physical benefit, such as improved range of motion, muscle strength, or cardiovascular function.

**thermotherapy** Applying heat to the body for therapeutic purposes.

**thoracalgia** Chest pain.

**thoracentesis** Surgical puncture of the chest wall for the removal of fluids.

**thoracic** Pertaining to the chest.

**thoracic cavity** A ventral body cavity in the chest area that contains the lungs and heart.

**thoracic duct** The largest lymph vessel. It drains the entire body except for the right arm, chest wall, and both lungs. It empties lymph into the left subclavian vein.

**thoracic surgeon** A physician specialized in treating conditions and diseases of the respiratory system by surgical teams.

**thoracic surgery** Branch of medicine specializing in surgery on the respiratory system and thoracic cavity.

**thoracic vertebrae** The 12 vertebrae in the chest region.

**thoracostomy** Insertion of a tube into the chest for the purpose of draining off fluid or air.

**thoracotomy** Incision into the chest.

**thrombectomy** Surgical removal of a thrombus or blood clot from a blood vessel.

**thrombin** A clotting enzyme that converts fibrinogen to fibrin.

**thrombocytes** Also called platelets. Platelets play a critical part in the blood-clotting process by agglutinating into small clusters and releasing thrombokinase.

**thrombocytopenia** Too few clotting cells (platelets).

**thrombocytosis** Too many clotting cells (platelets).

**thrombolytic** Able to dissolve existing blood clots.

**thrombolytic therapy** Drugs, such as streptokinase or tissue-type plasminogen activator, are injected into a blood vessel to dissolve clots and restore blood flow.

**thrombophlebitis** Inflammation of a vein that results in the formation of blood clots within the vein.

**thromboplastin** Substance released by platelets; reacts with prothrombin to form thrombin.

**thrombus** A blood clot.

**thymectomy** Removal of the thymus gland.

**thymoma** Malignant tumor of the thymus gland.

**thymosin** Hormone secreted by thymus gland. It causes lymphocytes to change into T-lymphocytes.

**thymus gland** An endocrine gland located in the upper mediastinum that assists the body with the immune function and the development of antibodies. As part of the immune response it secretes a hormone, thymosin, that changes lymphocytes to T cells.

**thyroid cartilage** A piece of cartilage associated with the larynx. It is also commonly called the Adam's apple and is larger in males.

**thyroid echogram** Ultrasound examination of the thyroid that can assist in distinguishing a thyroid nodule from a cyst.

**thyroid function tests (TFT)** Blood tests used to measure the levels of $T_3$, $T_4$, and TSH in the bloodstream to assist in determining thyroid function.

**thyroid gland** This endocrine gland is located on either side of the trachea. Its shape resembles a butterfly with a large left and right lobe connected by a narrow isthmus. This gland produces the hormones thyroxine (also known as $T_4$) and triiodothyronine (also known as $T_3$).

**thyroid replacement hormone** Given to replace thyroid in patients with hypothyroidism or who have had a thyroidectomy.

**thyroid scan** Test in which a radioactive element is administered that localizes in the thyroid gland. The gland can then be visualized with a scanning device to detect pathology such as tumors.

**thyroidectomy**   Removal of the entire thyroid or a portion (partial thyroidectomy) to treat a variety of conditions, including nodes, cancer, and hyperthyroidism.

**thyroidotomy**   Incision into the thyroid gland.

**thyroid-stimulating hormone**   A hormone secreted by the anterior pituitary. It regulates function of the thyroid gland.

**thyromegaly**   Enlarged thyroid.

**thyroparathyroidectomy**   Surgical removal (excision) of the thyroid and parathyroid glands.

**thyrotoxicosis**   Condition that results from overproduction of the thyroid glands. Symptoms include a rapid heart action, tremors, enlarged thyroid gland, exophthalmos, and weight loss.

**thyroxine ($T_4$)**   A hormone produced by the thyroid gland. It is also known as $T_4$ and requires iodine for its production. This hormone regulates the level of cell metabolism. The greater the level of hormone in the bloodstream, the higher cell metabolism will be.

**tibia**   Also called the shin bone. It is a lower extremity bone.

**tibial**   Pertaining to the tibia or shin bone.

**tic**   Spasmodic, involuntary muscular contraction involving the head, face, mouth, eyes, neck, and shoulders.

**tic douloureux**   Painful condition in which the trigeminal nerve is affected by pressure or degeneration. The pain is of a severe stabbing nature and radiates from the jaw and along the face.

**tinea**   Fungal skin disease resulting in itching, scaling lesions.

**tinea capitis**   Fungal infection of the scalp; commonly called ringworm.

**tinea pedis**   Fungal infection of the foot; commonly called athlete's foot.

**tinnitus**   Ringing in the ears.

**tissues**   Tissues are formed when cells of the same type are grouped to perform one activity. For example, nerve cells combine to form nerve fibers. There are four types of tissue: nerve, muscle, epithelial, and connective.

**tolerance**   Development of a capacity for withstanding a large amount of a substance, such as foods, drugs, or poison, without any adverse effect. A decreased sensitivity to further doses will develop.

**tongue**   A muscular organ in the floor of the mouth. Works to move food around inside the mouth and is also necessary for speech.

**tonometry**   Measurement of the intraocular pressure of the eye using a tonometer to check for the condition of glaucoma. After a local anesthetic is applied, the physician places the tonometer lightly upon the eyeball and a pressure measurement is taken. Generally part of a normal eye exam for adults.

**tonsillectomy**   Surgical removal of the tonsils.

**tonsillitis**   Inflammation of the tonsils.

**tonsils**   The collections of lymphatic tissue located in the pharynx to combat microorganisms entering the body through the nose or mouth. The tonsils are the pharyngeal tonsils, the palatine tonsils, and the lingual tonsils.

**topical**   Applied directly to the skin or mucous membranes. They are distributed in ointment, cream, or lotion form. Used to treat skin infections and eruptions.

**topical anesthesia**   Topical anesthesia is applied using either a liquid or gel placed directly onto a specific area. The patient remains conscious. This type of anesthetic is used on the skin, the cornea, and mucous membranes in dental work.

**torticollis**   Severe neck spasms pulling the head to one side; commonly called wryneck or a crick in the neck.

**total abdominal hysterectomy–bilateral salpingo-oophorectomy (TAH-BSO)**   Removal of the entire uterus, cervix, both ovaries, and both fallopian tubes.

**total calcium**   Blood test to measure the total amount of calcium to assist in detecting parathyroid and bone disorders.

**total hip replacement (THR)**   Surgical reconstruction of a hip by implanting a prosthetic or artificial hip joint.

**total knee replacement (TKR)**   Surgical reconstruction of a knee joint by implanting a prosthetic knee joint; also called total knee arthroplasty.

**toxic shock syndrome (TSS)**   Rare and sometimes fatal staphylococcus infection that generally occurs in menstruating women.

**toxicity**   Extent or degree to which a substance is poisonous.

**toxins**   Substances poisonous to the body. Many are filtered out of the blood by the kidney.

**trachea**   Also called the windpipe. It conducts air from the larynx down to the main bronchi in the chest.

**tracheostenosis**   Narrowing and stenosis of the lumen or opening into the trachea.

**tracheostomy**   Surgical procedure used to make an opening in the trachea to create an airway. A tracheostomy tube can be inserted to keep the opening patent.

**tracheotomy**   Surgical incision into the trachea to provide an airway.

**trachoma**   Chronic infectious disease of the conjunctiva and cornea caused by bacteria. Occurs more commonly in people living in hot, dry climates. Untreated, it may lead to blindness when the scarring invades the cornea. Trachoma can be treated with antibiotics.

**tract**   A bundle of fibers located within the central nervous system.

**traction**   Process of pulling or drawing, usually with a mechanical device. Used in treating orthopedic (bone and joint) problems and injuries.

**trade name**   The name a pharmaceutical company chooses as the trademark or market name for its drug. Also called proprietary or brand name.

**transcutaneous electrical nerve stimulation (TENS)**   Application of a mild electrical stimulation to skin via electrodes placed over a painful area, causing interference with the transmission of the painful stimuli. Can be used in pain management to interfere with the normal pain mechanism.

**transdermal**   Route of drug administration; medication coats the underside of a patch that is applied to the skin. The medication is then absorbed across the skin.

**transient ischemic attack (TIA)**   Temporary interference with blood supply to the brain, causing neurological symptoms such as dizziness, numbness, and hemiparesis. May lead eventually to a full-blown stroke (CVA).

**transurethral resection of the prostate (TUR)** Surgical removal of the prostate gland by inserting a device through the urethra and removing prostate tissue.

**transverse colon** The section of colon that crosses the upper abdomen from the right side of the body to the left.

**transverse fracture** Complete fracture that is straight across the bone at right angles to the long axis of the bone.

**transverse plane** A horizontal plane that divides the body into upper (superior) and lower (inferior) sections. Also called the horizontal plane.

**tremor** Involuntary quivering movement of a part of the body.

**Trendelenburg position** A surgical position in which the patient is lying face up and on an incline with the head lower than the legs.

**trephination** Process of cutting out a piece of bone in the skull to gain entry into the brain or relieve pressure.

**trephine** A surgical saw used to remove a disk-shaped piece of tissue.

**trichomoniasis** Genitourinary infection that is usually without symptoms (asymptomatic) in both males and females. In women the disease can produce itching and/or burning and a foul-smelling discharge, and can result in vaginitis.

**trichomycosis** Abnormal condition of hair fungus.

**tricuspid valve** A valve between the right atrium and ventricle of the heart. It prevents blood from flowing backwards into the atrium. A tricuspid valve has three cusps or flaps.

**triglycerides** Simple nutrient molecules absorbed from the intestines and circulated throughout the body.

**triiodothyronine (T₃)** A hormone produced by the thyroid gland known as $T_3$ that requires iodine for its production. This hormone regulates the level of cell metabolism. The greater the level of hormone in the blood stream, the higher cell metabolism will be.

**trochanter** The large blunt process that provides the attachment for tendons and muscles.

**tubal ligation** Surgical tying off of the fallopain tubes to prevent conception from taking place. Results in sterilization of the female.

**tubal pregnancy** Implantation of a fetus within the fallopian tube instead of the uterus. Requires immediate surgery.

**tubercle** A small, rounded process that provides the attachment for tendons and muscles.

**tuberculin skin tests (TB test)** Applying a chemical agent (Tine or Mantoux tests) under the surface of the skin to determine if the patient has been exposed to tuberculosis.

**tuberculosis (TB)** Infectious disease caused by the tubercle bacillus, *Myocobacterium tuberculosis*. Most commonly affects the respiratory system and causes inflammation and calcification of the system. Tuberculosis is again on the uprise and is seen in many patients who have AIDS.

**tuberosity** A large, rounded process that provides the attachment to tendons and muscles.

**tumor** Abnormal growth of tissue that may be benign or malignant. Also called a neoplasm.

**two-hour postprandial glucose tolerance test** Blood test to assist in evaluating glucose metabolism. The patient eats a high-carbohydrate diet and fasts overnight before the test. A blood sample is then taken 2 hours after a meal.

**tympanectomy** Excision of the eardrum.

**tympanic** Pertaining to the eardrum.

**tympanic membrane** Also called the eardrum. As sound moves along the auditory canal, it strikes the tympanic membrane causing it to vibrate. This conducts the sound wave into the middle ear.

**tympanitis** Eardrum inflammation.

**tympanometer** Instrument to measure the eardrum.

**tympanometry** Measurement of the movement of the tympanic membrane. Can indicate the presence of pressure in the middle ear.

**tympanoplasty** Another term for the surgical reconstruction of the eardrum. Also called myringoplasty.

**tympanorrhexis** Ruptured eardrum.

**tympanotomy** Incision into the eardrum.

**type 1 diabetes mellitus** Also called insulin-dependent diabetes mellitus (IDDM). It develops early in life when the pancreas stops insulin production. Therefore, persons with IDDM must take daily insulin injections.

**type 2 diabetes mellitus** Also called non–insulin-dependent diabetes mellitus (NIDDM). It develops later in life when the pancreas produces insufficient insulin. Persons may take oral hypoglycemics to stimulate insulin secretion, or may eventually have to take insulin.

**Type A** One of the ABO blood types. A person with type A markers on his or her RBCs. Type A blood will make anti-B antibodies.

**Type AB** One of the ABO blood types. A person with both type A and type B markers on his or her RBCs. Since it has both markers, it will not make antibodies against either A or B blood.

**type and crossmatch** Lab test performed before a person receives a blood transfusion; double checks the blood type of both the donor's and recipient's blood.

**Type B** One of the ABO blood types. A person with type B markers on his or her RBCs. Type B blood will make anti-A antibodies.

**Type O** One of the ABO blood types. A person with no markers on his or her RBCs. Type O blood will not react with anti-A or anti-B antibodies. Therefore, it is considered the universal donor.

**ulcer** Open sore or lesion in skin or mucous membrane.

**ulcerative colitis** Ulceration of unknown origin of the mucous membranes of the colon. Also known as inflammatory bowel disease (IBD).

**ulna** One of the forearm bones in the upper extremity.

**ulnar** Pertaining to the ulna, one of the lower arm bones.

**ultrasound (US)** The use of high-frequency sound waves to create heat in soft tissues under the skin. It is particularly useful for treating injuries to muscles, tendons, and ligaments, as well as muscle spasms. In radiology, ultrasound waves can be used to outline shapes of tissues, organs, and the fetus.

**umbilical** An anatomical division of the abdomen; the middle section of the middle row.

**umbilical cord** A cord extending from the baby's umbilicus (navel) to the placenta. It contains blood vessels that carry oxygen and nutrients from the mother to the baby and carbon dioxide and wastes from the baby to the mother.

**unconscious** Condition or state of being unaware of surroundings with the inability to respond to stimuli.

**ungual** Pertaining to the nails.

**unit dose** Drug dosage system that provides prepackaged, prelabeled, individual medications that are ready for immediate use by the patient.

**universal donor** Type O blood is considered the universal donor. Since it has no markers on the RBC surface, it will not trigger a reaction with anti-A or anti-B antibodies.

**universal recipient** A person with type AB blood has no antibodies against the other blood types and therefore, in an emergency, can receive any type of blood.

**upper extremity (UE)** The arm.

**upper gastrointestinal (UGI) series** Administering a barium contrast material orally and then taking an X-ray to visualize the esophagus, stomach, and duodenum.

**uptake** Absorption of radioactive material and medicines into an organ or tissue.

**urea** A waste product of protein metabolism. It diffuses through the tissues in lymph and is returned to the circulatory system for transport to the kidneys.

**uremia** An excess of urea and other nitrogenous waste in the blood.

**ureterectasis** Dilation of the ureter.

**ureterolith** A calculus in the ureter.

**ureterostenosis** Narrowing of the ureter.

**ureters** Organs in the urinary system that transport urine from the kidney to the bladder.

**urethra** The tube that leads from the urinary bladder to the outside of the body. In the male it is also used by the reproductive system to release semen.

**urethralgia** Urethral pain.

**urethritis** Inflammation of the urethra.

**urethrorrhagia** Rapid bleeding from the urethra.

**urethroscope** Instrument to view inside the urethra.

**urethrostenosis** Narrowing of the urethra.

**urgency** Feeling the need to urinate immediately.

**urinalysis (U/A, UA)** Laboratory test that consists of the physical, chemical, and microscopic examination of urine.

**urinary** Pertaining to urine.

**urinary bladder** Organ in the urinary system that stores urine.

**urinary incontinence** Involuntary release of urine. In some patients an indwelling catheter is inserted into the bladder for continuous urine drainage.

**urinary meatus** The external opening of the urethra.

**urinary retention** An inability to fully empty the bladder, often indicates a blockage in the urethra.

**urinary system** System that filters wastes from the blood and excretes the waste products in the form of urine. Organs include the kidneys, ureters, urinary bladder, and urethra.

**urinary tract infection (UTI)** Infection, usually from bacteria such as *E. coli*, of any organ of the urinary system; most often begins with cystitis and may ascend into the ureters and kidneys; most common in women because of their shorter urethra.

**urination** The release of urine from the urinary bladder.

**urine** It is the fluid that remains in the urinary system following the three stages of urine production: filtration, reabsorption, and secretion.

**urine culture and sensitivity** Laboratory test of urine for bacterial infection; attempt to grow bacteria on a culture medium in order to identify it and determine which antibiotics it is sensitive to.

**urinometer** Instrument to measure urine.

**urologist** A physician specialized in treating conditions and diseases of the urinary system and male reproductive system.

**urology** Branch of medicine specializing in conditions of the urinary system and male reproductive system.

**urticaria** Hives, a skin eruption of pale reddish wheals (circular elevations of the skin) with severe itching. Usually associated with food allergy, stress, or drug reactions.

**uterine tubes** Tubes that carry the ovum from the ovary to the uterus; also called fallopian tubes or oviducts.

**uterus** Also called the womb. An internal organ of the female reproductive system. This hollow, pear-shaped organ is located in the lower pelvic cavity between the urinary bladder and rectum. The uterus receives the fertilized ovum and it becomes implanted in the uterine wall, which provides nourishment and protection for the developing fetus. The uterus is divided into three regions: fundus, corpus, and cervix.

**utricle** Found in the inner ear. It plays a role in equilibrium.

**uvea** An alternate name for the choroid layer of the eye.

**uvula** Structure that hangs down from the posterior edge of the soft palate and helps in the production of speech and is the location of the gag reflex.

**vaccination** Providing protection against communicable diseases by stimulating the immune system to produce antibodies against that disease. Children can now be immunized for the following diseases: hepatitis B, diphtheria, tetanus, pertussis, tetanus, *Haemophilus influenzae* type b, polio, measles, mumps, rubella, and chickenpox. Also called immunization.

**vagina** Organ in the female reproductive system that receives the penis and semen.

**vaginal** Tablets and suppositories inserted vaginally and used to treat vaginal yeast infections and other irritations.

**vaginal hysterectomy** Removal of the uterus through the vagina rather than through an abdominal incision.

**vaginal orifice** The external vaginal opening. It may be covered by a hymen.

**vagotomy** Surgical resection of the vagus nerve in an attempt to decrease the amount of acid secretion into the stomach. Used as a method of treatment for patients with ulcers.

**valve replacement** Excision of a diseased heart valve and replacement with an artificial valve.

**valves** A flap-like structure found within the tubular organs such as lymph vessels, veins, and the heart. They function to prevent the backflow of fluid.

**valvular** Pertaining to a valve.

**valvulitis** Inflammation of a valve.

**varicella** Contagious viral skin infection; commonly called chickenpox.

**varicocele** Enlargement of the veins of the spermatic cord, which commonly occurs on the left side of adolescent males. Seldom needs treatment.

**varicose veins** Swollen and distended veins, usually in the legs.

**vas deferens** Also called ductus deferens. The vas deferens is a long, straight tube that carries sperm from the epididymis up into the pelvic cavity, where it continues around the bladder and empties into the urethra. It is one of the components, along with nerves and blood vessels, of the spermatic cord.

**vasectomy** Removal of a segment or all of the vas deferens to prevent sperm from leaving the male body. Used for contraception purposes.

**vasoconstrictor** Contracts smooth muscle in walls of blood vessels; raises blood pressure.

**vasodilator** Produces a relaxation of blood vessels to lower blood pressure.

**vasopressin** Given to control diabetes insipidus and promote reabsorption of water in the kidney tubules.

**vasovasostomy** Creation of a new opening between two sections of vas deferens. Used to reverse a vasectomy.

**veins** Blood vessels of the cardiovascular system that carry blood toward the heart.

**venereal disease (VD)** Disease usually acquired as the result of sexual intercourse; more commonly referred to as sexually transmitted disease.

**venipuncture** Puncture into a vein to withdraw fluids or to insert medication and fluids.

**venography** Process of taking an X-ray tracing of a vein.

**venotomy** Surgical incision into a vein.

**venous** Pertaining to a vein.

**ventilation and perfusion scan** A nuclear medicine diagnostic test that is especially useful in identifying pulmonary emboli. Radioactive air is inhaled for the ventilation portion to determine if air is filling the entire lung. Radioactive intravenous injection shows whether or not blood is flowing to all parts of the lung.

**ventral** Directional term meaning near or on the front or belly side of the body.

**ventricles** The two lower chambers of the heart that receive blood from the atria and pump it back out of the heart. The left ventricle pumps blood to the body, and the right ventricle pumps blood to the lungs. Also fluid-filled spaces within the cerebrum. These contain cerebrospinal fluid, which is the watery, clear fluid that provides a protection from shock or sudden motion to the brain.

**ventricular** Pertaining to a ventricle.

**venule** The smallest veins. Venules receive deoxygenated blood leaving the capillaries.

**verruca** Warts; a benign neoplasm (tumor) caused by a virus. Has a rough surface that is removed by chemicals and/or laser therapy.

**vertebral canal** The bony canal through the vertebrate that contains the spinal cord.

**vertebral column** The vertebral column is part of the axial skeleton. It is a column of 26 vertebra that forms the backbone and protects the spinal cord. It is divided into five sections: cervical vertebrae, thoracic vertebrae, lumbar vertebrae, sacrum, and coccyx. Also called spinal column.

**vertigo** Dizziness.

**vesicle** Small, fluid-filled raised spot on the skin.

**vestibular nerve** The branch of the vestibulocochlear nerve responsible for sending equilibrium information to the brain.

**vestibulocochlear nerve** The eighth cranial nerve. It is responsible for hearing and balance.

**viable** A fetus developed sufficiently to live outside the uterus.

**viruses** A group of infectious particles that cause disease.

**viscera** The name for the internal organs of the body, such as the lungs, stomach, and liver.

**visceral** Pertaining to the viscera or internal organs.

**visceral layer** The inner pleural layer. It adheres to the surface of the lung.

**visceral pericardium** The inner layer of the pericardium surrounding the heart.

**visceral peritoneum** The inner layer of the serous membrane sac encasing the abdominopelvic viscera.

**visceral pleura** The inner layer of the serous membrane sac encasing the thoracic viscera.

**visual acuity (VA)** Measurement of the sharpness of a patient's vision. Usually, a Snellen's chart is used for this test and the patient identifies letters from a distance of 20 feet.

**visual field** The size of the area perceived by one eye when it is stationary.

**vital signs (VS)** Respiration, pulse, temperature, skin color, blood pressure, and reaction of pupils. These are signs of the condition of body functions.

**Vitamin D therapy** Maintaining high blood levels of calcium in association with vitamin D helps maintain bone density and treats osteomalacia, osteoporosis, and rickets.

**vitiligo** Disappearance of pigment from the skin in patches, causing a milk-white appearance. Also called leukoderma.

**vitreous humor** The transparent jelly-like substance inside the eyeball.

**vocal cords** The structures within the larynx that vibrate to produce sound and speech.

**voiding** Another term for urination.

**voiding cystourethrography (VCUG)** X-ray taken to visualize the urethra while the patient is voiding after a contrast dye has been placed in the bladder.

**volvulus** Condition in which the bowel twists upon itself and causes a painful obstruction that requires immediate surgery.

**vomer bone** A facial bone.

**von Recklinghausen's disease** Excessive production of parathyroid hormone, which results in degeneration of the bones. Named for Friedrich von Recklinghausen, a German histologist.

**voyeurism** A sexual disorder characterized by receiving sexual gratification from observing others engaged in sexual acts.

**vulva** A general term meaning the external female genitalia. It consists of the Bartholin's glands, labia major, labia minora, and clitoris.

**waste products** Substances no longer needed by the body that are removed by the kidney during urine formation.

**Western blot** Test used as a backup to the ELISA blood test to detect the presence of the antibody to HIV (AIDS virus) in the blood.

**wet gangrene** Area of gangrene becoming infected by pus-producing bacteria.

**wheal** Small, round raised area on the skin that may be accompanied by itching.

**whiplash** Injury to the bones in the cervical spine as a result of a sudden movement forward and backward of the head and neck. Can occur as a result of a rear-end auto collision.

**whirlpool** Bath in which there are continuous jets of hot water reaching the body surfaces.

**white blood cell differential (diff)** Blood test to determine the number of each variety of leukocyte.

**white blood cells** Blood cells that provide protection against the invasion of bacteria and other foreign material.

**white blood count (WBC)** Blood test to measure the number of leukocytes in a volume of blood. An increase may indicate the presence of infection or a disease such as leukemia. A decrease in WBCs is caused by X-ray therapy and chemotherapy.

**white matter** Tissue in the central nervous system. It consists of myelinated nerve fibers.

**whole blood** Refers to the mixture of both plasma and formed elements.

**Wilm's tumor** Malignant kidney tumor found most often in children.

**word root** The foundation of a medical term that provides the basic meaning of the word. In general, the word root will indicate the body system or part of the body that is being discussed. A word may have more than one word root.

**xanthoderma** Yellow skin.

**xenograft** Skin graft from an animal of another species (usually pig); also called heterograft.

**xeroderma** Dry skin.

**xerophthalmia** Dry eyes.

**X-ray** High-energy wave that can penetrate most solid matter and present the image on photographic film.

**yellow bone marrow** Yellow bone marrow is located mainly in the center of the diaphysis of long bones. It contains mainly fat cells.

**zygomatic bone** A facial bone.

# A

Abbreviations, 12, 484–491. *See also* individual subject headings
Abdomen, 39–41
Abdominal, 41
Abdominal aortic aneurysm, 148*f*
Abdominal cavity, 38, 38*f*, 39
Abdominal ultrasonography, 253
Abdominopelvic cavity, 38, 38*f*, 39
Abducens nerve, 374*t*
Abduction, 111, 111*f*
ABGs, 216
Abnormal psychology, 445
ABO system, 169
Abortion, 302
Abrasion, 61
Abruptio placentae, 308
Abscess, 61
Absence seizure, 378
Acapnia, 210
Accessory nerve, 374*t*
Accommodation, 405
Achromatopsia, 406
Acidosis, 349
Acne, 65
Acne rosacea, 65
Acne vulgaris, 65
Acoustic, 415
Acoustic neuroma, 417
Acquired immunity, 182
Acquired immunodeficiency syndrome (AIDS), 186
Acromegaly, 349
Action, 110
Active acquired immunity, 182
Active exercises, 461
Active range of motion (AROM), 461
Active-resistive exercises, 461
Activities of daily living (ADL), 460
Acute care hospitals, 14
Acute tubular necrosis (ATN), 281
Adam's apple, 205
Adaptive equipment, 460, 462*f*
Addiction, 441
Addison's disease, 349
Additive, 441
Adduction, 111, 111*f*
Adductor longus, 109
Adenocarcinoma, 349
Adenoidectomy, 184, 203
Adenoiditis, 184
Adenoids, 181
Adenoma, 347
ADH, 338*t*

Adhesion, 113
Adipectomy, 70
Adipose tissue, 27
Adjective suffixes, 9–10
ADL, 460
Adrenal cortex, 339
Adrenal feminization, 349
Adrenal glands, 339–340
Adrenal medulla, 339
Adrenal virilism, 349
Adrenalectomy, 347
Adrenaline, 338*t*, 340
Adrenalitis, 347
Adrenocorticotropic hormone (ACTH), 338*t*, 343
Adrenomegaly, 347
Adrenopathy, 347
Adult respiratory syndrome (ARDS), 213
Adverse reaction, 441
Aerosol sprays, 439, 439*f*
Afferent, 274
Afferent arteriole, 273*f*, 274
Afferent neurons, 374
Afterbirth, 303
Agglutinate, 169
Agranulocytes, 167, 168*t*
AIDS, 186
AIDS-related complex (ARC), 186
Alanine transaminase (ALT), 253
Albino, 61
Albumin, 167, 277
Albuminuria, 279
Aldosterone, 338*t*, 339
Alimentary canal, 235
Allergen, 185
Allergist, 185
Allergy, 185
Allograft, 70
Alopecia, 61
ALS, 378
ALT, 253
Alveolar sac, 205*f*
Alveoli, 205, 205*f*
Alzheimer's disease, 378
Amblyopia, 406
Ambulatory care, 15
Amenorrhea, 306
American Sign Language (ASL), 416, 417
Amnesia, 446
Amniocentesis, 311
Amnion, 303
Amniorrhea, 305
Amniotic fluid, 302*f*, 303
Amniotomy, 305

Amplification, 419
Amputation, 105
Amylase, 243
Amyotrophic lateral sclerosis (ALS), 378
Anacusis, 417
Anal fissure, 249
Anal fistula, 249
Anal sphincter, 242
Analgesia, 377
Analgesic, 385, 467
Anaphylactic shock, 186
Anaphylaxis, 185
Anastomosis, 256
Anatomical position, 34, 35
Ancillary reports, 13
Androgen, 317, 321, 339, 347
Andropathy, 317
Anemia, 171
Anesthesia, 377, 464–465
Anesthesiologist, 464, 465*f*
Anesthesiologist's report, 14
Anesthetic, 71, 385, 467
Anesthetic ophthalmic solution, 409
Aneurysm, 146
Aneurysmectomy, 150
Angina pectoris, 146
Angiocarditis, 146
Angiography, 143, 149
Angioma, 146
Angioplasty, 150, 151–152*f*
Angiorrhaphy, 143
Angiospasm, 143, 146
Angiostenosis, 143
Anhidrosis, 58
Ankylosing spondylitis, 101
Anorchism, 317
Anorexia, 247, 248
Anorexia nervosa, 446, 447*f*
Anorexiant, 257
Anosmia, 210
Anoxia, 209
ANS, 137, 375
Answers/chapter review questions, 499–506
Antacid, 257
Antagonistic pairs, 110
Anteflexion, 297
Antepartum, 306
Anterior, 36, 37*f*, 41
Anterior tibial artery, 139*f*
Anterior tibial vein, 141*f*
Anteroposterior view (AP view), 451
Anthracosis, 213
Anti-inflammatory, 188
Anti-inflammatory drugs, 71

---

*Note:* Italic letters *f* and *t* indicate a figure or table.

561